TENTH EDITION

Medical Terminology

for Healthcare Professionals

Jane Rice, **RN,CMA-C**

Medical Assisting Program Director, Retired

Georgia Northwestern Technical College

Rome, Georgia

Dedication

To Charles Larry Rice, my husband and partner in life. In special memory of my parents, Warren Galileo and Elizabeth Styles Justice, and my sister, Betty Sue Nelson.

Please contact https://support.pearson.com/getsupport/s/ with any queries on this content

Cover Image: ramcreations/Shutterstock

Library of Congress Control Number: 2019952641

2 2020

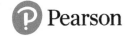 Pearson

ISBN-10: 0-13-574514-4
ISBN-13: 978-0-13-574514-4

Contents *in* Brief

CHAPTER 1	Introduction to Medical Terminology	1
CHAPTER 2	Suffixes and Prefixes	33
CHAPTER 3	Organization of the Body	59
CHAPTER 4	Integumentary System	94
CHAPTER 5	Skeletal System	139
CHAPTER 6	Muscular System	186
CHAPTER 7	Digestive System	223
CHAPTER 8	Cardiovascular System	274
CHAPTER 9	Blood and Lymphatic System	335
CHAPTER 10	Respiratory System	379
CHAPTER 11	Urinary System	424
CHAPTER 12	Endocrine System	464
CHAPTER 13	Nervous System	508
CHAPTER 14	Special Senses: The Ear	562
CHAPTER 15	Special Senses: The Eye	592
CHAPTER 16	Female Reproductive System with an Overview of Obstetrics	632
CHAPTER 17	Male Reproductive System	685
CHAPTER 18	Mental Health	719
Appendix I	Answer Key	748
Appendix II	Glossary of Word Parts	775
Appendix III	Abbreviations, Acronyms, and Symbols	789
Index		799

The 10th edition of *Medical Terminology for Healthcare Professionals* introduces the vocabulary of the art and science of medicine. Chapter 1 shows how to build medical words by using their component parts and how to spell, pronounce, and define medical words. Chapter 2 presents essential suffixes and prefixes that link with word roots and combining forms to build and expand the medical vocabulary. In Chapter 3, the organization of the amazing human body is introduced. In Chapters 4–17, the body systems are presented, working from the outside (skin) to the inside, and from less complex to more complex. Chapter 18 discusses aspects of mental health; it follows the *Diagnostic and Statistical Manual of Mental Disorders*, Fifth Edition (DSM-5), which is the standard classification of mental disorders used by mental health professionals in the United States. Every chapter is built around an alphabetical word list showing how word parts are built, pronounced, and defined. In these Building Your Vocabulary sections, a table of combining forms and word roots that pertain to the chapter being studied are included to assist in learning new component parts.

The text's strengths include:

1. **The Rice Method.** The ease with which students learn medical terminology using the Rice approach has made this text a popular seller, with over 780,000 books in print. It is written in a clear, concise style that focuses on the learner and provides a solid foundation for developing an understanding of the technical language of medicine. All of the information concerning each medical word that you will be introduced to is included in one place: **Building Your Medical Vocabulary**. The medical terminology words are in alphabetical order with a pronunciation guide found beneath the word. Word parts are identified and defined and then the general meaning of the term is described. Prefixes and suffixes are repeated throughout the text while word roots and combining forms are presented according to the system or specialty area to which they relate. To build a medical vocabulary, all you have to do is to recall the word parts that have been learned and link them with the new component parts presented in the next chapter. The word-building technique is unique to this text and, while not complicated, is the key to the classic design and popularity of *Medical Terminology for Healthcare Professionals*.

2. **Accurate and complete coverage of human anatomy and physiology.** This text presents concise coverage of all major body structures and functions, organized by body system. The anatomy and physiology sections have been reviewed by many medical and healthcare professionals and updated according to the offered suggestions.

3. **Study and Review.** These sections, which appear multiple times in each chapter, have been expanded to provide learners with the opportunity to "review as they go." The revised format and types of questions are placed to follow a segment of information so that learners may check their progress before moving on to the next section.

4. **Visually appealing with new art and photos.** In this edition the art collection has increased to approximately 470 images with an updating of corresponding material. Included in the new artwork are examples of "Building Blocks" for the component parts of words. Also a number of new medical photographs have been provided by Jason Smith, MD, a longtime contributor to this text. We are so pleased and excited about supplying more art to enhance the written word. If the statement "a picture is worth a thousand words" can be counted on, then we might say that we have added about 470,000 words to the learning experience!

A Special Feature New to This Edition:

GOOD TO KNOW ▶

A Note from the Author

A new feature, **GOOD TO KNOW**, brings to light some interesting information about current happenings concerning health and medicine. With the advent of the surge in infectious diseases affecting the United States and the world, it is very good to know and be aware of these conditions. During my lifetime I have seen many infectious diseases all but eliminated, and when they began to appear again, I became most concerned. I was sure it would be **GOOD** for students to know about what is happening in the United States and worldwide with infectious diseases and how to protect themselves and others, and so this new feature was created.

— Jane Rice

Features at a Glance

Let's take a look at what makes *Medical Terminology for Healthcare Professionals* so appealing and reliable as a learning resource.

Building Your Medical Vocabulary

This section provides the foundation for learning medical terminology. Review the alphabetized list of medical terms in the following pages. Note how common prefixes and suffixes are repeatedly applied to word roots and combining forms to create different meanings. A combining form is a word root plus a vowel. The chart below lists the combining forms and word roots used in this chapter and can help to strengthen your understanding of how medical words are built and spelled.

You will find that some terms have not been divided into word parts. These are common words or specialized terms that are included to enhance your medical vocabulary.

Combining Forms

agor/a	marketplace	path/o	disease
aut/o	self	phob/o	fear
centr/o	center	phren/o	mind
compuls/o	compel, drive	psych/o	mind
cycl/o	circle, cycle	schiz/o	to divide
delus/o	to cheat	somat/o	body
eg/o	I, self	thym/o	mind, emotion
neur/o	nerve	trop/o	turning
obsess/o	besieged by thoughts		

Word Roots

hallucinat	to wander in mind	iatr	treatment

Medical Word	Word Parts		Definition
	Part	Meaning	
affect (ăf´ fĕkt)			In psychology, observable evidence of an individual's emotional reaction associated with an experience
affective disorder (ăf-fĕk´ tĭv)			Characterized by a disturbance of mood accompanied by a manic or depressive syndrome; this syndrome is not caused by any other physical or mental disorder
agoraphobia (ăg´ ŏ-ră-fō´ bē-ă)	agor/a -phobia	marketplace fear	An anxiety disorder; agoraphobia involves intense fear and anxiety in any place or situation where escape might be difficult, leading to avoidance of being alone outside of the home; traveling in a car, bus, or airplane; or being in a crowded area.
anorexia nervosa (ăn-ŏ-rĕk´ sē-ă nĕr-vō´ să)	an- -orexia	lack of, without appetite	Complex psychological disorder in which the individual refuses to eat or has an abnormally limited eating pattern. People with eating disorders may engage in self-induced vomiting and abuse of laxatives, diuretics, or prolonged exercise to control their weight. The condition could lead them to become excessively thin or even emaciated. In severe cases, this condition can be life-threatening.

Building Your Medical Vocabulary—Think of this section as being like having a blueprint to build a house, but in this case the blueprint can be used to construct a solid and well-designed medical vocabulary. Progressing through each chapter, a solid foundation in the art of medical word building is acquired and understanding medical terminology becomes much easier. The design is simple and easy to follow. The same format is used for each chapter. Knowledge builds and accumulates as the learning process becomes comfortable and familiar. The learning process can be taken to any level desired because, in the medical field, learning never stops.

▶ **ANATOMY LABELING**   Identify the structures shown below by filling in the blanks.

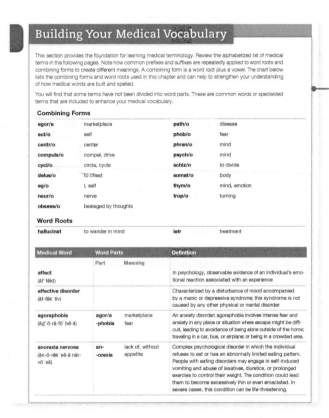

Designed for Visual Learners—Most pages are highlighted by a vibrant and instructive image. Examples include anatomically precise diagrams, authentic medical photographs, and engaging labeling activities.

! ALERT!
How many words can you build using the root **opt** and the combining form **opt/o**?

✓ RULE REMINDER
The **o** has been removed from the combining form because the suffix begins with a vowel.

ALERT!—Designed to help in the identification, building, and spelling of medical words, as well as the formation of plural endings and in the recall of word parts.

RULE REMINDER—Helps to reinforce the rules that govern medical terminology and includes helpful hints.

fyi The use of dichoptic therapy (simultaneous training of both eyes), which presents different images to each eye separately, using popular children's movies, has produced improved visual acuity in young children. Dichoptic techniques combined with perceptual-learning tasks or certain video games have been shown to improve visual acuity significantly in people with amblyopia.

FYI—Contains interesting medical information that will broaden knowledge and pique interest.

GOOD TO KNOW ▶

According to the American Society of Plastic Surgeons, regenerative medicine is the science of using adipose-derived stem cells harvested from fat to regenerate cells and tissues in the human body. Fat tissue is an important source of adult mesenchymal stem cells. (The term *mesenchymal* refers to the diffuse network of cells forming the embryonic mesoderm and giving rise to connective tissue, blood and blood vessels, the lymphatic system, and cells of the mononuclear phagocyte system.) Discovered by plastic surgeons, adipose-derived stem cells are easy to isolate from fat tissue and hold tremendous promise for treating many disorders across the body.

A significant advance in surgical regenerative medicine has been the development and refinement of techniques to transfer fat tissue in a minimally invasive manner, using a patient's own extra fat tissue, thus allowing the regeneration of fat tissue in other parts of the body. This technique is revolutionizing many reconstructive procedures, such as breast reconstruction.

Good to Know—Spotlights new research, current trends, and other medical issues in healthcare and medicine.

Drug Highlights

Classification of Drug	Description and Examples
antacids	Neutralize hydrochloric acid in the stomach; classified as nonsystemic and systemic.
nonsystemic	EXAMPLES: Amphojel (aluminum hydroxide), Tums (calcium carbonate), Riopan (magaldrate), and Milk of Magnesia (magnesium hydroxide)
systemic	EXAMPLE: sodium bicarbonate
antacid mixtures	Products that combine aluminum (may cause constipation) and/or calcium compounds with magnesium salts (may cause diarrhea). By combining the antacid properties of two single-entity agents, these products provide the antacid action of both yet tend to counter the adverse effects of each other. EXAMPLES: Gaviscon, Gelusil, Maalox Plus, and Mylanta
histamine H_2-receptor antagonists	Inhibit both daytime and nocturnal basal gastric acid secretion and inhibit gastric acid stimulated by food, histamines, caffeine, and insulin used in the treatment of active duodenal ulcer. EXAMPLES: Tagamet (cimetidine), Pepcid (famotidine), Axid (nizatidine), and Zantac (ranitidine)

Drug Highlights—Presents essential pharmacology information that relates to the subject of the chapter. The trade names of drugs and their availability were verified at the time of this text's publication, in order to provide the most up-to-date information possible.

Diagnostic *and* Laboratory Tests

Test	Description
color vision tests	Use of polychromatic (multicolored) charts or an *anomaloscope* (a device for detecting color blindness) to assess an individual's ability to recognize differences in color. A person who is color blind will not see the number 27 in the circle in Figure 15.21.

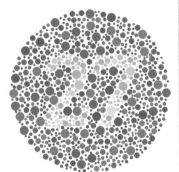

FIGURE 15.21 Color vision chart. Color-blind individuals cannot see the number *27* in the circle.

Diagnostic *and* Laboratory Tests—Provides an overview of current tests and procedures that are used in the physical assessment and diagnosis of certain conditions/diseases.

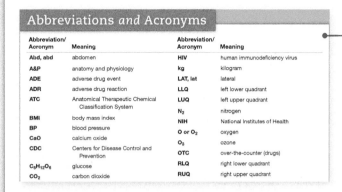

Abbreviations *and* Acronyms

Abbreviation/ Acronym	Meaning	Abbreviation/ Acronym	Meaning
Abd, abd	abdomen	HIV	human immunodeficiency virus
A&P	anatomy and physiology	kg	kilogram
ADE	adverse drug event	LAT, lat	lateral
ADR	adverse drug reaction	LLQ	left lower quadrant
ATC	Anatomical Therapeutic Chemical Classification System	LUQ	left upper quadrant
		N_2	nitrogen
BMI	body mass index	NIH	National Institutes of Health
BP	blood pressure	O or O_2	oxygen
CaO	calcium oxide	O_3	ozone
CDC	Centers for Disease Control and Prevention	OTC	over-the-counter (drugs)
		RLQ	right lower quadrant
$C_6H_{12}O_6$	glucose	RUQ	right upper quadrant
CO_2	carbon dioxide		

Abbreviations *and* Acronyms—Provides commonly used abbreviations and acronyms, specific to each chapter's content, with their meanings in an at-a-glance table format.

Study *and* Review II

Word Parts

Prefixes   Give the definitions of the following prefixes.

1. a- _____
2. bi- _____
3. en- _____
4. em- _____
5. eso- _____
6. hyper- _____

7. intra- _____
8. tri- _____
9. ex(o)- _____
10. hemi- _____
11. an- _____
12. retro- _____

Combining Forms   Give the definitions of the following combining forms.

1. ambly/o _____
2. anis/o _____
3. blephar/o _____
4. choroid/o _____
5. conjunctiv/o _____
6. cor/o _____
7. corne/o _____
8. cry/o _____
9. cycl/o _____
10. dacry/o _____
11. dipl/o _____
12. irid/o _____

13. kerat/o _____
14. lacrim/o _____
15. lent/o _____
16. mi/o _____
17. ophthalm/o _____
18. opt/o _____
19. orth/o _____
20. phac/o _____
21. phot/o _____
22. retin/o _____
23. xen/o _____
24. xer/o _____

Suffixes   Give the definitions of the following suffixes.

1. -al _____
2. -ar _____

3. -ary _____
4. -blast _____

Study *and* Review—Self-paced study guide sections featuring a wide variety of exercises, including **Case Snapshots**, which are case study vignettes that provide an opportunity to relate medical terminology to specific patient care presentations.

Practical Application

Medical Record Analysis

This exercise contains information, abbreviations/acronyms, and medical terminology from an actual medical record or case study that has been adapted for this text. The names and any personal information have been created by the author. Read and study each form or case study and then answer the questions that follow. You may refer to Appendix III, *Abbreviations, Acronyms, and Symbols*.

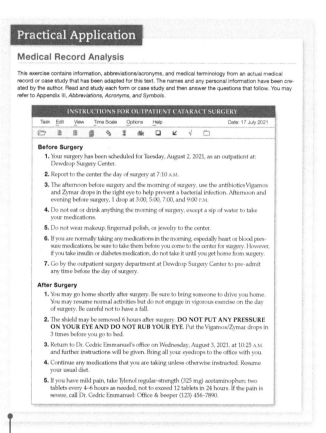

INSTRUCTIONS FOR OUTPATIENT CATARACT SURGERY

Task   Edit   View   Time Scale   Options   Help   Date: 17 July 2021

Before Surgery

1. Your surgery has been scheduled for Tuesday, August 2, 2021, as an outpatient at: Dewdrop Surgery Center.
2. Report to the center the day of surgery at 7:10 A.M.
3. The afternoon before surgery and the morning of surgery, use the antibiotics Vigamox and Zymar drops in the right eye to help prevent a bacterial infection. Afternoon and evening before surgery, 1 drop at 3:00, 5:00, 7:00, and 9:00 P.M.
4. Do not eat or drink anything the morning of surgery, except a sip of water to take your medications.
5. Do not wear makeup, fingernail polish, or jewelry to the center.
6. If you are normally taking any medications in the morning, especially heart or blood pressure medications, be sure to take them before you come to the center for surgery. However, if you take insulin or diabetes medication, do not take it until you get home from surgery.
7. Go by the outpatient surgery department at Dewdrop Surgery Center to pre-admit any time before the day of surgery.

After Surgery

1. You may go home shortly after surgery. Be sure to bring someone to drive you home. You may resume normal activities but do not engage in vigorous exercise on the day of surgery. Be careful not to have a fall.
2. The shield may be removed 6 hours after surgery. **DO NOT PUT ANY PRESSURE ON YOUR EYE AND DO NOT RUB YOUR EYE.** Put the Vigamox/Zymar drops in 3 times before you go to bed.
3. Return to Dr. Cedric Emmanuel's office on Wednesday, August 3, 2021, at 10:25 A.M. and further instructions will be given. Bring all your eyedrops to the office with you.
4. Continue any medications that you are taking unless otherwise instructed. Resume your usual diet.
5. If you have mild pain, take Tylenol regular-strength (325 mg) acetaminophen: two tablets every 4–6 hours as needed, not to exceed 12 tablets in 24 hours. If the pain is severe, call Dr. Cedric Emmanuel: Office & beeper (123) 456-7890.

Practical Application—Real-world medical practice sections that challenge readers to apply their understanding of each chapter while interacting with medical records.

MyLab Medical Terminology™

WHAT IS MYLAB MEDICAL TERMINOLOGY?

MyLab Medical Terminology is a comprehensive online testing program that gives you, the student, the opportunity to test your understanding of information, concepts, and medical language to see how well you know the material. From the test results, MyLab Medical Terminology builds a self-paced, personalized study plan unique to your needs. Remediation in the form of exercises, audio segments, and video clips is provided for those areas in which you may need additional instruction, review, or reinforcement. You can then work through the program until your study plan is complete and you have mastered the content. MyLab Medical Terminology is available with an embedded etext.

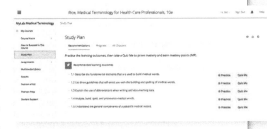

MyLab Medical Terminology is organized to follow the chapters and learning outcomes in *Medical Terminology for Healthcare Professionals*, **Tenth Edition**. With MyLab Medical Terminology, you can track your own progress through your entire medical terminology course.

HOW DO STUDENTS BENEFIT?

Here's how MyLab Medical Terminology helps you:

- Keep up with information presented in the text and lectures.
- Save time by focusing your study to review just the content you need.
- Increase your understanding of difficult concepts with study material that is appropriate for different learning styles.
- Remediate in areas in which you need additional review.

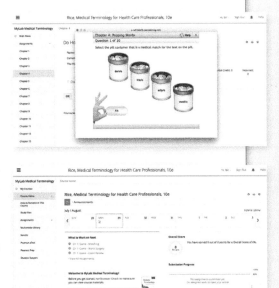

KEY FEATURES OF MYLAB MEDICAL TERMINOLOGY

Pre-Tests and Post-Tests. Using questions aligned to the learning outcomes in *Medical Terminology for Healthcare Professionals* multiple tests measure your understanding of topics.

Personalized Study Material. Based on the topic pre-test results, you receive a personalized study plan, highlighting areas where you may need improvement. It includes these study tools:

- Images for review
- Interactive exercises
- Animations and video clips
- Access to full Personalized Study Material.

HOW DO INSTRUCTORS BENEFIT?

- Save time by providing students with a comprehensive, media-rich study program.
- Track student understanding of course content in the program gradebook.
- Monitor student activity with viewable student assignments.

About the Author

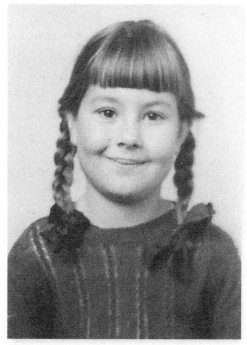

Source: Jane Rice

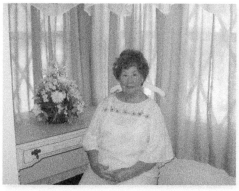

Source: Jane Rice

The year is 1947 and I am a little girl with brown hair that is braided into pigtails. I am very shy and afraid, for, you see, I am in the second grade and I cannot read. Not one little word. The teacher discovered this and made me sit on a tall metal stool in front of the classroom with a dunce cap on my head. Still to this day, I get very nervous when I have to get up in front of a crowd of people.

My mother taught me to read because back then, there were no special classes for children with learning disabilities. I did not learn "phonetics" but memorized everything. I still have trouble pronouncing words, but I can tell you all you want to know about a medical word.

After the death of two brothers, my father, and the impending death of my mother, I prayed for something else to do, something that would help take away the pain and the hurt. In 1982, my prayers were answered with a most precious gift: *Medical Terminology with Human Anatomy*, which was first published in September 1985, and is now titled *Medical Terminology for Healthcare Professionals*.

I owe so much to God and my best friend and husband, Charles Larry Rice. God continues to guide me in my writing. He provides me the knowledge and ability to organize, research, develop, and then to write. Larry, my husband of 54 years, is supportive and gives me the freedom to be an author. He is my love and hero.

I had a wonderful teaching career, and I am forever beholden to the many wonderful students who taught me so much and touched my life with their unique qualities. I hope and pray that this 10th edition of *Medical Terminology for Healthcare Professionals* will enable you, the learner, to become the professional that you choose to be.

— *Jane Rice, RN, CMA-C*

Acknowledgments

First, I would like to offer my warmest thanks to all of the individuals who have accepted my medical terminology text as their book of choice. Over the past 34 years, I have been blessed with the gift of writing. It is my desire for this edition to make learning a wonderful experience for you, the learner and educator.

I want to express my gratitude to each person who worked so hard on this project and provided his or her unique talents to create and develop this edition. A sincere thank you to all the exceptional people at Pearson, especially John Goucher, Derril Trakalo, Melissa Bashe, Cara Schaurer, and Rachele M. Strober. To Lynda Hatch—you are still with me all the way. Through your guidance and excellent work, this 10th edition of my "dream" has reached a new dimension. To Garnet Tomich—for your expert work in making sure that all the *t*'s are crossed and the *i*'s are dotted. To Jason Smith, MD, and Kristi Ware, CMA, Northwest Georgia Dermatology, Rome, Georgia—a special thank you for providing new photographs for this edition.

Editorial Development Team

The content and format of *Medical Terminology for Healthcare Professionals* are the result of an incredible collaboration of expert educators from all around. This book represents the collective insights, experience, and thousands of hours of work performed by members of this development team. Their influence will continue to have an impact for decades to come. Let us introduce the members of our team.

Karen Dal Poggetto, BA, MSHI
Santa Rosa Junior College
Santa Rosa, CA

Darlene Dulin, RN, MSN
Ivy Tech Community College, Valparaiso Campus
Valparaiso, IN

Robert Hawkes, MSPA
Florida Gulf Coast University
Fort Myers, FL

Angela Hess, PhD
Bloomsburg University of Pennsylvania
Bloomsburg, PA

Lina Jawad, Ed.D, MS, BS
University of Michigan
Dearborn, MI

Crystal Kitchens, MA, CHDS, RHIT
Richland Community College
Decatur, IL

Marissa Lajaunie, MBA, RHIA
University of Louisiana at Lafayette
Lafayette, LA

Mesfin Negia, MBS
Minneapolis Community and Technical College
Minneapolis, MN

Jennifer Peterson, RHIA, CTR
Illinois State University
Normal, IL

Travis Price, PhD, MLS(ASCP)
Weber State University
Ogden, UT

Adrienne Reaves, RMA, ASCP, AAS, BS, M.ED, Ed.D
South Suburban College
South Holland, IL

David Sullivan, PhD, NRP, NCEE
Pasco Hernando Community College
New Port Richey, FL

A Commitment to Accuracy

As a learner embarking on a career in healthcare you probably already know how critically important it is to be precise in your work. Patients and coworkers will be counting on you to avoid errors on a daily basis. Likewise, we owe it to you—the reader—to ensure accuracy in this book. We have gone to great lengths to verify that the information provided in *Medical Terminology for Healthcare Professionals* is complete and correct.

While our intent and actions have been directed at creating an error-free text, we have established a process for correcting any mistakes that may have slipped past our editors. Pearson takes this issue seriously and therefore welcomes any and all feedback that you can provide along the lines of helping us enhance the accuracy of this text. If you identify any errors that need to be corrected in a subsequent printing, please send them to:

Pearson Health Science Editorial
Medical Terminology Corrections
221 River Street
Hoboken, NJ 07030

Thank you for helping Pearson reach its goal of providing the most accurate medical terminology textbooks available.

Detailed Contents

CHAPTER 1

Introduction to Medical Terminology   1

Learning Outcomes   1
Comprehension of Fundamental Word Structure   2
Fundamentals of Word Structure   2
Principles of Component Parts   4
Identification of Medical Words   5
Vocabulary Words   5
Spelling   5
Formation of Plural Endings   7
Use of Abbreviations and Acronyms   7
Pronunciation   8
Study and Review I   9
Building Your Medical Vocabulary   11
Study and Review II   20
Medical Records   24
Methods of Documentation and Tools for
   Effective Communication   26
Abbreviations and Acronyms   28
Study and Review III   29
Practical Application   31

CHAPTER 2

Suffixes and Prefixes   33

Learning Outcomes   33
Overview of Suffixes   34
General-Use Suffixes   34
Study and Review I   36
Grammatical Suffixes   37
Suffixes That Pertain to Pathological Conditions   38
Suffixes Associated with Surgical and Diagnostic
   Procedures   40
Study and Review II   41
Overview of Prefixes   43
General-Use Prefixes   43
Prefixes That Have More Than One Meaning   45
Study and Review III   45
Prefixes That Pertain to Position or Placement   47
Prefixes That Pertain to Numbers and Amounts   48
Study and Review IV   49

Building Your Medical Vocabulary   51
Study and Review V   56

CHAPTER 3

Organization of the Body   59

Learning Outcomes   59
Anatomy and Physiology   60
Human Body: Levels of Organization   60
Anatomical Locations and Positions   68
Head-to-Toe Assessment   74
Study and Review I   75
Anatomy Labeling   77
The Body in Health and Disease   78
Study and Review II   80
Building Your Medical Vocabulary   81
Study and Review III   85
Drug Highlights   87
Abbreviations and Acronyms   89
Study and Review IV   90
Practical Application   92

CHAPTER 4

Integumentary System   94

Learning Outcomes   94
Anatomy and Physiology   95
Functions of the Skin   95
Layers of the Skin   97
Accessory Structures of the Skin   98
Study and Review I   100
Anatomy Labeling   101
Building Your Medical Vocabulary   102
Study and Review II   127
Drug Highlights   130
Diagnostic and Laboratory Tests   131
Abbreviations and Acronyms   132
Study and Review III   133
Practical Application   137

CHAPTER 5

Skeletal System   139

Learning Outcomes   139

Anatomy and Physiology   140
Bones   140
Joints and Movement   146
Vertebral Column   148
Anatomical Differences in the Male
    and Female Pelvis   149
Fractures   150
Study and Review I   151
Anatomy Labeling   154
Building Your Medical Vocabulary   155
Study and Review II   171
Drug Highlights   174
Diagnostic and Laboratory Tests   176
Abbreviations and Acronyms   179
Study and Review III   180
Practical Application   184

CHAPTER 6

Muscular System   186
Learning Outcomes   186
Anatomy and Physiology   187
Types of Muscles   188
Functions of Muscles   192
Study and Review I   192
Anatomy Labeling   194
Building Your Medical Vocabulary   195
Study and Review II   211
Drug Highlights   215
Diagnostic and Laboratory Tests   216
Abbreviations and Acronyms   216
Study and Review III   217
Practical Application   221

CHAPTER 7

Digestive System   223
Learning Outcomes   223
Anatomy and Physiology   224
Mouth   226
Teeth   227
Pharynx   229
Esophagus   229

Stomach   230
Small Intestine   231
Large Intestine   232
Accessory Organs   233
Study and Review I   235
Anatomy Labeling   237
Building Your Medical Vocabulary   238
Study and Review II   258
Drug Highlights   262
Diagnostic and Laboratory Tests   264
Abbreviations and Acronyms   266
Study and Review III   267
Practical Application   271

CHAPTER 8

Cardiovascular System   274
Learning Outcomes   274
Anatomy and Physiology   275
Heart   276
Blood Vessels   283
Study and Review I   289
Anatomy Labeling   290
Building Your Medical Vocabulary   291
Study and Review II   318
Drug Highlights   321
Diagnostic and Laboratory Tests   323
Abbreviations and Acronyms   327
Study and Review III   329
Practical Application   333

CHAPTER 9

Blood and Lymphatic System   335
Learning Outcomes   335
Anatomy and Physiology   336
Blood   336
Study and Review I   341
Lymphatic System   342
Accessory Organs   344
Immune System   345
Study and Review II   348
Anatomy Labeling   350

Building Your Medical Vocabulary   351
Study *and* Review III   367
Drug Highlights   370
Diagnostic *and* Laboratory Tests   371
Abbreviations *and* Acronyms   372
Study *and* Review IV   373
Practical Application   377

CHAPTER 10
Respiratory System   379

Learning Outcomes   379
Anatomy and Physiology   380
Nose   381
Pharynx   383
Larynx   384
Trachea   386
Bronchi   386
Lungs   387
Respiration   389
Study *and* Review I   390
Anatomy Labeling   392
Building Your Medical Vocabulary   393
Study *and* Review II   410
Drug Highlights   414
Diagnostic *and* Laboratory Tests   415
Abbreviations *and* Acronyms   417
Study *and* Review III   418
Practical Application   422

CHAPTER 11
Urinary System   424

Learning Outcomes   424
Anatomy and Physiology   425
Kidneys   425
Ureters   429
Urinary Bladder   430
Urethra   430
Urine   431
Study *and* Review I   434
Anatomy Labeling   435
Building Your Medical Vocabulary   436

Study *and* Review II   451
Drug Highlights   454
Diagnostic *and* Laboratory Tests   455
Abbreviations *and* Acronyms   457
Study *and* Review III   458
Practical Application   462

CHAPTER 12
Endocrine System   464

Learning Outcomes   464
Anatomy and Physiology   465
Hormonal Function of the Endocrine System   466
Pituitary Gland (Hypophysis)   469
Pineal Gland   469
Thyroid Gland   470
Parathyroid Glands   471
Pancreas   472
Adrenal Glands (Suprarenals)   473
Ovaries   475
Testes   476
Placenta   476
Gastrointestinal Mucosa   476
Thymus   476
Leptin and Ghrelin: Different Types of Hormones   477
Study *and* Review I   477
Anatomy Labeling   480
Building Your Medical Vocabulary   481
Study *and* Review II   495
Drug Highlights   498
Diagnostic *and* Laboratory Tests   499
Abbreviations *and* Acronyms   501
Study *and* Review III   502
Practical Application   506

CHAPTER 13
Nervous System   508

Learning Outcomes   508
Anatomy and Physiology   509
Tissues of the Nervous System   510
Nerve Fibers, Nerves, and Tracts   512
Transmission of Nerve Impulses   512

Central Nervous System   512
Peripheral Nervous System   519
Autonomic Nervous System   522
Study *and* Review I   523
Anatomy Labeling   525
Building Your Medical Vocabulary   526
Study *and* Review II   547
Drug Highlights   551
Diagnostic *and* Laboratory Tests   554
Abbreviations *and* Acronyms   555
Study *and* Review III   556
Practical Application   560

CHAPTER 14
Special Senses: The Ear   562
Learning Outcomes   562
Anatomy and Physiology   563
External Ear   564
Inner Ear   565
Study *and* Review I   568
Anatomy Labeling   570
Building Your Medical Vocabulary   571
Study *and* Review II   579
Drug Highlights   582
Diagnostic *and* Laboratory Tests   583
Abbreviations *and* Acronyms   586
Study *and* Review III   586
Practical Application   590

CHAPTER 15
Special Senses: The Eye   592
Learning Outcomes   592
Anatomy and Physiology   593
External Structures of the Eye   594
Internal Structures of the Eye   597
How Sight Occurs   598
Study *and* Review I   599
Anatomy Labeling   600
Building Your Medical Vocabulary   601
Study *and* Review II   619
Drug Highlights   622

Diagnostic *and* Laboratory Tests   623
Abbreviations *and* Acronyms   625
Study *and* Review III   626
Practical Application   630

CHAPTER 16
Female Reproductive System with an Overview of Obstetrics   632
Learning Outcomes   632
Anatomy and Physiology   633
Uterus   634
Fallopian Tubes   636
Fertilization   637
Ovaries   639
Vagina   640
Vulva   640
Breasts   641
Menstrual Cycle   643
Overview of Obstetrics   644
Pregnancy   644
Labor and Delivery   646
Study *and* Review I   649
Anatomy Labeling   651
Building Your Medical Vocabulary   652
Study *and* Review II   668
Drug Highlights   671
Diagnostic *and* Laboratory Tests   673
Abbreviations *and* Acronyms   678
Study *and* Review III   679
Practical Application   682

CHAPTER 17
Male Reproductive System   685
Learning Outcomes   685
Anatomy and Physiology   686
External Organs   686
Internal Organs   689
Sexually Transmitted Infections   691
Study *and* Review I   694
Anatomy Labeling   696
Building Your Medical Vocabulary   697

Study *and* Review II   708
Drug Highlights   711
Diagnostic *and* Laboratory Tests   712
Abbreviations *and* Acronyms   712
Study *and* Review III   713
Practical Application   717

CHAPTER 18

Mental Health   719

Learning Outcomes   719
Mental Health and Mental Disorders   720
Study *and* Review I   725
Building Your Medical Vocabulary   726

Study *and* Review II   740
Drug Highlights   742
Abbreviations *and* Acronyms   744
Study *and* Review III   744
Practical Application   746

Appendix I   Answer Key   748
Appendix II   Glossary of Word Parts   775
Appendix III Abbreviations, Acronyms, and Symbols   789
Index   799

Introduction to Medical Terminology

plural suffix
combining form
abbreviation **root**
spelling pronunciation
prefix

 ## Learning Outcomes

On completion of this chapter, you will be able to:

1. Describe the fundamental elements that are used to build medical words.
2. List four guidelines that will assist you with the building and spelling of medical words.
3. State the importance of correct spelling in medical terminology.
4. Explain the use of abbreviations when writing and documenting data.
5. Analyze, build, spell, and pronounce medical words.
6. Describe the general components of a patient's medical record.
7. List and describe the four parts of the SOAP chart note record.
8. State the meaning and purpose of the communication tools AIDET® and SBAR.
9. Identify and define selected abbreviations and acronyms.

*AIDET® is a registered trademark of The Studer Group L.L.C. All rights reserved. For more information, please visit www.studergroup.com/aidet.

Comprehension of Fundamental Word Structure

Medical terminology is the study of terms that are used in the art and science of medicine. It is a specialized language with its origin arising from the Greek influence on medicine. Hippocrates was a Greek physician who lived from 460 to 377 BC and whose vital role in medicine is still recognized today. He is called the "Father of Medicine" and is credited with establishing early ethical standards for physicians. Because of advances in scientific computerized technology, many new terms are coined daily; however, most of these terms are composed of word parts that have their origins in ancient Greek or Latin. Because of this foreign origin, it is necessary to learn the English translation of terms when learning the fundamentals of word structure.

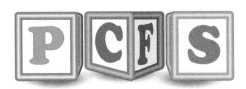

Fundamentals of Word Structure

The fundamental elements in medical terminology are the component parts used to build medical words. The abbreviations used for component parts in this text are **P (prefix)**, **R (root)**, **CF (combining form)**, and **S (suffix)**. The key to learning medical terminology is through the word-building technique used in this text. Combining forms and word roots are integrated into each chapter of the text, according to body system or specialty area. Suffixes and prefixes are presented in Chapter 2 and then will continue to be repeated throughout the text. To build your medical vocabulary, all you have to do is recall the word parts that you have learned and then link them with the new component parts presented in each chapter.

Presented throughout the Building Your Medical Vocabulary sections, which are the heart of every chapter, are special boxes designed to make your learning process the best it can be. These boxes include **Rule Reminder, Alert, fyi**, and **Good to Know**. The Rule Reminder boxes reinforce the rules that govern medical terminology and include helpful hints. The Alert boxes are designed to help you in the identification, building, and spelling of medical words. You will be assisted in the formation of plural endings and in the recall of word parts. The fyi boxes (fyi is an acronym meaning *for your information*) are filled with interesting medical information that will broaden your knowledge. The Good to Know boxes spotlight medical issues in healthcare and medicine. Through researching current trends, happenings, and just plain interesting material, we found so many things that we wanted to share with you, so we did. Of particular interest is the resurgence of infectious diseases that in the past were all but eliminated in the United States and many parts of the world.

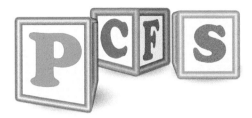

Prefix

The term *prefix* means *to fix before* or *to fix to the beginning* of a word. A prefix can be a syllable or a group of syllables. Prefixes are united with or placed at the beginning of words to alter or modify their meanings or to create entirely new words. For example, the word **ex / cis / ion** means *the process of cutting out; surgical removal*. Note its component parts:

ex-	**P** (prefix) meaning *out*
cis	**R** (root) meaning *to cut*
-ion	**S** (suffix) meaning *process*

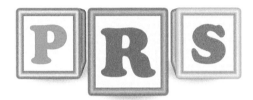

Word Root

A *root* is a word or word element from which other words are formed. It is the foundation of the word. The root conveys the central meaning of the word and forms the base to which prefixes and suffixes are attached for word modification.

For example, the word **mal / format / ion** means *the process of being badly shaped; deformed*. Note its component parts:

mal-	**P** (prefix) meaning *bad*
format	**R** (root) meaning *shaping*
-ion	**S** (suffix) meaning *process*

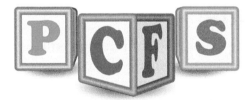

Combining Form

A *combining form* is a word root to which a vowel has been added. A combining vowel (*a, e, i, o, u,* and sometimes *y*) links the root to the suffix or the word root to another root. The combining vowel does not have a meaning of its own. The vowel *o* is used more often than any other to make combining forms. Combining forms can be found at the beginning of a word or within the word.

For example, the word **chem / o / therapy** means *treatment of disease by using chemical agents*. Note the relationship of its component parts:

chem/o	**CF** (combining form) meaning *chemical*
-therapy	**S** (suffix) meaning *treatment*

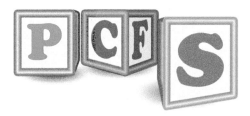

Suffix

The term *suffix* means *to fasten on, beneath, or under*. A suffix can be a syllable or group of syllables united with or placed at the end of a word to alter or modify the meaning of the word or to create a new word. Please note that sometimes a medical word is formed by attaching a suffix directly to a prefix, such as in the example words below, *centigrade* and *centimeter*. When you break down a word to understand it or when you give the meaning of the word or read its definition, you usually begin with the meaning of the suffix.

For example, the word **centi / grade** means *having 100 steps or degrees; unit of temperature measurement* (Celsius scale), and the word **centi / meter** means *unit of measurement in the metric system; one hundredth of a meter*:

centi-	**P** (prefix) meaning *one hundred, one hundredth*	
-grade	**S** (suffix) meaning *a step*	
centi-	**P** (prefix) meaning *one hundred, one hundredth*	
-meter	**S** (suffix) meaning *measure*	

Word roots and combining forms, together with their definitions, are included in each chapter according to the cell, tissue, organ, system, or element they describe. This arrangement makes it possible for you to form associations between medical terms and the various body systems. To reinforce the learning process, the text provides a general anatomy and physiology overview for each of the body systems.

This text presents an alphabetical listing of each chapter's medical words within the Building Your Medical Vocabulary sections. The alphabetical format groups together those terms with the same prefix, word root, and/or combining form, thereby reinforcing the ease of learning medical terminology using the Rice approach.

Principles of Component Parts

As you learn definitions for prefixes, roots, combining forms, and suffixes, you will discover that some component parts have the same meanings as others. This occurs most often with words that relate to the organs of the body and the diseases that affect them. The existence of more than one component part for a particular meaning can be traced to differences in the Greek or Latin words from which they originated. Most of the terms for the body's organs originated from Latin words, whereas terms describing diseases that affect these organs have their origins in Greek. For example:

- **Uterus.** Latin word for one of the organs of the female reproductive system, the womb
- **Metr/i.** Greek **CF** (combining form) for uterus (womb)
- **Endometriosis.** Pathological condition in which endometrial tissue has been displaced to various sites in the abdominal or pelvic cavity: **endo- (P)**, meaning *within*; **metr/i (CF)**, meaning *uterus*; and **-osis (S)**, meaning *condition*

In this text, definitions are worded in an attempt to establish a relationship with the meanings given for each word part. For example, the medical term **adhesion** is divided into two word parts: **adhes (R)**, meaning *stuck to,* and **-ion (S)**, meaning *process.* The definition given is *process of being stuck together.*

Identification of Medical Words

When identifying medical words, you learn to distinguish among and select the appropriate component parts for the meaning of the word. For example, the word **microscope** means *an instrument for examining small objects.* Note the following: *micro-* + *-scope;* not *-scope* + *micro.* With the proper placement of component parts (**P** + **S**) the definition translates **micro-** (*small*) and **-scope** (*instrument for examining*).

Vocabulary Words

You will find that some terms have not been divided into word parts. These are common words or specialized terms that are included to enhance your medical vocabulary. These terms were selected because of their usage in medical records/reports, case studies, and in various medical and surgical specialty areas. For example, **abate**, which means *to lessen, decrease, or cease.* This term is used to note the lessening of pain or the decrease in severity of symptoms. *The patient's arthritic pain did not* abate, *even though she followed the prescribed treatment plan.*

Spelling

Medical words of Greek origin are often difficult to spell because many of them begin with a silent letter or have a silent letter within the word. The following are examples of words that begin with silent letters:

Silent Beginning	Pronounced	Medical Term	Pronunciation Guide
gn	n	gnathic	(năth´ ĭk)
kn	n	knuckle	(nŭk´ ĕl)
mn	n	mnemonic	(nĭ-mŏn´ ĭk)
pn	n	pneumonia	(nū-mō´ nē-ă)
ps	s	psychiatrist	(sī-kī´ ă-trĭst)
pt	t	ptosis	(tō´ sĭs)

The following example is a medical term that contains a silent letter within the word:

Silent Letter	Medical Term	Pronunciation Guide
g	phlegm	(flĕm)

Correct spelling is extremely important in medical terminology because the addition or omission of a single letter can change the meaning of a word to something entirely different. The following examples illustrate this point:

Term/Letter Change	Meaning of Term	Term/Letter Change	Meaning of Term
abduct	To lead **away** from the middle	arteritis	Inflammation of an **artery**
adduct	To lead **toward** the middle	arthritis	Inflammation of a **joint**

Prefixes and Suffixes That Are Frequently Misspelled

Following are some of the prefixes and suffixes that often contribute to spelling errors:

Prefix	Meaning	Suffix	Meaning
ante-	before, forward	-poiesis	formation
anti-	against	-ptosis	prolapse, drooping, sagging, falling down
ecto-	out, outside, outer	-ptysis	spitting
endo-	within, inner	-rrhage	to burst forth, bursting forth
hyper-	above, beyond, excessive	-rrhagia	to burst forth, bursting forth
hypo-	below, under, deficient	-rrhaphy	suture
inter-	between	-rrhea	flow, discharge
intra-	within	-rrhexis	rupture
para-	beside, alongside, abnormal	-scope	instrument for examining
per-	through	-scopy	visual examination, to view, examine
peri-	around	-tome	instrument to cut
pre-	before, in front of	-tomy	incision
pro-	before	-tripsy	crushing
super-	above, beyond	-trophy	nourishment, development
supra-	above, beyond		

! ALERT!

Suffixes such as **-ectomy, -stomy**, and **-tomy** look very much alike, but have different meanings. For example, **-ectomy** means *surgical excision, surgical removal, resection*; **-stomy** means *new opening*; and **-tomy** means *incision*. For example words with these suffixes, *vasectomy, ileostomy,* and *myringotomy*, refer to Chapter 2, Table 2.6. Note how these words are divided into their component parts and their word definitions.

Building and Spelling Medical Words

Follow these guidelines for building and spelling medical words.

1. If the suffix begins with a vowel, drop the combining vowel from the combining form and add the suffix. For example, **necr/o** (*death*) + **-osis** (*condition*) becomes *necrosis* when we drop the **o** from **necr/o**.

2. If the suffix begins with a consonant, keep the combining vowel and add the suffix to the combining form. For example, **cardi/o** (*heart*) + **-logy** (*study of*) becomes *cardiology*; we keep the **o** on the combining form **cardi/o**.

3. Keep the combining vowel between two or more roots in a term. For example, **gastr/o** (*stomach*) + **enter/o** (*intestine*) + **-logy** (*study of*) becomes *gastroenterology* and we keep the two combining vowels.

4. When the medical word has two combining forms, drop the combining vowel from the second combining form and add the suffix. For example, **psych/o** (*mind*) + **somat/o** (*body*) + **-ic** (*pertaining to*) becomes *psychosomatic,* when we drop the **o** from **somat/o**. If the medical word has more than two combining forms, drop the combining vowel

from the combining form next to the suffix. For example, **stern/o** (*sternum*) + **cleid/o** (*clavicle*) + **mast/o** (*mastoid process*) + **-oid** (*resemble*) becomes *sternocleidomastoid*, when we drop the **o** from **mast/o**.

Formation of Plural Endings

To change the following singular endings to plural endings, substitute the plural endings as illustrated:

Singular Ending	Plural Ending	Singular Ending	Plural Ending
a as in bursa	to ae as in bursae	ix as in appendix	to ices as in appendices
a as in gingiva	to ae as in gingivae		
a as in vertebra	to ae as in vertebrae		
ax as in thorax	to aces as in thoraces or es as in thoraxes	nx as in phalanx	to ges as in phalanges
en as in foramen	to ina as in foramina	on as in spermatozoon	to a as in spermatozoa
		on as in ganglion	to a as in ganglia
is as in crisis	to es as in crises	um as in ovum	to a as in ova
is as in diagnosis	to es as in diagnoses	um as in serum	to a as in sera
is as in iris	to ides as in irides	us as in nucleus	to i as in nuclei
		us as in thrombus	to i as in thrombi
		us as in fungus	to i as in fungi
is as in femoris	to a as in femora	y as in artery	to i and add es as in arteries

Use of Abbreviations and Acronyms

An **abbreviation** is a process of shortening a word or phrase into appropriate letters. It is used as a form of communication in writing and documenting data. The Institute for Safe Medication Practices (ISMP) and The Joint Commission (TJC) developed a list of abbreviations considered to be dangerous because of the potential for misinterpretation. It is recommended that facilities using abbreviations for documentation keep a list of approved and unapproved abbreviations on hand and readily accessible.

 fyi To view the list of unapproved abbreviations from the ISMP and TJC, go to *https://www.ismp.org/ recommendations/error-prone-abbreviations-list* or *https://www.jointcommission.org/assets/1/18/ Do_Not_Use_List_9_14_18.pdf*.

When using abbreviations, caution must be exercised. Many have more than one meaning, such as *ER*, which means *emergency room* and *endoplasmic reticulum*, and *PA*, which means *physician assistant, posteroanterior*, and *pernicious anemia*. It is essential that you use or translate the correct meaning for the abbreviation being used. If there is any question about which abbreviation to use, it is best to spell out the word or phrase and not use an abbreviation.

An **acronym** is a word formed by the combining of initial letters, or syllables and letters, of a series of words or a compound term. Any shortened form of a word is an abbreviation, but an acronym is a special type of abbreviation that can be pronounced as a word. For example: HIPAA is an acronym for Health Insurance Portability and Accountability Act.

An **initialism** is another type of abbreviation. It is formed by the initial letters of a series of words or a compound term, but is not pronounced as a word. For example, for DOB (date of birth), each letter is pronounced.

In each chapter of this text, you will find selected abbreviations with their meanings. These abbreviations are in current use and are directly associated with the subject of the chapter. In the appendices, you will find an expanded alphabetical list of commonly used abbreviations and symbols. The abbreviations are presented using capital letters without periods except in those cases where lowercase letters and periods represent the norm or preferred method.

fyi An **eponym** is a disease, structure, operation, or procedure named for the person who discovered or described it first. For example, Alzheimer disease (AD) is named for Alois Alzheimer, a neuropathologist who in 1906 identified an unusual disease of the cerebral cortex and described the amyloid plaques and neurofibrillary tangles that are its characteristics.

Pronunciation

Pronunciation of medical words may seem difficult; however, it is very important to correctly pronounce medical words with the same or very similar sounds in order to convey their correct meanings. As in spelling, one mispronounced syllable can change the meaning of a medical word. The following guide will help you to pronounce each medical word in this text correctly.

PRONUNCIATION GUIDE

This text uses a *phonetic* type of pronunciation guide adapted from *Taber's Cyclopedic Medical Dictionary*. This system uses symbols called *diacritics* (shown in the table below) to help you pronounce the word correctly. You should practice speaking each term aloud when working with the various lists of medical terms or vocabulary words.

ACCENT MARKS	Marks used to indicate stress on certain syllables. *Example:* ăn″ tĭ-sĕp′ tĭk (antiseptic)
Single ′	Used to indicate stress on certain syllables; a single accent mark is called a *primary accent* and is used with the syllable that has the strongest stress (primary syllable).
Double ″	Used to indicate syllables that are stressed less than primary syllables; a double accent mark is called a *secondary accent*.
DIACRITICS	Marks placed over or under vowels to indicate the long or short sound of the vowel.
Macron ‾	Indicates the long sound of the vowel. *Example:* mī′ krō-skōp (microscope)
Breve ˘	Indicates the short sound of the vowel. *Example:* măks′ ĭ-măl (maximal)

Study *and* Review I

Word Parts

Prefixes   Write the correctly spelled prefix for each definition in the space provided.

1. against _____

   a. ante-   **b.** anti-

2. within, inner _____

   a. ecto-   **b.** endo-

3. through _____

   a. per-   **b.** peri-

4. between _____

   a. inter-   **b.** intra-

5. below, under, deficient _____

   a. hyper-   **b.** hypo-

Suffixes   Write the correctly spelled suffix for each definition in the space provided.

1. formation _____

   a. -ptosis   **b.** -poiesis

2. suture _____

   a. -rrhaphy   **b.** -rrhagia

3. visual examination, to view _____

   a. -scopy   **b.** -scope

4. incision _____

   a. -tomy   **b.** -tome

5. nourishment, development _____

   a. -tripsy   **b.** -trophy

Formation of Plural Endings

Write the plural form of these singular words in the space provided.

1. bursa _____

2. thorax _____

3. foramen _____

4. crisis _____

5. iris _____

6. femoris _____

7. appendix _____

8. phalanx _____

9. spermatozoon _____

10. ovum _____

Building Your Medical Vocabulary

This section provides the foundation for learning medical terminology. Review the alphabetized list of medical terms in the following pages. Note how common prefixes and suffixes are repeatedly applied to word roots and combining forms to create different meanings. A combining form is a word root plus a vowel. The chart below lists the combining forms and word roots used in this chapter and can help to strengthen your understanding of how medical words are built and spelled.

You will find that some terms have not been divided into word parts. These are common words or specialized terms that are included to enhance your medical vocabulary.

Combining Forms

bi/o	life	necr/o	death
chem/o	chemical	organ/o	organ
cis/o	to cut	onc/o	tumor
eti/o	cause	path/o	disease
kil/o	a thousand	pyr/o	heat, fire
macr/o	large	radi/o	ray, x-ray
malign/o	bad kind	therm/o	hot, heat

Word Roots

adhes	stuck to	mortal	human being
axill	armpit	norm	rule
dem	people	palm	palm
format	shaping	prophylact	guarding
gen, gene	formation, produce	pyret	fever
infect	to infect	scop	to examine
maxim	greatest	sept	putrefaction
minim	least	tuss	cough
morbid	sick		

Medical Word	Word Parts		Definition
	Part	Meaning	
abate (ă-bāt´)			To lessen, ease, decrease, or cease. Used to note the lessening of pain or the decrease in severity of symptoms.
abnormal (ăb-nōr´ măl)	ab- norm -al	away from rule pertaining to	Pertaining to away from the norm or rule. A condition that is considered to be not normal.

Medical Word	Word Parts		Definition
	Part	Meaning	
abscess (ăb´ sĕs)			Localized collection of pus, which may occur in any part of the body
acute (ă-cūt´)			Sudden, sharp, severe; used to describe a disease that has a sudden onset, severe symptoms, and a short course
adhesion (ăd´ hē-zhŭn)	adhes -ion	stuck to process	Literally means *a process of being stuck together*. An abdominal adhesion usually involves the intestines and is caused by inflammation or trauma. This type of adhesion may cause an intestinal obstruction and require surgery.
afferent (ăf´ ĕ-rĕnt)			Carrying impulses toward a center
ambulatory (ăm´ bū-lăh-tōr´ ē)			Condition of being able to walk, not confined to bed. See Figure 1.1.

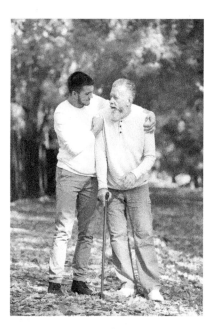

FIGURE 1.1 A young man helps his grandfather walk (*ambulate*) through the park on an autumn day.
Source: Africa Studio/Shutterstock

antidote (ăn´ tĭ-dōt)			Substance given to counteract poisons and their effects
antipyretic (ăn´´ tĭ-pī-rĕt´ ĭk)	anti- pyret -ic	against fever pertaining to	Pertaining to an agent that is used to lower an elevated body temperature (fever)

Medical Word	Word Parts		Definition
	Part	**Meaning**	
antiseptic (ăn″ tĭ-sĕp′ tĭk)	**anti-** **sept** **-ic**	against putrefaction pertaining to	Pertaining to an agent that works against sepsis (*putrefaction*); a technique or product used to prevent or limit infections. See Figures 1.2 and 1.3.

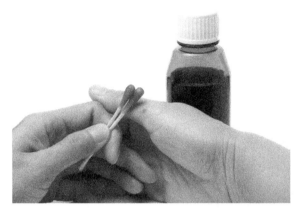

FIGURE 1.2 Betadine (povidone-iodine, also known as iodopovidone), is an antiseptic used for skin disinfection in the home and before and after surgery.
Source: jiangdi/Shutterstock

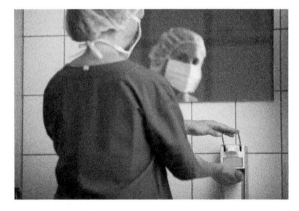

FIGURE 1.3 Antiseptics are used to disinfect both the skin of the patient and the hands of the healthcare professional.
Source: stockfour/Shutterstock

Medical Word	Word Parts		Definition
antitussive (ăn″ tĭ-tŭs′ ĭv)	**anti-** **tuss** **-ive**	against cough nature of, quality of	Pertaining to an agent that works against coughing
apathy (ăp′ ă-thē)			Condition in which one lacks feelings and emotions and is indifferent
asepsis (ā-sĕp′ sĭs)	**a-** **-sepsis**	without decay	Without decay; *sterile*, free from all living microorganisms
axillary (ax) (ăk′ sĭ-lār-ē)	**axill** **-ary**	armpit pertaining to	Pertaining to the armpit

Medical Word	Word Parts		Definition
	Part	**Meaning**	
biopsy (Bx) (bī′ ŏp-sē)	**bi(o)** **-opsy**	life to view	Surgical removal of a small piece of tissue for microscopic examination; used to determine a diagnosis of cancer or other disease processes in the body. See Figure 1.4.

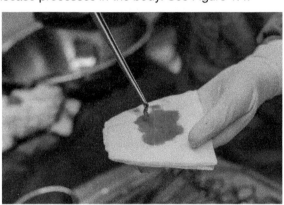

FIGURE 1.4 A surgical biopsy specimen will be placed in a specimen container and labeled with date and time of removal, patient's name, surgeon's name, and location of body area from where the specimen was removed.
Source: Chaikom/Shutterstock

! ALERT!

To change *biopsy* to its plural form, you change the **y** to **i** and add **es** to make *biopsies*.

Medical Word	Word Parts		Definition
cachexia (kă-kĕks′ ē-ă)	**cac-** **-hexia**	bad condition	Condition of ill health, malnutrition, and wasting. It may occur in chronic diseases such as cancer and pulmonary tuberculosis.
centigrade (C) (sĕn′ tĭ-grād)	**centi-** **-grade**	one hundred, one hundredth a step	Literally means *having 100 steps* or *degrees*; unit of temperature measurement (Celsius scale) with a boiling point at 100° and a freezing point at 0°. Each degree of temperature change is 0.01 (1/100) of the scale.
centimeter (cm) (sĕn′ tĭ-mē-tĕr)	**centi-** **-meter**	one hundred, one hundredth measure	Unit of measurement in the metric system; one hundredth of a meter
chemotherapy (kē″ mō-thĕr′ ă-pē)	**chem/o** **-therapy**	chemical treatment	The use of chemical agents in the treatment of disease, specifically drugs used in cancer therapy
chronic (krŏn′ ĭk)			Pertaining to time; denotes a disease with little change or of slow progression; the opposite of acute
diagnosis (Dx) (dī″ ăg-nō′ sĭs)	**dia-** **-gnosis**	through knowledge	The process of identifying a disease or disorder, which is generally determined through the use of scientific and skillful methods of knowledge. Several types of information are used for diagnosis, including signs and symptoms.

! ALERT!

To change *diagnosis* to its plural form, you change **is** to **es** to create *diagnoses*.

Medical Word	Word Parts		Definition
	Part	**Meaning**	
diaphoresis (dī″ă-fō-rē′sĭs)	**dia-** **-phoresis**	through to carry	To carry through sweat glands; *profuse sweating*
disease (dĭ-zēz′)			Literally means *lack of ease*; a pathological condition of the body that presents with a series of symptoms, signs, and laboratory findings peculiar to it and sets it apart from normal or other abnormal body states; a disruption of normal functioning of the body by a process that can be congenital or infectious, or the failure of normal activity to maintain and sustain health
disinfectant (dĭs″ĭn-fĕk′tănt)	**dis-** **infect** **-ant**	apart to infect forming	Chemical substance that can be applied to objects to destroy pathogenic microorganisms, such as bacteria. See Figure 1.5.

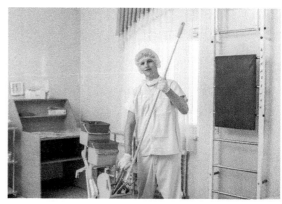

FIGURE 1.5 The cleaning and disinfecting of areas in a healthcare facility is vital for patient safety.
Source: nata-lunata/Shutterstock

Medical Word	Word Parts		Definition
efferent (ĕf′ĕr-ĕnt)			Carrying impulses away from a center
empathy (ĕm′pă-thē)			The ability to sense intellectually and emotionally the feelings of another person
epidemic (ĕp″ĭ-dĕm′ik)	**epi-** **dem** **-ic**	upon people pertaining to	Pertaining to upon the people; the rapid, widespread occurrence of an infectious disease that can be spread by any pathological organism transmitted by and to humans, birds, insects, and other living things. It is a term that may be used to describe any problem that has grown out of control.

 fyi The *opioid epidemic* is the name given to the rapid increase in the use of prescription and non-prescription opioid drugs in the United States and Canada beginning in the late 1990s and continuing throughout the next two decades. According to the Centers for Disease Control and Prevention (CDC), 70,237 drug overdose deaths occurred in the United States in 2017 and 48.5 million Americans have used illicit drugs or misused prescription drugs.

Medical Word	Word Parts		Definition
	Part	**Meaning**	
etiology (ē″ tē-ŏl′ ō-jē)	**eti/o** **-logy**	cause study of	Study of the cause(s) of disease

> **! ALERT!**
>
> In the language of health and medicine, **-logy**
> is a common suffix. It is used to describe things
> that are studied.

Medical Word	Word Parts		Definition
excision (ĕk-sĭ′ zhŭn)	**ex-** **cis** **-ion**	out to cut process	Process of cutting out, surgical removal
febrile (fē′ brĭl)			Pertaining to fever, a sustained body temperature (T) above 98.6°F
gram (g) (grăm)			Unit of weight in the metric system; a cubic centimeter or a milliliter of water is equal to the weight of a gram
heterogeneous (hĕt″ ĕr-ō-jē′ nē-ŭs)	**hetero-** **gene** **-ous**	different formation, produce pertaining to	Literally means *pertaining to a different formation*; composed of unlike substances; the opposite of homogeneous
illness (ĭl′ nĭs)			State of being sick
incision (ĭn-sĭzh′ ŭn)	**in-** **cis** **-ion**	in, into to cut process	Process of cutting into. See Figure 1.6.

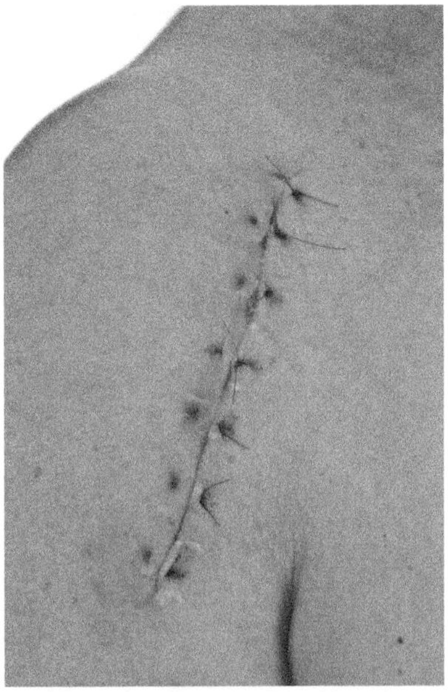

FIGURE 1.6 This incision line has been closed
with nonabsorbable 4-0 nylon suture material
that will stay in place for 10–14 days and then be
removed by a healthcare professional.
Source: Birgit Reitz-Hofmann/Shutterstock

Medical Word	Word Parts		Definition
	Part	**Meaning**	
kilogram (kg) (kĭl´ ō-grăm)	**kil/o** **-gram**	a thousand a weight	Unit of weight in the metric system; 1000 g; a kilogram is equal to 2.2 lb

✓ **RULE REMINDER**
> This term keeps the combining vowel **o** because the suffix begins with a consonant.

Medical Word	Word Parts		Definition
liter (L) (lē´ tĕr)			Unit of volume in the metric system; 1000 mL; a liter is equal to 33.8 fl oz or 1.0567 qt
macroscopic (măk˝ rō-skŏp´ ĭk)	**macr/o** **scop** **-ic**	large to examine pertaining to	Pertaining to objects large enough to be examined by the naked eye
malaise (mă-lāz´)			A general feeling of discomfort, uneasiness; often felt by a patient who has a chronic disease
malformation (măl˝ fōr-mā´ shŭn)	**mal-** **format** **-ion**	bad shaping process	Literally means *a process of being badly shaped, deformed*; a structural defect that fails to form normal shape and therefore can affect the function (e.g., *cleft palate*)

✓ **RULE REMINDER**
> The **o** has been removed from the combining form because the suffix begins with a vowel.

Medical Word	Word Parts		Definition
malignant (mă-lĭg´ nănt)	**malign** **-ant**	bad kind forming	Literally means *formation of a bad kind*; growing worse, harmful, cancerous
maximal (măks´ ĭ-măl)	**maxim** **-al**	greatest pertaining to	Pertaining to the greatest possible quantity, number, or degree
microgram (mcg) (mī´ krō-grăm)	**micro-** **-gram**	small a weight	Unit of weight in the metric system; one millionth of a gram or one thousandth of a milligram (0.001 mg)
microorganism (mī˝ krō-ōr´ găn-ĭzm)	**micro-** **organ** **-ism**	small organ condition	Small living organisms that are not visible to the naked eye

Medical Word	Word Parts		Definition
	Part	Meaning	
microscope (mī′ krō-skōp)	**micro-** **-scope**	small instrument for examining	Scientific instrument designed to view small objects that are not visible to the naked eye. With its magnification, we can see cells and even tiny structures within cells. See Figure 1.7.

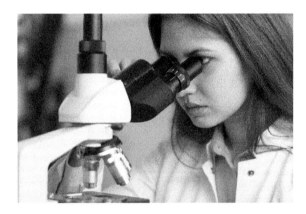

FIGURE 1.7 This young woman is using a microscope to view a laboratory specimen.
Source: science photo/Shutterstock

Medical Word	Word Parts		Definition
milligram (mg) (mĭl′ ĭ-grăm)	**milli-** **-gram**	one thousandth a weight	Unit of weight in the metric system; 0.001 g
milliliter (mL) (mĭl′ ĭ-lē″ tĕr)	**milli-** **-liter**	one thousandth liter	Unit of volume in the metric system; 0.001 L
minimal (mĭn′ ĭ-măl)	**minim** **-al**	least pertaining to	Pertaining to the least possible quantity, number, or degree
morbidity (mōr-bĭd′ ĭ-tē)	**morbid** **-ity**	sick condition	State of being diseased; ill, sick; refers to the disease rate or number of cases of a particular disease in a given age range, gender, occupation, or other relevant population-based grouping
mortality (mōr-tăl′ ĭ-tē)	**mortal** **-ity**	human being condition	Being human, subject to death; refers to the death rate reflected by the population in a given region, age range, or other relevant statistical grouping

GOOD TO KNOW ▶

Top 10 Leading Causes of Death/Mortality in the United States in 2017

1. Heart disease
2. Cancer (CA)
3. Chronic lower respiratory disease (infectious diseases)
4. Accidents (unintentional injuries)
5. Stroke (cerebrovascular accident [CVA])
6. Alzheimer disease (AD)
7. Diabetes (diabetes mellitus [DM])
8. Influenza and pneumonia
9. Kidney disease (nephritis, nephrotic syndrome, nephrosis)
10. Suicide (intentional self-harm)

Medical Word	Word Parts		Definition
	Part	Meaning	
multiform (mŭl´ tĭ-form)	multi- -form	many, much shape	Occurring in or having many shapes; an object that has more than one defined shape
necrosis (nĕ-krō´ sis)	necr -osis	death condition	Abnormal condition of tissue death
oncology (ŏng-kŏl´ ō-jē)	onc/o -logy	tumor study of	Literally means *the study of tumors*; medical specialty that studies the etiology, the characteristics, the treatments, etc., of cancer

 fyi   Tumors of various types are the focus of study by *oncologists*. Tumors can be classified as *benign* or *malignant*. Benign means the tumor is not cancerous. Malignant means that the tumor is cancerous.

Medical Word	Word Parts		Definition
pallor (păl´ or)			Paleness, a lack of color
palmar (păl´ măr)	palm -ar	palm pertaining to	Pertaining to the palm of the hand
paracentesis (păr˝ ă-sĕn-tē´ sĭs)	para- -centesis	beside surgical puncture	Surgical puncture of a body cavity for fluid removal
pathogenic (path´ ŏ-jĕn´ ĭk)	path/o gen -ic	disease produce pertaining to	Pertaining to producing disease
prognosis (prŏg-nō´ sĭs)	pro- -gnosis	before knowledge	Literally means *a state of foreknowledge*; prediction of the course of a disease and the recovery rate of the affected person
prophylactic (prō-fĭ-lăk´ tĭk)	prophylact -ic	guarding pertaining to	Pertaining to preventing or protecting against disease or pregnancy
pyrogenic (pī˝ rō-jĕn´ ĭk)	pyr/o -genic	heat, fire formation, produce	Pertaining to the production of heat; *a fever*
radiology (rā˝ dē-ŏl´ ō-jē)	radi/o -logy	ray, x-ray study of	Study of x-rays and other imaging modalities that use x-rays
rapport (ră-pōr´)			Relationship of understanding between two individuals, especially between the patient and the physician
sequela (sē-kwĕ´ lă)			The late or residual effect (condition produced) after the acute phase of an illness or injury has ended, such as deafness after treatment with an ototoxic drug

!   **ALERT!**

To change *sequela* to its plural form, you add an *e* to create *sequelae*.

Medical Word	Word Parts		Definition
	Part	Meaning	
sign (sīn)			Any objective clinical evidence of an illness or disordered function of the body. A sign can be seen, heard, measured, or felt by the examiner. For example, a nosebleed can be seen, a hiccup can be heard, vital signs TPR, P, and B/P can be measured, and a lump in the breast can be felt by a patient and/or an examiner.
syndrome (sĭn´ drōm)	**syn-** **-drome**	together, with that which runs together	A group of signs and symptoms occurring together that characterize a specific disease or pathological condition
thermometer (thĕr-mŏm´ ĕ-tĕr)	**therm/o** **-meter**	hot, heat instrument to measure	An instrument used to measure degree of heat, especially the temperature of a person

✓ RULE REMINDER

This term keeps the combining vowel **o** because the suffix begins with a consonant.

triage (trē-ahzh´)			A system of prioritizing and classifying patient injuries to determine priority of need and treatment

Study *and* Review II

Word Parts

Prefixes Give the definitions of the following prefixes.

1. a- _____

2. ab- _____

3. anti- _____

4. cac- _____

5. centi- _____

6. dia- _____

7. dis- _____

8. epi- _____

9. ex- _____

10. hetero- _____

11. in- _____   **15.** multi- _____

12. mal- _____   **16.** para- _____

13. micro- _____   **17.** pro- _____

14. milli- _____   **18.** syn- _____

Roots and Combining Forms   Give the definitions of the following roots and combining forms.

1. adhes _____   **15.** scop _____

2. axill _____   **16.** sept _____

3. chem/o _____   **17.** therm/o _____

4. format _____   **18.** tuss _____

5. gene _____   **19.** infect _____

6. kil/o _____   **20.** dem _____

7. macr/o _____   **21.** eti/o _____

8. necr _____   **22.** cis _____

9. norm _____   **23.** malign _____

10. onc/o _____   **24.** maxim _____

11. organ _____   **25.** minim _____

12. pyret _____   **26.** palm _____

13. pyr/o _____   **27.** prophylact _____

14. radi/o _____

Suffixes   Give the definitions of the following suffixes.

1. -al _____   **6.** -form _____

2. -ar _____   **7.** -genic _____

3. -ary _____   **8.** -gnosis _____

4. -centesis _____   **9.** -grade _____

5. -drome _____   **10.** -gram _____

11. -hexia _____

12. -ic _____

13. -ion _____

14. -ism _____

15. -ive _____

16. -liter _____

17. -logy _____

18. -meter _____

19. -osis _____

20. -ous _____

21. -phoresis _____

22. -scope _____

23. -sepsis _____

24. -therapy _____

Identifying Medical Terms

In the spaces provided, write the medical terms for the following meanings.

1. _____ Process of being stuck together

2. _____ Without decay

3. _____ Pertaining to the armpit

4. _____ Use of chemical agents in the treatment of disease

5. _____ Pertaining to a different formation

6. _____ Process of being badly shaped, deformed

7. _____ Scientific instrument designed to view small objects

8. _____ Occurring in or having many shapes

9. _____ Study of tumors

Using Component Parts to Build Medical Words

Write in the component part for each of the following:

1. The component parts that make up the term *anti/pyret/ic* are:

_____ prefix that means *against*

_____ root that means *fever*

_____ suffix that means *pertaining to*

2. The component parts that make up the term *epi/dem/ic* are:

_____ prefix that means *upon*

_____ root that means *people*

_____ suffix that means *pertaining to*

3. The component parts that make up the term *ex/cis/ion* are:

_____ prefix that means *out*

_____ root that means *to cut*

_____ suffix that means *process*

4. The component parts that make up the term *eti/o/logy* are:

_____ combining form that means *cause*

_____ suffix that means *study of*

5. The component parts that make up the term *onc/o/logy* are:

_____ combining form that means *tumor*

_____ suffix that means *study of*

Matching

Select the appropriate lettered meaning for each of the following words.

_____ **1.** abate

_____ **2.** antipyretic

_____ **3.** cachexia

_____ **4.** diagnosis

_____ **5.** disease

_____ **6.** etiology

_____ **7.** illness

_____ **8.** prognosis

_____ **9.** prophylactic

_____ **10.** triage

a. Literally means *lack of ease*

b. State of being sick

c. Pertaining to protecting against disease or pregnancy

d. Pertaining to an agent that is used to lower an elevated body temperature (fever)

e. A system of prioritizing and classifying patient injuries to determine priority of need and treatment

f. To lessen, ease, decrease, or cease

g. Determination of the cause and nature of a disease

h. Study of the cause(s) of disease

i. Literally means *a state of foreknowledge*

j. Condition of ill health, malnutrition, and wasting

Medical Records

Electronic Health Record

The **electronic health record (EHR)** is an electronic record of health-related information for an individual that is created, gathered, managed, and consulted by authorized healthcare clinicians and staff. Included in this information are patient demographics, progress notes, problems, medications, vital signs, past medical history, immunizations, laboratory data, radiology images, and personal data such as age, weight, and billing information. The EHR automates and streamlines the clinician's workflow. The EHR has the ability to generate a complete record of a clinical patient encounter, as well as supporting other care-related activities directly or indirectly via interface, including evidence-based decision support, quality management, and outcomes reporting. See Figure 1.8.

An EHR is generated and maintained within an institution, such as a hospital, clinic, or physician's office. Its purpose is to give patients, physicians, and other healthcare providers, employers, or insurers access to a patient's medical records across facilities.

Sections contained within the medical record will vary according to the physician's preference, type of practice, cost, and regulatory requirements. Many of the EHR software programs have a prescription component that can be accessed by clicking on the prescription tab. This program can store thousands of drug names with their usual dosages. With just a few clicks, an entire prescription can be created.

A patient's medical record, electronic or paper, is often referred to as a *chart* or *file*. The general components of a patient's medical record include the following:

- **Patient Data.** Information that is provided by the patient and then updated as necessary. It is data that relates directly to the patient, including last name, first name, gender, date of birth (DOB), marital status, street address, city, state, zip code, telephone number, insurance information, employment status, address and phone number of employer, name and contact information for the person who is responsible for the patient's bill, and vital information concerning who should be contacted in case of an emergency.

- **Medical History (Hx).** Document describing past and current history of all medical conditions experienced by the patient.

- **Physical Examination (PE).** Record that includes a current head-to-toe assessment of the patient's physical condition. It is prudent for the healthcare professional to establish rapport and obtain permission from the patient before beginning the physical exam. An explanation of what will be involved in the exam and the involvement of touch during the process should be given to the patient. Healthcare professionals should always show respect for patients, be courteous, speak slowly and clearly, answer questions, and encourage patients to participate during the exam by talking when appropriate. An

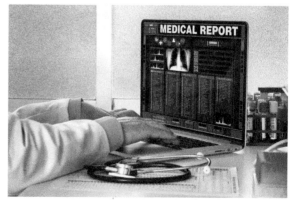

FIGURE 1.8 This authorized healthcare professional is checking health-related information of an individual patient. Note the image of a chest x-ray film showing the lungs (in dark shade) and the shape of the heart (in light shade).
Source: angellodeco/123RF

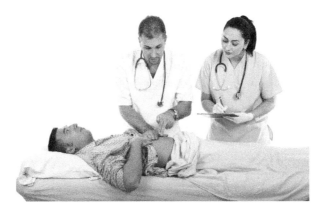

FIGURE 1.9 Palpation is using the hands to feel an area of masses, lumps, or enlarged organs. The physician is using his fingertips to palpate the patient's abdomen and also noting signs of tenderness or pain due to the patient's reaction.
Source: Blaj Gabriel/Shutterstock

evaluation of parts and areas of the body are made by the healthcare professional, who uses techniques of inspection (looking), palpation (feeling with the hands) (Figure 1.9), percussion (tapping with the fingers or an instrument) (Figure 1.10), and auscultation (listening to the sounds of the body, usually with a stethoscope) (Figure 1.11). The patient should be reassured that the privacy of the information being provided is protected by the Health Insurance Portability and Accountability Act (HIPAA).

- **Consent Form.** Signed document by the patient or legal guardian giving permission for treatment.

- **Informed Consent Form.** Signed document by the patient or legal guardian that explains the purpose, risks, and benefits of a procedure and serves as proof that the patient was properly informed before undergoing a procedure.

- **Physician's Orders.** Record of the prescribed care, medications, tests, and treatments for a given patient.

- **Nurse's Notes.** Record of a patient's care that includes vital signs, particularly temperature (T), pulse (P), respiration (R) [TPR], and blood pressure (BP). The nurse's notes can also include treatments, procedures, and patient's responses to such care.

- **Physician's Progress Notes.** Documentation given by the physician regarding the patient's condition, results of the physician's examination, summary of test results, plan of treatment, and updating of data as appropriate (assessment and diagnosis [Dx]).

- **Consultation Reports.** Documentation given by specialists whom the physician has asked to evaluate the patient.

- **Ancillary/Miscellaneous Reports.** Documentation of procedures or therapies provided during a patient's care, such as physical therapy, respiratory therapy, or chemotherapy.

- **Diagnostic Tests/Laboratory Reports.** Documents providing the results of all diagnostic and laboratory tests performed on the patient.

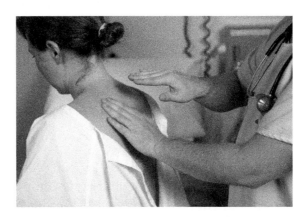

FIGURE 1.10 Percussion is using the fingers or an instrument for tapping on a body area. In this photo, the physician will use the fingers of the right hand to tap on the fingers of the left hand to percuss an area on the patient's upper back. After a few taps the fingers are moved to another area of the upper back.
Source: Sian Bradfield/Pearson Education Australia Pty Ltd.

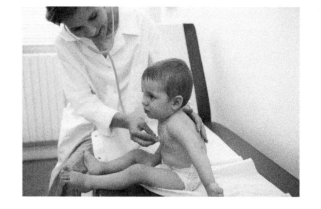

FIGURE 1.11 Auscultation is listening to the sounds of the body, usually with a stethoscope. The doctor is using a stethoscope to listen to sounds of this little boy's lungs and heart.
Source: Image Point Fr/Shutterstock

- **Operative Report.** Documentation from the surgeon detailing the operation, including the preoperative and postoperative diagnosis, specific details of the surgical procedure, how well the patient tolerated the procedure, and any complications that occurred.

- **Anesthesiology Report.** Documentation from the attending anesthesiologist or nurse anesthetist that includes a detailed account of anesthesia during surgery, which drugs were used, dose and time given, patient response, monitoring of vital signs, how well the patient tolerated the anesthesia, and any complications that occurred.

- **Pathology Report.** Documentation from the pathologist regarding the findings or results of samples taken from the patient, such as bone marrow, blood, or tissue.

- **Discharge Summary (also called Clinical Résumé, Clinical Summary, or Discharge Abstract).** Outline summary of the patient's care at the healthcare facility, including date of admission, diagnosis, course of treatment and patient's response(s), results of tests, final diagnosis, follow-up plans, and date of discharge.

Health Insurance Portability and Accountability Act

In 1996 the Health Insurance Portability and Accountability Act (HIPAA) was passed and in 2002 the U.S. Department of Health and Human Services (HHS) issued the Privacy Rule to implement the requirement of HIPAA. HIPAA is a set of rules that doctors, healthcare facilities, and other healthcare providers must follow to help ensure that all medical records, medical billing, and patient accounts meet certain consistent standards with regard to documentation, handling, and privacy. In addition, HIPAA requires that all patients be able to access their own medical records, correct errors or omissions, and be informed about how personal information is shared or used and about privacy procedures.

HIPAA also includes provisions designed to encourage electronic transactions and requires safeguards to protect the security and confidentiality of health information. It covers health plans, healthcare clearinghouses, and those healthcare providers who conduct certain financial and administrative transactions (e.g., enrollment, billing, and eligibility verification) electronically.

Methods of Documentation and Tools for Effective Communication

SOAP: Chart Note

The acronym **SOAP** stands for subjective, objective, assessment, plan. The SOAP chart note is a method of documentation employed by healthcare providers to write out notes in a patient's chart, along with other common formats, such as the admission note.

Documenting patient encounters in the medical record is an integral part of medical/surgical practice workflow, starting with patient appointment scheduling, to writing out notes, to medical billing. The SOAP note is a method of displaying patient data in a concise, organized format and is written to improve communication among those caring for the patient. The length and focus of each component of a SOAP note varies depending on the specialty area. The four parts of a SOAP chart note follow.

1. **Subjective.** This describes the patient's current condition in narrative form and is information provided by the patient. It includes symptoms that the subject (patient) feels and describes to the healthcare professional. These symptoms arise within the individual and are not perceptible to an observer. Examples include pain, nausea, dizziness, tightness in the chest, lump in the throat, weakness of the legs, and "butterflies" in the stomach. The healthcare professional can see the physical reaction of the patient to the symptom but not the actual symptom. Subjective symptoms can be expressed verbally by a parent or a significant other. Also included in the subjective section is the patient's chief complaint (CC), presenting symptom, or presenting complaint stated by the patient and described in the patient's own words. This includes the concern that brings a patient to a doctor. See Figure 1.12.

2. **Objective.** This section documents the objective data from the healthcare provider's encounter with the patient. This includes the vital signs (TPR and BP) and data relating to the physical examination (PE) such as height (Ht); weight (Wt); general appearance; and condition of the lungs, heart, abdomen, musculoskeletal and nervous systems, and the skin. The results of laboratory and diagnostic tests may also be included. *Please note that it may be common practice for the nurse or other medical professional assisting the physician to record the patient's vital signs, allergies, and chief complaint at the top of the chart, instead of within the SOAP chart note.*

3. **Assessment.** Interpretation of the subjective and objective findings. Generally includes a diagnosis, sometimes including a *differential diagnosis* (the process of differentiating between two or more conditions that share similar signs or symptoms), or in some cases will rule out a disease/condition.

4. **Plan.** Includes the management and treatment regimen for the patient; may include laboratory tests, radiological tests, physical therapy, diet therapy, medications, medical and surgical interventions, patient referrals such as counseling and finding a support group, patient teaching, and follow-up directions.

A SOAP chart note should express current patient data, including the date of the visit, patient's name, date of birth, age, and gender.

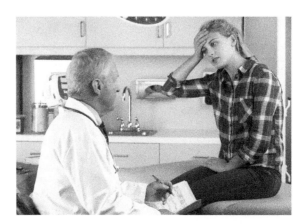

FIGURE 1.12 This patient is describing her symptoms to the physician.
Source: Cathy Yeulet/123RF

Tools for Effective Communication

AIDET®

AIDET® is an acronym (Acknowledge, Introduce, Duration, Explanation, Thank you) that represents the components of an effective communication framework to leverage during interactions, especially with people who might be nervous, anxious, or vulnerable. Developed by Studer Group as the "Five Fundamentals of Patient Communication" in the mid-1990s and later registered by Studer Group as AIDET®, it is most often used by healthcare professionals to communicate with patients and their families, as well as with each other. Research studies confirm that this approach appears to improve communication between healthcare professionals and their patients. The tenets of the AIDET® framework are as follows:

A **Acknowledge.** Greet people using appropriate tone and body language and use their names if you know them.

I **Introduce.** Introduce yourself to others. Tell them who you are (including skills set, experience and qualifications, if appropriate) and how you are going to help them. Escort people where they need to go rather than pointing or giving directions.

D **Duration.** Provide a time estimate and identify next steps. Keep in touch to ease waiting times. Let others know if there is a delay and how long it will be. When this is not possible, provide a time by which you will provide an update.

E **Explanation.** Explain step-by-step what to expect next, answer questions, and let the other person know how to contact you. Assess comprehension using the teach-back method. Listen and respond with compassion if needed.

T **Thank you.** Foster an attitude of gratitude. Thank people for their patronage, help, or assistance.

THE SBAR TECHNIQUE

The **SBAR** (Situation, Background, Assessment, Recommendation) technique, created by clinical staff at Kaiser Permanente in Colorado, provides a framework for communication between members of the healthcare team about a patient's condition. It is an acronym that represents a more efficient way for healthcare professionals to communicate, promotes effective collaboration, increases patient satisfaction, and improves patient outcomes. SBAR stands for:

S **Situation.** Clearly and briefly define the situation.

B **Background.** Provide clear, relevant background information that relates to the situation, such as the patient's diagnosis, the prescribing physicians, and the dates and dosages of medications.

A **Assessment.** A statement of your professional conclusion.

R **Recommendation.** What do you need for this individual? What action is requested and recommended?

Abbreviations *and* Acronyms

Abbreviation/Acronym	Meaning	Abbreviation/Acronym	Meaning
AD	Alzheimer disease	**C**	centigrade, Celsius
AIDET®	Acknowledge, Introduce, Duration, Explanation, Thank you	**CA**	cancer
		CC	chief complaint
ax	axillary	**CDC**	Centers for Disease Control and Prevention
BP	blood pressure		
Bx	biopsy	**cm**	centimeter

Abbreviation/ Acronym	Meaning	Abbreviation/ Acronym	Meaning
CVA	cerebrovascular accident	mg	milligram
DM	diabetes mellitus	mL	milliliter
DOB	date of birth	ng	nanogram
Dx	diagnosis	P	pulse
EHR	electronic health record	Path	pathology
g	gram	PE	physical examination
HIPAA	Health Insurance Portability and Accountability Act	R	respiration
		SOAP	subjective, objective, assessment, plan
Ht	height	SBAR	Situation, Background, Assessment, Recommendation
Hx	history		
ISMP	Institute for Safe Medication Practices	T	temperature
kg	kilogram	TJC	The Joint Commission
L	liter	TPR	temperature, pulse, respiration
mcg	microgram	Wt	weight

Study *and* Review III

Abbreviations

Place the correct word phrase or abbreviation in the space provided

1. CC _____

2. ax _____

3. biopsy _____

4. weight _____

5. Alzheimer disease _____

6. height _____

7. milliliter _____

8. gram _____

9. diagnosis _____

10. physical examination _____

Medical Case Snapshot

Note: There are certain qualifications for various conditions/diseases that must be met before patients who come to emergency departments on their own are admitted to hospitals. In the case that follows, the qualifications for chest pain admission are: (1) vital signs not within the normal range, (2) abnormal ECG/EKG, and (3) abnormal cardiac troponin positive. Cardiac troponin consists of proteins whose levels become elevated when the heart muscle has been damaged, such as occurs with a heart attack. The more damage there is to the heart, the greater the amount of troponin there will be in the blood. (See *Diagnostic and Laboratory Tests* in Chapter 8 for more information.)

Effective Ways to Communicate With a Patient

On the previous night, a 70-year-old female, Sarah Elizabeth Styles, came into the emergency department at 11:45 PM. She stated that she lives alone and awoke around 11:00 PM with sharp, burning pain in her chest, down her left arm, and up into her left jaw. When the pain did not go away, she drove herself to the hospital. The following tests and assessments were done:

Initial assessment: Vital signs, electrocardiogram (EKG), and a cardiac troponin blood test.

EKG Report: Abnormal. An abnormal EKG can signal a medical emergency, such as a myocardial infarction (heart attack) or a dangerous arrhythmia.

Laboratory Report: Cardiac troponin blood test, high—0.48 ng/mL. A nanogram (ng) is one billionth of a gram. The level of troponin that indicates a heart attack is the level above the reference range. For troponin concentrations 0.40 ng/mL and higher, the underlying cardiac injury is usually a myocardial infarction.

    The patient was admitted to the hospital for further evaluation and treatment. The next morning, a registered nurse enters the patient's room and says, "Hello, Ms. Styles, I am Sally Jones, your caregiver for this morning. I understand that you were admitted last evening with chest pain. How are you feeling now? Is there anything that I can get for you? I want to check your name band and then check your vital signs. What is your full name? Now, let's check your temperature, pulse, respirations, and blood pressure."

    The nurse records the following:

Name: Sarah Elizabeth Styles

T	98.6°F
P	96
R	20
B/P	154/92

"Your physician has ordered some follow-up lab tests and an EKG. These are used to check on your state of health at this time and help the doctor in planning his treatment for you. The lab technician will be here before breakfast.

"Let me help make you more comfortable, Ms. Styles. Shall I adjust the bed so you can sit up? You can have water or ice chips now, if you like.

"I will be back to check on you in a little while. If you need anything before then or change your mind about the ice chips, please use your call button. You have been very helpful this morning, and I thank you."

Note: The patient was glad to see the nurse and answered all of the questions that were asked and thanked Ms. Jones for her care.

Questions

Using the acronym AIDET, identify each letter's meaning and how it has been met by the nurse. Write in your answers.

A _____

I _____

D _____

E _____

T _____

Practical Application

Methods of Documentation and Tools for Effective Communication

Write your answers to the following questions.

1. The _____ note is a method of displaying patient data in a concise, organized format and is written to improve communication among those caring for the patient.

2. Pain, nausea, dizziness, tightness in the chest, lump in the throat, weakness of the legs, and "butterflies" in the stomach are examples of which part of a chart note? _____

3. The vital signs are included in which part of a chart note? _____

4. What is the acronym that is used to describe a way to communicate with people who are often nervous, anxious, and feeling vulnerable? _____

5. What part of the above-mentioned acronym is used when you "Greet people with a smile and use their names if you know them"? _____

6. What part of the above-mentioned acronym is used when you "Advise others what you are doing, how procedures work, and whom to contact if they need assistance"? _____

7. What part of the above-mentioned acronym is used when you "Foster an attitude of gratitude"? _____ _____

8. What is the technique, created by clinical staff at Kaiser Permanente in Colorado, that provides a framework for communication between members of the healthcare team about a patient's condition? _____

9. In the above-mentioned technique, included in the relevant background information are situations, such as the patient's _____, the prescribing physicians, and the dates and _____ of medications.

10. What part of the above-mentioned technique is "A statement of your professional conclusion"? _____

MyLab Medical Terminology™

MyLab Medical Terminology is a premium online homework management system that includes a host of features to help you study. Registered users will find:

- A multitude of activities and assignments built within the MyLab platform
- Powerful tools that track and analyze your results—allowing you to create a personalized learning experience
- Videos and audio pronunciations to help enrich your progress
- Streaming lesson presentations (guided lectures) and self-paced learning modules
- A space where you and your instructor can check your progress and manage your assignments

Suffixes and Prefixes

-rrhea
-oma intra-
-genesis mono-
anti- -itis
-uria
hyper-

Learning Outcomes

On completion of this chapter, you will be able to:

1. Describe how suffixes are used when building medical words.
2. Name adjective, noun, and diminutive suffixes.
3. Recognize suffixes that pertain to pathological conditions.
4. Identify selected suffixes common to surgical and diagnostic procedures.
5. Describe how prefixes are used when building medical words.
6. Name prefixes that are commonly used in medical terminology.
7. Identify prefixes that have more than one meaning.
8. Recognize prefixes that pertain to position or placement.
9. Identify selected prefixes that pertain to numbers and amounts.
10. Analyze, build, spell, and pronounce medical words.

Overview of Suffixes

The term **suffix** means *to fasten on, beneath, or under*. A suffix can be a syllable or group of syllables united with or placed at the end of a word to alter or modify the meaning of the word or to create a new word. A suffix can be connected to a prefix, a root, or to a combining form to make new words. For example, the suffix **-ic** (*pertaining to*) can be combined with the word root **gastr** (*stomach*) to make the medical word **gastr/ic** (*pertaining to the stomach*) or the suffix **-itis** (*inflammation*) can be combined with the word root **gastr** to make another medical word, **gastr/itis** (*inflammation of the stomach*).

A compound suffix is made up of more than one word component. It too is added to a root or a combining form to modify its meaning. For example, look at the suffix **-ectomy** (*surgical excision*). It is a combination of three word elements: **ec-**, a prefix meaning *out*; **tom**, a word root meaning *to cut*; and **-y**, a suffix meaning *process*. When the resulting suffix **-ectomy** is added to the root **gastr**, it forms the medical word **gastr/ectomy**, which means *surgical excision of the stomach* or literally *the process to cut out the stomach*.

Whenever you change the suffix, you alter the meaning of the word to which it is attached. For example, adding the suffix **-tomy** (*incision*) to the combining form **gastr/o** forms the medical word **gastr/o/tomy** (*incision into the stomach*). Notice that in the definition, the meaning associated with the suffix (*incision*) precedes the meaning associated with the combining form (*stomach*) to which it is attached. The term **gastr/o/tomy** means or can be read as *incision into* (the suffix) *the stomach* (the combining form).

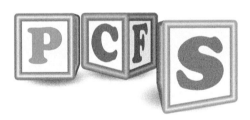

General-Use Suffixes

A collection of suffixes common to medical terminology is listed in Table 2.1. Note that all are preceded by a hyphen (-) to signify that they are to be linked to the end of a word root, combining form, or, in some cases, a prefix. Example words are included for each suffix along with their definition. As you progress through this text, the understanding of word parts and the process of building medical words will become easier and easier for you. You do not need to learn all the word parts at one time or the definition of each example word. Start with 10 and then add 10 more and soon you will be surprised at how much you have learned. In each chapter, the medical terms are divided into their component parts, and you will see the same word parts over and over. Before you know it, you are mastering the language of medicine.

TABLE 2.1 Selected Suffixes for General Use

Suffix	Meaning	Example Word	Word Definition
-algesia	condition of pain	an/*algesia*	Condition in which there is a lack of the sense of pain
-ase	enzyme	amyl/*ase*	Enzyme that breaks down starch
-ate	use, action	exud/*ate*	An oozing of pus or serum
-blast	immature cell, germ cell	oste/o/*blast*	Bone-forming cell
-cide	to kill	sperm/i/*cide*	Agent that kills sperm
-crit	to separate	hemat/o/*crit*	Blood test that separates solids from plasma in the blood by centrifuging the blood sample
-cuspid	point	bi/*cuspid*	Having two points or cusps
-cyst	bladder, sac	blast/o/*cyst*	A structure formed in the early embryogenesis of mammals, after the formation of the morula but before implantation
-cyte	cell	neur/o/*cyte*	Nerve cell, more commonly known as a neuron
-drome	that which runs together	syn/*drome*	A group of signs and symptoms occurring together that characterize a specific disease or pathological condition
-gen	formation, produce	muta/*gen*	Agent that causes a change in the genetic structure of an organism
-genesis	formation, produce	spermat/o/*genesis*	Formation of spermatozoa
-ive	nature of, quality of	connect/*ive*	Having the nature of connecting or binding together
-liter	liter	milli/*liter*	Unit of volume in the metric system; 0.001 L
-logy	study of	gynec/o/*logy*	Study of the female, especially the diseases of the female reproductive organs and the breasts
-lymph	clear fluid, serum, pale fluid	peri/*lymph*	Serous fluid of the inner ear
-or	one who, a doer	doct/*or*	Literally means to teach; one who is a recipient of an advanced degree, such as doctor of medicine (MD)
-phil	attraction	bas/o/*phil*	White blood cell that has an attraction for a base dye
-stasis	control, stop, stand still	hem/o/*stasis*	To stop bleeding
-therapy	treatment	hydro/*therapy*	Treatment using scientific application of water
-thermy	heat	dia/*thermy*	Treatment using high-frequency current to produce heat within a part of the body
-um	structure	epi/thel/i/*um*	Structure that covers the internal and external organs of the body and the lining of vessels, body cavities, glands, and organs

! ALERT!
The suffix **-um** also identifies the singular form of certain words, such as *ovum* (plural: *ova*).

| **-uria** | urination, condition of urine | hemat/*uria* | Blood in the urine |

Study *and* Review I

General-Use Suffixes

Write the correct answers in the spaces provided.

1. Why are suffixes preceded by a hyphen? _____
_____

2. Identify the suffix in the example word **analgesia** and give its meaning. _____
_____

3. Connect the combining form **neur/o** with the suffix **-cyte** and build a medical word. _____

4. What is a medical word that means blood in the urine? Use the suffix **-uria** and the word root **hemat** to build this word. _____

5. Form a medical word that means a blood test that separates solids from plasma in the blood by centrifuging the blood sample. Use the suffix **-crit** and the combining form **hemat/o**. _____

Matching

Select the appropriate lettered meaning for each of the following suffixes.

_____ **1.** -ase	**a.**	bladder, sac
_____ **2.** -cide	**b.**	formation, produce
_____ **3.** -cyst	**c.**	enzyme
_____ **4.** -genesis	**d.**	study of
_____ **5.** -ive	**e.**	to kill
_____ **6.** -logy	**f.**	heat
_____ **7.** -therapy	**g.**	urination, condition of urine
_____ **8.** -thermy	**h.**	structure
_____ **9.** -um	**i.**	nature of, quality
_____ **10.** -uria	**j.**	treatment

Grammatical Suffixes

Grammatical suffixes are those that can be attached to a word root to form a part of speech, especially a noun or an adjective, or to make a medical word singular or plural in its form. They are also used to indicate a diminutive form of a word that specifies a smaller version of the object indicated by the word root. You will find that many of these suffixes are the same as those used in the English language. See Tables 2.2, 2.3, and 2.4.

TABLE 2.2	Adjective Suffixes That Mean *Pertaining To*	
Suffix	**Word Analysis**	**Word Definition**
-ac	cardi/*ac*	Pertaining to the heart
-al	con/genit/*al*	Pertaining to presence at birth
-ar	muscul/*ar*	Pertaining to the muscles
-ary	integument/*ary*	Pertaining to the skin (a covering)
-ic	norm/o/cephal/*ic*	Pertaining to a normal appearance of the head as used in the objective description during a physical examination
-ile	pen/*ile*	Pertaining to the penis
-ior	anter/*ior*	Pertaining to a surface or part situated toward the front of the body
-ose	grandi/*ose*	Pertaining to a feeling of greatness
-ous	edemat/*ous*	Pertaining to an abnormal condition in which the body tissues contain an accumulation of fluid
-tic	cyan/o/*tic*	Pertaining to an abnormal condition of the skin and mucous membranes caused by oxygen deficiency in the blood
-us	de/cubit/*us*	Pertaining to a bedsore
-y	a/ton/*y*	Pertaining to a lack of normal tone or tension

TABLE 2.3	Noun Suffixes That Mean *Condition, Treatment,* or *Specialist*	
Suffix	**Word Analysis**	**Word Definition**
-esis	enur/*esis*	Condition of involuntary emission of urine; bedwetting
-ia	a/lopec/*ia*	Condition of loss of hair; baldness
-iatry	pod/*iatry*	Treatment of diseases and disorders of the foot
-ician	obstetr/*ician*	Physician who specializes in treating the female during pregnancy, childbirth, and postpartum
-ism	embol/*ism*	Condition in which a blood clot obstructs a blood vessel
-ist	cardi/o/log/*ist*	Physician who specializes in the study of the heart
-osis	hyper/hidr/*osis*	Condition of excessive sweating
-y	an/encephal/*y*	Congenital condition in which there is a lack of development of the brain

TABLE 2.4 Diminutive Suffixes That Mean *Small* or *Minute*

Suffix	Word Analysis	Word Definition
-icle	ventr/*icle*	Literally means *little belly*; a small cavity or chamber within a body or organ
-ole	bronchi/*ole*	One of the smaller subdivisions of the bronchial tubes
-ula	mac/*ula*	Small spot or discolored area of the skin
-ule	pust/*ule*	Small, elevated, circumscribed lesion of the skin that is filled with pus

Suffixes That Pertain to Pathological Conditions

Suffixes that carry meanings such as pain, weakness, swelling, softening, inflammation, and tumor are often combined with roots or combining forms to describe pathological conditions. Table 2.5 is an alphabetical listing of some of the more frequently used suffixes associated with disease conditions and disorders.

TABLE 2.5 Selected Suffixes That Pertain to Pathological Conditions

Suffix	Meaning	Pathological Condition	Definition of Condition
-algia	pain, ache	dent/*algia*	Pain in a tooth; toothache

> **! ALERT!**
> Other medical terms that mean *toothache* are odont/*algia* and odont/o/*dynia*.

Suffix	Meaning	Pathological Condition	Definition of Condition
-asthenia	weakness	my/*asthenia*	Muscular weakness and abnormal fatigue
-betes	to go	dia/*betes*	General term used to describe diseases characterized by excessive discharge of urine
-cele	hernia, tumor, swelling	cyst/o/*cele*	Hernia of the bladder that protrudes into the vagina
-cusis	hearing	presby/*cusis*	Impairment of hearing that occurs with aging
-derma	skin	xer/o/*derma*	Dry skin
-dynia	pain, ache	ot/o/*dynia*	Pain in the ear, earache
-ectasis	dilation, distention	bronch/i/*ectasis*	Chronic dilation of a bronchus or bronchi, with a secondary infection that usually involves the lower portion of a lung
-edema	swelling	papill/*edema*	Swelling of the optic disk, usually caused by increased intracranial pressure (ICP)
-emesis	vomiting	hyper/*emesis*	Excessive vomiting
-ion	process	in/fect/*ion*	Process whereby a pathogenic (*disease-producing*) microorganism invades the body, reproduces, multiplies, and causes disease
-itis	inflammation	burs/*itis*	Inflammation of a bursa (*padlike sac between muscles, tendons, and bones*)
-kinesis	motion	hyper/*kinesis*	Excessive muscular movement and motion; inability to be still; also known as hyperactivity
-lepsy	seizure	narc/o/*lepsy*	Chronic condition with recurrent attacks of uncontrollable drowsiness and sleep
-lexia	diction, word, phrase	dys/*lexia*	Condition in which an individual has difficulty in reading and comprehending written language

(continued)

TABLE 2.5   Selected Suffixes That Pertain to Pathological Conditions (continued)

Suffix	Meaning	Pathological Condition	Definition of Condition
-malacia	softening	oste/o/*malacia*	Softening of the bones
-mania	madness	pyro/*mania*	Impulse-control disorder consisting of a compulsion to set fires or to watch fires
-megaly	enlargement, large	acr/o/*megaly*	Characterized (in the adult) by marked enlargement and elongation of the bones of the face, jaw, and extremities
-mnesia	memory	a/*mnesia*	Condition in which there is a loss or lack of memory
-noia	mind	para/*noia*	Mental disorder characterized by highly exaggerated or unwarranted mistrust or suspiciousness
-oid	resemble	carcin/*oid*	Slow-growing type of cancer that typically begins in the lining of the digestive tract
-oma	tumor	carcin/*oma*	Malignant tumor arising in epithelial tissue
-opia	sight, vision	presby/*opia*	Vision defect in which parallel rays come to a focus beyond the retina; occurs normally with aging; farsightedness
-oxia	oxygen	hyp/*oxia*	Deficient amount of oxygen in the blood cells and tissues
-pathy	disease, emotion	retin/o/*pathy*	Any disease of the retina
-penia	deficiency	oste/o/*penia*	Deficiency of bone tissue, regardless of the cause
-pepsia	to digest	dys/*pepsia*	Difficulty in digestion; indigestion
-phagia	to eat, to swallow	a/*phagia*	Loss or lack of the ability to eat or swallow
-phasia	to speak, speech	dys/*phasia*	Impairment of speech caused by a brain lesion
-phobia	fear	acr/o/*phobia*	Fear of heights
-plasia	formation, produce	hyper/*plasia*	Excessive formation and growth of normal cells
-plasm	a thing formed, plasma	neo/*plasm*	New thing formed, such as an abnormal growth or tumor
-plegia	paralysis, stroke	hemi/*plegia*	Paralysis that affects one side of the body
-pnea	breathing	sleep a/*pnea*	Temporary cessation of breathing during sleep
-ptosis	drooping, prolapse, sagging	blephar/o/*ptosis*	Drooping of the upper eyelid(s)
-ptysis	spitting, coughing up	hem/o/*ptysis*	Spitting or coughing up blood
-rrhage	bursting forth	hem/o/*rrhage*	Excessive bleeding; bursting forth of blood
-rrhea	flow, discharge	rhin/o/*rrhea*	Discharge from the nose
-rrhexis	rupture	my/o/*rrhexis*	Rupture of a muscle

! ALERT!

Memorize these suffixes that begin with **rrh:** **-rrhage** (*bursting forth*), **-rrhea** (*flow, discharge*), **-rrhexis** (*rupture*), and the surgical procedure suffix **-rrhaphy** (*suture*).

Suffix	Meaning	Pathological Condition	Definition of Condition
-spasm	tension, spasm, contraction	my/o/*spasm*	Spasmodic contraction of a muscle
-trophy	nourishment, development	hyper/*trophy*	Literally means *excessive nourishment*

Suffixes Associated with Surgical and Diagnostic Procedures

Suffixes with meanings such as puncture, surgical excision, instrument to measure, and new opening are often combined with roots or combining forms to describe surgical and/ or diagnostic procedures. See Table 2.6 for an alphabetical listing of some of the more frequently used suffixes associated with surgery and diagnosis.

TABLE 2.6	Selected Suffixes Used in Surgical and Diagnostic Procedures		
Suffix	**Meaning**	**Example Word**	**Word Definition**
-centesis	surgical puncture	amni/o/*centesis*	Surgical puncture of the amniotic sac to obtain a sample of amniotic fluid containing fetal cells that are examined
-clasis	a break	oste/o/*clasis*	The intentional surgical fracture of a bone to correct a deformity
-desis	binding	arthr/o/*desis*	Surgical binding of a joint; surgical fixation of a joint
-ectomy	surgical excision, surgical removal, resection	vas/*ectomy*	Surgical procedure in which both of the vas deferens are clamped, cut, or otherwise sealed providing permanent sterility by preventing transport of sperm out of the testes
-gram	a weight, mark, record	dactyl/o/*gram*	Fingerprint
-graph	instrument for recording	electr/o/cardi/o/*graph*	Medical diagnostic device used for recording the electrical impulses of the heart muscle
-graphy	recording	mamm/o/*graphy*	Process of obtaining x-ray pictures of the breast using a low-dose x-ray system
-ize	to make, treat, or combine with	an/esthet/*ize*	To induce a loss of feeling or sensation with the administration of an anesthetic
-lysis	destruction, separation, breakdown, loosening	lip/o/*lysis*	Destruction of fat
-meter	instrument to measure, measure	audi/o/*meter*	Medical instrument used to measure hearing
-metry	measurement	pelvi/*metry*	Measurement of the expectant mother's pelvic dimensions to determine whether it will be possible to deliver a fetus through the normal vaginal route
-opsy	to view	bi/*opsy*	Surgical removal of a small piece of tissue for microscopic examination
-pexy	surgical fixation	gastr/o/*pexy*	Surgical fixation of the stomach to the abdominal wall for correction of displacement
-pheresis	remove	plasma/*pheresis*	Removal of blood from the body and centrifuging it to separate the plasma from the blood and reinfusing the cellular elements back into the patient
-plasty	surgical repair	rhin/o/*plasty*	Surgical repair of the nose
-rrhaphy	suture	my/o/*rrhaphy*	Suture of a muscle wound
-scope	instrument for examining	ophthalm/o/*scope*	Medical instrument used to examine the interior of the eye

(continued)

TABLE 2.6	Selected Suffixes Used in Surgical and Diagnostic Procedures *(continued)*		
Suffix	**Meaning**	**Example Word**	**Word Definition**
-scopy	visual examination, to view, examine	lapar/o/*scopy*	Visual examination of the abdominal cavity
-stomy	new opening	ile/o/*stomy*	Creation of a new opening through the abdominal wall into the ileum

> **! ALERT!**
> Be sure that you see the difference: **-stomy** means *new opening* and **-tomy** means *incision*.

-tome	instrument to cut	derma/*tome*	Instrument used to cut the skin for grafting
-tomy	incision	myring/o/*tomy*	Surgical incision of the tympanic membrane to remove unwanted fluids from the ear
-tripsy	crushing	lith/o/*tripsy*	Crushing of a kidney stone.

Study *and* Review II

Suffixes That Pertain to Pathological Conditions

Multiple Choice Select the correct suffix for the meaning.

1. weakness
   - **a.** -algia
   - **b.** -asthenia
   - **c.** -ectasis
   - **d.** -emesis

2. inflammation
   - **a.** -edema
   - **b.** -emesis
   - **c.** -ion
   - **d.** -itis

3. softening
   - **a.** -lepsy
   - **b.** -lexia
   - **c.** -malacia
   - **d.** -mania

4. disease, emotion
   - **a.** -pathy
   - **b.** -penia
   - **c.** -pnea
   - **d.** -plegia

5. spitting/coughing up
   - **a.** -rrhage
   - **b.** -rrhea
   - **c.** -rrhexis
   - **d.** -ptysis

Suffixes That Pertain to Surgical and Diagnostic Procedures

True / False Select true or false for the following statements.

1. The suffix *-centesis* means surgical puncture.

_____ True _____ False

2. The meaning of *-graphy* is an instrument for recording.

_____ True _____ False

3. The suffix *-plasty* means surgical puncture.

_____ True _____ False

4. A medical word that means a new opening through the abdominal wall into the ileum uses the suffix *-stomy*.

_____ True _____ False

5. An instrument used to cut the skin for grafting is called a *dermatome*.

_____ True _____ False

Overview of Prefixes

The term **prefix** means *to fix before* or *to fix to the beginning* of a word. A prefix can be a syllable or a group of syllables. Prefixes are united with or placed at the beginning of words to alter or modify their meanings or to create entirely new words. For example, by adding the prefix **ab-** to the root **norm** and the suffix **-al**, the word ***ab/norm/al*** is created. As you know, there is a big difference between normal and abnormal. Ab/norm/al means *pertaining to away from the norm*. Remember that when giving the meaning of the word or reading its definition, you usually begin with the meaning of the suffix. Note the component parts of the word *abnormal*:

ab-	**P** or prefix meaning	*away from*
norm	**R** or root meaning	*norm*
-al	**S** or suffix meaning	*pertaining to*

Not all medical words have a prefix, but when they do, the prefix will alter or modify the meaning of the word. For example, see the following list of medical words that were formed by uniting various prefixes with a single suffix (**-pnea**).

Prefix	Suffix	Medical Word	Word Definition
a- (lack of)	-pnea (breathing)	*a*/pnea	Temporary absence of (lack of) breathing
brady- (slow)	-pnea (breathing)	*brady*/pnea	Slow breathing
dys- (difficult)	-pnea (breathing)	*dys*/pnea	Difficult breathing
eu- (good, normal)	-pnea (breathing)	*eu*/pnea	Good, normal breathing
hyper- (excessive)	-pnea (breathing)	*hyper*/pnea	Excessive breathing
hypo- (deficient)	-pnea (breathing)	*hypo*/pnea	Deficient breathing
tachy- (rapid)	-pnea (breathing)	*tachy*/pnea	Rapid breathing

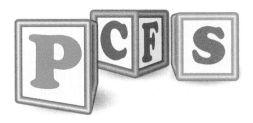

General-Use Prefixes

See Table 2.7 for a collection of prefixes that are commonly used in medical terminology. These prefixes can be linked with a word root, combining form, or suffix.

TABLE 2.7 Selected Prefixes for General Use

Prefix	Meanings	Example Words	Word Definitions
a-, an-	no, without, lack of, apart	a/mnes/ia	Condition in which there is a loss or lack of memory
		an/emia	Literally *a lack of red blood cells*; it is a reduction in the number of circulating red blood cells, the amount of hemoglobin, or the volume of packed red blood cells
anti-, contra-	against	anti/vir/al	Agent that works against viruses
		contra/indicat/ion	The process against the giving of a drug or treatment because it could be unsafe or inappropriate
auto-	self	auto/trans/fus/ion	Process of infusing a patient's own blood
brachy-	short	brachy/therapy	Radiation therapy in which the radioactive substance is inserted into a body cavity or organ. The source of radiation is located a short distance from the body area being treated.
brady-	slow	brady/card/ia	Abnormally slow heartbeat defined as less than 60 beats per minute
cac-, mal-	bad	cac/hexia	Condition of ill health, malnutrition, and wasting; may occur in chronic diseases such as cancer and pulmonary tuberculosis
		mal/format/ion	The process of being badly shaped, deformed
dia-	through, between	dia/gnosis	Determination of the cause and nature of a disease
dys-	bad, difficult, painful, abnormal	dys/men/o/rrhea	Difficulty or painful monthly flow (menses or menstruation)
eu-	good, normal	eu/pnea	Good or normal breathing
ex-, exo-	out, away from	ex/cis/ion	Process of cutting out, surgical removal
		exo/crine	Pertains to a type of gland that secretes into ducts (duct glands); examples include sweat glands, salivary glands, and mammary glands and also organs such as the stomach, liver, and pancreas
hetero-	different	hetero/sexu/al	Pertaining to the opposite sex; refers to an individual who has a sexual preference and relationship with the opposite sex
homeo-	similar, same, likeness, constant	homeo/stasis	State of equilibrium maintained in the body's internal environment; an important fundamental principle of physiology that permits a body to maintain a constant internal environment despite changes in the external environment
hydro-	water	hydro/cele	Accumulation of fluid in a saclike cavity
micro-	small	micro/cephal/us	Abnormally small head
oligo-	scanty, little	oligo/men/o/rrhea	Scanty monthly flow (menses, menstruation)
pan-	all	pan/cyt/o/penia	Lack of the cellular elements of the blood
pseudo-	false	pseudo/cyesis	False pregnancy
sym-, syn-	together, with	sym/physis	State of growing together
		syn/erget/ic	Pertaining to certain muscles that work together

Prefixes That Have More Than One Meaning

Just like suffixes, many prefixes have more than one meaning. See Table 2.8. To be able to identify the correct meaning of the prefix, you will need to analyze the definition of the medical word. For example, in the medical word **dyspnea** (*difficult breathing*), **dys-** means *difficult*. Note that **dys-** also means *bad, painful,* or *abnormal,* but in dyspnea these meanings do not apply. As you learn the various component parts that are used to build medical words, you will acquire the knowledge to select and use the correct meaning for each word.

TABLE 2.8	Selected Prefixes That Have More Than One Meaning		
Prefix	**Meanings**	**Prefix**	**Meanings**
a-, an-	no, not, without, lack of, apart	**extra-**	outside, beyond
ad-	toward, near	**hyper-**	above, beyond, excessive
bi-	two, double	**hypo-**	below, under, deficient
de-	down, away from	**in-**	in, into, not
di-	two, double	**mega-**	large, great
dia-	through, between, complete	**meta-**	beyond, over, between, change
dif-, dis-	apart, free from, separate	**para-**	beside, alongside, abnormal
dys-	bad, difficult, painful, abnormal	**poly-**	many, much, excessive
ec-, ecto-	out, outside, outer	**post-**	after, behind
end-, endo-	within, inner	**pre-**	before, in front of
ep-, epi-	upon, over, above	**pro-**	before, in front of
eu-	good, normal	**super-**	upper, above
ex-, exo-	out, away from	**supra-**	above, beyond

Study *and* Review III

Prefixes for General Use

Multiple Choice   Select the correct prefix for the meaning.

1. against

   a. an-

   b. auto-

   c. anti-

   d. dys-

2. slow

    a. brachy-   **c.** micro-

    b. brady-   **d.** pan-

3. small

    a. dys-   **c.** hetero-

    b. pan-   **d.** micro-

4. together, with

    a. homeo-   **c.** exo-

    b. sym-   **d.** an-

5. good, normal

    a. ex-   **c.** eu-

    b. dia-   **d.** dia-

Prefixes That Have More Than One Meaning

Matching   Select the appropriate lettered meanings for each of the prefixes.

_____ **1.** an-	**a.**	upon, over, above
_____ **2.** ad-	**b.**	many, much, excessive
_____ **3.** dia-	**c.**	good, normal
_____ **4.** epi-	**d.**	upper, above
_____ **5.** eu-	**e.**	above, beyond
_____ **6.** mega-	**f.**	no, not, without, lack of, apart
_____ **7.** poly-	**g.**	toward, near
_____ **8.** pre-	**h.**	through, between, complete
_____ **9.** super-	**i.**	large, great
_____ **10.** supra-	**j.**	before, in front of

Prefixes That Pertain to Position or Placement

Prefixes that carry meanings such as *away from, toward, before, above,* and *below* are often combined with roots and suffixes to describe a position or placement. See Table 2.9 for an alphabetical listing of some of the more frequently used prefixes associated with position or placements.

TABLE 2.9	Prefixes That Pertain to Position or Placement		
Prefix	**Meanings**	**Example Words**	**Word Definitions**
ab-	away from	*ab*/duct/ion	Process of moving a body part away from the middle
ad-	toward, near	*ad*/duct/or	Muscle that draws a part toward the middle
ana-	up, apart, backward	*ana*/trop/ia	Tendency of eyeballs to turn upward
ante-	before, forward	*ante*/flex/ion	The process of bending forward of an organ or part
cata-	down	*cata*/bol/ism	Literally *a casting down*; a breaking of complex substances into more basic elements
circum-, peri-	around	*circum*/cis/ion	Surgical process of removing (a cutting around) the foreskin of the penis
		peri/cardi/al	Pertaining to the pericardium, the sac surrounding the heart
endo-	within, inner	*endo*/card/itis	Inflammation of the endocardium (inner lining of the heart)
epi-	upon, above, over	*epi*/gastr/ic	Pertaining to the region above the stomach
ex-	out, away from	*ex*/cis/ion	Process of cutting out; surgical removal
extra-	outside, beyond	*extra*/corpor/eal	Pertaining to a medical procedure that is performed outside the body; for example, the circulation of the blood outside the body via a heart-lung machine or hemodialyzer
hyper-	above, beyond, excessive	*hyper*/tens/ion	High blood pressure
hypo-	below, under, deficient	*hypo*/tens/ion	Low blood pressure
inter-	between	*inter*/cost/al	Pertaining to between the ribs
intra-	within, into	*intra*/uter/ine	Pertaining to within the uterus
meso-	middle	*meso*/derm	A middle layer of the embryo lying between the ectoderm and endoderm
para-	beside, alongside	*para*/plegia	Paralysis of the lower part of the body and of both legs
retro-	backward	*retro*/vers/ion	Process of being turned backward, such as the displacement of the uterus with the cervix pointed forward
sub-	below, under, beneath	*sub*/lingu/al	Pertaining to below the tongue
supra-	above, beyond, superior	*supra*/ren/al	Two small glands located on top (above) of each kidney, also called adrenal glands

Prefixes That Pertain to Numbers and Amounts

Prefixes with meanings such as *both, ten, double, many, half,* and *none* are often combined with roots or suffixes to describe numbers or amounts. See Table 2.10 for an alphabetical list of some of the more frequently used prefixes associated with numbers and amounts.

TABLE 2.10	Prefixes That Pertain to Numbers and Amounts		
Prefix	**Meanings**	**Example Word**	**Word Definitions**
ambi-	both	*ambi*/later/al	Pertaining to both sides
bi-	two, double	*bi*/later/al	Pertaining to two sides
bin-	twice, two	*bin*/aur/al	Pertaining to both ears
centi-	one hundredth	*centi*/meter	Unit of measurement in the metric system; one hundredth of a meter
deca-	ten	*deca*/gram	A weight of 10 grams
di(s)-	two, apart	*dis*/locat/ion	Displacement of a bone from a joint
milli-	one thousandth	*milli*/liter	Unit of volume in the metric system; 0.001 L
mono-	one	*mono*/nucle/osis	Condition of excessive amounts of mononuclear leukocytes in the blood
multi-	many, much	*multi*/para	Refers to a woman who has given birth to two or more children and is written as para 2 (3, 4, 5, etc.)
nulli-	none	*nulli*/para	Refers to a woman who has never delivered a viable offspring and is written as para 0
poly-	many	*poly*/uria	Excessive urination
primi-	first	*primi*/para	Refers to a woman who has had one birth at more than 20 weeks' gestation, regardless of whether the infant is born alive or dead and is written as para 1
quadri-	four	*quadri*/plegia	Paralysis of all four extremities and usually the trunk due to injury to the spinal cord in the cervical spine
semi-, hemi-	half	*semi*/lun/ar	Valves of the aorta and pulmonary artery; shaped like a crescent (half-moon)
		hemi/plegia	Paralysis of one half of the body when it is divided along the midsagittal plane
tri-	three	*tri*/som/y	Genetic condition of having three chromosomes instead of two that causes birth defects, such as Down syndrome
uni-	one	*uni*/later/al	Pertaining to one side

Study *and* Review IV

Prefixes That Pertain to Position or Placement

Matching   Select the appropriate lettered meaning for each of the following.

_____ 1. ab-	**a.** above, beyond, excessive
_____ 2. ad-	**b.** within, inner
_____ 3. peri-	**c.** away from
_____ 4. endo-	**d.** below, under, deficient
_____ 5. hyper-	**e.** around
_____ 6. hypo-	**f.** backward
_____ 7. inter-	**g.** between
_____ 8. intra-	**h.** below, under, beneath
_____ 9. retro-	**i.** toward, near
_____ 10. sub-	**j.** within, into

Prefixes That Pertain to Numbers and Amounts

Multiple Choice Select the correct prefix for the meaning.

1. two, double

    a. ambi-   **c.** deca-

    b. bi-   **d.** centi-

2. many, much

    a. milli-   **c.** nulli-

    b. tri-   **d.** multi-

3. four

    a. bin-   **c.** quadri-

    b. primi-   **d.** nulli-

4. three

    a. tri-   **c.** milli-

    b. uni-   **d.** deca-

5. one

    a. nulli-   **c.** uni-

    b. primi-   **d.** hemi-

Building Your Medical Vocabulary

This section provides the foundation for learning medical terminology. Review the alphabetized list of medical terms in the following pages. Note how common prefixes and suffixes are repeatedly applied to word roots and combining forms to create different meanings. A combining form is a word root plus a vowel. The chart below lists the combining forms and word roots used in this chapter and can help to strengthen your understanding of how medical words are built and spelled.

You will find that some terms have not been divided into word parts. These are common words or specialized terms that are included to enhance your medical vocabulary.

Combining Forms

act/o	acting, act	**later/o**	side
cardi/o	heart	**somn/o**	sleep
dactyl/o	fingers or toes	**ven/o**	vein
gynec/o	female		

Word Roots

comat	a deep sleep	**palp**	touch
consci	aware	**ras**	to scrape off
esthet	feeling, sensation	**ster**	solid
infect	to infect	**symmetric**	symmetry
menstru	to discharge the menses	**turg**	swelling

Medical Word	Word Parts		Definition
	Part	**Meaning**	
abrasion (ă-brā′ zhŭn)	**ab-** **ras** **-ion**	away from to scrape off process	Process of scraping away from a surface, such as skin or teeth, by friction. See Figure 2.1. An abrasion may be the result of trauma, such as a "skinned knee," or from a therapy, such as dermabrasion of the skin for removal of scar tissue. It can also occur from the wearing-down of a tooth from mastication (*chewing*).

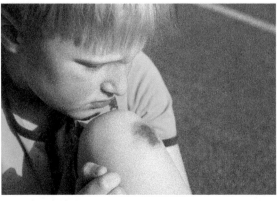

FIGURE 2.1 This young soccer player has an abrasion on his knee.
Source: Oksana Bratanova/123RF

Medical Word	Word Parts		Definition
	Part	Meaning	
anesthetize (ă-nĕs´ thĕ-tīz)	an- esthet -ize	without, lack of feeling, sensation to make	To induce a loss of feeling or sensation with the administration of an anesthetic agent. See Figure 2.2. 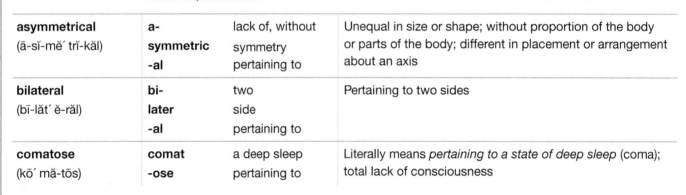 **FIGURE 2.2** A patient is being anesthetized before undergoing surgery. Source: herjua/Shutterstock
asymmetrical (ā-sǐ-mĕ´ trǐ-kăl)	a- symmetric -al	lack of, without symmetry pertaining to	Unequal in size or shape; without proportion of the body or parts of the body; different in placement or arrangement about an axis
bilateral (bī-lăt´ ĕ-răl)	bi- later -al	two side pertaining to	Pertaining to two sides
comatose (kō´ mă-tōs)	comat -ose	a deep sleep pertaining to	Literally means *pertaining to a state of deep sleep* (coma); total lack of consciousness

✓ **RULE REMINDER**

The **o** has been removed from the combining form because the suffix begins with a vowel.

gynecoid (gī´ nǐ-koyd)	gynec -oid	female resemble	Literally means *to resemble a female*; gynecoid pelvis is the normal shape of the birth canal that allows for the exit of the average-size fetus
hyperactive (hī˝ pĕr-ăk´ tǐv)	hyper- act -ive	excessive acting, act nature of, quality of	Nature or quality of excessive activity; this can refer to the entire organism or to a particular entity such as the thyroid, heart, or muscles. It may also describe an individual who exhibits constant overactivity.
hypoplasia (hī˝ pō-plā´ zhē-ă)	hypo- -plasia	under formation	Underdevelopment of a tissue, organ, or body
infection (ĭn-fĕk´ shŭn)	infect -ion	to infect process	Process whereby a pathogenic (*disease-producing*) microorganism invades the body, reproduces, multiplies, and causes disease

Medical Word	Word Parts		Definition
	Part	Meaning	
insomnia (ĭn-sŏm′ nē-ă)	in- somn -ia	not sleep condition	Condition of not being able to sleep. People with insomnia can have difficulty falling asleep, wake up often during the night and have trouble going back to sleep, wake up too early in the morning, or experience unrefreshing sleep.
intravenous (in′ tră-vē′ nŭs)	intra- ven -ous	within vein pertaining to	Pertaining to within a vein

GOOD TO KNOW ▶

According to the Centers for Disease Control and Prevention, vaccines are available for many dangerous or deadly infectious diseases. Over the years, vaccines have prevented countless cases of disease and saved millions of lives. Everyone, from infant to adult, needs to be vaccinated for certain diseases, depending on their age, location, job, lifestyle, travel schedule, health conditions, or previous vaccinations. See Figure 2.3.

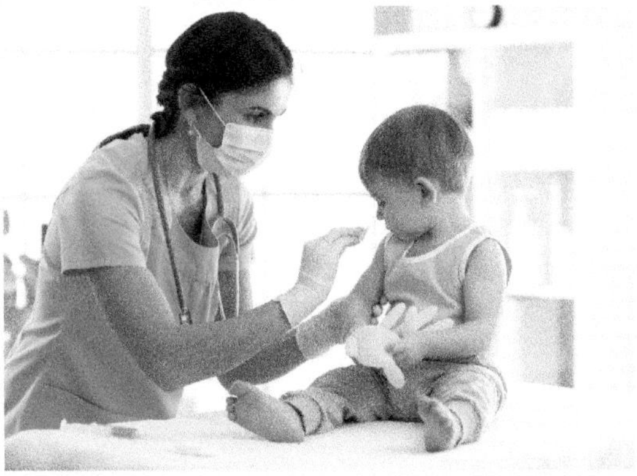

Vaccines are available for the following diseases, many of which are discussed throughout this text.

- Chickenpox (Varicella)
- Diphtheria
- Flu (Influenza)
- Hepatitis A
- Hepatitis B
- Hib (Haemophilus influenzae type b)
- HPV (Human Papillomavirus)
- Measles
- Meningococcal
- Mumps
- Pneumococcal
- Polio (Poliomyelitis)
- Rotavirus
- Rubella (German Measles)
- Shingles (Herpes Zoster)
- Tetanus (Lockjaw)
- Whooping Cough (Pertussis)

FIGURE 2.3 The healthcare professional is preparing to administer the DTaP vaccine to a young boy. DTaP is a vaccine that helps children younger than age 7 to develop immunity to three deadly diseases caused by bacteria: diphtheria, tetanus, and pertussis (whooping cough).
Source: Oksana Kuzmina/123RF

| latent
(lāt′ ĕnt) | | | Lying hidden; quiet, not active; for example, tuberculosis (TB) may be latent for extended periods of time and become active under certain conditions |

Medical Word	Word Parts		Definition
	Part	**Meaning**	
lumen (loo′ mĕn)			Space within an artery, vein, intestine, or tube; it is also the hollow core of a hypodermic needle, which forms an oval-shaped opening when exposed at the beveled (flat, slanted surface) point
palpate (păl′ pāt)	**palp** **-ate**	touch use, action	To use the hands or fingers to examine by touch; to feel. See Figure 2.4 and refer to Figure 1.9.

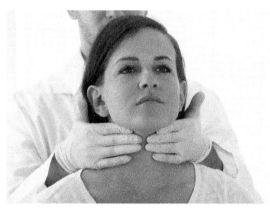

FIGURE 2.4 The physician is palpating the patient's thyroid gland, checking its size and location.
Source: Andriy Popov/123RF

Medical Word	Word Parts		Definition
patent (pat′ ĕnt)			Wide open; freely open; for example, a lumen would be patent (opposite of occlusion)
pericardial (pĕr-ĭ-kăr′ dē-ăl)	**peri-** **cardi** **-al**	around heart pertaining to	Pertaining to the pericardium (a fibrous sac surrounding the heart)
polydactyly (pŏl″ ē-dăk′ tĭ-lē)	**poly-** **dactyl** **-y**	many fingers or toes pertaining to	Pertaining to having more than the normal number of fingers and toes; for example, a person having six fingers or toes

✓ **RULE REMINDER**

The **o** has been removed from the combining form because the suffix **-y** is a vowel.

Medical Word	Word Parts		Definition
premenstrual (prē-mĕn′ stroo-ăl)	**pre-** **menstru** **-al**	before to discharge the menses pertaining to	Pertaining to the number of days before the discharge of the menses (the monthly flow of bloody fluid from the endometrium via the vagina)

Medical Word	Word Parts		Definition
	Part	Meaning	
steroid (stĕr´ oyd)	ster -oid	solid resemble	Literally means *resembling a solid substance*; applies to any one of a large group of substances chemically related to sterols; natural steroid hormones include androgens, estrogens, and adrenal cortex secretions
superinfection (soo˝ pĕr-ĭn-fĕk´ shŭn)	super- infect -ion	upper, above to infect process	An infection following a previous infection produced by an overgrowth of a resistant strain of bacteria, fungi, or yeast. It can occur as an adverse effect of antibiotic usage or overusage.
trauma (traw´ mă)			Physical injury or wound caused by external force, violence, or a toxic substance; also refers to psychological injury resulting from a severe emotional shock, which can cause disordered feelings and/or behavior. See Figure 2.5.

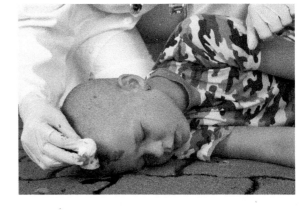

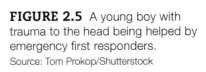

FIGURE 2.5 A young boy with trauma to the head being helped by emergency first responders.
Source: Tom Prokop/Shutterstock

Medical Word	Word Parts		Definition
turgor (tur´ gor)	turg -or	swelling one who	Generally refers to the expected resiliency of the skin caused by the outward pressure of the cells and interstitial fluid. An evaluation of the skin turgor is an essential part of physical assessment.
unconscious (ŭn-kŏn´ shŭs)	un- consci -ous	not aware pertaining to	An abnormal state in which the person is not aware of his or her environment. In this state the person experiences no sensory impressions and is unresponsive neurologically.

Study *and* Review V

Using Suffixes to Build Medical Words

Using a suffix from the following list, build the appropriate medical word.

-al	-ior	-ar	-ile	-icle
-ary	-osis	-ia	-ula	-us

1. Condition of excessive sweating   hyper/hidr/_____

2. Pertaining to muscles   muscul/_____

3. Small spot or discolored area of the skin   mac/_____

4. Condition of loss of hair   a/lopec/_____

5. Literally means *little belly*   ventr/_____

6. Pertaining to a bedsore   de/cubit/_____

7. Pertaining to the skin   integument/_____

8. Pertaining to the penis   pen/_____

9. Pertaining to present at birth   con/genit/_____

10. Pertaining to toward the front of the body   anter/_____

Using Prefixes to Build Medical Words

Using a prefix from the following list and the suffix -pnea (*breathing*), build the appropriate medical word.

a-	brady-	dys-	eu-
hyper-	hypo-	tachy-	

1. Temporary lack of breathing   _____ /pnea

2. Rapid breathing   _____ /pnea

3. Good, normal breathing   _____ /pnea

4. Difficult breathing   _____ /pnea

5. Excessive breathing   _____ /pnea

6. Slow breathing   _____ /pnea

7. Deficient breathing   _____ /pnea

Identifying Medical Terms—Suffixes

In the spaces provided, write the medical terms for the following meanings.

1. _____ Process of scraping away from a surface

2. _____ To induce a loss of feeling or sensation

3. _____ Pertaining to a state of alertness or consciousness

4. _____ Unequal in size or shape

5. _____ The process whereby a pathogenic organism invades the body and causes disease

6. _____ Pertaining to a state of deep sleep

7. _____ Refers to the expected resiliency of the skin

8. _____ Pertaining to a feeling of greatness

9. _____ To resemble a female

10. _____ To use the hands or fingers to examine by touch

Identifying Medical Terms—Prefixes

In the spaces provided, write the medical terms for the following meanings.

1. _____ Pertaining to two sides

2. _____ Nature or quality of excessive activity

3. _____ Underdevelopment of a tissue, organ, or body

4. _____ Condition of not being able to sleep

5. _____ Pertaining to within a vein

6. _____ Pertaining to the pericardium (the sac surrounding the heart)

7. _____ Pertaining to having more than the normal number of fingers and/or toes

8. _____ Pertaining to the number of days before the discharge of the menses (monthly menstrual flow)

9. _____ An infection following a previous infection produced by an overgrowth of a resistant strain of bacteria, fungi, or yeast

10. _____ An abnormal state in which the person is not aware of his or her environment

MyLab Medical Terminology™

MyLab MedicalTerminology is a premium online homework management system that includes a host of features to help you study. Registered users will find:

- A multitude of quizzes and activities built within the MyLab platform
- Powerful tools that track and analyze your results—allowing you to create a personalized learning experience
- Videos and audio pronunciations to help enrich your progress
- Streaming lesson presentations (guided lectures) and self-paced learning modules
- A space where you and your instructor can check your progress and manage your assignments

Organization of the Body

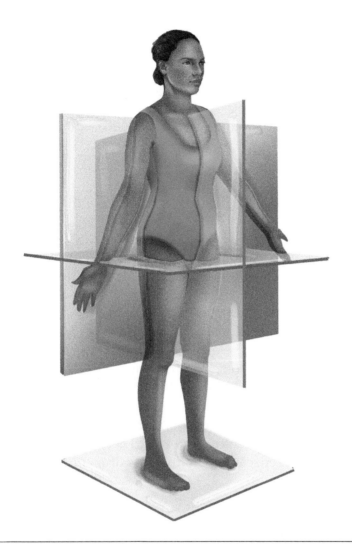

 ## Learning Outcomes

On completion of this chapter, you will be able to:

1. Define terms that describe the body and its structural units.
2. List the systems of the body and the organs in each system.
3. Define terms that are used to describe direction, planes, and cavities of the body.
4. Describe word analysis as it relates to head-to-toe assessment.
5. Analyze, build, spell, and pronounce medical words.
6. Describe the drugs highlighted in this chapter.
7. Identify and define selected abbreviations and acronyms.

Anatomy and Physiology

This chapter introduces you to terms describing the body and its structural units. To aid you, these terms have been grouped into two major sections: The first offers an overview of the units that make up the human body, and the second covers terms used to describe anatomical positions and locations.

The human body is made up of atoms, molecules, organelles, cells, tissues, organs, and systems. See Figure 3.1. All of these parts normally function together in a unified and complex process known as **homeostasis** (a state of equilibrium that is maintained within the body's internal environment). This means that the body's fluid composition, its volume and characteristics, and its temperature (T), blood pressure (BP), and the exchange of oxygen (O_2) and carbon dioxide (CO_2) remain within normal limits. By maintaining homeostasis, the cells of the body are in an environment that meets their needs and permits them to function optimally under changing conditions.

Human Body: Levels of Organization

Atoms

An **atom** is the smallest, most basic chemical unit of an element. It consists of a nucleus that contains protons and neutrons and is surrounded by electrons. A **proton** is a positively charged particle; a **neutron** is without any electrical charge. An **electron** is a negatively charged particle that revolves around the nucleus of an atom.

Chemical elements are made up of atoms, which can be classified on the basis of their atomic number into groups called elements. An **element** is a substance that cannot be broken down by chemical means into any other substance. There are 118 elements listed on the Periodic Table from atomic numbers 1 (hydrogen) to 118 (ununoctium).

Elements found in the human body include aluminum, carbon, calcium, chlorine, cobalt, copper, fluorine, hydrogen, iodine, iron, manganese, magnesium, nitrogen, oxygen, phosphorus, potassium, sodium, sulfur, and zinc. The mass of the human body is made up of just six elements: oxygen, carbon, hydrogen, nitrogen, calcium, and phosphorus.

Molecules

A **molecule** is a chemical combination of two or more atoms that form a chemical bond with each other. It does not matter if the atoms are the same or are different from each other. Molecules may be simple or complex. Examples of molecules include H_2O (water), N_2 (nitrogen), O_3 (ozone), CaO (calcium oxide), and $C_6H_{12}O_6$ (glucose, a type of sugar).

In a water molecule (H_2O), oxygen forms polar covalent (sharing of electrons) bonds with two hydrogen atoms. **Water** is a tasteless, clear, odorless liquid that makes up 65% of a male's body weight and 55% of a female's body weight. Water is the most important constituent of all body fluids, secretions, and excretions. It is an ideal transportation medium for inorganic and organic compounds.

Cells

The body consists of millions of cells working individually and with each other to sustain life. For the purposes of this text, **cells** are considered the basic building blocks for the various structures that together make up a human being. There are several types of

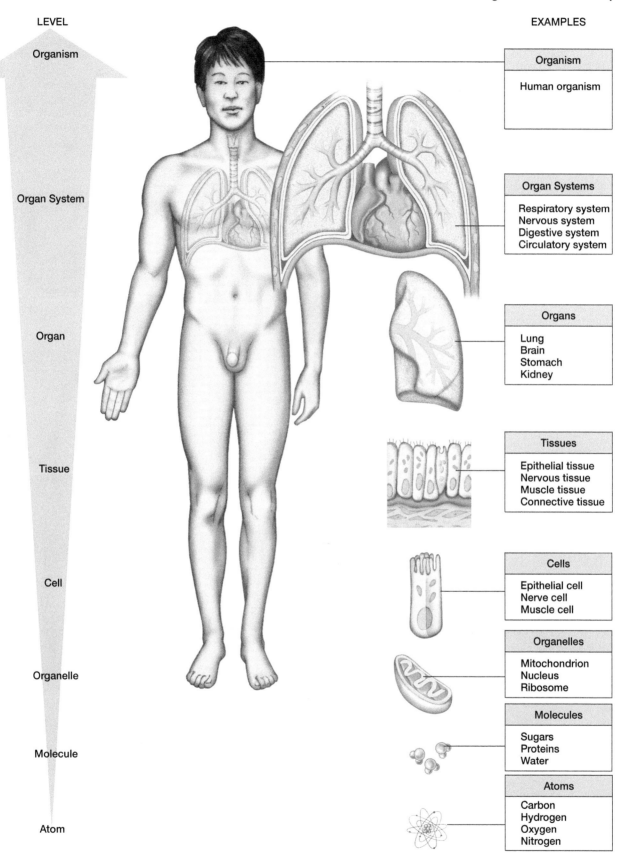

LEVEL

Organism

Organ System

Organ

Tissue

Cell

Organelle

Molecule

Atom

EXAMPLES

Organism

Human organism

Organ Systems

Respiratory system
Nervous system
Digestive system
Circulatory system

Organs

Lung
Brain
Stomach
Kidney

Tissues

Epithelial tissue
Nervous tissue
Muscle tissue
Connective tissue

Cells

Epithelial cell
Nerve cell
Muscle cell

Organelles

Mitochondrion
Nucleus
Ribosome

Molecules

Sugars
Proteins
Water

Atoms

Carbon
Hydrogen
Oxygen
Nitrogen

FIGURE 3.1 Human body: levels of organization.

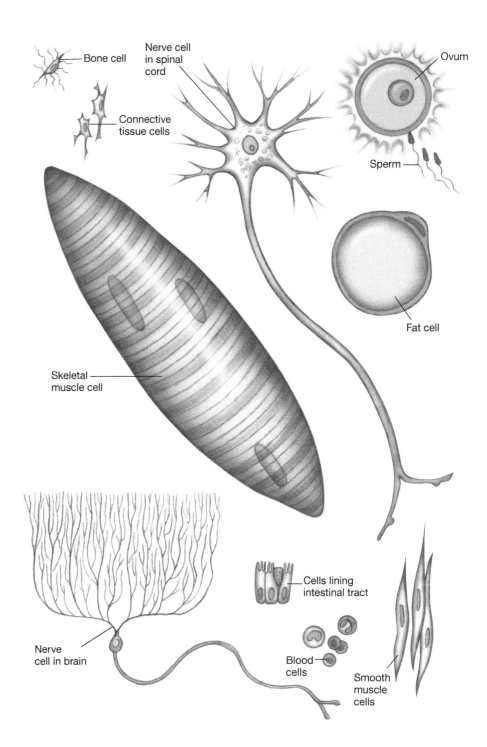

FIGURE 3.2 Cells are the basic building blocks of the human body. They have many different shapes and vary in size and function. These examples show the range of forms and sizes with the dimensions they would have if magnified approximately 500 times.

cells, with each specialized to perform specific functions. The size and shape of a cell are generally related directly to its function. See Figure 3.2.

For example, cells forming the skin overlap each other to form a protective barrier, whereas nerve cells are usually elongated with branches connecting to other cells for the transmission of sensory impulses. Despite these differences, however, cells can generally be said to have a number of common components. The major parts of the cell are the cell membrane, cytoplasm, and nucleus. See Figure 3.3 and Table 3.1.

CELL MEMBRANE

The outer covering of the cell is called the *cell membrane*. Cell membranes have the capability of allowing some substances to pass into and out of the cell while denying passage

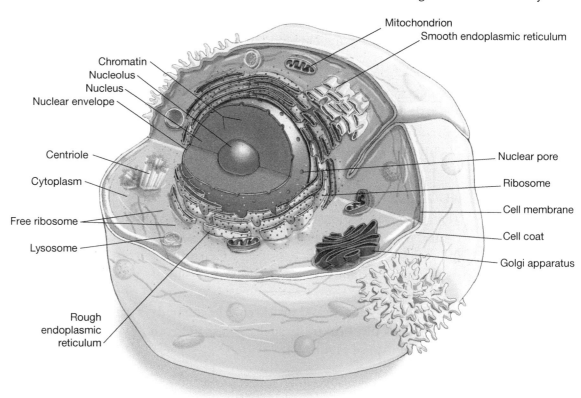

FIGURE 3.3 Major parts of a cell.

TABLE 3.1	**Major Cell Structures and Primary Functions**
Cell Structures	**Primary Functions**
Cell membrane	Protects the cell; provides for communication via receptor proteins; surface proteins serve as positive identification tags; allows some substances to pass into and out of the cell while denying passage to other substances; this selectivity allows cells to receive nutrition and dispose of waste
Cytoplasm	Provides storage and work areas for the cell; the work and storage elements of the cell, called *organelles*, are the ribosomes, endoplasmic reticulum, Golgi apparatus, mitochondria, lysosomes, and centrioles
Ribosomes	Make enzymes and other proteins; nicknamed "protein factories"
Endoplasmic reticulum (ER)	Carries proteins and other substances through the cytoplasm
Golgi apparatus	Chemically processes the molecules from the endoplasmic reticulum and then packages them into vesicles; nicknamed "chemical processing and packaging center"
Mitochondria	Involved in cellular metabolism and respiration; provide the principal source of cellular energy and are the place where complex, energy-releasing chemical reactions occur continuously; nicknamed "power plants"
Lysosomes	Contain enzymes that can digest food compounds; nicknamed "digestive bags"
Centrioles	Play an important role in cell reproduction
Cilia	Hairlike processes that project from epithelial cells; help propel mucus, dust particles, and other foreign substances from the respiratory tract
Flagellum	"Tail" of the sperm that enables the sperm to "swim" or move toward the ovum
Nucleus	Controls every *organelle* (little organ) in the cytoplasm; contains the genetic matter necessary for cell reproduction as well as control over activity within the cell's cytoplasm; responsible for the cell's metabolism, growth, and reproduction

to other substances. This selectivity allows cells to receive nutrition and dispose of waste just as a human being eats food and disposes of waste.

CYTOPLASM

The substance between the cell membrane and the nuclear membrane is called the *cytoplasm*. It is a jelly-like material that is mostly water. The cytoplasm provides storage and work areas for the cell. The work and storage elements of the cell, called *organelles* (little organs), are the endoplasmic reticulum (ER), ribosomes, Golgi apparatus, mitochondria, lysosomes, and centrioles.

NUCLEUS

The nucleus is responsible for the cell's metabolism, growth, and reproduction. It is the central portion of the cell that contains the chromosomes (microscopic bodies that carry the genes that determine hereditary characteristics). A single gene makes up each segment of deoxyribonucleic acid (DNA) and is located in a specific site on the chromosome. The human body has 23 pairs of chromosomes. A genome is the complete set of genes and chromosomes tucked inside each of the body's trillions of cells. Genes determine an individual's physical traits such as hair, skin, and eye color, body structure, and metabolic activity. See Figure 3.4.

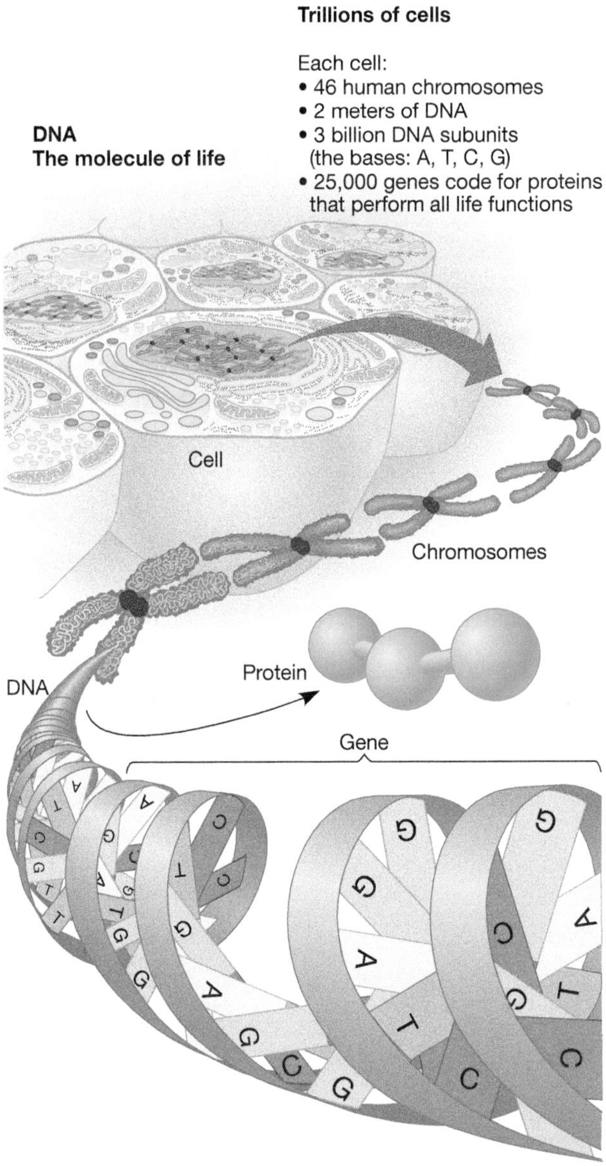

Trillions of cells

Each cell:
• 46 human chromosomes
• 2 meters of DNA
• 3 billion DNA subunits (the bases: A, T, C, G)
• 25,000 genes code for proteins that perform all life functions

DNA
The molecule of life

Cell

Chromosomes

Protein

Gene

DNA

FIGURE 3.4 Each cell nucleus throughout the body contains the genes, DNA, and chromosomes that make up the majority of an individual's genome.

Source: Zelman, Mark; Tompary, Elaine; Raymond, Jill; Holdaway, Paul; Mulvihill, Mary Lou E., Human Diseases, 8th Ed., ©2015. Reprinted and Electronically reproduced by permission of Pearson Education, Inc., New York, NY.

Stem Cells

Stem cells are the precursors of all body cells. Stem cells have three general properties: They are capable of dividing and renewing themselves for long periods, they are unspecialized, and they can give rise to specialized cell types. Some primary sources of stem cells include embryos, adult tissues, and umbilical cord blood. An embryonic cell is an unspecialized cell that can turn itself into any type of tissue. Embryonic stem cells are derived primarily from frozen **in vitro** (in glass, as in a test tube) fertilized embryos. An adult stem cell is a more specialized cell found in many kinds of tissue, such as bone marrow, skin, and the liver. An umbilical cord cell is a rich source of precursors of mature blood cells. It is obtained from cord blood at the time of birth.

Stem cells can now be grown and transformed into specialized cells with characteristics consistent with cells of various tissues such as muscles or nerves through cell culture. Highly plastic adult stem cells from a variety of sources, including umbilical cord blood and bone marrow, are used in medical therapies, which are often referred to as *regenerative medicine*.

GOOD TO KNOW ▶

According to the American Society of Plastic Surgeons, regenerative medicine is the science of using adipose-derived stem cells harvested from fat to regenerate cells and tissues in the human body. Fat tissue is an important source of adult mesenchymal stem cells. (The term *mesenchymal* refers to the diffuse network of cells forming the embryonic mesoderm and giving rise to connective tissue, blood and blood vessels, the lymphatic system, and cells of the mononuclear phagocyte system.) Discovered by plastic surgeons, adipose-derived stem cells are easy to isolate from fat tissue and hold tremendous promise for treating many disorders across the body.

A significant advance in surgical regenerative medicine has been the development and refinement of techniques to transfer fat tissue in a minimally invasive manner, using a patient's own extra fat tissue, thus allowing the regeneration of fat tissue in other parts of the body. This technique is revolutionizing many reconstructive procedures, such as breast reconstruction.

Tissues

A **tissue** is a grouping of similar cells that together perform specialized functions. There are four basic types of tissue in the body: epithelial, connective, muscle, and nerve. Each of the four basic tissues has several subtypes named for their shape, appearance, arrangement, or function. The following sections describe the four basic types of tissue. See Figure 3.5.

EPITHELIAL TISSUE

Epithelial tissue appears as sheetlike arrangements of cells, sometimes several layers thick, that form the outer surfaces of the body and line the body cavities and the principal tubes and passageways leading to the exterior. These cells form the secreting portions

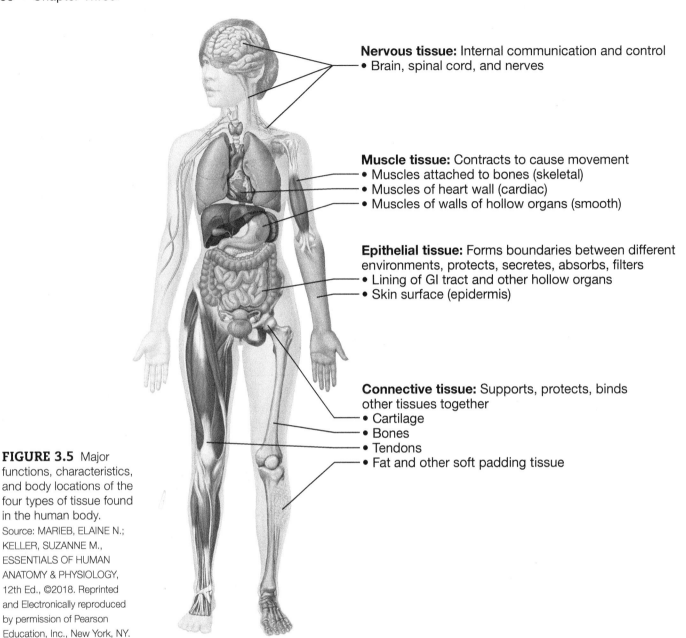

Nervous tissue: Internal communication and control
• Brain, spinal cord, and nerves

Muscle tissue: Contracts to cause movement
• Muscles attached to bones (skeletal)
• Muscles of heart wall (cardiac)
• Muscles of walls of hollow organs (smooth)

Epithelial tissue: Forms boundaries between different environments, protects, secretes, absorbs, filters
• Lining of GI tract and other hollow organs
• Skin surface (epidermis)

Connective tissue: Supports, protects, binds other tissues together
• Cartilage
• Bones
• Tendons
• Fat and other soft padding tissue

FIGURE 3.5 Major functions, characteristics, and body locations of the four types of tissue found in the human body.
Source: MARIEB, ELAINE N.; KELLER, SUZANNE M., ESSENTIALS OF HUMAN ANATOMY & PHYSIOLOGY, 12th Ed., ©2018. Reprinted and Electronically reproduced by permission of Pearson Education, Inc., New York, NY.

of glands and their ducts and are important parts of certain sense organs. There are six main functions of epithelial tissue:

1. *Protection.* Protects underlying tissue from mechanical injury, harmful chemicals and **pathogens**, and excessive water loss.

2. *Sensation.* Sensory stimuli are detected by specialized epithelial cells found in the skin, eyes, ears, and nose and on the tongue.

3. *Secretion.* In glands, epithelial tissue is specialized to secrete specific chemical substances such as enzymes, hormones, and lubricating fluids.

4. *Absorption.* Certain epithelial cells lining the small intestine absorb nutrients from the digestion of food.

5. *Excretion.* Epithelial tissues in the kidney excrete waste products from the body and reabsorb needed materials from the urine. Sweat is also excreted from the body by epithelial cells in the sweat glands.

6. *Diffusion.* Simple epithelium (found in the walls of capillaries and lungs) promotes the diffusion of gases, liquids, and nutrients.

CONNECTIVE TISSUE

The most widespread and abundant of the body tissues, **connective tissue** forms the supporting network for the organs of the body, sheaths the muscles, and connects muscles to bones and bones to joints. Bone is a dense form of connective tissue.

MUSCLE TISSUE

There are three types of **muscle tissue**:

1. **Skeletal muscle** or *voluntary muscle* is striated in appearance and is anchored by tendons to bone. They are used to effect skeletal movement such as locomotion and in maintaining posture. An average adult male is made up of 42% skeletal muscle and an average adult female is made up of 36% (as a percentage of body mass).

2. **Smooth muscle** or *involuntary muscle* is found within the walls of organs and structures such as the esophagus, stomach, intestines, bronchi, uterus, urethra, bladder, blood vessels, and the arrector pili in the skin. Unlike skeletal muscle, smooth muscle is not under conscious control and is under the control of the autonomic nervous system.

3. **Cardiac muscle** is also an involuntary muscle and is a specialized form of striated tissue found only in the heart. Cardiac muscle is under the control of the autonomic nervous system.

NERVE TISSUE

Nerve tissue (also called *nervous tissue*) consists of nerve cells (neurons) and supporting cells called *neuroglia*. It has the properties of excitability and conductivity and functions to control and coordinate the activities of the body.

Organs

Multiple different tissues serving a common purpose or function make up structures called **organs**. Examples are the brain, skin, or heart.

Systems

A group of different organs functioning together for a common purpose is called a **system**. The various body systems function in support of the body as a whole. Figure 3.6 shows the organ systems of the body. Each body system is discussed in the following chapters.

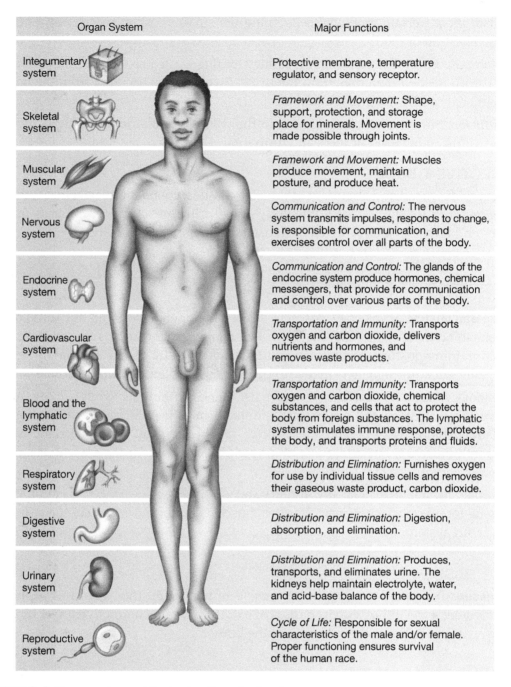

Organ System	Major Functions
Integumentary system	Protective membrane, temperature regulator, and sensory receptor.
Skeletal system	*Framework and Movement:* Shape, support, protection, and storage place for minerals. Movement is made possible through joints.
Muscular system	*Framework and Movement:* Muscles produce movement, maintain posture, and produce heat.
Nervous system	*Communication and Control:* The nervous system transmits impulses, responds to change, is responsible for communication, and exercises control over all parts of the body.
Endocrine system	*Communication and Control:* The glands of the endocrine system produce hormones, chemical messengers, that provide for communication and control over various parts of the body.
Cardiovascular system	*Transportation and Immunity:* Transports oxygen and carbon dioxide, delivers nutrients and hormones, and removes waste products.
Blood and the lymphatic system	*Transportation and Immunity:* Transports oxygen and carbon dioxide, chemical substances, and cells that act to protect the body from foreign substances. The lymphatic system stimulates immune response, protects the body, and transports proteins and fluids.
Respiratory system	*Distribution and Elimination:* Furnishes oxygen for use by individual tissue cells and removes their gaseous waste product, carbon dioxide.
Digestive system	*Distribution and Elimination:* Digestion, absorption, and elimination.
Urinary system	*Distribution and Elimination:* Produces, transports, and eliminates urine. The kidneys help maintain electrolyte, water, and acid-base balance of the body.
Reproductive system	*Cycle of Life:* Responsible for sexual characteristics of the male and/or female. Proper functioning ensures survival of the human race.

FIGURE 3.6 Organ systems of the body with major functions.

Anatomical Locations and Positions

Four primary reference systems have been adopted to provide uniformity to the anatomical description of the body. These reference systems are **direction**, **planes**, **cavities**, and **structural unit**. The standard **anatomical position** for the body is erect, head facing forward, arms by the sides with palms to the front. Left and right are from the subject's point of view, not from the point of view of the person doing the examination. See Figure 3.7.

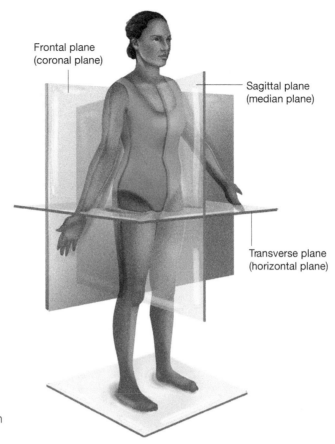

Frontal plane
(coronal plane)

Sagittal plane
(median plane)

Transverse plane
(horizontal plane)

FIGURE 3.7 Standard anatomical position
and planes of the body.

Direction

Directional and positional terms describe the location of organs or body parts in relationship to one another. See Figure 3.8. They are used in describing physical assessment of a patient's presenting complaints and in pinpointing the location of a given sign or symptom. Table 3.2 lists the terms used to describe direction and position, including their combining forms (CFs).

Planes

The following terms are used to describe the imaginary planes that are depicted in Figure 3.7 as passing through the body and dividing it into various sections.

- **Sagittal plane.** Vertically divides the body or structure into *right* and *left sides*.
- **Midsagittal plane.** Divides the body or structure into *right* and *left halves*.
- **Transverse** or **horizontal plane.** Any plane that divides the body into *superior* and *inferior* portions.
- **Coronal** or **frontal plane.** Any plane that divides the body at right angles to the midsagittal plane. The coronal plane divides the body into *anterior* (ventral) and *posterior* (dorsal) portions.

Cavities

A *cavity* is a hollow space containing body organs. Body cavities are classified into two groups according to their location. On the front is the **ventral cavity** (also called the *anterior cavity*) and on the back is the **dorsal cavity** (also called the *posterior cavity*). Various cavities found in the human body are depicted in Figure 3.9.

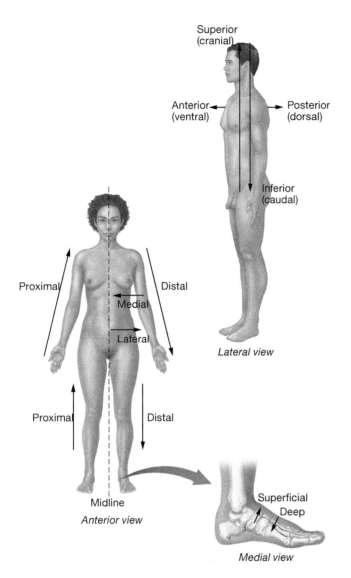

TERM	DEFINITION	EXAMPLES
Anterior (ventral)	Toward the front	• The palms are on the anterior side of the body. • The esophagus is anterior to the spinal cord.
Posterior (dorsal)	Toward the back	• The occipital bone is on the posterior cranium (skull). • The spinal cord is posterior to the esophagus.
Superior (cranial)	Toward the head	• The nose is superior to the mouth. • The neck is superior to the chest.
Inferior (caudal)	Toward the tail	• The nose is inferior to the forehead. • The umbilicus (belly button) is inferior to the chest.
Proximal	Closer to the point of origin (generally the trunk)	• The knee is proximal to the ankle. • The shoulder is proximal to the elbow.
Distal	Farther away from the point of origin (generally the trunk)	• The foot is distal to the hip. • The wrist is distal to the elbow.
Medial	Closer to the midline of the body or a body part; on the inner side of	• The ear is medial to the shoulder. • The index finger is medial to the thumb.
Lateral	Farther away from the midline of the body or a body part; on the outer side of	• The shoulder is lateral to the chest. • The thumb is lateral to the index finger.
Superficial	Closer to the surface	• The skin is superficial to the muscle. • Muscle is superficial to bone.
Deep	Farther below the surface	• Bone is deep to the skin. • Bone is deep to muscle.

FIGURE 3.8 Directional terms.

Source: AMERMAN, ERIN C., HUMAN ANATOMY & PHYSIOLOGY, 2nd Ed., ©2019. Reprinted and Electronically reproduced by permission of Pearson Education, Inc., New York, NY.

TABLE 3.2	Directional and Positional Terms		
Term	**Combining Form (CF)**	**Description**	**Example**
superior		Above, in an upward direction, toward the head. *Note:* **super-** is a prefix (P) that means *upper, above.*	The head is superior to the neck of the body.
inferior	(infer/o)	Below or in a downward direction; more toward the feet or tail	The feet are inferior to the head of the body.
anterior	(anter/o)	In front of or before, the front side of the body	The breasts are located on the anterior side of the body.
posterior	(poster/o)	Toward the back, back side of the body	The nape is the back of the neck and is located on the posterior side of the body.

(continued)

TABLE 3.2 Directional and Positional Terms *(continued)*

Term	Combining Form (CF)	Description	Example
cephalic	(cephal/o)	Pertaining to the head; superior in position	A cephalic presentation is one in which any part of the head of the fetus is presented during delivery.
caudal	(caud/o)	Pertaining to the tail; inferior in position	The cauda equina (horse's tail) is a bundle of spinal nerves below the end of the spinal cord.
medial	(medi/o)	Nearest the midline or middle	The umbilicus is a depressed point in the medial area of the abdomen.
lateral	(later/o)	To the side, away from the middle	In the anatomical position, the arm is located on the lateral side of the body.
proximal	(proxim/o)	Nearest the point of attachment or near the point of origin	The proximal end of the humerus (upper bone of the arm) joins with part of the shoulder bone.
distal	(dist/o)	Away from the point of attachment or far from the point of origin	The distal end of the humerus joins with part of the elbow.

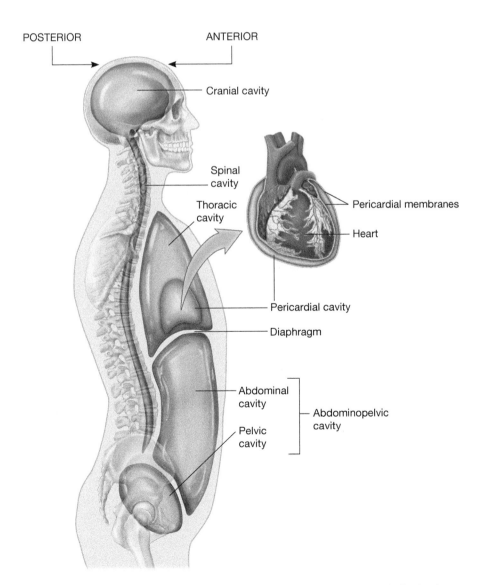

FIGURE 3.9 Body cavities. Lateral view of a sagittal section through the body.

VENTRAL CAVITY

The ventral cavity is the hollow portion of the human torso extending from the neck to the pelvis and containing the heart and the organs of respiration, digestion, reproduction, and elimination. The ventral cavity can be subdivided into three distinct areas: thoracic, abdominal, and pelvic.

- **Thoracic cavity.** The area of the chest containing the heart and the lungs. Within this cavity, the space containing the **heart** is called the **pericardial cavity** and the spaces surrounding each **lung** are known as the **pleural cavities**. Other organs located in the thoracic cavity are the esophagus, trachea, thymus, and certain large blood and lymph vessels.
- **Abdominal cavity.** The space below the diaphragm, commonly referred to as the *belly*; contains the stomach, intestines, and other organs of digestion.
- **Pelvic cavity.** The space formed by the bones of the pelvic area; contains the organs of reproduction and elimination.

DORSAL CAVITY

The dorsal cavity contains the structures of the nervous system and is subdivided into the cranial cavity and the spinal cavity.

- **Cranial cavity.** The space in the skull containing the brain.
- **Spinal cavity.** The space within the bony spinal column that contains the spinal cord and spinal fluid.

ABDOMINOPELVIC CAVITY

The abdominopelvic cavity is the combination of the abdominal and pelvic cavities. It is divided into nine regions.

Nine Regions of the Abdominopelvic Cavity. As a ready reference for locating visceral organs, anatomists divided the abdominopelvic cavity into nine regions (see Figure 3.10B). A grid pattern drawn across the abdominopelvic cavity delineates these regions:

- **Right hypochondriac.** Upper right region at the level of the ninth rib cartilage
- **Left hypochondriac.** Upper left region at the level of the ninth rib cartilage
- **Epigastric.** Region over the stomach
- **Right lumbar.** Right middle lateral region
- **Left lumbar.** Left middle lateral region
- **Umbilical.** In the center, between the right and left lumbar regions; at the navel
- **Right iliac (inguinal).** Right lower lateral region
- **Left iliac (inguinal).** Left lower lateral region
- **Hypogastric.** Lower middle region below the navel

Abdomen Divided into Quadrants

The **abdomen (Abd, abd)** is divided into four corresponding regions (quadrants) that are used for descriptive and diagnostic purposes. By using these regions, one may describe the exact location of pain, a skin lesion, surgical incision, and/or abdominal tumor. See Figure 3.10A.

- **Right upper quadrant (RUQ).** Contains the right lobe of the liver, gallbladder, part of the pancreas, and part of the small and large intestines

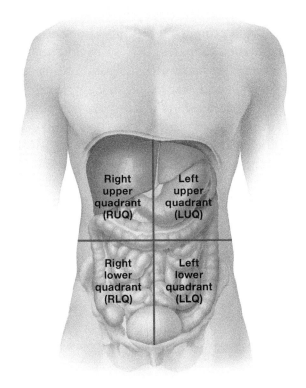

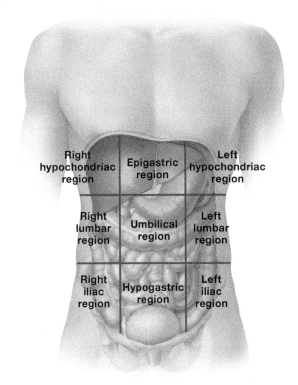

A The four abdominopelvic quadrants

B The nine abdominopelvic regions

FIGURE 3.10 A The four regions of the abdomen, which are referred to as quadrants. **B** The nine regions of the abdominopelvic cavity.

- **Left upper quadrant (LUQ).** Contains the left lobe of the liver, stomach, spleen, part of the pancreas, and part of the small and large intestines
- **Right lower quadrant (RLQ).** Contains part of the small and large intestines, appendix, right ovary, right fallopian tube, right ureter
- **Left lower quadrant (LLQ).** Contains part of the small and large intestines, left ovary, left fallopian tube, left ureter

Note: Some organs, such as the urinary bladder and uterus, are located half in the right quadrant and half in the left quadrant. These organs are generally referred to as being in the *midline* of the body.

Trunk

The **trunk**, also called the *torso*, is an anatomical term for the central part of the human body, not including the head and extremities (arms and legs). The trunk includes the chest, the back, the shoulders, and the abdomen (Abd, abd). The trunk is also described as that part of the body defined by the length of the vertebral column with reference to the posterior or back of the body. The trunk also contains many of the main groups of muscles in the body, including the pectoral, abdominal, and lateral groups. The muscles and organs mainly originating from thoracic vertebral segments are innervated by various peripheral nerves. The internal organs within the trunk are the heart, the lungs, the stomach, the liver, the gallbladder, the pancreas, the spleen, the kidneys, and the small and large intestine (bowel).

In the upper chest, the heart and lungs are protected by the rib cage. The abdomen contains the majority of organs responsible for digestion. The liver plays an essential role in the normal metabolism of carbohydrates, fats, and proteins. It produces bile necessary for the breakdown of large fat globules into smaller particles. Digestion and absorption take place chiefly in the small intestine where digested nutrients pass into the villi through diffusion and, in the large intestine, digestion and absorption are completed. The gallbladder stores and concentrates bile. Other organs found in the trunk are the kidneys, which produce urine; the ureters, which drain urine from the kidneys to the bladder; and the urethra, which conveys urine out of the body in the female and conveys urine and semen out of the body in the male. The pelvic region contains the male or female reproductive organs.

Head-to-Toe Assessment

The terminology associated with head-to-toe assessment can be useful when studying the organization of the body and in understanding information contained in a patient's medical record. Body areas, along with their word parts, are listed in Table 3.3.

TABLE 3.3	Body Area Terminology		
Body Area	**Word Part(s)**	**Body Area**	**Word Part(s)**
abdomen (belly)	abdomin/o	liver	hepat/o
ankle (tarsus)	tars/o	lungs	pulm/o, pulmon/o, pneum/o, pneumon/o
arm	brach/i, brachi/o	mouth	or/o
back	poster/o	muscles	muscul/o, my/o
bones	oste/o	navel	umbilic/o, omphal/o
breast	mast/o, mamm/o	neck	cervic/o
cheek	bucc/o	nerves	neur/o
chest	thorac/o	nose	rhin/o, nas/o
ear	aur/i, ot/o	ribs	cost/o
elbow	cubit/o, olecran/o	skin	derm/a, dermat/o, derm/o, cutane/o
eye	ophthalm/o, ocul/o, opt/o	skull	crani/o
finger	dactyl/o	stomach	gastr/o
foot	pod/o	tooth	dent/i, dent/o
gums	gingiv/o	temples	tempor/o
hand (manus)	chir/o	thigh bone	femor/o
head	cephal/o	throat	pharyng/o
heart	cardi/o	tongue	lingu/o, gloss/o
hip (ischium, coxa)	isch/i	wrist (carpus)	carp/o
leg	crur/o		

Study *and* Review I

Anatomy and Physiology

Write your answers to the following questions.

1. The _____ consist of millions of _____ working individually and with each other to _____ life.

2. The outer covering of the cell is known as the _____, which has the capability of allowing some substances to pass into and out of the cell.

3. The common parts of the cell are the _____, _____, and _____.

4. The cell's nucleus is responsible for these three functions: _____, _____, and _____.

5. An _____ is an unspecialized cell that can turn itself into any type of tissue.

6. List the six functions of epithelial tissue.

   a. _____   d. _____

   b. _____   e. _____

   c. _____   f. _____

7. _____ tissue is the most widespread and abundant of the four body tissues.

8. Name the three types of muscle tissue.

   a. _____   c. _____

   b. _____

9. Two properties of nerve tissue are _____ and _____.

10. Define *organ*. _____.

11. Define *body system*. _____.

Matching

Write in the lettered function that goes with the numbered organ system.

_____ 1. integumentary

_____ 2. skeletal

_____ 3. muscular

_____ 4. nervous

_____ 5. endocrine

_____ 6. cardiovascular

_____ 7. respiratory

_____ 8. digestive

_____ 9. urinary

_____ 10. reproductive

a. Produces hormones, provides for communication and control over various parts of the body

b. Furnishes oxygen and removes carbon dioxide

c. Produces urine, transports urine, eliminates urine

d. Shape, support, protection, storage of minerals

e. Responsible for sexual characteristics of male and/or female

f. Protective membrane, regulates temperature, sensory receptor

g. Transmits impulses, responds to change, responsible for communication, control over all parts of the body

h. Transports oxygen and carbon dioxide, delivers nutrients and hormones, removes waste products

i. Digestion, absorption, elimination

j. Produces movement, maintains posture, produces heat

Anatomical Locations and Positions

Write your answers to the following questions.

1. Define the following directional terms.

   a. superior _____

   b. anterior _____

   c. posterior _____

   d. cephalic _____

   e. medial _____

   f. lateral _____

   g. proximal _____

   h. distal _____

2. The _____ vertically divides the body. It passes through the midline to form a right and left half.

3. The _____ plane is any plane that divides the body into superior and inferior portions.

4. The _____ plane is any plane that divides the body at right angles to the plane described in question 2.

5. List the three distinct cavities that are located in the ventral cavity.

   a. _____   **c.** _____

   b. _____

6. Name the two distinct cavities located in the dorsal cavity.

   a. _____   **b.** _____

7. The _____ cavity is the combination of the abdominal and pelvic cavities.

8. There are _____ regions of the above cavity.

9. The abdomen is divided into _____ corresponding regions (quadrants) that are used for descriptive and diagnostic purposes.

10. What is the anatomical term for the central part of the human body? _____
(*Note:* This area of the body is also called the torso.)

▶ **ANATOMY LABELING**   Identify the structures shown below by filling in the blanks.

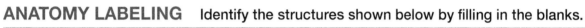

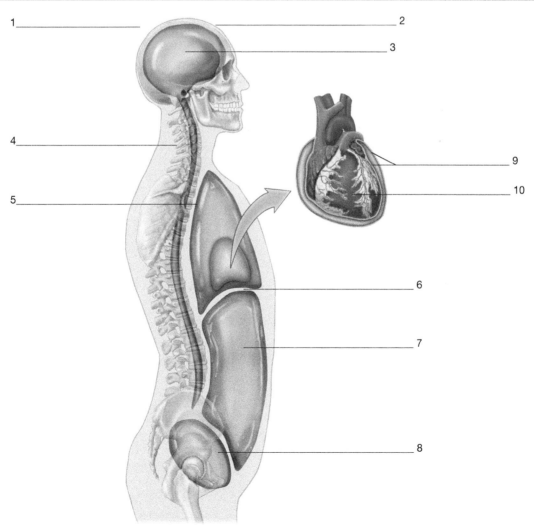

The Body in Health and Disease

Health is defined by the World Health Organization (WHO) as a state of complete physical, mental, and social well-being. When a deviation from normal occurs in any of these states, a process known as disease, illness, or disorder generally appears.

Infectious Diseases

Infectious diseases are the third leading cause of death in human beings and are caused by *pathogenic* (pertaining to producing disease) microorganisms such as bacteria, viruses, parasites, and fungi that can be spread, directly or indirectly, from one person to another. See Figure 3.11. Some are transmitted through bites from insects while others are caused by ingesting contaminated food or water. Over 80 infectious diseases have been identified.

A variety of disease-producing bacteria and viruses are carried in the mouth, nose, throat, and respiratory tract. Conditions such as pertussis (whooping cough), tuberculosis (TB), and different strains of influenza (flu) can be spread by coughing, sneezing, and saliva or mucus on unwashed hands.

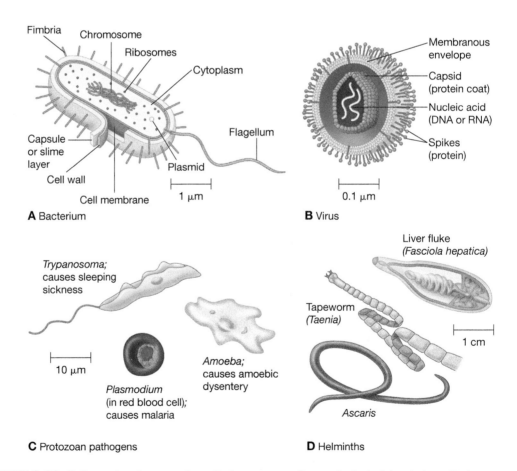

FIGURE 3.11 Pathogenic microorganisms that can cause disease include **A** bacterium, **B** virus, **C** protozoan, and **D** helminths.

Source: Zelman, Mark; Tompary, Elaine; Raymond, Jill; Holdaway, Paul; Mulvihill, Mary Lou E., Human Diseases, 8th Ed., ©2015. Reprinted and Electronically reproduced by permission of Pearson Education, Inc., New York, NY.

Sexually transmitted infections (STIs) such as HIV (human immunodeficiency virus) and viral hepatitis are spread through the exposure to infective bodily fluids such as blood, vaginal secretions, and semen.

Insects play a significant role in the transmission of disease. Bites from certain species of mosquitoes can transmit West Nile virus (WNV) encephalitis, dengue (deng' gē) fever, chikungunya (chĭ″ kun-gun' yă) virus, and the Zika virus, which can cause microcephaly in newborns. In 2018, according to the Centers for Disease Control and Prevention (CDC), a total of 45 states and the District of Columbia reported WNV infections in people, birds, or mosquitoes. The CDC now recommends wearing insect repellent whenever you are outdoors.

GOOD TO KNOW ▶

The following terms are associated with the causative agents of some infections and diseases.

arthropods	Invertebrate animals (mosquitoes, ticks, mites, fleas, sand fleas, lice) that can transmit diseases to humans and animals. They function as hematophagous (hemat/o [*blood*], phag [*to eat*], -ous [*pertaining to*]) **vectors** (carriers) that transmit disease through their bite. Only female mosquitoes bite to get a blood meal for their growing eggs. Arthropods are the largest animal *phylum* (scientific way of grouping together related organisms), comprising about 85% of all known animals in the world. See Figure 3.12.

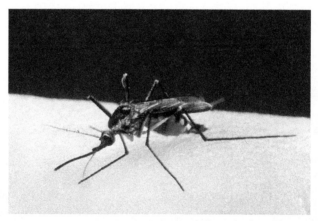

FIGURE 3.12 The *Aedes* species mosquito, the vector responsible for causing West Nile virus encephalitis, dengue fever, chikungunya virus, and Zika virus.
Source: Centers for Disease Control and Prevention (CDC)/Robert S. Craig

helminths	Wormlike animals (vermiform parasites) (refer to Figure 3.11D). Broadly classified into tapeworms, flukes, and roundworms, these parasites often live in the gastrointestinal tract of their hosts, but may also burrow into other organs, where they induce physiological damage. *Helminthiasis* is the term used for the patient having intestinal parasites or worms.
mycoses	Fungal infections
prion infections	Disease caused by a protein-like infectious particle (prion). Prions cause a number of diseases in animals and humans known as spongiform encephalopathies (brain diseases), in which the brain becomes damaged with holes. Mad cow disease in cattle is a prion infection.
protozoal	Pertaining to single-celled parasitic organisms (protozoa) with flexible membranes and the ability to move (refer to Figure 3.11C). They can cause amebic dysentery, sleeping sickness, and malaria.

(continued)

rickettsioses	Infection with rickettsiae, the most common being Rocky Mountain spotted fever and epidemic typhus. See Figure 3.13.

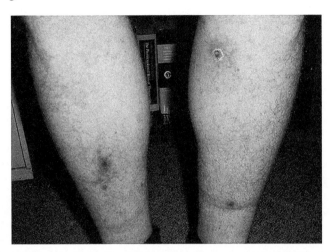

FIGURE 3.13 Inoculation eschars associated with the site of tick attachment in a patient infected with rickettsial infection *R. parkeri*.
Source: Centers for Disease Control and Prevention (CDC)

spirochetal	Pertaining to spirochetes, especially infections caused by them, such as syphilis.
zoonoses	Diseases that are communicable (transmissible) from animals to humans. Examples are viruses, bacteria, parasites, and mycoses.

Study *and* Review II

The Body in Health and Disease

Write the correct answers in the spaces provided.

1. _____ is defined by the World Health Organization (WHO) as a state of complete physical, mental, and social well-being.

2. Infectious diseases are the third leading cause of death in human beings and are caused by _____ (pertaining to producing disease) microorganisms.

3. The medical term for whooping cough is _____.

4. State how infectious diseases caused by certain microorganisms, such as bacteria, viruses, parasites, and fungi, are spread. _____

5. Insects play a significant role in the transmission of disease. Bites from certain species of mosquitoes can transmit _____ _____ _____ encephalitis, _____ fever, chikungunya virus, and the _____ virus.

Building Your Medical Vocabulary

This section provides the foundation for learning medical terminology. Review the alphabetized list of medical terms in the following pages. Note how common prefixes and suffixes are repeatedly applied to word roots and combining forms to create different meanings. A combining form is a word root plus a vowel. The chart below lists the combining forms and word roots used in this chapter and can help to strengthen your understanding of how medical words are built and spelled.

You will find that some terms have not been divided into word parts. These are common words or specialized terms that are included to enhance your medical vocabulary.

Combining Forms

adip/o	fat	later/o	side
andr/o	man	medi/o	toward the middle
anter/o	toward the front	organ/o	organ
bi/o	life	path/o	disease
caud/o	tail	phen/o	to show
cyt/o	cell	physi/o	nature
dist/o	away from the point of origin	poster/o	behind, toward the back, back
dors/o	backward	proxim/o	near the point of origin
filtrat/o	to strain through	somat/o	body
fus/o	to pour	system/o	composite, whole
hist/o	tissue	troph/o	nourishment, development
hydr/o	water	ventr/o	near or on the belly side of the body
infer/o	below	somat/o	body
inguin/o	groin	viscer/o	body organs
kary/o	cell's nucleus		

Word Roots

horizont	horizon	topic	place
intern	within		

Medical Word	Word Parts		Definition
	Part	Meaning	
adipose (ăd´ ĭ-pōs)	adip -ose	fat pertaining to	Pertaining to fatty tissue throughout the body

 Adiposity is the condition of being obese. The recommended measurement of **obesity** is the body mass index (BMI), a key index for relating weight to height. To determine a person's BMI, weight in kilograms (kg) is divided by height in meters squared. The National Institutes of Health (NIH) now defines normal weight, overweight, and obesity according to BMI rather than the traditional height/weight charts. Overweight is a BMI of 27.3 or more for women and 27.8 or more for men. Obesity is a BMI of 30 or more for both males and females (about 30 pounds overweight).

Medical Word	Word Parts		Definition
ambilateral (ăm˝ bĭ-lăt´ ěr-ăl)	ambi- later -al	both side pertaining to	Pertaining to both sides
anatomy (ăn-ăt´ ō-mē)	ana-´ -tomy	up, apart incision	Literally means *to cut up* or *to cut apart*; the study of the structure of an organism such as humans.

 A method that can be used to learn about the anatomy of the body of a once-living thing is termed *dissection*. To *dissect* means to separate tissues and parts of a cadaver for anatomical study. In anatomy and physiology lab, a frog may be dissected for learning purposes.

Medical Word	Word Parts		Definition
android (ăn´ droyd)	andr -oid	man resemble	To resemble man
apex (ā´ pěks)			Pointed end of a cone-shaped structure
base (bās)			Lower part or foundation of a structure
bilateral (bī-lăt´ ěr-ăl)	bi- later -al	two side pertaining to	Pertaining to two sides
biology (bī-ŏl´ ō-jē)	bi/o -logy	life study of	Study of life
center (sěn´ těr)			Middle or midpoint of a body
chromosome (krō´ mō-sōm)	chromo- -some	color body	Microscopic bodies in the nucleus that carry the genes that determine hereditary characteristics
cytology (sī-tŏl´ ō-jē)	cyt/o -logy	cell study of	Study of cells

Medical Word	Word Parts		Definition
	Part	Meaning	
dehydrate (dē-hī′ drāt)	de- hydr -ate	down, away from water use, action	To remove water; to lose or be deprived of water from the body; to become dry
diffusion (dǐ-fū′ zhŭn)	dif- fus -ion	apart to pour process	The process whereby particles in a fluid move from an area of high concentration to an area of lower concentration, resulting in an even distribution of the particles in the fluid
ectomorph (ĕk′ tō-morf)	ecto- -morph	outside form, shape	Slender physical body form; linear physique

! ALERT!

Note that **ecto-** means *outside*, while **endo-** means *within*.

endomorph (ĕn′ dō-morf)	endo- -morph	within form, shape	Round and soft physical body form
filtration (fĭl-trā′ shŭn)	filtrat -ion	to strain through process	Process of filtering or straining particles from a solution
gene (jēn)			Hereditary unit that transmits and determines one's characteristics or hereditary traits
histology (hĭs-tŏl′ ō-jē)	hist/o -logy	tissue study of	Study of tissue

✓ RULE REMINDER

This term keeps the combining vowel **o** because the suffix begins with a consonant.

homeostasis (hō″ mē-ō-stā′ sĭs)	homeo- -stasis	similar, same control, stop, stand still	State of equilibrium maintained in the body's internal environment; an important fundamental principle of physiology that permits a body to maintain a constant internal environment despite changes in the external environment
horizontal (hŏr′ ă-zŏn′ tăl)	horizont -al	horizon pertaining to	Pertaining to the horizon, of or near the horizon, lying flat, even, level
human genome (hū′ măn jē′ nōm)			Complete set of genes and chromosomes tucked inside each of the body's trillions of cells
inguinal (ĭng′ gwĭ-năl)	inguin -al	groin pertaining to	Pertaining to the groin, of or near the groin

Medical Word	Word Parts		Definition
	Part	**Meaning**	
internal (ĭn-tĕr´ nal)	**intern** **-al**	within pertaining to	Pertaining to within or the inside
karyogenesis (kăr″ ē-ō-jĕn´ ĕ-sĭs)	**kary/o** **-genesis**	cell's nucleus formation, produce	Formation of a cell's nucleus
lateral (LAT, lat) (lăt´ ĕr-ăl)	**later** **-al**	side pertaining to	Pertaining to the side

✓ RULE REMINDER

The **o** has been removed from the combining form because the suffix begins with a vowel.

medial (mē´ dē-ăl)	**medi** **-al**	toward the middle pertaining to	Pertaining to the middle or midline
mesomorph (mĕs´ ō-morf)	**meso-** **-morph**	middle form, shape	Well-proportioned body form marked by predominance of tissue derived from the mesoderm (the middle layer of cells in the developing embryo)

! ALERT!

Meso- means *middle*. Using the suffix **-morph** and the prefixes **ecto-**, **endo-**, and **meso-**, build three medical terms that describe body forms.

organic (or-găn´ ĭk)	**organ** **-ic**	organ pertaining to	Pertaining to an organ or organs; pertaining to or derived from vegetable or animal forms of life
pathology (pă-thŏl´ ō-jē)	**path/o** **-logy**	disease study of	Study of disease
perfusion (pĕr-fū´ zhŭn)	**per-** **fus** **-ion**	through to pour process	Literally means *a process of pouring through*; as passing of a fluid through spaces; to supply the body with nutritive fluid via the bloodstream
phenotype (fē´ nō-tīp)	**phen/o** **-type**	to show type	Physical appearance or type of makeup of an individual
physiology (fĭz″ ē-ŏl´ ō-jē)	**physi/o** **-logy**	nature study of	Study of the function (nature) of living organisms; anatomy and physiology (A&P) is the combination of the study of the anatomy and physiology of the human body
protoplasm prō´ tō-plăzm	**proto-** **-plasm**	first a thing formed, plasma	Essential matter inside of a living cell

Medical Word	Word Parts		Definition
	Part	**Meaning**	
somatotrophic (sō˝ mă-tō-trŏf´ ĭk)	**somat/o**	body	Pertaining to stimulation of body growth
	troph	nourishment, development	
	-ic	pertaining to	
superficial (soo˝ pĕr-físh´ ăl)			Pertaining to the surface, on or near the surface
systemic (sĭs-tĕm´ ĭk)	**system**	composite, whole	Pertaining to the body as a whole
	-ic	pertaining to	
topical (tŏp´ ĭ-kăl)	**topic**	place	Pertaining to a place, definite locale
	-al	pertaining to	
unilateral (ū˝ nĭ-lăt´ ĕr-ăl)	**uni-**	one	Pertaining to one side
	later	side	
	-al	pertaining to	
ventral (vĕn´ trăl)	**ventr**	near the belly side	Pertaining to the belly side, abdomen; front side of the body (same as anterior)
	-al	pertaining to	
vertex (vĕr´ tĕks)			Top or highest point; top or crown of the head
visceral (vĭs´ ĕr-ăl)	**viscer**	body organs	Pertaining to body organs enclosed within a cavity, especially abdominal organs
	-al	pertaining to	

Study *and* Review III

Word Parts

Prefixes   Give the definitions of the following prefixes.

1. ambi- _____

2. ana- _____

3. bi- _____

4. chromo- _____

5. de- _____

6. dif- _____

7. ecto- _____

8. endo- _____

9. homeo- _____

10. meso- _____

11. per _____

12. proto- _____

13. uni- _____

Combining Forms   Give the definitions of the following combining forms.

1. adip/o _____

2. andr/o _____

3. anter/o _____

4. bi/o _____

5. caud/o _____

6. cyt/o _____

7. dist/o _____

8. dors/o _____

9. hist/o _____

10. hydr/o _____

11. infer/o _____

12. inguin/o _____

13. kary/o _____

14. later/o _____

15. medi/o _____

16. organ/o _____

17. path/o _____

18. phen/o _____

19. physi/o _____

20. poster/o _____

21. proxim/o _____

22. somat/o _____

23. ventr/o _____

24. viscer/o _____

Suffixes   Give the definitions of the following suffixes.

1. -al _____

2. -ate _____

3. -genesis _____

4. -ic _____

5. -ion _____

6. -logy _____

7. -morph _____

8. -oid _____

9. -ose _____

10. -plasm _____

11. -some _____

12. -stasis _____

13. -tomy _____

14. -type _____

Identifying Medical Terms In the spaces provided, write the medical terms for the following meanings.

1. _____ To resemble man

2. _____ Pertaining to two sides

3. _____ Study of cells

4. _____ Slender physical body form

5. _____ Formation of a cell's nucleus

6. _____ Pertaining to the stimulation of body growth

7. _____ Pertaining to one side

Matching Select the appropriate lettered meaning for each of the numbered words.

_____ 1. ambilateral

_____ 2. anatomy

_____ 3. atom

_____ 4. chromosome

_____ 5. cilia

_____ 6. homeostasis

_____ 7. human genome

_____ 8. phenotype

_____ 9. physiology

_____ 10. vertex

a. Hairlike processes that project from epithelial cells

b. Top or highest point

c. Pertaining to both sides

d. Study of the structure of an organism such as a human

e. Smallest, most basic chemical unit of an element

f. Microscopic bodies that carry the genes that determine hereditary characteristics

g. Complete set of genes and chromosomes

h. Physical appearance or type of makeup of an individual

i. State of equilibrium maintained in the body's internal environment

j. Study of the nature of a living organism

Drug Highlights

A **drug** is a chemical substance that can alter or modify the functions of a living organism. It may be classified by the chemical type of the active ingredient or by the way it is used to treat a particular condition. Each drug can be classified into one or more drug classes. The Anatomical Therapeutic Chemical Classification System (ATC) is used to classify the active ingredients of drugs according to the organ or system on which they act and their therapeutic, pharmacological, and chemical properties. It is controlled by the World Health Organization Collaborating Centre (WHOCC) for Drug Statistics Methodology and was first published in 1976.

Drugs are classified chemically, according to how they affect the brain and the body. Common classifications include stimulants, depressants, hallucinogens, and opioids. Additionally, the United States Drug Enforcement Administration (DEA) legally classifies drugs into schedules (I, II, III, IV, and V) based on their medical use and potential for abuse and dependence.

Drugs are also classified in many other ways, such as by preparation and by therapeutic action. The therapeutic action of the drug involves the process of treating, relieving, or obtaining results through the action of the medication on the body. Examples of this type of action include analgesic (agent that relieves pain), antibiotic (agent that is destructive to or inhibits growth of microorganisms), and antidote (agent that counteracts poisons and their effects). In Chapters 4 through 18, Drug Highlights present classifications of drugs according to preparation and therapeutic effect.

There are thousands of drugs that are available as over-the-counter (OTC) medicines and do not require a prescription. A prescription is a written legal document that gives directions for compounding, dispensing, and administering a medication to a patient.

In general, there are five medical uses for drugs:

- **Therapeutic use.** Used in the treatment of a disease or condition, such as an allergy, to relieve the symptoms or to sustain the patient until other measures are instituted.
- **Diagnostic use.** Certain drugs are used in conjunction with radiology to allow the physician to pinpoint the location of a disease process.
- **Curative use.** Certain drugs, such as antibiotics, kill or remove the causative agent of a disease.
- **Replacement use.** Certain drugs, such as hormones and vitamins, are used to replace or supplement substances normally found in the body.
- **Preventive** or **prophylactic use.** Certain drugs, such as immunizing agents, are used to ward off or lessen the severity of a disease.

Drug names	A drug can have multiple different names. The **chemical name** specifies the formula that denotes the composition of the drug. It is made up of letters and numbers that represent the drug's molecular structure. The **generic name** is the drug's official name and is descriptive of its chemical structure and is written in lowercase letters. A generic drug is generally more economical (costs less) than a brand name drug and is often preferred by insurance companies for patients. A generic drug can be manufactured by more than one pharmaceutical company. When this is the case, each company markets the drug under its own unique brand name. For example, the antibiotic drug amoxicillin (generic name) can have several brand names, such as Amoxil, Polymox, and Trimox. A **brand name** is the private property of the drug manufacturer that makes the drug and is registered by the U.S. Patent Office as well as approved by the U.S. Food and Drug Administration (FDA). A brand name is capitalized and is also called a *trade name*. See the following example of a nonsteroidal anti-inflammatory drug:

- Chemical name: 4-hydroxyl-2-methyl-N-2-pyridinyl-2H-1, 2-benzothiazine3-carboxamide 1, 1-dioxide
- Generic name: piroxicam
- Brand or trade name: Feldene

Undesirable actions of drugs	Most drugs have the potential for causing an action other than the intended action. A *side effect* is an undesirable action of a drug and may limit its usefulness. For example, antibiotics that are administered orally may disrupt the normal bacterial flora of the gastrointestinal (GI) tract and cause gastric discomfort.
	An *adverse drug reaction (ADR)* is defined by the World Health Organization (WHO) as "any response to a drug which is noxious and unintended, and which occurs at doses normally used in man." For example, an adverse reaction to Demerol may be light-headedness, dizziness, sedation, nausea, and sweating. A *drug interaction* can occur when one drug potentiates (increases the action) or diminishes the action of another drug. Drugs can also interact with foods, alcohol, tobacco, and other substances.
	An *adverse drug event (ADE)* can be a medication error, adverse drug reaction, allergic reaction, or overdose. With concurrent use of multiple medications, the potential for adverse drug reactions and drug interactions increases.

fyi A significant change to the classification of drugs occurred with the 2015 publication of the *ICD-10-CM* (*International Classification of Diseases, Tenth Revision, Clinical Modification*), which is published by the WHO. This change was made to include poisonings, adverse effects of drugs, underdosing of drugs, medicaments (substances used for medical treatment), and biological substances. Also, poisonings are further classified as accidental (unintentional), intentional (self-harm), assault, and undetermined.

Medication order and dosage

- The **medication order** is given for a specific patient and denotes the name of the drug, the dosage, the form of the drug, the time for or frequency of administration, and the route by which the drug is to be given.
- The **dosage** is the amount of medicine that is prescribed for administration. The form of the drug can be liquid, solid, semisolid, tablet, capsule, transdermal therapeutic patch, etc.
- *Underdosing* is a new term that is defined as taking less of a medication than is prescribed by a physician or the manufacturer's instructions with a resulting negative health consequence.
- The **route of administration** can be by mouth, by injection, into the eye(s), ear(s), nostril(s), rectum, vagina, etc. It is important for the patient to know when and how to take a medication.

Abbreviations *and* Acronyms

Abbreviation/Acronym	Meaning	Abbreviation/Acronym	Meaning
Abd, abd	abdomen	HIV	human immunodeficiency virus
A&P	anatomy and physiology	kg	kilogram
ADE	adverse drug event	LAT, lat	lateral
ADR	adverse drug reaction	LLQ	left lower quadrant
ATC	Anatomical Therapeutic Chemical Classification System	LUQ	left upper quadrant
		N_2	nitrogen
BMI	body mass index	NIH	National Institutes of Health
BP	blood pressure	O or O_2	oxygen
CaO	calcium oxide	O_3	ozone
CDC	Centers for Disease Control and Prevention	OTC	over-the-counter (drugs)
$C_6H_{12}O_6$	glucose	RLQ	right lower quadrant
CO_2	carbon dioxide	RUQ	right upper quadrant
DEA	Drug Enforcement Administration	STIs	sexually transmitted infections
DNA	deoxyribonucleic acid	T	temperature
ER	endoplasmic reticulum (as used in this chapter); also means emergency room	TB	tuberculosis
		WHO	World Health Organization
FDA	Food and Drug Administration	WHOCC	World Health Organization Collaborating Centre
GI	gastrointestinal		
H_2O	water	WNV	West Nile virus

Study *and* Review IV

Building Medical Terms

Using the following word parts, fill in the blanks to build the correct medical terms.

bi-	bi/o	path/o	-al	-logy
uni-	inguin	physi/o	-ic	

Definition	Medical Term
1. Pertaining to two sides	_____lateral
2. Study of life	_____logy
3. Farthest from the point of origin	dist_____
4. Pertaining to the groin	_____al
5. Pertaining to the side	later_____
6. Study of disease	_____logy
7. Study of the function of living organisms	_____logy
8. Pertaining to the body as a whole	system_____
9. Pertaining to one side	_____lateral
10. Pertaining to body organs enclosed within a cavity	viscer_____

Combining Form Challenge

Using the combining forms provided, write the medical term correctly.

adip/o	hist/o	phen/o
andr/o	kary/o	somat/o

1. Pertaining to fatty tissue throughout the body: _____ose

2. To resemble man: _____oid

3. Study of tissue: _____logy

4. Formation of a cell's nucleus: _____genesis

5. Physical appearance or type of makeup of an individual: _____type

6. Pertaining to stimulation of body growth: _____trophic

Select the Right Term

Select the correct answer, and write it on the line provided.

1. Literally means *to cut up* or *to cut apart* is _____.

   physiology　　　　anatomy　　　　homeostasis　　　　topical

2. A surface or part situated toward the front of the body is _____.

   caudal　　　　cranial　　　　anterior　　　　medical

3. A well-proportioned body form is _____.

   endomorph　　　　phenotype　　　　somatotrophic　　　　mesomorph

4. The lower part or foundation of a structure is _____.

   apex　　　　base　　　　dorsal　　　　vertex

5. Nearest the center or point of origin is _____.

   superior　　　　ventral　　　　topical　　　　proximal

6. Pertaining to lying flat, even, level is _____.

   inguinal　　　　horizontal　　　　medial　　　　dorsal

Drug Highlights

Match the appropriate lettered description or examples of drug(s) with the class of drug.

_____ 1. analgesic

_____ 2. antibiotic

_____ 3. antidote

_____ 4. prescription

_____ 5. dosage

_____ 6. underdosing

_____ 7. side effect

_____ 8. adverse drug event

_____ 9. chemical name of drug

_____ 10. generic name of drug

a. Official name of a drug

b. Amount of a drug that is prescribed for administration

c. Written legal document that gives directions for compounding, dispensing, and administering a medication to a patient

d. Undesirable action of a drug

e. Agent that is destructive to or inhibits growth of microorganisms

f. Medication error, adverse drug reaction, allergic reaction, or overdose

g. Specifies the formula that denotes composition of the drug

h. Agent that relieves pain

i. Taking less of a medication than prescribed

j. Agent that counteracts poisons and their effects

Abbreviations and Acronyms

Write the correct word, phrase, or abbreviation/acronym in the space provided.

1. Abd, abd _____

2. A&P _____

3. DNA _____

4. body mass index _____

5. gastrointestinal _____

6. H_2O _____

7. LLQ _____

8. oxygen _____

9. over-the-counter (drugs) _____

10. RUQ _____

Practical Application

This exercise is adapted from the CDC's *Whooping Cough: A True Story*. The names and personal information have been created by the author. After reading the overview and story, please answer the questions that follow.

Overview

Since 2010, the CDC has seen between 10,000 and 50,000 cases of pertussis (whooping cough) every year in the United States. Whooping cough, caused by the *Bordetella pertussis bacterium*, is very serious for babies because it can cause them to stop breathing. About half of babies younger than 1 year old who get whooping cough need care in a hospital. Babies are at high risk for complications such as pneumonia, convulsions, and brain damage from whooping cough. Although death from whooping cough is rare, most deaths are among babies who are too young to be protected by their own vaccinations, which are not given until infants are 2 months old or older. However, by getting the whooping cough vaccine during the third trimester of pregnancy, the mother can pass antibodies to her fetus, so that after birth the infant is protected against whooping cough until the baby can be vaccinated. There are two vaccines that include protection against whooping cough:

- The DTaP vaccine protects young babies (beginning at 2 months old) and children from diphtheria, tetanus, and whooping cough.
- The Tdap vaccine protects preteens, teens, and adults from tetanus, diphtheria, and whooping cough.

When Tamara was 5 weeks old, her mother, Ellen, thought that she had a cold. Several days later she noticed that her baby had a strange cough. Twenty-four hours later, Tamara started having trouble breathing. She had periods of many rapid coughs, followed by a high-pitched "whooping" sound.

"Tamara was turning different shades of blue and her breathing was very difficult. I was so afraid," said Ellen. "My husband and I immediately drove Tamara to the emergency room. Once we got to the ER and she was checked in and put in a room, she got worse. IV medications were started and she was hooked up to a ventilator. The nurse explained that this was a machine to help her breathe. When the doctor came in, she said Tamara had whooping cough."

Case Study Questions

Write the correct answer in the space provided.

1. What is the name of the bacteria that causes "whooping cough"? _____

2. Why is pertussis very serious for babies? _____

   _____

3. A _____ is a machine to help with breathing.

4. Why are babies younger than 2 months old at high risk for complications from pertussis? _____

   _____

5. The whooping cough vaccine for babies is called _____.

MyLab Medical Terminology™

MyLab Medical Terminology is a premium online homework management system that includes a host of features to help you study. Registered users will find:

- A multitude of activities and assignments built within the MyLab platform
- Powerful tools that track and analyze your results—allowing you to create a personalized learning experience
- Videos and audio pronunciations to help enrich your progress
- Streaming lesson presentations (guided lectures) and self-paced learning modules
- A space where you and your instructor can check your progress and manage your assignments

4 Integumentary System

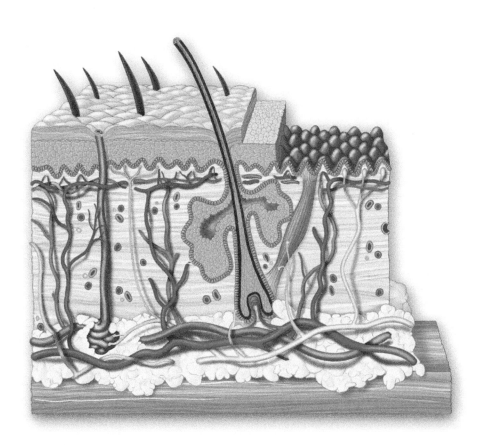

Learning Outcomes

On completion of this chapter, you will be able to:

1. Describe the integumentary system and its accessory structures.
2. List the functions of the skin.
3. Analyze, build, spell, and pronounce medical words.
4. Classify the drugs highlighted in this chapter.
5. Describe diagnostic and laboratory tests related to the integumentary system.
6. Identify and define selected abbreviations and acronyms.

Anatomy and Physiology

The integumentary system is composed of the skin, the largest organ of the body, and its accessory structures, the hair, nails, sebaceous glands, and sweat glands. Table 4.1 provides an at-a-glance look at the integumentary system.

TABLE 4.1 Integumentary System at-a-Glance	
Organ/Structure	**Primary Functions/Description**
Skin	Protection, regulation, sensation, and secretion
Epidermis	Outer protective covering of the body that can be divided into five strata (*in order as the layers evolve and mature*). See Figure 4.1.
stratum basale (basal layer)	Innermost epidermal layer responsible for regeneration of the epidermis. Damage to this layer, as in severe burns, necessitates the use of skin grafts (SG). **Melanin**, the pigment that gives color to the skin, is formed in this layer. The more abundant the melanin, the darker the color of the skin.
stratum spinosum	Means "spiny layer." Each time a stem cell divides, one of the daughter cells is pushed into this layer. Contains Langerhans cells, which are responsible for stimulating a defense against invading microorganisms and superficial skin cancers.
stratum granulosum	Large amounts of **keratin**, a protein substance, are made here. In humans, keratin is the basic structural component of hair and nails.
stratum lucidum	Present in thick skin of the palms and soles. Cells are flattened, densely packed, and filled with keratin.
stratum corneum	Outermost, horny layer, consisting of dead cells. Cells are active in the **keratinization** process, during which the cells lose their nuclei and become hard or horny. Forms protective covering for the body.
Dermis	Nourishes the epidermis, provides strength, and supports blood vessels
Papillae	Produce ridges that are one's fingerprints
Subcutaneous tissue	Supports, nourishes, insulates, and cushions the skin
Hair	Provides sensation and some protection for the head. Hair around the eyes, in the nose, and in the ears filters out foreign particles.
Nails	Protect ends of fingers and toes
Sebaceous (oil) glands	Lubricate the hair and skin
Sweat glands	Secrete sweat or perspiration, which helps to cool the body by evaporation. Sweat also rids the body of waste. Also referred to as *sudoriferous glands*.

Functions of the Skin

The **skin** is the external covering of the body. In an average adult, it covers more than 3,000 square inches of surface area, weighs more than 6 pounds, and is the largest organ of the body. The skin is well supplied with blood vessels and nerves and has four main functions: protection, regulation, sensation, and secretion.

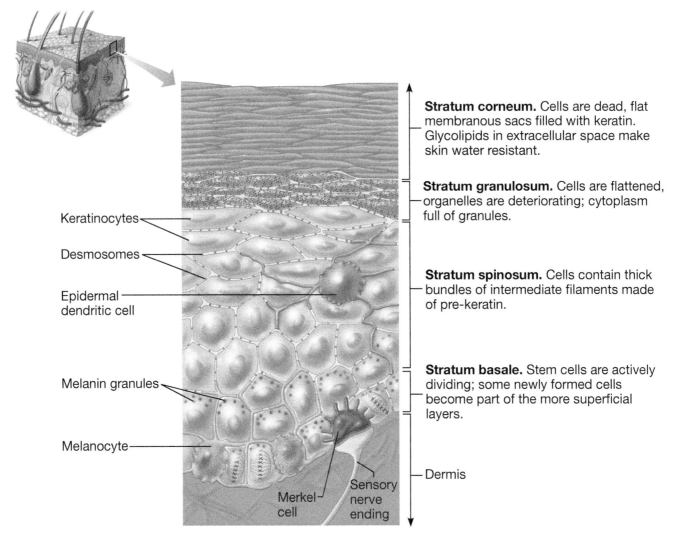

Keratinocytes

Desmosomes

Epidermal dendritic cell

Melanin granules

Melanocyte

Stratum corneum. Cells are dead, flat membranous sacs filled with keratin. Glycolipids in extracellular space make skin water resistant.

Stratum granulosum. Cells are flattened, organelles are deteriorating; cytoplasm full of granules.

Stratum spinosum. Cells contain thick bundles of intermediate filaments made of pre-keratin.

Stratum basale. Stem cells are actively dividing; some newly formed cells become part of the more superficial layers.

Dermis

Merkel cell

Sensory nerve ending

FIGURE 4.1 The main structural features of the epidermis.

Source: MARIEB, ELAINE N.; KELLER, SUZANNE M., ESSENTIALS OF HUMAN ANATOMY & PHYSIOLOGY, 12th Ed., ©2018. Reprinted and Electronically reproduced by permission of Pearson Education, Inc., New York, NY.

Protection

The skin serves as a protective membrane against invasion by bacteria and other potentially harmful agents that could try to penetrate into deeper tissues. It protects against mechanical injury of delicate cells located beneath its epidermis or outer covering. The skin also serves to inhibit excessive loss of water and electrolytes and provides a reservoir for storing food and water. The skin guards the body against excessive exposure to the sun's ultraviolet (UV) rays by producing a protective pigmentation, and it helps to produce the body's supply of vitamin D.

Regulation

The skin serves to raise or lower body temperature as necessary. When the body needs to lose heat, the blood vessels in the skin dilate, bringing more blood to the surface for cooling by **radiation**. At the same time, the sweat glands are secreting more sweat for cooling by means of **evaporation**. Conversely, when the body needs to conserve heat, the reflex actions of the nervous system cause the skin's blood vessels to constrict, thereby allowing more heat-carrying blood to circulate to the muscles and vital organs.

Sensation

The skin contains millions of microscopic nerve endings that act as **sensory receptors** for pain, touch, heat, cold, and pressure. When stimulation occurs, nerve impulses are sent to the cerebral cortex of the brain. The nerve endings in the skin are specialized according to the type of sensory information transmitted and, once this information reaches the brain, it triggers any necessary response. For example, touching a hot surface with the hand causes the brain to recognize the senses of *touch*, *heat*, and *pain* and results in the immediate removal of the hand from the hot surface.

Secretion

The skin contains millions of sweat glands, which secrete **perspiration** or **sweat**, and **sebaceous glands**, which secrete oil (sebum) for lubrication. Perspiration is largely water with a small amount of salt and other chemical compounds. This secretion, when left to accumulate, causes body odor, especially where it is trapped among hairs in the axillary region. **Sebum** is an oily secretion that acts to protect the body from dehydration and possible absorption of harmful substances.

fyi Before birth, **vernix caseosa**, a cheeselike substance, covers the fetus. At birth, the skin may be a dark red to purple color. As the baby begins to breathe air into the lungs, the color changes to red. This redness normally begins to fade in the first day. A baby's hands and feet may stay bluish in color for several days. This is a normal response to a baby's immature blood circulation. A baby's skin coloring can vary, depending on the baby's age, race or ethnic group, temperature, and whether or not the baby is crying. Skin color in babies often changes depending on both the baby's environment and health status.

In about 13–16 weeks, downy lanugo hair begins to develop, especially on the head. At 21–24 weeks, the skin is wrinkled and has little subcutaneous fat. Newborns have less subcutaneous fat than adults; therefore, they are more sensitive to heat and cold.

Layers of the Skin

The skin is essentially composed of two layers, the epidermis and the dermis. See Figure 4.2.

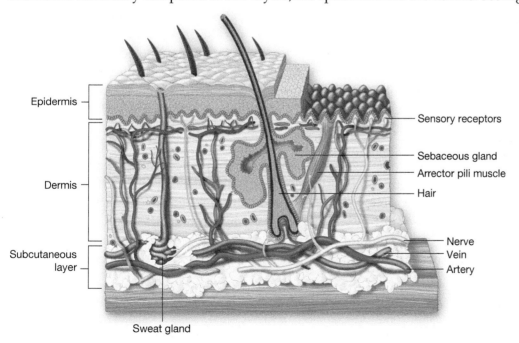

FIGURE 4.2 Skin structure. Microscopic view of the epidermis, dermis, underlying subcutaneous tissue, and accessory structures.

Epidermis

The **epidermis** is the outer layer of skin. The thickness of the epidermis varies in different types of skin. It is the thinnest on the eyelids at 0.05 mm and the thickest on the palms and soles at 1.5 mm.

The epidermis can be divided into five strata: *stratum basale*, *stratum spinosum*, *stratum granulosum*, *stratum lucidum*, and *stratum corneum*. Refer to Table 4.1 and Figure 4.1 for the functions, descriptions, and locations of these strata within the epidermis.

Dermis

Sometimes called the **corium** or **true skin**, the **dermis** is composed of connective tissue containing lymphatics, nerves and nerve endings, blood vessels, sebaceous and sweat glands, elastic fibers, and hair follicles (refer to Figure 4.2). It is divided into two layers: the *upper layer* or **papillary layer** and the *lower layer* or **reticular layer**. The papillary layer is arranged into parallel rows of microscopic structures called **papillae**, which produce the ridges of the skin that are one's fingerprints or footprints. The reticular layer is composed of white fibrous tissue that supports the blood vessels. The dermis is attached to underlying structures by the **subcutaneous tissue**. This tissue supports, nourishes, insulates, and cushions the skin.

fyi As a person ages, the skin becomes looser as the dermal papillae become thinner. Collagen and elastic fibers of the upper dermis decrease and skin loses its elastic tone and wrinkles more easily.

Accessory Structures of the Skin

The hair, nails, sebaceous glands, and sweat glands are the accessory structures of the skin.

Hair

A **hair** is a thin, threadlike structure formed by a group of cells that develop within a hair **follicle** or *socket* (refer to Figure 4.2). Each hair is composed of a **shaft**, which is the visible portion, and a **root**, which is embedded within the follicle. At the base of each follicle is a loop of capillaries enclosed within connective tissue called the **hair papilla**. The **arrector pili muscle** attaches to the side of each follicle. When the skin is cooled or the individual has an emotional reaction, the skin often forms "gooseflesh" as a result of contraction by these muscles. Hair is distributed over the whole body with the exception of the palms of the hands, soles of the feet, and the penis. It is thicker on the scalp and thinner on the other parts of the body. Hair around the eyes, in the nose, and in the ears serves to filter out foreign particles. Hair grows at approximately 0.5 inch a month, and its growth is not affected by cutting. Hair color is determined by the differences in the type and amount of melanin (pigment) produced by melanocytes at the hair papilla. Different types of melanin give dark-brown, yellow-brown, or red coloration to the hair. The color of hair is genetically determined, but the condition of the hair can be affected by hormonal or environmental factors. As pigment production decreases with age, the color of the hair lightens, and the process of graying occurs.

fyi By age 50, approximately half of all people have some gray hair. Scalp hair thins in women and men. The hair becomes dry and often brittle. Some older women may have an increase in facial hair due to hormonal changes. Some men may have an increase in hair of the nares (nostrils), eyebrows, or helix of the ear. In addition to the changes in the skin and hair, nails can flatten and become discolored, dry, and brittle.

Nails

Fingernails and **toenails** are horny cell structures of the epidermis and are composed of hard keratin. A nail consists of a **nail body** (the visible dense mass of dead keratinized cells) that covers the ends of fingers and toes. The body of the nail covers an area of epidermis known as the **nail bed**. The **nail root** is an epithelial fold not visible from the surface. The **eponychium** or *cuticle* is a portion of the epithelial fold that extends over the exposed nail adjacent to the root. The underlying blood vessels give the nail its pink color. Near the nail root these vessels are obscured, leaving a pale crescent-shaped area known as the **lunula** (from *luna*, Latin for moon). The **free edge** of the nail is the extension of the nail plate that protects the tip of the finger or toe. It is the portion that can be trimmed. See Figure 4.3.

Nail growth may vary with age, disease, and hormone deficiency. Average growth is 1 mm per week, and a lost fingernail usually regenerates in 3½ to 5½ months. A lost toenail may require 6–8 months for regeneration.

Sebaceous (Oil) Glands

The oil-secreting glands of the skin are called *sebaceous glands* (refer to Figure 4.2). They have tiny ducts that open into the hair follicles, and their secretion, *sebum*, lubricates the hair as well as the skin. The amount of secretion is controlled by the endocrine system and varies with age, puberty, and pregnancy.

Sweat Glands

The skin has two major types of **sweat glands**: eccrine and apocrine. Derived from embryonic ectoderm, millions of eccrine glands are distributed across the human skin and occur over most of the body; they open directly onto the surface of the skin (refer to Figure 4.2). **Eccrine sweat glands** help to maintain homeostasis, primarily by stabilizing body temperature. An individual can secrete up to 4 liters of eccrine sweat in an hour, thus cooling down body temperature as necessary. Evaporation of sweat from the skin surface effectively dissipates heat generated by physical activity, fever, or hot environments.

Apocrine sweat glands open into the hair follicle, leading to the surface of the skin. They are found in the skin of the areola (pigmented area) of the breast, armpit, groin, eyelid, and ear. Apocrine glands in the areola secrete fat droplets into breast milk, and those in the ear help form earwax. Apocrine glands in the skin are scent glands. They secrete fluid containing water, proteins, and lipids. When skin bacteria proliferate in the presence of apocrine gland secretions, a distinctive scent may be released that we call body odor.

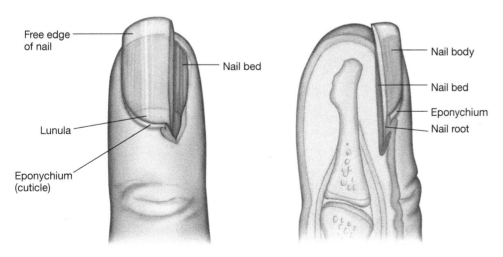

FIGURE 4.3 Structure of the fingernail, an appendage of the integument.
Source: Courtesy of Jason L. Smith, MD

Sweat gland dysfunction, such as the inability to sweat (called *hypohydrosis*) often seen in the older adult, is linked to heat stroke, which kills approximately 1,000 people annually in the United States. Sweat is essential to human survival because it serves as the body's coolant, getting rid of excess body heat and protecting the body from overheating. By contrast, overactive sweat glands can cause local *hyperhidrosis*, a chronic condition of excessive sweating that affects the quality of life for approximately 2.8% of the U.S. population.

Study *and* Review I

Anatomy and Physiology

Write your answers to the following questions.

1. Name the primary organ of the integumentary system. _____ _____

2. Name the four accessory structures of the integumentary system.

  a. _____   **c.** _____

  b. _____   **d.** _____

3. State the four main functions of the skin.

  a. _____   **c.** _____

  b. _____   **d.** _____

4. The skin is essentially composed of two layers, the _____ and the _____.

5. Name the five strata of the epidermis.

  a. _____   **d.** _____

  b. _____   **e.** _____

  c. _____

6. _____ is a protein substance that is the basic structural component of hair and nails.

7. _____ is a pigment that gives color to the skin.

8. The _____ is known as the *corium* or *true skin*.

9. Name the two layers of the part of the skin described in question 8.

  a. _____   **b.** _____

10. The crescent-shaped white area of the nail is the _____.

ANATOMY LABELING   Identify the structures shown below by filling in the blanks.

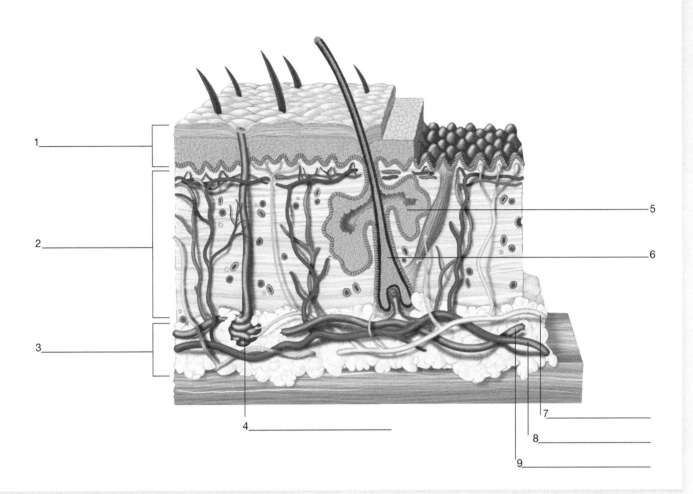

1 _____

2 _____

3 _____

4 _____

5 _____

6 _____

7 _____

8 _____

9 _____

Building Your Medical Vocabulary

This section provides the foundation for learning medical terminology. Review the alphabetized list of medical terms in the following pages. Note how common prefixes and suffixes are repeatedly applied to word roots and combining forms to create different meanings. A combining form is a word root plus a vowel. The chart below lists the combining forms and word roots used in this chapter and can help to strengthen your understanding of how medical words are built and spelled.

You will find that some terms have not been divided into word parts. These are common words or specialized terms that are included to enhance your medical vocabulary.

Combining Forms

acr/o	extremity	kerat/o	horn
aden/o	gland	leuk/o	white
albin/o	white	melan/o	black
ang/i	vessel	myc/o	fungus
carcin/o	cancer	onych/o	nail
caus/o	burn, burning	pachy/o	thick
cellul/o	little cell	pedicul/o	a louse
cutane/o	skin	plak/o	plate
derm/a	skin	prurit/o	itching
derm/o	skin	rhytid/o	wrinkle
dermat/o	skin	scler/o	hard, hardening
erythr/o	red	seb/o	oil
follicul/o	little bag	therm/o	hot, heat
hidr/o	sweat	trich/o	hair
icter/o	jaundice	ungu/o	nail
integument/o	a covering	vuls/o	to pull
jaund/o	yellow	xanth/o	yellow
kel/o	tumor	xer/o	dry

Word Roots

actin	ray, light	log	study
chym	juice	lopec	fox mange
chord	cord	miliar	millet (tiny)
coriat	corium	pannicul	fat cells
cubit	to lie	tel	end, distant

Medical Word	Word Parts		Definition
	Part	Meaning	
acne (ăk´ nē)			Inflammatory condition of the sebaceous glands and the hair follicles; *pimples*. See Figure 4.4.

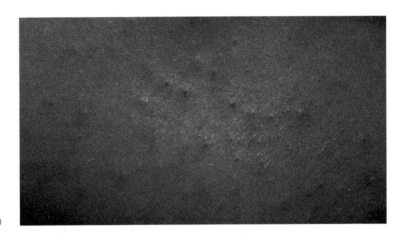

FIGURE 4.4 Acne.
Source: Courtesy of Jason L. Smith, MD

fyi Acne fulminans is a rare type of acne in teenage boys, marked by inflamed, tender, ulcerative, and crusting lesions of the upper trunk and face. It has a sudden onset and is characterized by fever, leukocytosis (elevated white blood cell count), and an elevated sedimentation rate. About 50% of the cases have inflammation of several joints. See Figure 4.5.

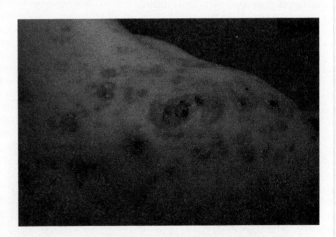

FIGURE 4.5 Acne fulminans.
Source: Courtesy of Jason L. Smith, MD

Medical Word	Word Parts		Definition
acrochordon (ăk´ rō-kor´ dŏn)	**acr/o** **chord** **-on**	extremity cord pertaining to	Small outgrowth of epidermal and dermal tissue; *skin tags*

Medical Word	Word Parts		Definition
	Part	Meaning	
actinic dermatitis (ăk-tĭn´ ĭk děr˝ mă-tī´ tĭs)	**actin** **-ic** **dermat** **-itis**	ray pertaining to skin inflammation	Inflammation of the skin caused by exposure to radiant energy, such as x-rays, ultraviolet light, and sunlight. See Figure 4.6.

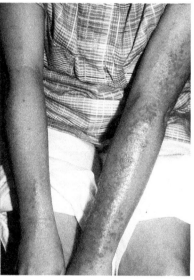

FIGURE 4.6 Photodermatitis.
Source: Courtesy of Jason L. Smith, MD

albinism (ăl´ bĭn-ĭsm)	**albin** **-ism**	white condition	Genetic condition in which there is partial or total absence of pigment in skin, hair, and eyes
alopecia (al˝ ō-pē´ shē-ă)	**a-** **lopec** **-ia**	without, lack of fox mange condition	Absence or loss of hair, especially of the head; baldness; *alopecia areata* is loss of hair in defined patches usually involving the scalp. See Figure 4.7. Androgenetic (formerly called *male pattern*) alopecia is a common form of hair loss in both men and women. In men, hair is lost in a well-defined pattern, beginning above both temples and receding to form a characteristic "M" shape. In women, the hair becomes thinner all over the head and the hairline does not recede. See Figure 4.8.

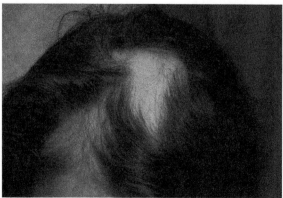

FIGURE 4.7 Alopecia areata.
Source: Courtesy of Jason L. Smith, MD

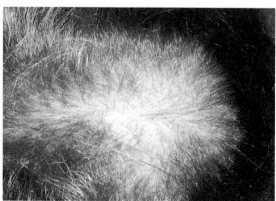

FIGURE 4.8 Androgenetic alopecia.
Source: Courtesy of Jason L. Smith, MD

Medical Word	Word Parts		Definition
	Part	Meaning	
anhidrosis (ăn″ hī-drō′ sĭs)	**an-** **hidr** **-osis**	without, lack of sweat condition	Abnormal condition in which there is a lack of or complete absence of sweating. May be congenital or disease related, generalized or localized, temporary or permanent.
autograft (ŏ′ tō-grăft)	**auto-** **-graft**	self grafting knife	Graft taken from one part of the patient's body and transferred to another part of that same patient

 fyi Patients who undergo an autograft procedure may experience increased postoperative pain from the second surgical (autograft) site. They may also require longer periods of rehabilitation. Other types of skin grafts are *allograft*, in which skin is taken from a cadaver and comes from a skin bank; and *xenograft*, in which the skin comes from a pig and is temporarily used to cover a severe burn.

avulsion (ă-vŭl′ shŭn)	**a-** **vuls** **-ion**	apart to pull process	Process of forcibly tearing off a part or structure of the body, such as a finger or toe
basal cell carcinoma (BCC) (bā′ săl sĕl kăr″ sĭ-nō′ mă)	**carcin** **-oma**	cancer tumor	Epithelial malignant tumor of the skin that rarely metastasizes. It usually begins as a small, shiny papule and enlarges to form a whitish border around a central depression. See Figure 4.9.

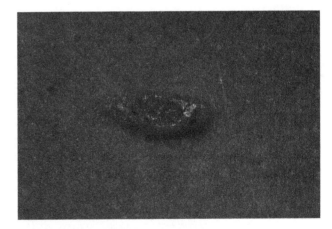

FIGURE 4.9 Basal cell carcinoma.
Source: Courtesy of Jason L. Smith, MD

fyi Premalignant and malignant skin lesions increase with aging and with overexposure to the sun. Carcinomas (the plural form *carcinomata* is also used) appear frequently on the nose, eyelid, or cheek. Basal cell carcinomas (BCC) account for 80% of the skin cancers seen in the older adult. These cancers are generally slow growing but should be surgically removed as soon as possible (ASAP).

Medical Word	Word Parts		Definition
	Part	Meaning	
bite			Injury in which a part of the skin is torn by an insect, animal, or human, resulting in a combination of an abrasion, puncture, or laceration. See Figures 4.10, 4.11, and 4.12.

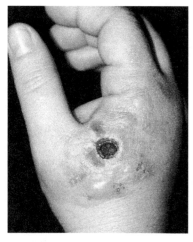

FIGURE 4.10 Brown recluse spider bites.
Source: Courtesy of Jason L. Smith, MD

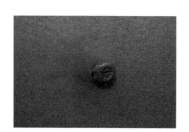

FIGURE 4.11 Tick bite.
Source: Courtesy of Jason L. Smith, MD

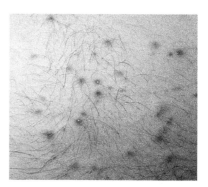

FIGURE 4.12 Flea bites.
Source: Courtesy of Jason L. Smith, MD

GOOD TO KNOW ▶

Lyme disease is caused by the bacterium *Borrelia burgdorferi* and is transmitted to humans through the bite of infected black-legged ticks. Typical symptoms include fever, headache, fatigue, and a characteristic skin rash called *erythema migrans*. If left untreated, infection can spread to joints, the heart, and the nervous system. Lyme disease is diagnosed based on symptoms; physical findings, especially a rash; and the possibility of exposure to infected ticks. Most cases of Lyme disease can be treated successfully with antibiotics. Take these steps to prevent Lyme disease:

• Apply insect repellent/pesticide.
• Use a tick-preventive product on your pets.
• Remove ticks promptly.
• Reduce tick habitat in your yard.

| boil | | | Acute, infected, painful nodule formed in the subcutaneous layers of the skin, gland, or hair follicle; most often caused by the invasion of staphylococci; *furuncle* |

Medical Word	Word Parts		Definition
	Part	Meaning	
bulla (bŭl´ lă)			Larger blister; *bleb*. See Figure 4.13.

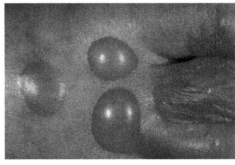

FIGURE 4.13 Bulla.
Source: Courtesy of Jason L. Smith, MD

| burn | | | Injury to tissue caused by heat, fire, chemical agents, electricity, lightning, or radiation; classified according to degree or depth of skin damage. The three classifications are first degree, second degree, and third degree. See Figures 4.14 and 4.15. |

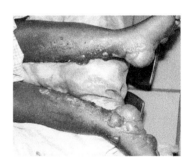

FIGURE 4.14 Burn, second degree.
Source: Courtesy of Jason L. Smith, MD

Superficial Partial Thickness (first degree) Damages only outer layer of skin; burn is painful and red; heals in a few days (e.g., sunburn)

Partial Thickness (second degree) Involves epidermis and upper layers of dermis; may have sparing of sweat glands and sebaceous glands; heals in 10–14 days

Full Thickness (third degree) Involves all of epidermis and dermis; may also involve underlying tissue; nerve ending usually destroyed; requires skin grafting

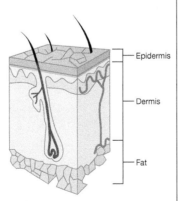

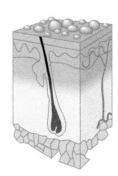

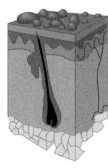

FIGURE 4.15 Characteristics of burns by depth of thermal injury.
Source: Pearson Education, Inc.

Erythema, blanches on pressure, no bullae, peeling after a few days due to premature cell death

Blisters or bullae, erythema, blanches on pressure, pain and sensitivity to cold air, minimal scar formation

Skin may appear brown, black, deep cherry red, white to gray, waxy or translucent, usually no pain, injured area may appear sunken

Medical Word	Word Parts		Definition
	Part	Meaning	
candidiasis (kăn″ dĭ-dī′ ă -sĭs)			Infection of the skin or mucous membranes with any species of *Candida* but chiefly *Candida albicans*. *Candida* is a genus of yeasts. See Figure 4.16.

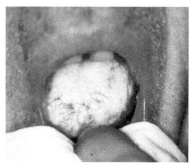

FIGURE 4.16 Candidiasis.
Source: Courtesy of Jason L. Smith, MD

Medical Word	Word Parts		Definition
carbuncle (kăr′ bŭng″ kl)			Infection of the subcutaneous tissue, usually composed of a cluster of boils. See Figure 4.17.

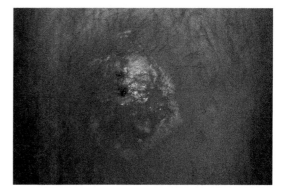

FIGURE 4.17 Carbuncle.
Source: Courtesy of Jason L. Smith, MD

Medical Word	Word Parts		Definition
causalgia (kŏ-săl′ jē-ă)	caus -algia	burning pain	Intense burning pain associated with trophic skin changes such as thinning of hair and loss of sweat glands due to peripheral nerve damage
cellulitis (sĕl-ū-lī′ tĭs)	cellul -itis	little cell inflammation	An acute, diffuse inflammation of the skin and subcutaneous tissue characterized by local heat, redness, pain, and swelling. See Figure 4.18.

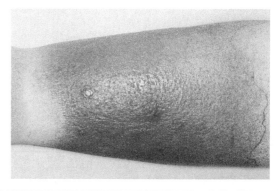

FIGURE 4.18 Cellulitis.
Source: Courtesy of Jason L. Smith, MD

Medical Word	Word Parts		Definition
	Part	Meaning	
cicatrix (sĭk´ ă-trĭks)			Scar left after the healing of a wound
comedo (kŏm´ ă-dō)			Blackhead
corn (korn)			Thickening of the skin that may be soft or hard depending on location; caused by local pressure, friction, or both that irritates tissue over a bony prominence, such as from ill-fitting shoes
cryosurgery (krī˝ ō-sĕr´ jĕr-ē)			Technique of using subfreezing temperature (usually with liquid nitrogen) to produce well-demarcated areas of cell injury and destruction
cutaneous (kū-tā´ nē-ŭs)	cutane -ous	skin pertaining to	Pertaining to the skin
cyst (sĭst)			Closed sac that contains fluid, semifluid, or solid material
debridement (dā-brēd-mŏn´)			Removal of foreign material or damaged or dead tissue, especially in a wound. It is used to promote healing and to prevent infection.
decubitus (decub) ulcer (dē-kū´ bĭ-tŭs ŭl´ sĕr)	de- cubit -us	down to lie pertaining to	An area of skin and tissue that becomes injured or broken down. Also known as a *bedsore* or *pressure ulcer*. The literal meaning of the word *decubitus* is *a lying down*. (See types of skin signs in Figure 4.42.)
dehiscence (dē-hĭs´ ĕns)			Surgical complication where there is separation or bursting open of a surgical wound. See Figure 4.19.

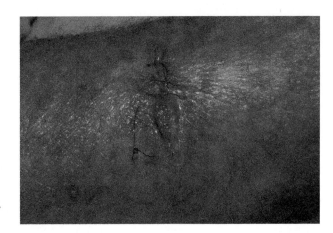

FIGURE 4.19 Wound dehiscence, back.
Source: Courtesy of Jason L. Smith, MD

Medical Word	Word Parts		Definition
dermabrasion (dĕrm´ ă-brā˝ zhŭn)			Skin resurfacing procedure to remove acne scars, nevi, tattoos, or fine wrinkles by using a rapidly rotating device to sand the outer layers of skin

Medical Word	Word Parts		Definition
	Part	Meaning	
dermatitis (děr″ mă-tī′ tĭs)	dermat -itis	skin inflammation	Inflammation of the skin. See Figure 4.20.

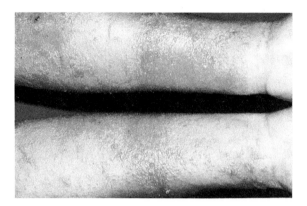

FIGURE 4.20 Dermatitis; poison ivy.
Source: Courtesy of Jason L. Smith, MD

fyi To help prevent contact dermatitis with poison ivy, learn to recognize and avoid poison ivy. One form of poison ivy is a low plant usually found in groups of many plants and looks like weeds growing from 6 to 30 inches high. The other form is a "hairy" vine that grows up a tree. Each form has stems with three leaves. See Figure 4.21. There is an old saying people should remember: "Leaflets three, let it be." If in contact with poison ivy, oak, or sumac, wash skin immediately with soap and water to remove oleoresin within 15 minutes of exposure. Also, wash all clothing including gloves, jackets, shoes, and shoelaces as soon as possible. Oleoresin, the extract of the plant, can be active for 6 months on surfaces such as clothing.

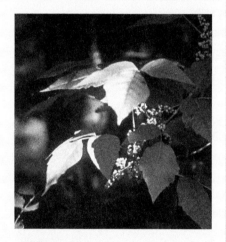

FIGURE 4.21 Poison ivy plant.
Source: Pearson Education, Inc.

Medical Word	Word Parts		Definition
dermatologist (děr″ mă-tŏl′ ŏ-jĭst)	dermat/o log -ist	skin study one who specializes	Physician who specializes in the study of the skin
dermatology (Derm) (děr″ mă-tŏl′ ŏ-jē)	dermat/o -logy	skin study of	Study of the skin
dermatome (děr′ mă-tōm)	derm/a -tome	skin instrument to cut	Surgical instrument used to produce thin slices of skin (*Note:* Dermatome also means an area of skin that is supplied by a single pair of dorsal roots or the portion of the embryonic mesoderm that gives rise to the dermis.)

Medical Word	Word Parts		Definition
	Part	Meaning	
dermomycosis (dĕr″ mō-mī-kō´ sĭs)	**derm/o** **myc** **-osis**	skin fungus condition	Skin condition caused by a fungus; also called *dermatomycosis* or *tinea*
ecchymosis (ĕk-ĭ-mō´ sĭs)	**ec-** **chym** **-osis**	out juice condition	Abnormal condition in which the blood seeps into the skin causing discolorations ranging from blue-black to greenish yellow; *bruise*. See Figure 4.22.
			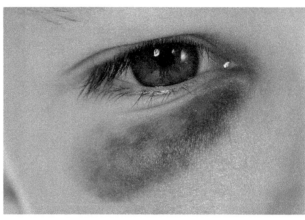

FIGURE 4.22 A child with a bruise under the eye.
Source: Nataliia Prokofyeva/123RF

Medical Word	Word Parts		Definition
eczema (ĕk´ zĕ-mă)			An acute or chronic inflammatory skin disorder characterized by erythema, papules, vesicles, pustules, scales, crusts, or scabs alone or in combination. The most promising treatment involves nonsteroidal skin medications classified as topical immunomodulators (TIMs) or topical calcineurin (a protein phosphatase) inhibitor.
erythema (ĕr″ ĭ-thē´ mă)			Redness of the skin; may be caused by capillary congestion, inflammation, heat, sunlight, or cold temperature. *Erythema infectiosum* is known as fifth disease, a mild, moderately contagious disease caused by the human parvovirus B-19. It is most commonly seen in school-age children and is thought to be spread via respiratory secretions from infected persons. See Figure 4.23.

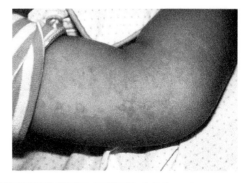

FIGURE 4.23 Erythema infectiosum; fifth disease.
Source: Courtesy of Jason L. Smith, MD

Medical Word	Word Parts		Definition
	Part	Meaning	
erythroderma (ĕ-rĭth″ rō-dĕr′ mă)	**erythr/o** **-derma**	red skin	Abnormal redness of the skin occurring over widespread areas of the body
eschar (ĕs′ kăr)			Slough, scab
excoriation (ĕks-kō″ rē-ā′ shŭn)	**ex-** **coriat** **-ion**	out corium process	Abrasion of the epidermis by scratching, trauma, chemicals, or burns
exudate (ĕks′ ū-dāt)			An oozing of pus or serum
folliculitis (fō-lĭk″ ū-lī′ tĭs)	**follicul** **-itis**	little bag inflammation	Inflammation of a follicle or follicles. See Figure 4.24.

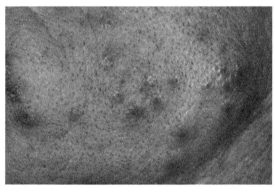

FIGURE 4.24 Staphylococcal folliculitis.
Source: Courtesy of Jason L. Smith, MD

gangrene (găng′ grēn)			Literally means *an eating sore*. It is a necrosis, or death, of tissue or bone that usually results from a deficient or absent blood supply to the area.
herpes simplex (hĕr′ pēz sĭm′ plĕks)			An inflammatory skin disease caused by a herpes virus (type I); *cold sore* or *fever blister*. See Figure 4.25.

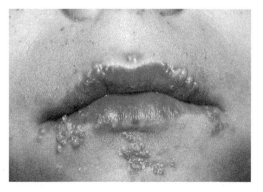

FIGURE 4.25 Herpes labialis.
Source: Courtesy of Jason L. Smith, MD

hidradenitis (hī-drăd-ĕ-nī′ tĭs)	**hidr** **aden** **-itis**	sweat gland inflammation	Inflammation of the sweat glands

Medical Word	Word Parts		Definition
	Part	Meaning	
hives (hīvz)			Eruption of itching and burning swellings on the skin; *urticaria*. See Figure 4.26.

FIGURE 4.26 Urticaria; hives.
Source: Courtesy of Jason L. Smith, MD

Medical Word	Word Parts		Definition
hyperhidrosis (hī″ pĕr-hī-drō′ sĭs)	**hyper-** **hidr** **-osis**	excessive sweat condition	Abnormal condition of excessive sweating
hypodermic (hī″ pō-dĕr′mĭk)	**hypo-** **derm** **-ic**	under skin pertaining to	Pertaining to under the skin or inserted under the skin, as a hypodermic injection
hypohidrosis (hī″ pō-hī-drō′ sĭs)	**hypo-** **hidr** **-osis**	deficient, under sweat condition	Abnormal condition of the inability to sweat; also called *anhidrosis*
icteric (ĭk-tĕr′ ĭk)	**icter** **-ic**	jaundice pertaining to	Pertaining to jaundice
impetigo (ĭm″ pĕ-tī′ gō)			Skin infection marked by vesicles or bullae; usually caused by streptococcus (strep) or staphylococcus (staph). See Figure 4.27.

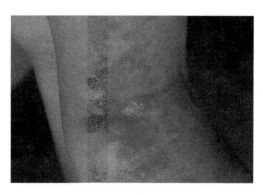

FIGURE 4.27 Impetigo.
Source: Courtesy of Jason L. Smith, MD

Medical Word	Word Parts		Definition
	Part	Meaning	
integumentary (ĭn-tĕg″ ū-mĕn′ tă-rē)	**integument** **-ary**	a covering pertaining to	Covering; the skin, consisting of the dermis and the epidermis
intradermal (ID) (in″ tră-dĕr′ măl)	**intra-** **derm** **-al**	within skin pertaining to	Pertaining to within the skin, as an intradermal injection
jaundice (jawn′ dĭs)	**jaund** **-ic(e)**	yellow pertaining to	Yellow; a symptom of a disease in which there is excessive bile in the blood; the skin, whites of the eyes, and mucous membranes are yellow; *icterus*
keloid (kē′ loyd)	**kel** **-oid**	tumor resemble	Overgrowth of scar tissue caused by excessive collagen formation. See Figure 4.28.

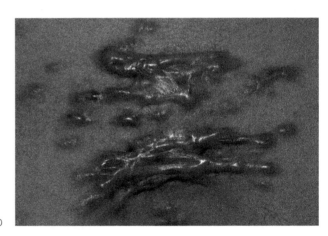

FIGURE 4.28 Keloid.
Source: Courtesy of Jason L. Smith, MD

lentigo (lĕn-tī′ gō)			A flat, brownish spot on the skin sometimes caused by exposure to the sun and weather
leukoderma (loo-kō-dĕr′ mă)	**leuk/o** **-derma**	white skin	Localized loss of pigmentation of the skin
leukoplakia (loo″ kō-plā′ kē-ă)	**leuk/o** **plak** **-ia**	white plate condition	White spots or patches formed on the mucous membrane of the tongue or cheek; the spots are smooth, hard, and irregular in shape and can become malignant
lupus (loo′ pŭs)			Originally used to describe a destructive type of skin lesion; current usage of the word is usually in combination with the words *vulgaris* or *erythematosus* (e.g., *lupus vulgaris* or *lupus erythematosus*)

Medical Word	Word Parts		Definition
	Part	Meaning	
measles (mē' zĕlz)			Highly contagious illness caused by the rubeola virus, which replicates in the nose and throat of an infected child or adult

GOOD TO KNOW ▶

When someone with measles coughs, sneezes, or talks, infected droplets spray into the air where other people can inhale them. The infected droplets may also land on a surface where they remain active and contagious for several hours. After touching the infected surface, individuals who have not been immunized with the MMR (measles, mumps, rubella) vaccine (a suspension of attenuated live or killed microorganisms) may contract the virus by putting their fingers in their mouths or noses or rubbing their eyes. About 90% of susceptible people who are exposed to the virus will be infected.

At one time, measles was virtually eliminated in the United States. Today, it is back and on the rise. The message is that *immunization* (the protection of individuals from specific diseases by vaccination) is the best protection against diseases such as measles. Signs and symptoms of measles include fever, malaise, sneezing, nasal congestion, brassy cough, conjunctivitis, spots on the buccal mucosa (Koplik spots), and a *maculopapular eruption* (type of rash) over the body.

Medical Word	Word Parts		Definition
melanoma (mĕl″ ă-nō′ mă)	melan -oma	black tumor	Cancer that develops in the pigment cells of the skin; malignant black mole or tumor. See Figures 4.29 and 4.30. Often the first sign of melanoma is change in the size, shape, or color of a mole. To describe the changes that can occur in a mole, use the **ABCDEs** Rule. **A**—**A**symmetry: one half of the mole does not match the other; irregularity. **B**—**B**order: edges are ragged, notched, or blurred. **C**—**C**olor: not uniform; shades of black, brown, or tan are present and areas of white, red, or blue may be seen. **D**—**D**iameter: greater than 6 mm (about the size of a pencil eraser) **E**—**E**volving: size, shape, or color may change

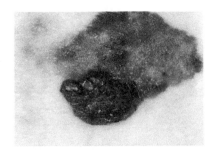

FIGURE 4.29
Melanoma, forearm.
Source: Courtesy of
Jason L. Smith, MD

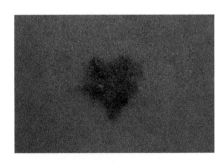

FIGURE 4.30
Melanoma, thigh.
Source: Courtesy of
Jason L. Smith, MD

Medical Word	Word Parts		Definition
	Part	Meaning	
miliaria (mĭl-ē-ā′ rē-ă)	**miliar** **-ia**	millet (tiny) condition	Rash with tiny pinhead-sized papules, vesicles, and/or pustules commonly seen in newborns and infants; *prickly heat*. It is caused by excessive body warmth. There is retention of sweat in the sweat glands, which have become blocked or inflamed, and then rupture or leak into the skin. See Figure 4.31.

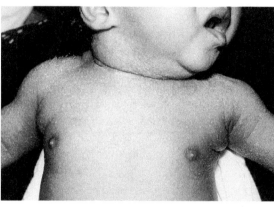

FIGURE 4.31 Miliaria.
Source: Courtesy of Jason L. Smith, MD

Medical Word	Word Parts		Definition
mole (mōl)			Pigmented, elevated spot above the surface of the skin; *nevus*. See Figure 4.32.

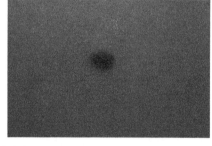

FIGURE 4.32 Nevus; benign mole.
Source: Courtesy of Jason L. Smith, MD

Medical Word	Word Parts		Definition
onychia (ō-nĭk′ ē-ă)	**onych** **-ia**	nail condition	Inflammation of the nail bed resulting in loss of nail
onychomycosis (ŏn″ ĭ-kō-mī-kō′ sĭs)	**onych/o** **myc** **-osis**	nail fungus condition	A fungal infection of the nails. See Figure 4.33.

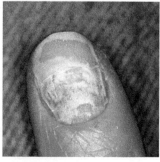

FIGURE 4.33 Onychomycosis.
Source: Courtesy of Jason L. Smith, MD

Medical Word	Word Parts		Definition
	Part	**Meaning**	
pachyderma (păk-ē-děr´ mă)	**pachy** **-derma**	thick skin	Thick skin; also called *pachydermia*
panniculectomy (păn-ĭk˝ ū-lĕk' tō-mē)	**pannicul** **-ectomy**	fat cells surgical excision	Surgical excision of fat cells in the superficial fascia; a body-contouring surgical procedure that removes hanging fat and skin, typically after massive weight loss; may be performed as a standalone procedure or combined with a tummy tuck (abdominoplasty)

 fyi CoolSculpting®, or *cryolipolysis*, is a nonsurgical body-contouring procedure approved by the Food and Drug Administration (FDA). A plastic surgeon uses a device to freeze fat cells under the skin. Once the fat cells have been destroyed, they are gradually broken down and removed from the body by the liver. Most people start to notice the effects a few days after the procedure, but it often takes 1–4 months for the full results to show.

paronychia (păr˝ ō-nĭk´ ē-ă)	**para-** **onych** **-ia**	next to nail condition	Infectious condition of the marginal structures surrounding the nail

✓ RULE REMINDER

The *a* has been dropped from the prefix **para-** to form the correct spelling of paronychia.

pediculosis (pĕ-dĭk˝ ū-lō´ sĭs)	**pedicul** **-osis**	a louse condition	Condition of infestation with lice. See Figure 4.34.

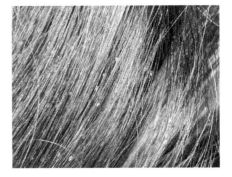

FIGURE 4.34 Pediculosis capitis.
Source: Courtesy of Jason L. Smith, MD

petechiae (pē-tē´ kē-ē)			Small, pinpoint, purplish hemorrhagic spots on the skin
pruritus (proo-rī´ tŭs)	**prurit** **-us**	itching pertaining to	Severe itching

Medical Word	Word Parts		Definition
	Part	Meaning	
psoriasis (sō-rī′ ă-sĭs)			Chronic skin condition characterized by frequent episodes of redness, itching, and thick, dry scales on the skin. See Figure 4.35.

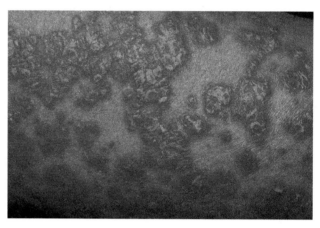

FIGURE 4.35 Psoriasis, lower extremities.
Source: Courtesy of Jason L. Smith, MD

Medical Word	Word Parts		Definition
purpura (pŭr′ pū-ră)			Purplish discoloration of the skin caused by extravasation of blood into the tissues. See Figure 4.36.

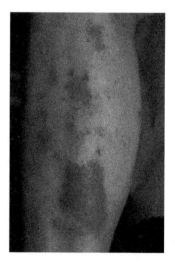

FIGURE 4.36 Purpura.
Source: Courtesy of Jason L. Smith, MD

Medical Word	Word Parts		Definition
rhytidoplasty (rĭt′ ĭ-dō-plăs″ tē)	**rhytid/o** **-plasty**	wrinkle surgical repair	Plastic surgery for the removal of wrinkles

Medical Word	Word Parts		Definition
	Part	Meaning	
rosacea (rō-zā´ shē-ă)			A chronic disease of the skin of the face marked by varying degrees of papules, pustules, erythema, telangiectasia, and hyperplasia of the soft tissues of the nose; usually occurs in middle-aged and older people. See Figure 4.37.

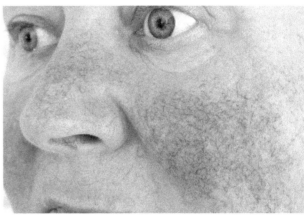

FIGURE 4.37 Rosacea.
Source: Lipowski Milan/Shutterstock

| **roseola**
(rō-zē´ ō-lă) | | | Any rose-colored rash marked by *maculae* or red spots on the skin. See Figure 4.38. |

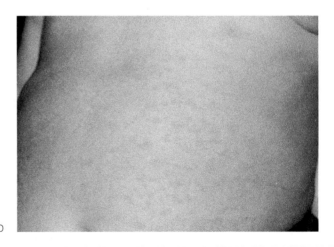

FIGURE 4.38 Roseola.
Source: Courtesy of Jason L. Smith, MD

Medical Word	Word Parts		Definition
	Part	Meaning	
rubella (roo-bĕl´ lă)			Contagious viral infection best known by its distinctive red rash; also called *German measles* and *three-day measles*. See Figure 4.39.

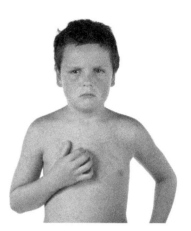

FIGURE 4.39 A boy with rash caused by the rubella virus.
Source: Stacy Barnett/123RF

GOOD TO KNOW ▶

Rubella is not the same as measles (rubeola) and is caused by a different virus (rubella virus). If contracted by the mother during pregnancy, the consequences for the unborn child may be severe and, in some cases, fatal. The highest risk to the fetus is during the first trimester, but exposure later in pregnancy is also dangerous. To help prevent the complications of rubella during pregnancy, the CDC recommends that women should update their vaccinations 3 months before attempting conception. The measles, mumps, and rubella (MMR) vaccine should be given to children beginning at 12–15 months of age with a booster vaccine at 4–6 years of age.

Medical Word	Word Parts		Definition
scabies (skā´ bēz)			Contagious skin disease characterized by papules, vesicles, pustules, burrows, and intense itching; it is caused by an arachnid, *Sarcoptes scabiei, variety hominis,* the itch mite; also called *the itch*. See Figure 4.40.

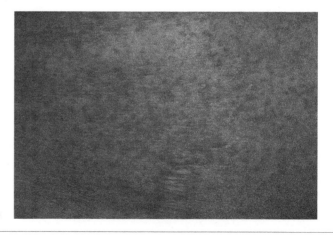

FIGURE 4.40 Scabies.
Source: Courtesy of Jason L. Smith, MD

Medical Word	Word Parts		Definition
	Part	Meaning	
scar			Mark left by the healing process of a wound, sore, or injury
scleroderma (sklĕr″ ă-dĕr′ mă)	**scler/o** **-derma**	hard, hardening skin	Chronic condition with hardening of the skin and other connective tissues of the body
seborrhea (sĕb″ or-ē′ ă)	**seb/o** **-rrhea**	oil flow	Excessive flow (secretion) of oil from the sebaceous glands
seborrheic keratosis (sĕb″ ō-rē′ ĭk kĕr″ ă-tō′ sĭs)	**seb/o** **-rrhe** **-ic** **kerat** **-osis**	sebum flow pertaining to horn condition	Condition occurring in older people wherein there is dry skin and localized scaling caused by excessive exposure to the sun. It usually appears as a brown, black, or light tan growth on the face, chest, shoulders, or back and has a waxy, scaly, slightly elevated appearance. See Figure 4.41.

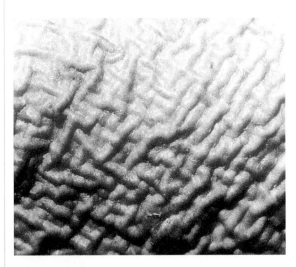

FIGURE 4.41 Photoaging solar elastosis; seborrheic keratosis.
Source: Courtesy of Jason L. Smith, MD

✓ RULE REMINDER

With the suffix **-rrhea**, the *a* has been dropped to add the suffix **-ic**, forming *seborrheic*.

sebum (sē′ bŭm)		Fatty or oily secretion produced by the sebaceous glands

Medical Word	Word Parts		Definition
	Part	Meaning	
skin signs			Objective evidence of an illness or disorder. They can be seen, measured, or felt. Types of skin signs are shown and described in Figure 4.42.

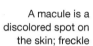

A macule is a discolored spot on the skin; freckle

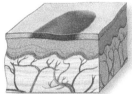

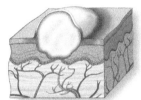

A pustule is a small, elevated, circumscribed lesion of the skin that is filled with pus; varicella (chickenpox)

A wheal is a localized, evanescent elevation of the skin that is often accompanied by itching; urticaria

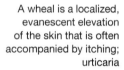

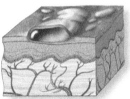

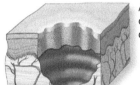

An erosion or ulcer is an eating or gnawing away of tissue; decubitus ulcer

A papule is a solid, circumscribed, elevated area on the skin; pimple

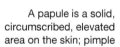

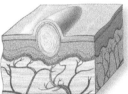

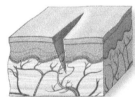

A fissure is a crack like sore or slit that extends through the epidermis into the dermis

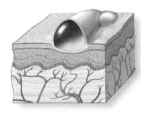

A vesicle is a small fluid-filled sac; blister. A bulla is a large vesicle.

FIGURE 4.42 Skin signs are objective evidence of an illness or disorder. They can be seen, measured, or felt.

Medical Word	Word Parts		Definition
	Part	Meaning	
squamous cell carcinoma (SCC) (skwā´ mŭs sĕl kăr˝ sĭ-nō´ mă)			Malignant tumor of squamous epithelial tissue. See Figures 4.43 and 4.44.

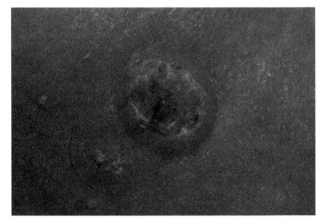

FIGURE 4.43 Squamous cell carcinoma.
Source: Courtesy of Jason L. Smith, MD

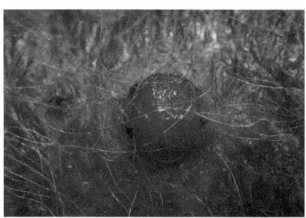

FIGURE 4.44 Squamous cell carcinoma on forearm.
Source: Courtesy of Jason L. Smith, MD

Medical Word	Word Parts		Definition
striae *(plural)* (strī´ ē)			Streaks or lines on the breasts, thighs, abdomen, or buttocks caused by weakening of elastic tissue; can be caused by obesity or as a result of pregnancy. See Figure 4.45.

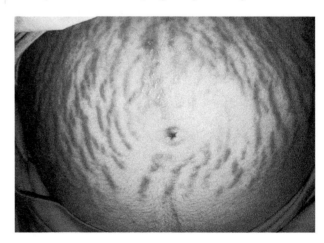

FIGURE 4.45 Striae.
Source: Courtesy of Jason L. Smith, MD

Medical Word	Word Parts		Definition
subcutaneous (sŭb˝ kū-tā´ nē-ŭs)	**sub-** **cutane** **-ous**	below skin pertaining to	Pertaining to below the skin, as a subcutaneous injection
subungual (sŭb-ŭng´ gwăl)	**sub-** **ungu** **-al**	below nail pertaining to	Pertaining to below the nail

Medical Word	Word Parts		Definition
	Part	Meaning	
taut (tŏt)			Tight, firm; to pull or draw tight a surface, such as the skin
telangiectasia (tĕl-ăn″ jē-ĕk-tā′ zē-ă)	**tel** **ang/i** **-ectasia**	end, distant vessel dilatation	Small dilated blood vessels that appear as small red or purple clusters, often spidery in appearance, and are visible near the surface of the skin; also called *spider veins*. See Figure 4.46.

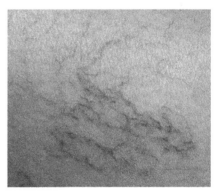

FIGURE 4.46 Close-up of leg with telangiectasia (spider veins).
Source: schankz/Shutterstock

! ALERT!

Note the spelling of *telangiectasia* and *thermoanesthesia*. The suffix -**ectasia** means *dilatation* and the suffix -**esthesia** means *sensation*.

Medical Word	Word Parts		Definition
thermoanesthesia (thĕr″ mō-ăn-ĕs-thē′ zhă)	**therm/o** **an-** **-esthesia**	hot, heat without, lack of sensation	Inability to distinguish between the sensations of heat and cold
tinea (tĭn′ē-ă)			Contagious skin diseases affecting both humans and domestic animals, caused by certain fungi and marked by the localized appearance of discolored, scaly patches on the skin; *ringworm*. See Figure 4.47.

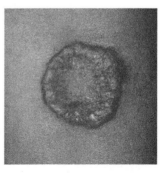

FIGURE 4.47 Tinea corporis.
Source: Courtesy of Jason L. Smith, MD

Medical Word	Word Parts		Definition
	Part	Meaning	
trichomycosis (trĭk″ ō-mī-kō′ sĭs)	**trich/o** **myc** **-osis**	hair fungus condition	Fungal condition of the hair
ulcer (ŭl′ sĕr)			Open lesion or sore of the epidermis or mucous membrane. See Figure 4.48.

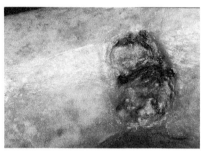

FIGURE 4.48 Leg ulcer radiation site.
Source: Courtesy of Jason L. Smith, MD

Medical Word	Word Parts		Definition
varicella (văr″ ĭ-sĕl′ ă)			Contagious viral disease characterized by fever, headache, and a crop of red spots that become macules, papules, vesicles, and crusts; *chickenpox*. See Figure 4.49.

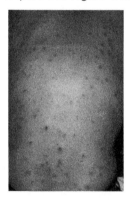

FIGURE 4.49 Varicella; chickenpox.
Source: Courtesy of Jason L. Smith, MD

Medical Word	Word Parts		Definition
vitiligo (vĭt-ĭl-ī′ gō)			Skin condition characterized by milk-white patches surrounded by areas of normal pigmentation
wart			A skin lesion with a rough papillomatous surface (of viral origin) on the epidermis; *verruca*. A plantar wart, *verruca plantaris*, occurs on a pressure-bearing area, especially the sole of the foot. See Figure 4.50.

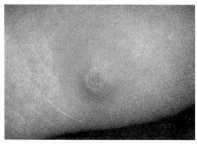

FIGURE 4.50 Plantar wart.
Source: Courtesy of Jason L. Smith, MD

Medical Word	Word Parts		Definition
	Part	**Meaning**	
wound (woond)			Injury to soft tissue caused by trauma; generally classified as open or closed
xanthoderma (zăn″ thō-dĕr′ mă)	**xanth/o** **-derma**	yellow skin	Yellowness of the skin
xanthoma (zăn-thō′ mă)	**xanth** **-oma**	yellow tumor	Literally means *yellow tumor*; a soft, rounded plaque or nodule, usually on the eyelids, especially near the inner canthus
xeroderma (zēr″ ō-dĕr′ mă)	**xer/o** **-derma**	dry skin	Dry skin
xerosis (zē″ rō′ sĭs)	**xer** **-osis**	dry condition	Abnormal dryness of skin, mucous membranes, or the conjunctiva

 fyi Sun exposure, skin disorders, aging, and heredity can contribute to skin irregularities on the face, arms, legs, and elsewhere on the body. These include textural irregularities like wrinkles and acne scars, pigmentation changes like freckles, sunspots, or telangiectasia (spider veins). In addition, skin may lose tone and feel less firm than it once did. Different treatment modalities are available to treat the different aspects of skin damage. These modalities are included in the specialty of skin rejuvenation and resurfacing, which can be performed by a board-certified plastic surgeon. The following are types of skin rejuvenation and resurfacing treatment modalities and their purposes:

Ablative laser (fractional, CO_2 lasers)	Smooth lines and wrinkles by removing outer layers of the skin
Botulinum toxin type A (Botox®)	Relax wrinkles by blocking nerve contractions in facial muscles
Chemical peels	Remove damaged outer skin layers through the use of various acid peels that can be used in different combinations
Dermal fillers	Improve skin contouring by injecting various soft tissue filler compounds
Intense pulsed light (IPL)	Remove discolorations and brown spots and/or tighten sagging skin through photorejuvenation
Mechanical ablations (dermabrasion, dermaplaning)	Soften skin surface irregularities by using surgical scraping/sanding methods
Minimally invasive ablative methods (microdermabrasion, microneedling, light acid peels)	Treat light scarring and discolorations using minimally invasive sanding methods
Sclerotherapy (spider vein treatment)	Collapse unsightly surface veins by injecting an irritant into them that causes inflammation, coagulation of blood, and narrowing of the blood vessel walls, making the veins less visible

Study *and* Review II

Word Parts

Prefixes   Give the definitions of the following prefixes.

1. a-, an- _____

2. auto- _____

3. ec- _____

4. de- _____

5. ex- _____

6. hyper- _____

7. hypo- _____

8. intra- _____

9. par- _____

10. sub- _____

Combining Forms   Give the definitions of the following combining forms.

1. albin/o _____

2. caus/o _____

3. cutane/o _____

4. derm/o _____

5. erythr/o _____

6. hidr/o _____

7. icter/o _____

8. kel/o _____

9. kerat/o _____

10. leuk/o _____

11. melan/o _____

12. onych/o _____

13. pachy/o _____

14. pedicul/o _____

15. plak/o _____

16. prurit/o _____

17. rhytid/o _____

18. scler/o _____

19. seb/o _____

20. therm/o _____

21. trich/o _____

22. vuls/o _____

23. xanth/o _____

24. xer/o _____

Suffixes   Give the definitions of the following suffixes.

1. -al _____

2. -algia _____

3. -on _____

4. -us _____

5. -derma _____

6. -ary _____

7. -esthesia _____

8. -graft _____

9. -ia _____

10. -ic _____

11. -ion _____

12. -ism _____

13. -ist _____

14. -itis _____

15. -logy _____

16. -ectasia _____

17. -oid _____

18. -oma _____

19. -osis _____

20. -ous _____

21. -plasty _____

22. -rrhea _____

23. -tome _____

Identifying Medical Terms

In the spaces provided, write the medical terms for the following meanings.

1. _____ Inflammation of the skin caused by exposure to actinic rays

2. _____ Pertaining to the skin

3. _____ Inflammation of the skin

4. _____ Study of the skin

5. _____ Severe itching

6. _____ Condition of excessive sweating

7. _____ Pertaining to under the skin

8. _____ Pertaining to jaundice

9. _____ Inflammation of the nail

10. _____ Thick skin

Matching

Select the appropriate lettered meaning for each of the following words.

_____ 1. acne

_____ 2. alopecia

_____ 3. cicatrix

_____ 4. comedo

_____ 5. decubitus

_____ 6. dehiscence

_____ 7. exudate

_____ 8. leukoplakia

_____ 9. petechiae

_____ 10. pruritus

a. Small, pinpoint, purplish hemorrhagic spots on the skin

b. Production of pus or serum

c. Severe itching

d. Inflammatory condition of the sebaceous glands and the hair follicles

e. Scar left after the healing of a wound

f. Loss of hair, baldness

g. White spots or patches formed on the mucous membrane of the tongue or cheek

h. Blackhead

i. Separation or bursting open of a surgical wound

j. Bedsore

Medical Case Snapshots

This learning activity provides an opportunity to relate the medical terminology you are learning to sample patient case presentations. In the spaces provided, write in your answers.

Case 1

A 36-year-old male is concerned about noticeable loss of scalp hair. The medical term for this condition is

_____ (loss of hair, especially on the scalp). In the androgenetic type

of this condition (formerly called *male-pattern baldness*), hair is lost in a well-defined pattern, beginning above both

temples and receding to form a characteristic "M" shape.

Case 2

When the 45-year-old female was asked about her chief complaint, she said, "I would like something done to

remove the wrinkles from around my eyes and mouth." Dr. Smith, a dermatologist, explained that he could either do a

_____ (surgical procedure to remove fine wrinkles) or he could perform a

_____ (type of plastic surgery).

Case 3

The 84-year-old bedridden patient is diagnosed with a large decubitus ulcer located on her right buttocks. The literal

meaning of the word *decubitus* is _____ _____ _____.

Drug Highlights

Classification of Drug	Description and Examples
emollients	Substances that are generally oily in nature. These substances are used for dry skin caused by aging, excessive bathing, and psoriasis. EXAMPLE: Desitin
keratolytics	Agents that cause or promote loosening of horny (keratin) layers of the skin. These agents may be used for acne, warts, psoriasis, corns, calluses (hardened skin), and fungal infections. EXAMPLES: Duofilm, Keralyt, and Compound W
local anesthetic agents	Agents that inhibit the conduction of nerve impulses from sensory nerves and thereby reduce pain and discomfort. These agents may be used topically to reduce discomfort associated with insect bites, burns, and poison ivy. EXAMPLES: Solarcaine and Xylocaine
antihistamine agents	Agents that act to prevent the action of histamine. Used to help relieve symptoms, such as itching, in allergic responses and contact dermatitis. EXAMPLE: Benadryl (diphenhydramine)
antipruritic agents	Agents that prevent or relieve itching EXAMPLES: Topical—tripelennamine HCl; Oral—Benadryl (diphenhydramine HCl) and hydroxyzine HCl
antibiotic agents	Agents that destroy or stop the growth of microorganisms (bacteria). These agents are used to prevent infection associated with minor skin abrasions and to treat superficial skin infections and acne. Several antibiotic agents are combined in a single product to take advantage of the different antimicrobial spectrum of each drug. EXAMPLES: Neosporin, Polysporin, and Mycitracin
antifungal agents	Agents that destroy or inhibit the growth of fungi and yeast. These agents are used to treat fungus and/or yeast infection of the skin, nails, and scalp. EXAMPLES: Equate antifungal cream (clotrimazole) and Lamisil (terbinafine)
antiviral agents	Agents that combat specific viral diseases. EXAMPLE: Zovirax (acyclovir) is used in the treatment of herpes simplex virus types 1 and 2, varicella zoster, Epstein–Barr, and cytomegalovirus
anti-inflammatory agents	Agents used to relieve the swelling, tenderness, redness, and pain of inflammation. Topically applied corticosteroids are used in the treatment of dermatitis and psoriasis. EXAMPLES: Dermolate (hydrocortisone) and Temovate (clobetasol propionate) Oral corticosteroids are used in the treatment of contact dermatitis, such as in poison ivy, when the symptoms are severe. EXAMPLE: Sterapred (prednisone 12-day unipak)
antiseptic agents	Agents that prevent or inhibit the growth of pathogens. Antiseptics are generally applied to the surface of living tissue to reduce the possibility of infection, sepsis, or putrefaction. EXAMPLE: Isopropyl alcohol

Classification of Drug	Description and Examples
other drugs	Retin-A (tretinoin) is available as a cream, gel, or liquid. It is used in the treatment of acne vulgaris.
	Rogaine® (minoxidil) is available as a topical solution to stimulate hair growth. It was first approved as a treatment for androgenetic (formerly called *male pattern*) alopecia.
	Botox® (onabotulinum toxin A), commonly called *botulinum toxin type A*, is approved by the FDA to temporarily improve the appearance of moderate to severe frown lines between the eyebrows (glabellar lines). Small doses of a sterile, purified botulinum toxin are injected into the affected muscles and block the release of the chemical acetylcholine that would otherwise signal the muscle to contract. The toxin thus temporarily paralyzes or weakens the injected muscle.

Diagnostic *and* Laboratory Tests

Test	Description
tuberculosis (TB) skin test (tū-bĕr″ kū-lō′ sĭs)	The Mantoux type of tuberculin skin test (TST) is the standard method of determining whether an individual is infected with *mycobacterium tuberculosis*. Reliable administration and reading of the TST requires standardization of procedures, training, supervision, and practice. In the Mantoux tests, 0.1 mL of purified protein derivative (PPD) tuberculin is injected intradermally. Test results are read 48–72 hours after administration. The result depends on the size of the raised, hard area or swelling. A positive skin test means the person's body was infected with TB bacteria. Additional tests are needed to determine if the person has latent TB infection or TB disease. A negative skin test means the person's body did not react to the test and that latent TB infection or TB disease is not likely. The TB skin test is the preferred TB test for children under the age of 5. See Figure 4.51.

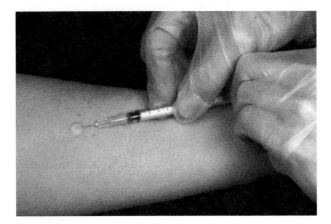

FIGURE 4.51 Mantoux tuberculin skin test.
Source: Centers for Disease Control and Prevention (CDC)

Test	Description
tuberculosis (TB) blood tests (tū-bĕr″ kū-lō′ sĭs)	Interferon-gamma release assays (IGRAs) are blood tests that may be used to determine whether an individual is infected with *mycobacterium tuberculosis*. IGRAs are the preferred tests for individuals who have received the TB vaccine bacille Calmette–Guérin (BCG).
scratch (epicutaneous) or prick test (skrăch)	Involves the placement of a suspected allergen in the uppermost layers of the epidermis. One technique used is to place a drop of the allergen on the skin of the forearm or back. A sterile lancet or needle is passed through the drop and pricks the skin no deeper than the uppermost layers of the epidermis. Redness or swelling at the scratch site within 10 minutes indicates allergy to the substance. This indicates that the test result is positive. If no reaction occurs, the test result is negative.
sweat test (chloride) (swĕt)	Performed on sweat to determine the level of chloride concentration on the skin. In **cystic fibrosis (CF)**, which is an inherited disease that affects the pancreas, respiratory system, and sweat glands, there is an increase in skin chloride.
Tzanck test (zonk)	Microscopic examination of a small piece of tissue that has been surgically scraped from a pustule. The specimen is placed on a slide and stained, and the type of viral infection can be identified.
wound culture (woond)	Performed on wound exudate to determine the presence of microorganisms and to identify the specific type. An effective antibiotic can be prescribed for identified microbes.
biopsy (Bx) (bī′ŏp-sē)	The obtaining of a small piece of living tissue for microscopic examination. May be obtained surgically, through a needle and syringe, hollow punch, brush, or stereotactically. Used to establish a diagnosis (Dx), especially to distinguish between benign and malignant conditions.
erythrocyte sedimentation rate (ESR, sed rate) (ĕ-rĭth′ rō-sīt sĕd″ ĭ-mĕn-tā′ shŭn rāt)	Blood test to determine the rate at which red blood cells (RBCs) settle in a long, narrow tube. The distance the RBCs settle in 1 hour is the rate. Higher or lower rate can indicate certain disease conditions.

Abbreviations *and* Acronyms

Abbreviation/ Acronym	Meaning	Abbreviation/ Acronym	Meaning
ASAP	as soon as possible	cm	centimeter
BCC	basal cell carcinoma	CO₂	carbon dioxide
BCG	bacille Calmette–Guérin	decub	decubitus
Botox®	botulinum toxin type A	Derm	dermatology
Bx	biopsy	Dx	diagnosis
CDC	Centers for Disease Control and Prevention	ESR, sed rate	erythrocyte sedimentation rate
		FDA	Food and Drug Administration
CF	cystic fibrosis	ID	intradermal

Abbreviation/ Acronym	Meaning	Abbreviation/ Acronym	Meaning
IGRAs	interferon-gamma release assays	SG	skin graft
IPL	intense pulsed light	staph	staphylococcus
mm	millimeter	strep	streptococcus
MMR	measles, mumps, and rubella	TB	tuberculosis
PPD	purified protein derivative	TIMs	topical immunomodulators
RBCs	red blood cells	TST	tuberculin skin test
SCC	squamous cell carcinoma	UV	ultraviolet

Study *and* Review III

Building Medical Terms

Using the following word parts, fill in the blanks to build the correct medical terms.

de-	xanth	-ic	pachy	xer
melan	xanth/o	-rrhea	onych	-logy

Definition	Medical Term
1. An area of skin and tissue that becomes broken down	_____cubitus
2. Study of the skin	dermato_____
3. Pertaining to jaundice	icter_____
4. Cancer that develops in the pigment cells of the skin	_____oma
5. Inflammation of the nail	_____itis
6. Thick skin	_____derma
7. Excessive flow of oil from the sebaceous glands	sebo_____
8. Yellowness of the skin	_____derma
9. Literally means yellow tumor	_____oma
10. Abnormal dryness of skin	_____osis

Combining Form Challenge

Using the combining forms provided, write the medical term correctly.

erythr/o	caus/o	albin/o
dermat/o	integument/o	cutane/o

1. Genetic condition in which there is a partial or total absence of pigment in skin, hair, and eyes: _____ism

2. Intense burning pain associated with trophic skin changes in the hand or foot after trauma to the part: _____algia

3. Pertaining to the skin: _____ous

4. Inflammation of the skin: _____itis

5. Abnormal redness of the skin occurring over widespread areas of the body: _____derma

6. Covering; the skin, consisting of the dermis and epidermis: _____ary

Select the Right Term

Select the correct answer and write it on the line provided.

1. Inflammatory condition of the sebaceous glands and hair follicles is _____.

    actinic dermatitis   bite   boil   acne

2. The absence or loss of hair, especially of the head, is _____.

    acrochordon   alopecia   anhidrosis   avulsion

3. Scar left after the healing of a wound is _____.

    boil   burn   corn   cicatrix

4. Slough, scab is _____.

    eschar   exudate   folliculitis   gangrene

5. A flat, brownish spot on the skin; freckle is _____.

    keloid   lupus   lentigo   mole

6. Any rose-colored rash marked by maculae or red spots on the skin is _____.

    rosacea   roseola   rubella   robeola

Drug Highlights

Match the appropriate lettered description or examples of drug(s) with the class of drug.

_____ 1. emollients

_____ 2. keratolytics

_____ 3. local anesthetics

_____ 4. antihistamines

_____ 5. examples of antipruritic agents

_____ 6. antibiotics

_____ 7. antifungals

_____ 8. examples of antiviral agents

_____ 9. anti-inflammatory agents

_____ 10. antiseptics

a. Treat fungus and/or yeast infection of the skin, nails, and scalp

b. Prevent infection associated with minor skin abrasions and to treat superficial skin infections by stopping the growth of microorganisms

c. Substances that are generally oily in nature and are used for dry skin

d. Zovirax (acyclovir), used in the treatment of herpes simplex virus types 1 and 2, varicella zoster, Epstein–Barr, and cytomegalovirus

e. Prevent or inhibit the growth of pathogens

f. Cause or promote loosening of horny (keratin) layers of the skin

g. Prevent the action of histamine, which helps relieve symptoms, such as itching, in allergic responses and contact dermatitis

h. Topical—tripelennamine HCl; Oral—Benadryl (diphenhydramine HCl) and hydroxyzine HCl

i. Relieve the swelling, tenderness, redness, and pain of inflammation

j. Inhibit the conduction of nerve impulses from sensory nerves and thereby reduce pain and discomfort

Diagnostic and Laboratory Tests

Select the best answer to each multiple-choice question. Circle the letter of your choice.

1. Which skin test is the standard method of determining whether an individual is infected with *mycobacterium* tuberculosis?

   a. sweat test

   b. Tzanck test

   c. Mantoux test

   d. interferon-gamma release assays (IGRAs)

2. A test done on wound exudate to determine the presence of microorganisms is called a

_____.

    a. sweat test   **c.** Tzanck test

    b. biopsy   **d.** wound culture

3. A microscopic examination of a small piece of tissue that has been surgically scraped from a pustule is called

a _____.

    a. Tzanck test   **c.** biopsy

    b. sweat test   **d.** wound culture

4. Which is the preferred TB test for individuals who have received the TB vaccine BCG?

    a. sweat test   **c.** Tzanck test

    b. interferon-gamma release assays (IGRAs)   **d.** scratch or prick test

5. The _____ test is used to determine the level of chloride concentration on the skin.

    a. sweat   **c.** scratch

    b. Tzanck   **d.** Mantoux

Abbreviations and Acronyms

Write the correct word, phrase, or abbreviation/acronyms in the space provided.

1. basal cell carcinoma _____

2. Bx _____

3. decub _____

4. ID _____

5. SCC _____

6. PPD _____

7. skin graft _____

8. staph _____

9. strep _____

10. topical immunomodulators _____

Practical Application

Medical Record Analysis

This exercise contains information, abbreviations/acronyms, and medical terminology from an actual medical record or case study that has been adapted for this text. The names and any personal information have been created by the author. Read and study each form or case study and then answer the questions that follow. You may refer to Appendix III, *Abbreviations, Acronyms, and Symbols*.

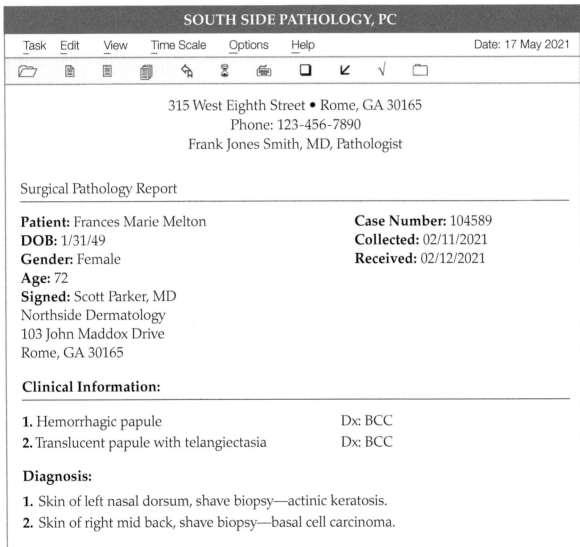

SOUTH SIDE PATHOLOGY, PC	

| Task | Edit | View | Time Scale | Options | Help | Date: 17 May 2021 |

315 West Eighth Street • Rome, GA 30165
Phone: 123-456-7890
Frank Jones Smith, MD, Pathologist

Surgical Pathology Report

Patient: Frances Marie Melton   **Case Number:** 104589
DOB: 1/31/49   **Collected:** 02/11/2021
Gender: Female   **Received:** 02/12/2021
Age: 72
Signed: Scott Parker, MD
Northside Dermatology
103 John Maddox Drive
Rome, GA 30165

Clinical Information:

1. Hemorrhagic papule   Dx: BCC
2. Translucent papule with telangiectasia   Dx: BCC

Diagnosis:

1. Skin of left nasal dorsum, shave biopsy—actinic keratosis.
2. Skin of right mid back, shave biopsy—basal cell carcinoma.

Gross Description:

1. Two containers, the first labeled "left nasal dorsum," have within a brown and white 4 × 5 mm superficial skin shave. With margins inked, this is bisected and entirely submitted.
2. The second, labeled "right mid back," has within a 0.5 × 0.7 cm superficial skin shave. With margins inked, this is trisected and entirely submitted.

Microscopic Description:

1. Sections show keratinocyte atypical involving the lower layers of the epidermis as well as solar elastosis (breakdown of elastic tissue due to apparent excessive sun exposure) and parakeratosis (incomplete keratinization due to apparent excessive sun exposure). The actinic keratosis has proliferative features.

2. Sections show a mixed superficial and micronodular form of basal cell carcinoma featuring focal pigmentation. The lesion extends to the base of the shave.

Frank Jones Smith, MD
Pathologist
(Case signed 02/14/2021)

Medical Record Questions

Write the correct answer in the space provided.

1. What is the abbreviation for diagnosis? _____

2. What does the abbreviation BCC mean? _____

3. What is the medical term for the small dilated blood vessels that appear as small red or purple clusters, often spidery in appearance, and are visible near the surface of the skin? _____

   a. keratosis   **c.** basal cell

   b. cellulitis   **d.** telangiectasia

4. Write in the diagnosis of the skin of the left nasal dorsum. _____

   _____

5. The diagnosis of basal cell carcinoma was identified from skin on the right side of what part of the body?

   _____

MyLab Medical Terminology™

MyLab Medical Terminology is a premium online homework management system that includes a host of features to help you study. Registered users will find:

- A multitude of quizzes and activities built within the MyLab platform

- Powerful tools that track and analyze your results—allowing you to create a personalized learning experience

- Videos and audio pronunciations to help enrich your progress

- Streaming lesson presentations (guided lectures) and self-paced learning modules

- A space where you and your instructor can check your progress and manage your assignments

Skeletal System

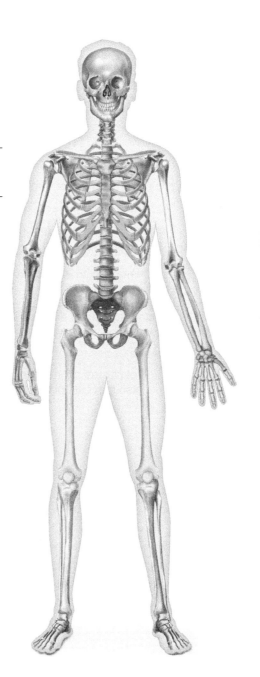

 Learning Outcomes

On completion of this chapter, you will be able to:

1. List the primary functions of bones.
2. Explain various types of body movements that occur at the freely movable joints.
3. Contrast the male pelvis to the female pelvis.
4. Define fracture and state the various types.
5. Analyze, build, spell, and pronounce medical words.
6. Classify the drugs highlighted in this chapter.
7. Describe diagnostic and laboratory tests related to the skeletal system.
8. Identify and define selected abbreviations and acronyms.

Anatomy and Physiology

The human adult skeletal system is composed of 206 bones that, with **cartilage**, **tendons**, and **ligaments**, make up the **framework** or skeleton of the body. The skeleton can be divided into two main groups of bones: the **axial skeleton**, consisting of 80 bones, and the **appendicular skeleton**, with the remaining 126 bones. The principal bones of the axial skeleton are the skull, spine, ribs, and sternum. The shoulder girdle, arms, and hands and the pelvic girdle, legs, and feet are the primary bones of the appendicular skeleton. Table 5.1 provides an at-a-glance look at the skeletal system. See Figure 5.1 for an anterior view of the skeleton.

TABLE 5.1 Skeletal System at-a-Glance

Organ/Structure	Primary Functions/Description
Bones	• Primary organs of the skeletal system, which are composed of water and solid matter • Provide shape, support, and the framework of the body • Provide protection for internal organs • Serve as a storage place for mineral salts, calcium, and phosphorus • Play an important role in the formation of blood cells (**hematopoiesis**) • Provide areas for the attachment of skeletal muscles • Help make movement possible through **articulation** See Figure 5.2.
Cartilage	• Specialized type of fibrous connective tissue found at the ends of bones; forms the major portion of the embryonic skeleton and part of the skeleton in adults
Tendons	• Attach muscles to bones; consist of connective tissue
Ligaments	• Bands of fibrous connective tissue that connect bones, cartilages, and other structures; also serve as places for the attachment of fascia

Bones

The **bones** are the primary organs of the skeletal system; they are composed of approximately 25% water and 75% solid matter. The solid matter in bone is a calcified, rigid substance known as **osseous tissue**. This tissue is a relatively hard and lightweight composite material, formed mostly of calcium phosphate. While bone is essentially brittle, it does have a significant degree of elasticity, contributed chiefly by collagen. All bones consist of living and dead cells embedded in the mineralized organic **matrix** (the intercellular substance of bone) that makes up the osseous tissue.

fyi Bone begins to develop during the second month of fetal life as cartilage cells enlarge, break down, disappear, and are replaced by bone-forming cells called **osteoblasts**. Most bones of the body are formed by this process, known as **endochondral ossification**. In this process, the bone cells deposit organic substances in the spaces vacated by cartilage to form bone matrix. As this process proceeds, blood vessels form within the bone and deposit salts such as calcium phosphate and phosphorus that serve to harden the developing bone. After age 35, both men and women will normally lose 0.3–0.5% of their bone density per year as part of the aging process.

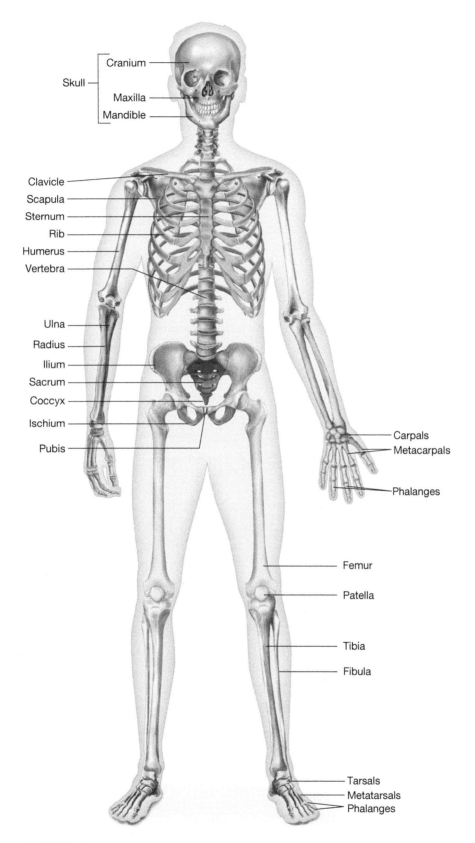

FIGURE 5.1 Anterior view of the human skeleton.

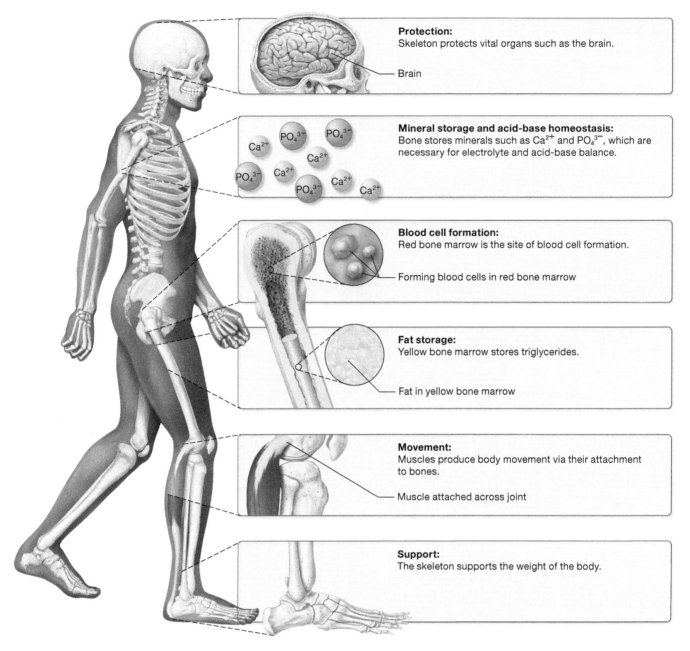

FIGURE 5.2 Functions of the skeletal system.
Source: AMERMAN, ERIN C., HUMAN ANATOMY & PHYSIOLOGY, 2nd Ed., ©2019. Reprinted and Electronically reproduced by permission of Pearson Education, Inc., New York, NY.

Classification of Bones

Bones are classified according to their shapes. See Figure 5.3. Table 5.2 classifies the bones and gives an example of each type.

TABLE 5.2 Classifications of Bone	
Bone	**Example**
Flat	Ribs, scapula (shoulder blade), parts of the pelvic girdle, bones of the skull
Long	Tibia (shin bone), femur (thigh bone), humerus, radius
Short	Carpals, tarsals
Irregular	Vertebrae, ossicles of the ear
Sesamoid	Patella (kneecap)
Sutural or wormian	Between the flat bones of the skull

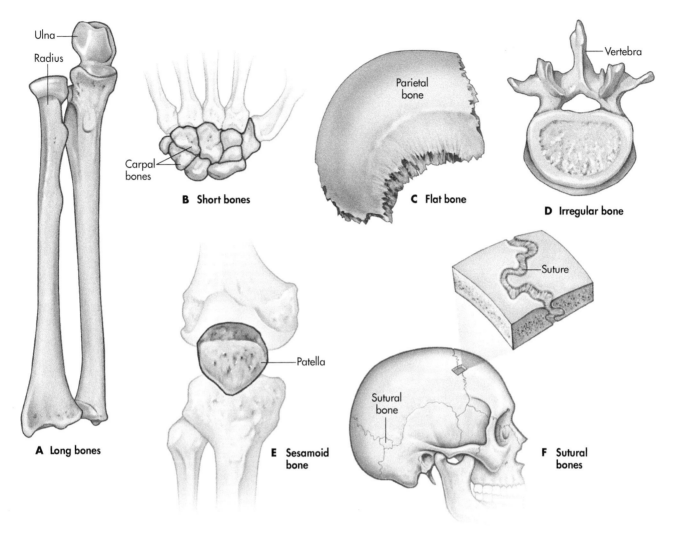

FIGURE 5.3 Classification of bones by shape.

Structure of a Long Bone

Long bones, such as the tibia, femur, humerus, or radius, have most of the features found in all bones. These features are listed here and shown in Figure 5.4.

- **Epiphysis.** The end of a developing bone. (When discussing the two ends of a long bone, the plural form *epiphyses* is used.)

- **Metaphysis.** The narrow portion of a long bone between the epiphysis and the diaphysis. It contains the *epiphyseal plate*, also called the *growth plate*, the part of the bone that grows during childhood, and as it grows it ossifies near the diaphysis and the epiphysis.

- **Diaphysis.** The shaft of a long bone.

- **Periosteum.** A fibrous vascular membrane that forms the covering of bones except at their articular (joint) surfaces.

- **Compact bone.** The dense, hard layer of bone tissue.

- **Medullary canal.** A narrow space or cavity throughout the length of the diaphysis.

- **Endosteum.** A tough, connective tissue membrane lining the medullary canal and containing the bone marrow.

- **Cancellous** or **spongy bone.** The reticular network that makes up most of the volume of bone.

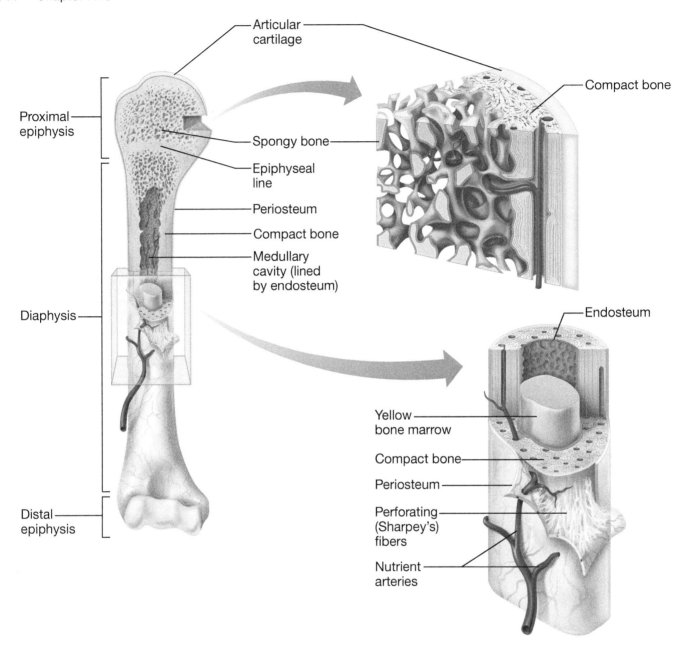

FIGURE 5.4 Features found in a long bone.

Bone Markings

Certain commonly used terms describe the **markings of bones**. These markings are listed and described in Table 5.3 so you can better understand their roles in joining bones together, providing areas for muscle attachments, and serving as a passageway for blood vessels, ligaments, and nerves.

TABLE 5.3 Bone Markings

Marking	Description of the Bone Structure
Condyle	Rounded projection that enters into the formation of a joint, articulation
Crest	Ridge on a bone
Fissure	Slitlike opening between two bones
Foramen	Opening in the bone for blood vessels, ligaments, and nerves
Fossa	Shallow depression in or on a bone
Head	Rounded end of a bone
Meatus	Tubelike passage or canal
Process	Enlargement or protrusion of a bone
Sinus	Air cavity within certain bones
Spine	Pointed, sharp, slender process
Sulcus	Groove, furrow, depression, or fissure
Trochanter	Either of the two bony projections below the neck of the femur
Tubercle	Small, rounded process
Tuberosity	Large, rounded process

fyi The **epiphyseal plate** (also called *physis* or *growth plate*) is a hyaline cartilage plate in the metaphysis at each end of a long bone. See Figure 5.5. In children, this is the center of longitudinal bone growth. The bone growth continues as mitosis is happening in the zone of proliferation, where chondrocytes (cartilage cells) divide. At about 12–15 years of age, the rate of mitosis slows, but the rate of ossification continues. At about age 18–21, the zone of proliferation completely ossifies and at this point, the ends of the long bones (*epiphyses*) knit securely to their shafts (*diaphyses*). Once growth is completed and an individual reaches full maturity and stature, the epiphyseal plate becomes the epiphyseal line.

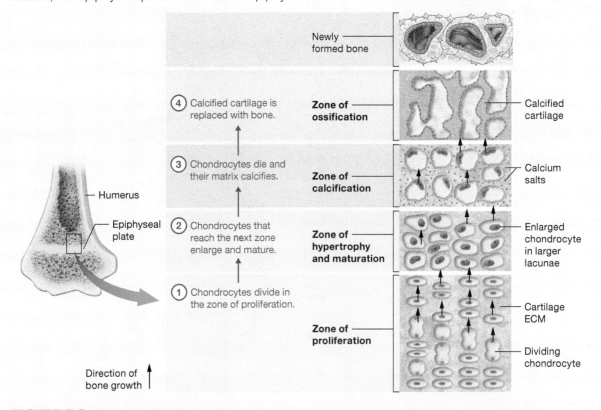

FIGURE 5.5 Bone growth at the epiphyseal plate.

Source: AMERMAN, ERIN C., HUMAN ANATOMY & PHYSIOLOGY, 2nd Ed., ©2019. Reprinted and Electronically reproduced by permission of Pearson Education, Inc., New York, NY.

Joints and Movement

A **joint (jt)** is an articulation, a place where two or more bones connect. Figure 5.6 shows the knee joint. The manner in which bones connect determines the type of movement possible at the joint.

 fyi Various age-related joint changes that occur in the older person are due to diminished viscosity of the synovial fluid, degeneration of collagen and elastin cells, outgrowth of cartilaginous clusters in response to continuous wear and tear, and formation of scar tissues and calcification in the joint capsules.

Classification of Joints

Joints are classified as follows:

- **Synarthrosis (fibrous).** Does not permit movement. The bones are in close contact with each other, but there is no joint cavity. An example is a *cranial suture*.
- **Amphiarthrosis (cartilaginous).** Permits very slight movement. An example of this type of joint is a *vertebra*.
- **Diarthrosis (synovial).** Allows free movement in a variety of directions. A synovial membrane lines the joint and produces synovial fluid, which lubricates the joint. Examples of this type of joint are the *knee, hip, elbow, wrist,* and *foot*.

Joint Movements

The following terms describe types of body movement that occur at the **freely movable joints**. See Figure 5.7.

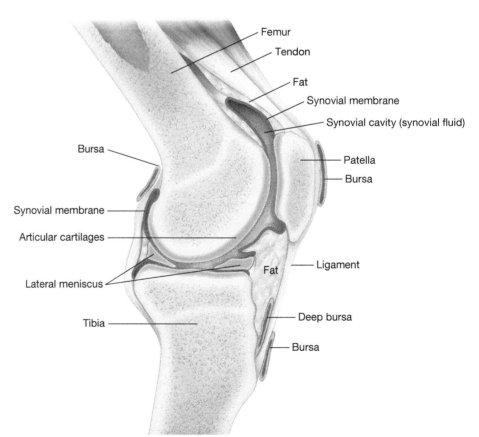

FIGURE 5.6 Knee joint.

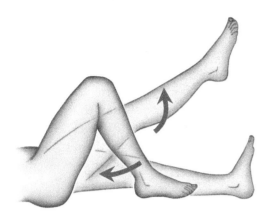

FIGURE 5.7A Flexion and extension
Flexion—Bending a limb.
Extension—Straightening a flexed limb.

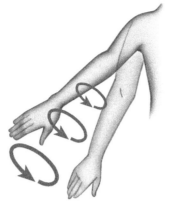

FIGURE 5.7B Circumduction
Circumduction—Moving a body part in a circular motion.

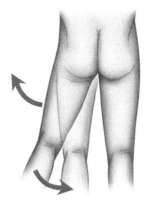

FIGURE 5.7C Abduction and adduction
Abduction—Moving a body part away from the middle.
Adduction—Moving a body part toward the middle.

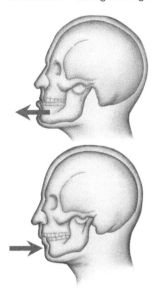

FIGURE 5.7D Protraction and retraction
Protraction—Moving a body part forward.
Retraction—Moving a body part backward.

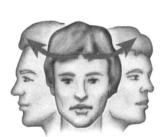

FIGURE 5.7E Rotation
Rotation—Moving a body part around a central axis.

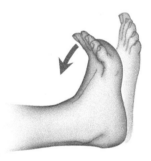

FIGURE 5.7F Dorsiflexion
Dorsiflexion—Bending a body part backward.

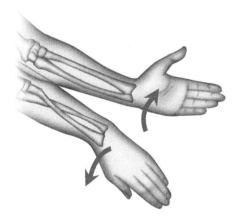

FIGURE 5.7G Pronation and supination
Pronation—Lying prone (face downward); also turning the palm downward.
Supination—Lying supine (face upward); also turning the palm or foot upward.

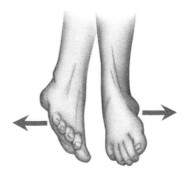

FIGURE 5.7H Eversion and inversion
Eversion—Turning outward.
Inversion—Turning inward.

Vertebral Column

The **vertebral column** is composed of a series of separate bones (**vertebrae**) connected in such a way as to form four spinal curves. These curves have been identified as the cervical, thoracic, lumbar, and sacral. The *cervical curve* consists of the first seven vertebrae, the *thoracic curve* consists of the next 12 vertebrae, the *lumbar curve* consists of the next five vertebrae, and the *sacral curve* consists of the sacrum and coccyx (tailbone). See Figure 5.8.

It is known that a curved structure has more strength than a straight structure. The spinal curves of the human body are most important because they help support the weight of the body and provide the balance that is necessary to walk on two feet.

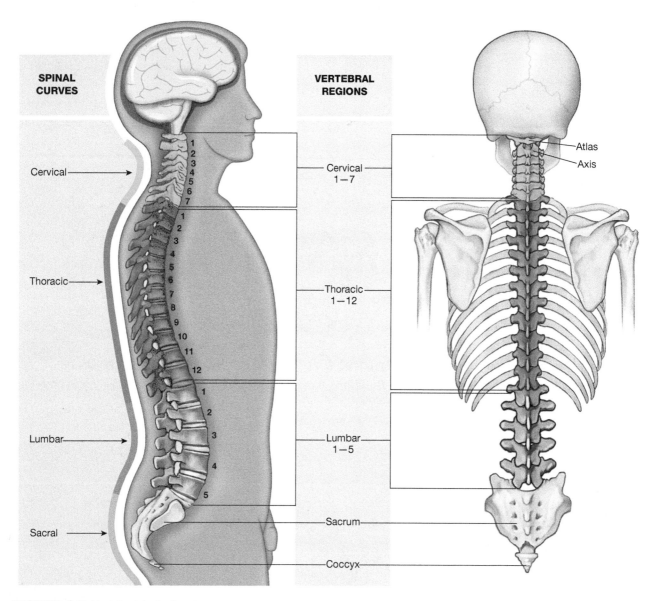

FIGURE 5.8 Vertebral (spinal) column.

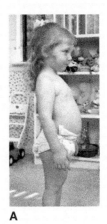 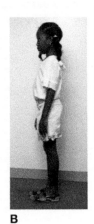

FIGURE 5.9 Normal development of posture and spinal curves. **A** Toddler: Protruding abdomen; lumbar lordosis. **B** School-age child: Height of shoulders and hips is level; balanced thoracic convex and lumbar concave curves.

Source: Pearson Education, Inc.

A   **B**

Anatomical Differences in the Male and Female Pelvis

The **pelvis** is the lower portion of the trunk of the body. It forms a basin bound anteriorly and laterally by the hip bones and posteriorly by the sacrum and coccyx.

The bony pelvis is formed by the sacrum, the coccyx, and the bones that form the hip and pubic arch—the ilium, pubis, and ischium. These bones are separate in the child but become fused in adulthood.

Male Pelvis

The **male pelvis** (android type) is shaped like a *funnel*, forming a narrower outlet than the female. The bones of the android pelvis are generally thick and heavy and more suited for lifting and running. See Figure 5.10A.

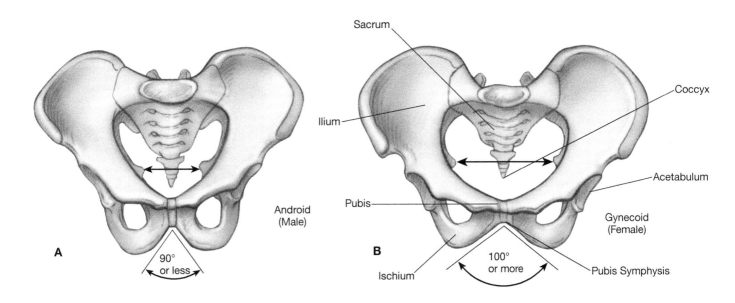

FIGURE 5.10 A The male pelvis (android) is shaped like a funnel, forming a narrower outlet than the female. **B** The female pelvis (gynecoid) is shaped like a basin.

Female Pelvis

The **female pelvis** (gynecoid type) is shaped like a *basin*. It can be oval to round, and it is wider than the male pelvis (Figure 5.10B). Its structure is designed to accommodate the average fetus during pregnancy and to facilitate the downward passage of the fetus through the birth canal during childbirth. The **gynecoid** pelvis is a type of pelvis characteristic of the normal female and is the ideal pelvic type for childbirth.

Fractures

A crack or break in the bone is called a **fracture (Fx)**. A fracture is classified according to its external appearance, the site of the fracture, and the nature of the crack or break in the bone. Many fractures fall into more than one category. For example, depending on the injury, a transverse fracture can also be categorized as a comminuted fracture, which can be either open or closed. Figure 5.11 provides a summary of the types of fractures.

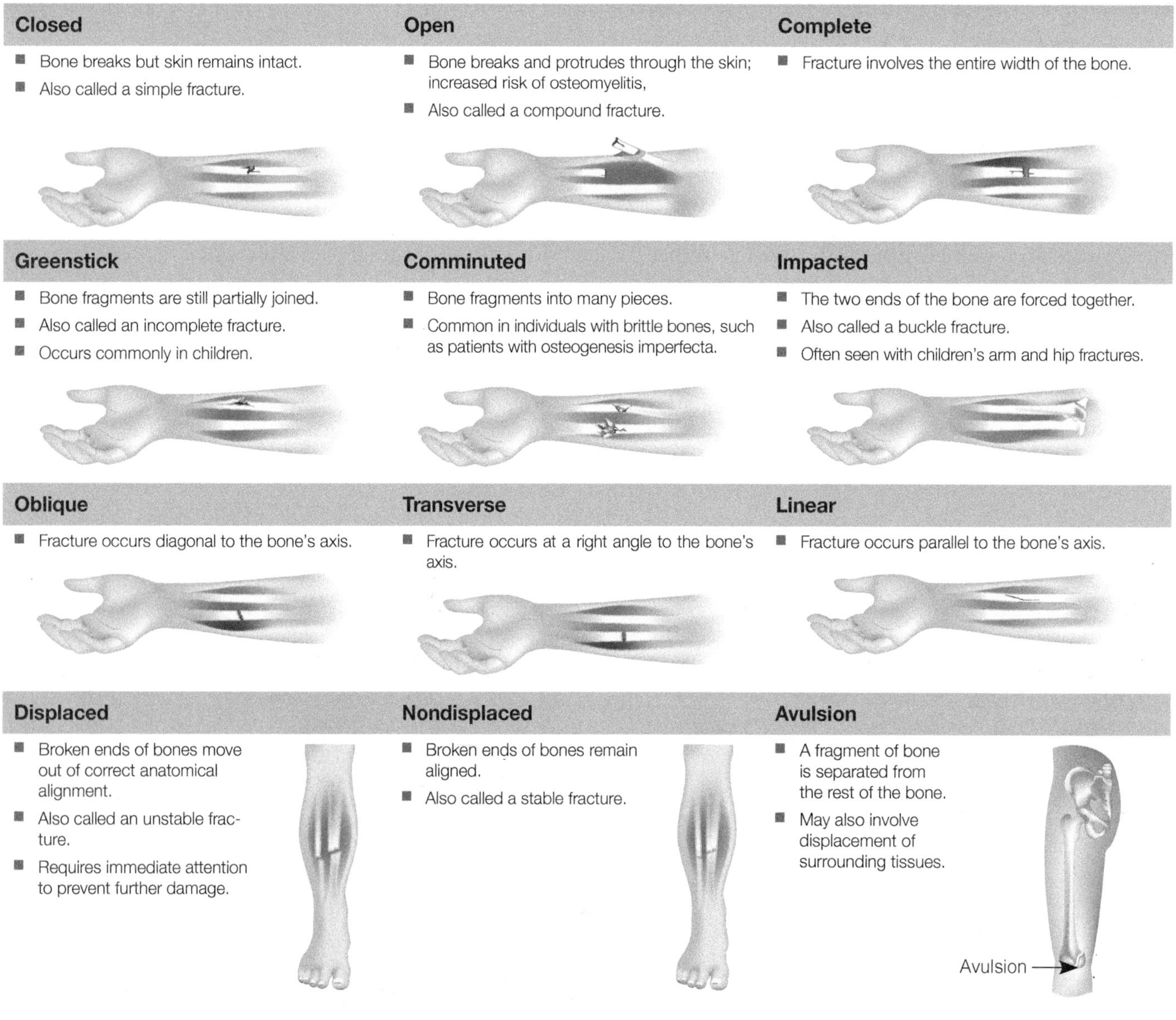
Closed
Bone breaks but skin remains intact.
Also called a simple fracture.
Open
Bone breaks and protrudes through the skin; increased risk of osteomyelitis,
Also called a compound fracture.
Complete
Fracture involves the entire width of the bone.
Greenstick
Bone fragments are still partially joined.
Also called an incomplete fracture.
Occurs commonly in children.
Comminuted
Bone fragments into many pieces.
Common in individuals with brittle bones, such as patients with osteogenesis imperfecta.
Impacted
The two ends of the bone are forced together.
Also called a buckle fracture.
Often seen with children's arm and hip fractures.
Oblique
Fracture occurs diagonal to the bone's axis.
Transverse
Fracture occurs at a right angle to the bone's axis.
Linear
Fracture occurs parallel to the bone's axis.
Displaced
Broken ends of bones move out of correct anatomical alignment.
Also called an unstable fracture.
Requires immediate attention to prevent further damage.
Nondisplaced
Broken ends of bones remain aligned.
Also called a stable fracture.
Avulsion
A fragment of bone is separated from the rest of the bone.
May also involve displacement of surrounding tissues.
Avulsion

FIGURE 5.11 Common fractures.

Source: PEARSON EDUCATION; SERVICES, PEARSON; PEARSON EDUCATION, . ., NURSING: A CONCEPT-BASED APPROACH TO LEARNING, VOLUME I, 1st Ed., ©2019. Reprinted and Electronically reproduced by permission of Pearson Education, Inc., New York, NY.

Stress	Spiral	Depression
■ Caused by small repetitive forces on the bone. ■ Often caused by participation in sports or exercise. 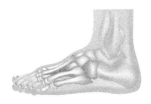	■ Fracture spirals around the bone. ■ Occurs as the result of a twisting force, often during sports. ■ Occurs commonly in children. 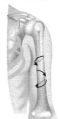	■ Bone is forced inward. ■ Occurs commonly in skull fractures. 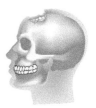

Pathologic	Compression
■ Caused by a disease that weakens the bone such as osteoporosis, bone cancer, and osteogenesis imperfecta. 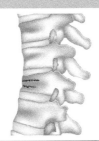	■ Bone is crushed; occurs most commonly in vertebrae. ■ Common in patients with osteoporosis. Compressed 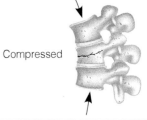

FIGURE 5.11 (*continued*)

Study *and* Review I

Anatomy and Physiology

Write your answers to the following questions.

1. The skeletal system is composed of _____ bones.

2. Name the two main divisions of the skeletal system.

a. _____   b. _____

3. Name five classifications of bone and give an example of each.

a. _____ Example: _____

b. _____ Example: _____

c. _____ Example: _____

d. _____ Example: _____

e. _____ Example: _____

4. State the six main functions of bones.

a. _____   d. _____

b. _____   e. _____

c. _____   f. _____

5. Define the following features of a long bone.

a. Epiphysis _____

b. Metaphysis _____

c. Diaphysis _____

d. Periosteum _____

e. Compact bone _____

f. Medullary canal _____

g. Endosteum _____

h. Cancellous or spongy bone _____

6. Match the term in the left column with its definition from the right. Place the correct letter from the right column in the space provided in the left column.

_____ 1. meatus

_____ 2. head

_____ 3. tuberosity

_____ 4. process

_____ 5. condyle

_____ 6. tubercle

_____ 7. crest

_____ 8. trochanter

_____ 9. sinus

_____ 10. fissure

a. Air cavity within certain bones

b. Enlargement or protrusion of a bone

c. Either of the two bony projections below the neck of the femur

d. Large, rounded process

e. Rounded end of a bone

f. Tubelike passage or canal

g. Slitlike opening between two bones

h. Rounded projection that enters into the formation of a joint, articulation

i. Ridge on a bone

j. Small, rounded process

7. Name the three classifications of joints.

    a. _____   **c.** _____

    b. _____

8. _____ is moving a body part away from the middle.

9. Adduction is _____.

10. _____ is moving a body part in a circular motion.

11. Dorsiflexion is _____.

12. _____ is turning outward.

13. Extension is _____.

14. _____ is bending a limb.

15. Inversion is _____.

16. _____ is lying face downward.

17. Protraction is _____.

18. _____ is moving a body part backward.

19. Rotation is _____.

20. _____ is lying face upward.

▶ **ANATOMY LABELING** Identify the structures shown below by filling in the blanks.

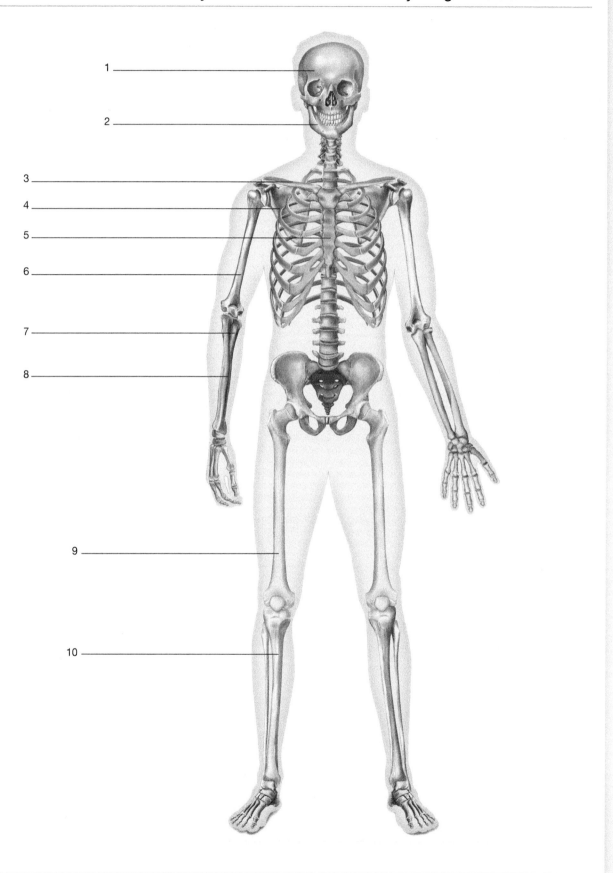

1 _____

2 _____

3 _____

4 _____

5 _____

6 _____

7 _____

8 _____

9 _____

10 _____

Building Your Medical Vocabulary

This section provides the foundation for learning medical terminology. Review the alphabetized list of medical terms in the following pages. Note how common prefixes and suffixes are repeatedly applied to word roots and combining forms to create different meanings. A combining form is a word root plus a vowel. The chart below lists the combining forms and word roots used in this chapter and can help to strengthen your understanding of how medical words are built and spelled.

You will find that some terms have not been divided into word parts. These are common words or specialized terms that are included to enhance your medical vocabulary.

Combining Forms

acetabul/o	acetabulum	menisc/i	crescent-shaped
acr/o	extremity	myel/o	bone marrow
ankyl/o	stiffening, crooked	olecran/o	elbow
arthr/o	joint	orth/o	straight
burs/o	pouch	oste/o	bone
calcan/e	heel bone	patell/o	kneecap
carp/o	wrist	ped/o	foot
chondr/o	cartilage	phalang/e phalang/o	phalanges (finger/toe bones)
clavicul/o	clavicle, collar bone		
coccyg/e coccyg/o	coccyx, tailbone	rad/i	radius
		radi/o	x-ray
coll/a	glue	rheumat/o	discharge
cost/o	rib	sacr/o	sacrum
crani/o	skull	sarc/o	flesh
dactyl/o	finger or toe	scapul/o	shoulder blade
femor/o	femur	scoli/o	curvature
fibul/o	fibula	spin/o	spine
fixat/o	fastened	spondyl/o	vertebra
humer/o	humerus	stern/o	sternum, breastbone
ili/o	ilium	tendin/o tendon/o	tendon
isch/i	ischium, hip		
kyph/o	a hump	tibi/o	tibia
lamin/o	lamina (thin plate)	tract/o	to draw
lord/o	bending, curve, swayback	uln/o	ulna
lumb/o	loin, lower back	vertebr/o	vertebra
mandibul/o	lower jawbone	xiph/o	sword
maxill/o	upper jawbone		

Word Roots

connect	to bind together	**omion**	shoulder
duct	to lead	**phor**	carrying
locat	to place	**phos**	light
maxilla	jaw	**por**	passage

Medical Word	Word Parts		Definition
	Part	**Meaning**	
acetabulum (ăs″ ĕ-tăb′ ū-lŭm)	**acetabul**	acetabulum, hip socket	Cup-shaped socket of the innominate bone (hip bone) into which the head of the femur (thigh bone) fits
	-um	structure, tissue	
achondroplasia (ă-kŏn″ drō-plā′ zhē-ă)	**a-**	without	Defect in the formation of cartilage at the epiphyses of long bones
	chondr/o	cartilage	
	-plasia	formation	
acroarthritis (ăk″ rō-ăr-thrī′ tĭs)	**acr/o**	extremity	Inflammation of the joints of the hands or feet (the extremities)
	arthr	joint	
	-itis	inflammation	
acromion (ă-krō′ mē-ŏn)	**acr**	extremity, point	Projection of the spine of the scapula that forms the point of the shoulder and articulates with the clavicle
	omion	shoulder	
ankylosis (ăng″ kĭ-lō′ sĭs)	**ankyl**	stiffening, crooked	Abnormal condition of stiffening of a joint
	-osis	condition	
arthralgia (ăr-thrăl′ jē-ă)	**arthr**	joint	Joint pain
	-algia	pain	
arthritis (ăr-thrī′ tĭs)	**arthr**	joint	Inflammation of a joint that can result from various disease processes, such as injury to a joint (including fracture), an attack on the joints by the body itself (caused by an auto-immune disease, such as rheumatoid arthritis), or general wear and tear on joints (osteoarthritis)
	-itis	inflammation	

fyi No matter the type of arthritis one has, the main symptoms are pain, swelling, and stiffness in the affected joint. Over time, the joint can become so stiff that movement is difficult or even impossible.

Total joint arthroplasty (TJA) is a surgical procedure in which parts of an arthritic or damaged joint are removed and replaced with a metal, plastic, or ceramic device called a *prosthesis*. The prosthesis is designed to replicate the movement of a normal, healthy joint.

More than 1 million total joint replacements are performed in the United States annually and that number is expected to increase to 4 million by 2030. Hip and knee replacements are the most commonly performed joint replacements, but replacement surgery can be performed on other joints, including the ankle, wrist, fingers, shoulder, and elbow.

Medical Word	Word Parts		Definition
	Part	Meaning	
arthrocentesis (ăr˝ thrō-sĕn-tē´ sĭs)	arthr/o -centesis	joint surgical puncture	Surgical procedure to remove joint fluid; may be used as a diagnostic tool or as part of a treatment regimen
arthrodesis (ăr˝ thrō-dē´ sĭs)	arthr/o -desis	joint binding	Surgical fusion of a joint
arthroplasty (ăr˝ thrō-plăs´ tē)	arthr/o -plasty	joint surgical repair	Surgical procedure used to repair a joint
arthroscope (ăr´ thrō-scōp)	arthr/o -scope	joint instrument for examining	Surgical instrument used to examine the interior of a joint
bone marrow transplant			Surgical procedure used to transfer bone marrow from a donor to a patient
bursa (bŭr´ să)			Padlike sac between muscles, tendons, and bones that is lined with synovial membrane and contains a fluid called synovia

! ALERT!

To change *bursa* to its plural form, you change the *a* to *ae* to create *bursae*.

bursitis (bŭr-sī´ tĭs)	burs -itis	pouch inflammation	Inflammation of a bursa
calcaneal (kăl-kā´ nē-ăl)	calcan/e -al	heel bone pertaining to	Pertaining to the heel bone
calcium (Ca) (kăl´ sē-ŭm)			Mineral that is essential for bone growth, teeth development, blood coagulation, and many other functions
carpal (kăr´ păl)	carp -al	wrist pertaining to	Pertaining to the wrist bones; there are two rows of four bones in the wrist for a total of eight wrist bones

Medical Word	Word Parts		Definition
	Part	Meaning	
carpal tunnel syndrome			Abnormal condition caused by compression of the median nerve by the carpal ligament due to injury or trauma to the area, including repetitive movement of the wrists; symptoms: soreness, tenderness, weakness, pain, tingling, and numbness at the wrist. See Figure 5.12.

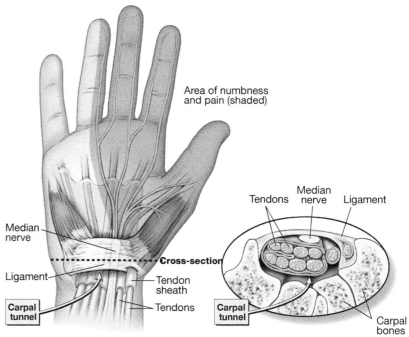

FIGURE 5.12 Cross-section of wrist showing tendons and nerves involved in carpal tunnel syndrome.

cast			Type of material made of plaster of Paris, fiberglass, sodium silicate, starch, or dextrin used to immobilize a fractured bone, a dislocation, a deformity, or a sprain. See Figure 5.13.

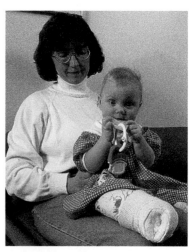

FIGURE 5.13 This girl has a long leg cast, which was applied after surgery to correct her clubfoot.
Source: Pearson Education, Inc.

Medical Word	Word Parts		Definition
	Part	Meaning	
chondral (kŏn´ drăl)	chondr -al	cartilage pertaining to	Pertaining to cartilage
chondrocostal (kŏn˝ drō-kŏs´ tăl)	chondr/o cost -al	cartilage rib pertaining to	Pertaining to the rib cartilage
clavicular (klă-vĭk´ ū-lăr)	clavicul -ar	clavicle, collar bone pertaining to	Pertaining to the clavicle (collar bone)
coccygeal (kŏk-sĭj´ ē-ăl)	coccyg/e -al	coccyx, tailbone pertaining to	Pertaining to the coccyx (tailbone)
coccygodynia (kŏk-sĭ-gō-dĭn´ ē-ă)	coccyg/o -dynia	coccyx, tailbone pain	Pain in the coccyx (tailbone)
collagen (kŏl´ ă-jĕn)	coll/a -gen	glue formation, produce	Fibrous insoluble protein found in the connective tissue, skin, ligaments, and cartilage
connective	connect -ive	to bind together nature of	Literally means the nature of connecting or binding together
costosternal (kŏs˝ tō-stĕr´ năl)	cost/o stern -al	rib sternum pertaining to	Pertaining to rib and sternum
craniectomy (krā˝ nē-ĕk´ tŏ-mē)	crani -ectomy	skull surgical excision	Surgical excision of a portion of the skull
craniotomy (krā˝ nē-ŏt´ ō-mē)	crani/o -tomy	skull incision	Surgical incision made into the skull

! ALERT!

The word parts **crani** and **crani/o** build different terms by using the suffixes **-ectomy** (*surgical excision*) and **-tomy** (*incision*).

dactylic (dăk-tĭl´ ĭk)	dactyl -ic	finger or toe pertaining to	Pertaining to a finger or toe
dactylogram (dăk-tĭl´ə grăm)	dactyl/o -gram	finger or toe mark, record	Medical term for fingerprint
dislocation (dĭs˝ lō-kā´ shŭn)	dis- locat -ion	apart to place process	Displacement of a bone from a joint

Medical Word	Word Parts		Definition
	Part	Meaning	
femoral (fĕm´ ŏr-ăl)	**femor** **-al**	femur pertaining to	Pertaining to the femur; the *thigh bone*, the longest bone in the body
fibular (fĭb´ ū-lăr)	**fibul** **-ar**	fibula pertaining to	Pertaining to the fibula; the smaller of the two lower leg bones
fixation (fĭks-ā´ shŭn)	**fixat** **-ion**	fastened process	Process of holding or fastening in a fixed position; making rigid, immobilizing
flatfoot			Abnormal flatness of the sole and arch of the foot; also known as *pes planus*
genu valgum (jē´ nū văl gŭm)			Medical term for knock-knee. See Figure 5.14A.

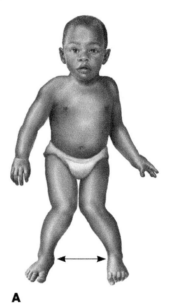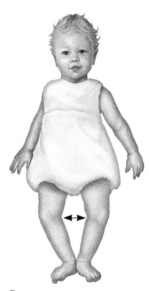

FIGURE 5.14 A Genu valgum, or knock-knee. Note that the ankles are far apart when the knees are together. **B** Genu varum, or bowleg. The legs are bowed so that the knees are far apart as the child stands.

A   **B**

genu varum (jē´ nū vā´ rŭm)			Medical term for bowleg. See Figure 5.14B.
gout (gowt)			Hereditary metabolic disease that is a form of acute arthritis, which is marked by joint inflammation. It is caused by hyperuricemia, excessive amounts of uric acid in the blood, and deposits of urates of sodium (uric acid crystals) in and around the joints. It usually affects the great toe first, but can be seen in the finger, knee, or foot joints.
hallux (hăl´ ŭks)			Medical term for the big or great toe

Medical Word	Word Parts		Definition
	Part	Meaning	
hammertoe (hăm´ er-tō)			An acquired flexion deformity of the interphalangeal joint. See Figure 5.15.

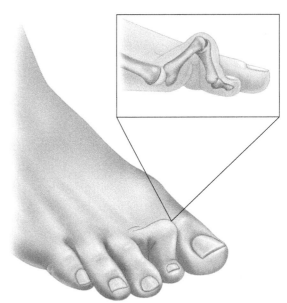

FIGURE 5.15 Hammertoe.

Medical Word	Word Parts		Definition
humeral (hū´ mĕr-ăl)	humer -al	humerus pertaining to	Pertaining to the humerus (*upper arm bone*)
hydrarthrosis (hī˝ drăr-thrō´ sĭs)	hydr- arthr -osis	water joint condition	An abnormal condition in which there is an accumulation of watery fluid in the cavity of a joint
iliac (ĭl´ ē-ăk)	ili -ac	ilium pertaining to	Pertaining to the ilium
iliosacral (ĭl˝ ē-ō-sā´ krăl)	ili/o sacr -al	ilium sacrum pertaining to	Pertaining to the ilium and the sacrum
intercostal (ĭn˝ tĕr-kŏs´ tăl)	inter- cost -al	between rib pertaining to	Pertaining to the space between two ribs
ischial (ĭs´ kē-al)	isch/i -al	ischium, hip pertaining to	Pertaining to the ischium, hip

Medical Word	Word Parts		Definition
	Part	Meaning	
ischialgia (ĭs″ kē-ăl′ jē-ă)	isch/i -algia	ischium, hip pain	Pain in the ischium, hip
kyphosis (kī-fō′ sĭs)	kyph -osis	hump condition	Condition in which the normal thoracic curvature becomes exaggerated, producing a "humpback" appearance. It can be caused by a congenital defect, a disease process such as tuberculosis and/or syphilis, malignancy, compression fracture, faulty posture, osteoarthritis, rheumatoid arthritis, rickets, osteoporosis, or other conditions. See Figure 5.16A.

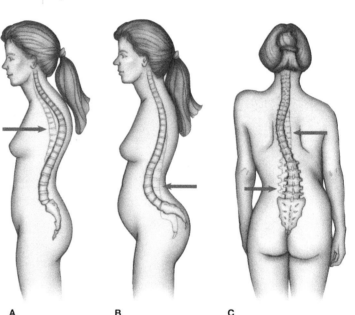

FIGURE 5.16 Abnormal curvatures of the spine: **A** kyphosis, **B** lordosis, and **C** scoliosis.

laminectomy (lăm″ ĭ-nĕk′ tō-mē)	lamin -ectomy	lamina (thin plate) surgical excision	Surgical excision of a vertebral posterior arch
lordosis (lor-dō′ sĭs)	lord -osis	bending, curve, swayback condition	An abnormal anterior curvature of the lumbar spine. This condition can be referred to as *swayback* because the abdomen and buttocks protrude due to an exaggerated lumbar curvature. See Figure 5.16B.
lumbar (lŭm′ băr)	lumb -ar	loin, lower back pertaining to	Pertaining to the loins (lower back)
lumbodynia (lŭm″ bō-dĭn′ ē-ă)	lumb/o -dynia	loin, lower back pain	Pain in the loins (lower back)

Medical Word	Word Parts		Definition
	Part	Meaning	
mandibular (măn-dĭb´ ū-lăr)	mandibul -ar	lower jawbone pertaining to	Pertaining to the lower jawbone
maxillary (măk´ sĭ-lĕr˝ ē)	maxill -ary	upper jawbone pertaining to	Pertaining to the upper jawbone
meniscus (měn-ĭs´ kŭs)	menisc -us	crescent-shaped structure	Crescent-shaped interarticular fibrocartilaginous structure found in certain joints, especially the lateral and medial *menisci* (semilunar cartilages) of the knee joint
metacarpals (mĕt˝ ă-kar´ păls)	meta- carp -al	beyond wrist pertaining to	Pertaining to the bones of the hand. There are five radiating bones in the fingers. *Note:* The bones of the foot are the *metatarsals*.
metacarpectomy (mĕt˝ ă-kăr-pĕk´ tō-mē)	meta- carp -ectomy	beyond wrist surgical excision	Surgical excision of one or more bones of the hand
myelitis (mī-ĕ-lī´ tĭs)	myel -itis	bone marrow inflammation	Inflammation of the bone marrow
myeloma (mī-ĕ-lō´ mă)	myel -oma	bone marrow tumor	Tumor of the bone marrow
myelopoiesis (mī˝ ĕl-ō-poy-ē´ sĭs)	myel/o -poiesis	bone marrow formation	Formation of bone marrow
olecranal (ō-lĕk´ răn-ăl)	olecran -al	elbow pertaining to	Pertaining to the elbow
orthopedics (Orth, ortho) (or˝ thō-pē´ dĭks)	orth/o ped -ic	straight foot pertaining to	Diseases and disorders involving locomotor structures of the body
orthopedist (or˝ thō-pē´ dĭst)	orth/o ped -ist	straight foot one who specializes	One who specializes in diseases and disorders involving locomotor structures of the body
osteoarthritis (OA) (ŏs˝ tē-ō-ăr-thrī´ tĭs)	oste/o arthr -itis	bone joint inflammation	Inflammation of the bone and joint; the most common type of arthritis in the United States in people over 50 years of age. It is often called *wear-and-tear disease* because the cartilage that cushions a joint wears away as one ages, so that bone rubs against bone.

Medical Word	Word Parts		Definition
	Part	Meaning	
osteoblast (ŏs´ tē-ō-blăst″)	**oste/o** **-blast**	bone immature cell, germ cell	Bone-forming cell
osteochondritis (ŏs″ tē-ō-kŏn-drī´ tĭs)	**oste/o** **chondr** **-itis**	bone cartilage inflammation	Inflammation of bone and cartilage
osteogenesis (ŏs″ tē-ō-jĕn´ ĕ-sĭs)	**oste/o** **-genesis**	bone formation	Formation of bone
osteomalacia (ŏs″ tē-ō-mă-lā´ shē-ă)	**oste/o** **-malacia**	bone softening	Softening of bones
osteomyelitis (ŏs″ tē-ō-mī″ ĕ-lī´ tĭs)	**oste/o** **myel** **-itis**	bone bone marrow inflammation	Inflammation of bone, especially the marrow, caused by a pathogenic organism. See Figure 5.17. *Note:* Frontal osteomyelitis is a rare complication of sinusitis. Common intracranial complications of frontal osteomyelitis are meningitis, epidural empyema, subdural empyema, and brain abscess caused by *Staphylococcus aureus*.

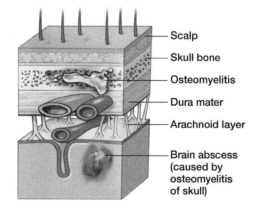 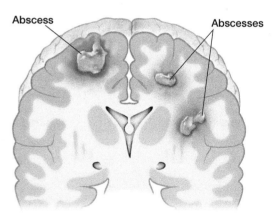

FIGURE 5.17 Abscess of the brain due to osteomyelitis.

Scalp
Skull bone
Osteomyelitis
Dura mater
Arachnoid layer
Brain abscess (caused by osteomyelitis of skull)

Abscess
Abscesses

Medical Word	Word Parts		Definition
osteopenia (ŏs″ tē-ō-pē´ nē-ă)	**oste/o** **-penia**	bone deficiency	Deficiency of bone tissue, regardless of the cause
osteoporosis (ŏs″ tē-ō-por-ō´ sĭs)	**oste/o** **por** **-osis**	bone passage condition	Abnormal condition characterized by a decrease in the density of bones, decreasing their strength and causing fragile bones, which can result in fractures. It is most common in women after menopause, when it is called *postmenopausal osteoporosis*, but may also develop in men. See Figure 5.18.

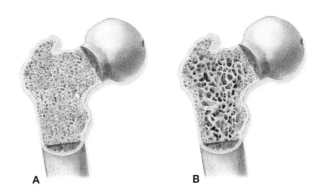

FIGURE 5.18 A Normal spongy bone. **B** Spongy bone with osteoporosis, which is characterized by a loss of bone density.

fyi With normal aging, individuals can lose 1.0–1.5 inches in height. Loss of more than 1.5 inches in height can be related to vertebral compression fractures and other issues due to osteoporosis. See Figure 5.19.

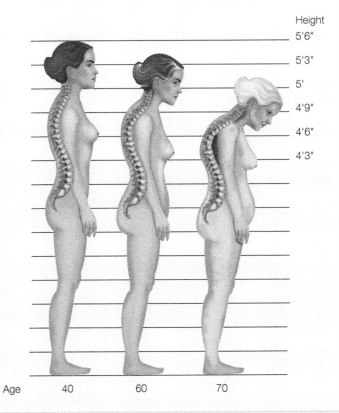

FIGURE 5.19 Spinal changes caused by osteoporosis.
Source: PEARSON EDUCATION; SERVICES, PEARSON; PEARSON EDUCATION, . ., NURSING: A CONCEPT-BASED APPROACH TO LEARNING, VOLUME I, 1st Ed., ©2019. Reprinted and Electronically reproduced by permission of Pearson Education, Inc., New York, NY.

Medical Word	Word Parts		Definition
	Part	**Meaning**	
osteosarcoma (ŏs″ tē-ō-săr-kō′ mă)	**oste/o** **sarc** **-oma**	bone flesh tumor	Malignant tumor of the bone; cancer growing from cells of "fleshy" connective tissue such as bone or muscle
osteotome (ŏs′ tē-ō-tōm)	**oste/o** **-tome**	bone instrument to cut	Surgical instrument used for cutting bone
patellar (pă-těl′ ăr)	**patell** **-ar**	kneecap pertaining to	Pertaining to the patella, the *kneecap*
pedal (pěd′ ăl)	**ped** **-al**	foot pertaining to	Pertaining to the foot
phalangeal (fă-lăn′ jē-ăl)	**phalang/e** **-al**	phalanges (finger/ toe bones) pertaining to	Pertaining to the bones of the fingers and the toes
phosphorus (P) (fŏs′ fă-rŭs)	**phos** **phor** **-us**	light carrying pertaining to	Mineral that is essential in bone formation, muscle contraction, and many other functions
polyarthritis (pŏl″ ē-ăr-thrī′ tĭs)	**poly-** **arthr** **-itis**	many, much joint inflammation	Inflammation of more than one joint
radial (rā′ dē-ăl)	**rad/i** **-al**	radius pertaining to	Pertaining to the radius (lateral lower arm bone in line with the thumb). A radial pulse can be found on the thumb side of the arm.
radiograph (rā′ dē-ō-grăf)	**radi/o** **-graph**	x-ray record	Film or record on which an x-ray image is produced
reduction (rē-dŭk′ shŭn)	**re-** **duct** **-ion**	back to lead process	Manipulative or surgical procedure used to correct a fracture or hernia

Medical Word	Word Parts		Definition
	Part	Meaning	
rheumatoid arthritis (RA) (roo´ mă-toyd ăr-thrī´ tĭs)	rheumat -oid arthr -itis	discharge resemble joint inflammation	Chronic autoimmune disease characterized by inflammation of the joints, stiffness, pain, and swelling, which results in crippling deformities. See Figure 5.20.

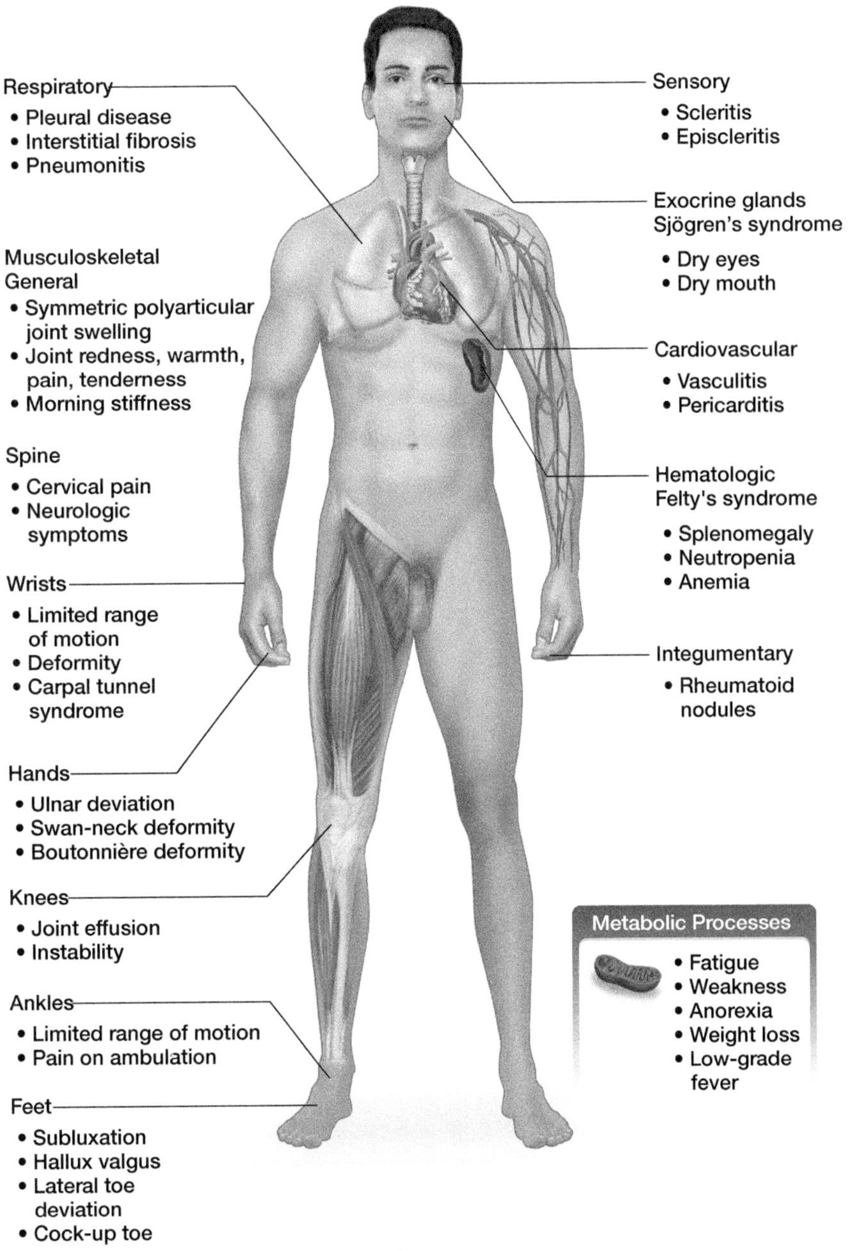

Respiratory
• Pleural disease
• Interstitial fibrosis
• Pneumonitis

Musculoskeletal
General
• Symmetric polyarticular joint swelling
• Joint redness, warmth, pain, tenderness
• Morning stiffness

Spine
• Cervical pain
• Neurologic symptoms

Wrists
• Limited range of motion
• Deformity
• Carpal tunnel syndrome

Hands
• Ulnar deviation
• Swan-neck deformity
• Boutonnière deformity

Knees
• Joint effusion
• Instability

Ankles
• Limited range of motion
• Pain on ambulation

Feet
• Subluxation
• Hallux valgus
• Lateral toe deviation
• Cock-up toe

Sensory
• Scleritis
• Episcleritis

Exocrine glands
Sjögren's syndrome
• Dry eyes
• Dry mouth

Cardiovascular
• Vasculitis
• Pericarditis

Hematologic
Felty's syndrome
• Splenomegaly
• Neutropenia
• Anemia

Integumentary
• Rheumatoid nodules

Metabolic Processes
• Fatigue
• Weakness
• Anorexia
• Weight loss
• Low-grade fever

FIGURE 5.20 Multisystem effects of rheumatoid arthritis.

Medical Word	Word Parts		Definition
	Part	**Meaning**	
rickets (rĭk´ ĕts)			Abnormal condition that can occur in children; caused by a lack of vitamin D
scapular (skăp´ ū-lăr)	**scapul** **-ar**	shoulder blade pertaining to	Pertaining to the shoulder blade
scoliosis (skō˝ lē-ō´ sĭs)	**scoli** **-osis**	curvature condition	An abnormal lateral curvature of the spine. The characteristic signs include asymmetry of the trunk, uneven shoulders and hips, a one-sided rib hump, and a prominent scapula. See Figure 5.21 and refer to Figure 5.16C.

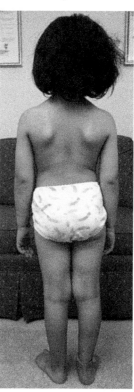

FIGURE 5.21 Does this child have legs of different lengths or scoliosis? Look at the level of the iliac crests and shoulders to see if they are level. See the more prominent crease at the waist on the right side? This child could have scoliosis.
Source: Pearson Education, Inc.

spinal (spī´ năl)	**spin** **-al**	spine pertaining to	Pertaining to the spine
splint			Appliance used for fixation, support, and rest of an injured body part

Medical Word	Word Parts		Definition
	Part	Meaning	
spondylodesis (spŏn″ dĭ-lō-dĕ′ sĭs)	spondyl/o -desis	vertebra binding	Surgery performed to permanently connect two or more vertebrae in the spine, eliminating motion between them. It involves techniques designed to mimic the normal healing process of broken bones. The surgeon places bone or a bonelike material within the space between two spinal vertebrae. Metal plates, screws, and rods may be used to hold the vertebrae together (binding), so they can heal into one solid unit. Also known as *spinal fusion* and *spondylo-syn*desis (**syn-** [P]), meaning *together*.

! ALERT!

To change *vertebra* to its plural form, you change the *a* to *ae* to create *vertebrae*.

Medical Word	Word Parts		Definition
sprain			A traumatic injury to the tendons, muscles, or ligaments around a joint characterized by pain, swelling, and discoloration
spur			Sharp or pointed projection, as on a bone
sternal (stĕr′ năl)	stern -al	sternum, breastbone pertaining to	Pertaining to the sternum, the *breastbone*
sternotomy (stĕr-nŏt′ ō-mē)	stern/o -tomy	sternum, breastbone incision	Surgical incision of the sternum, the *breastbone*
subclavicular (sŭb″ klă-vĭk′ ū-lăr)	sub- clavicul -ar	under, beneath clavicle, collar bone pertaining to	Pertaining to beneath the clavicle (*collar bone*)
subcostal (sŭb-kŏs′ tăl)	sub- cost -al	under, beneath rib pertaining to	Pertaining to beneath the ribs
submaxilla (sŭb″ măk-sĭl′ ă)	sub- maxilla	under, beneath jaw	Below the jaw or mandible
symphysis (sĭm′ fĭ-sĭs)	sym- -physis	together growth	Literally means *growing together*; a joint in which adjacent bony surfaces are firmly united by fibrocartilage. An example is the *symphysis pubis*, where the bones of the pelvis have grown together.
tendinitis (tĕn″ dĭn-ī′ tĭs)	tendin -itis	tendon inflammation	Inflammation of a tendon

Medical Word	Word Parts		Definition
	Part	**Meaning**	
tennis elbow			Chronic condition characterized by elbow pain caused by excessive pronation and supination activities of the forearm; usually caused by strain, as in playing tennis

> **fyi** The medical term used to denote tennis elbow is *lateral humeral epicondylitis*. Epi/condyl/itis is divided into **epi-** (*upon*) + **condyl** (*knuckle*) + **-itis** (*inflammation*). A "knuckle" is a rounded protuberance formed by the bones in a joint.

Medical Word	Word Parts		Definition
	Part	**Meaning**	
tibial (tĭb´ ē-ăl)	**tibi**	tibia	Pertaining to the tibia; the *shin bone*. Larger of the two bones of the lower leg.
	-al	pertaining to	
traction (Tx) (trăk´ shŭn)	**tract**	to draw	Process of drawing or pulling on bones or muscles to relieve displacement and facilitate healing. See Figure 5.22.
	-ion	process	

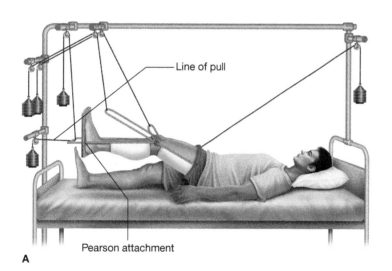
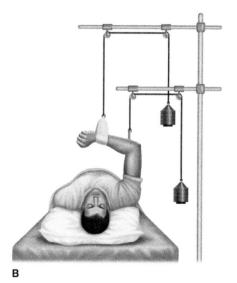

Line of pull

Pearson attachment

A

B

FIGURE 5.22 Traction is the application of a pulling force to maintain bone alignment during fracture healing. Different fractures require different types of traction. **A** Balanced suspension traction is commonly used for fractures of the femur. **B** Skeletal traction, in which the pulling force is applied directly to the bone, may be used to treat fractures of the humerus.

Medical Word	Word Parts		Definition
ulnar (ŭl´ năr)	**uln**	ulna	Pertaining to the ulna (the longer bone of the forearm between the wrist and elbow) or to the nerve or artery named from it. The ulna is located on the little-finger side of the arm.
	-ar	pertaining to	
ulnocarpal (ŭl´ nō-kăr´ păl)	**uln/o**	ulna	Pertaining to the ulna side of the wrist
	carp	wrist	
	-al	pertaining to	

Medical Word	Word Parts		Definition
	Part	Meaning	
vertebral (věr´ tě-brăl)	**vertebr** **-al**	vertebra pertaining to	Pertaining to a vertebra (any of the small bones linked together to form the backbone)
xiphoid (zīf´ oyd)	**xiph** **-oid**	sword resemble	Literally means *resembling a sword*. The xiphoid process is the lowest portion of the sternum; a sword-shaped cartilaginous process supported by bone.

Study *and* Review II

Word Parts

Prefixes   Give the definitions of the following prefixes.

1. a- _____

2. dis- _____

3. hydr- _____

4. inter- _____

5. meta- _____

6. poly- _____

7. sub- _____

8. sym- _____

9. re- _____

Combining Forms   Give the definitions of the following combining forms.

1. acr/o _____

2. ankyl/o _____

3. arthr/o _____

4. burs/o _____

5. calcan/e _____

6. carp/o _____

7. chondr/o _____

8. coccyg/o _____

9. cost/o _____

10. crani/o _____

11. dactyl/o _____

12. isch/i _____

13. kyph/o _____

14. lord/o _____

15. lumb/o _____

16. oste/o _____

17. patell/o _____

18. ped/o _____

19. sacr/o _____

20. scoli/o _____

21. spin/o _____

22. stern/o _____

23. uln/o _____

24. xiph/o _____

Suffixes   Give the definitions of the following suffixes.

1. -ac _____

2. -al _____

3. -algia _____

4. -ar _____

5. -ary _____

6. -blast _____

7. -centesis _____

8. -ion _____

9. -dynia _____

10. -ectomy _____

11. -edema _____

12. -gen _____

13. -genesis _____

14. -gram _____

15. -graph _____

16. -ic _____

17. -itis _____

18. -ive _____

19. -scope _____

20. -malacia _____

21. -us _____

22. -oid _____

23. -oma _____

24. -osis _____

25. -penia _____

26. -physis _____

27. -plasia _____

28. -plasty _____

29. -poiesis _____

30. -tome _____

31. -tomy _____

32. -um _____

Identifying Medical Terms

In the spaces provided, write the medical terms for the following meanings.

1. _____ Inflammation of the joints of the hands or feet

2. _____ Abnormal condition of stiffening of a joint

3. _____ Inflammation of a joint

4. _____ Pertaining to the heel bone

5. _____ Pertaining to cartilage

6. _____ Pain in the coccyx

7. _____ Pertaining to the rib cartilage

8. _____ Surgical excision of a portion of the skull

9. _____ Pertaining to a finger or toe

10. _____ Surgical instrument used for cutting bone

Matching

Select the appropriate lettered meaning for each of the following words.

_____ 1. arthroscope

_____ 2. carpal tunnel syndrome

_____ 3. fixation

_____ 4. gout

_____ 5. hammertoe

_____ 6. kyphosis

_____ 7. metacarpal

_____ 8. rickets

_____ 9. tennis elbow

_____ 10. ulnar

a. Abnormal condition that can occur in children and is caused by a lack of vitamin D

b. An acquired flexion deformity of the interphalangeal joint

c. Hereditary metabolic disease that is a form of acute arthritis

d. Chronic condition characterized by elbow pain that is caused by excessive pronation and supination activities of the forearm

e. Making rigid, immobilizing

f. Pertaining to the ulna (long bone of the forearm between the wrist and elbow) or to the nerve or artery named for it

g. Pertaining to the bones of the hand

h. In this condition, the normal thoracic curvature becomes exaggerated, producing a "humpback" appearance

i. Surgical instrument used to examine the interior of a joint

j. Abnormal condition caused by compression of the median nerve by the carpal ligament

Medical Case Snapshots

This learning activity provides an opportunity to relate the medical terminology you are learning to sample patient case presentations. In the spaces provided, write in your answers.

Case 1

A 66-year-old female is scheduled for a dual-energy x-ray absorptiometry (DXA) scan, to measure her bone mineral density. She is diagnosed with osteoarthritis. The results of her test show _____ (deficiency of bone tissue) and _____ (which is characterized by a decrease in bone density).

Case 2

A 4-year-old female is seen by an orthopedic specialist. Upon physical examination, an abnormal lateral curvature of the spine, known as _____, was noted. The characteristic signs of this condition include _____ of the trunk, uneven shoulders and hips, a one-sided rib hump, and a prominent _____.

Case 3

Upon a return visit to her physician, Ms. Anita Sinclair presented with symptoms of inflammation of the joints, stiffness, pain, and swelling, especially of both hands. This condition is referred to as _____ _____ (RA). The multisystem effects of this condition are varied. Refer to Figure 5.20.

Drug Highlights

Classification of Drug	Description and Examples
anti-inflammatory agents	Relieve the swelling, tenderness, redness, and pain of inflammation. Such agents can be classified as steroidal (corticosteroids) and nonsteroidal.
corticosteroids (glucocorticoids)	Steroid substances that have potent anti-inflammatory effects in disorders of many organ systems. Steroids have an array of serious side effects that may be caused by long-term use. EXAMPLES: Depo-Medrol (methylprednisolone acetate) and prednisone
nonsteroidal anti-inflammatory drugs (NSAIDs)	Agents used in the treatment of arthritis and related disorders EXAMPLES: Bayer aspirin (acetylsalicylic acid), Motrin IB (ibuprofen), Feldene (piroxicam), ketoprofen, and Naprosyn (naproxen)

(continued)

Classification of Drug	Description and Examples
disease-modifying antirheumatic drugs (DMARDs)	Can influence the course of the disease progression; therefore, their introduction in early rheumatoid arthritis is recommended to limit irreversible joint damage. EXAMPLES: gold preparation Ridaura (auranofin); antimalarial Plaquenil (hydroxychloroquine sulfate); a chelating agent Cuprimine (penicillamine); and the immunosuppressants Trexall (methotrexate sodium), Imuran (azathioprine), and Cytoxan (cyclophosphamide)
COX-2 inhibitors	Cyclooxygenase (COX) is an enzyme involved in many aspects of normal cellular function and in the inflammatory response. COX-2 is found in joints and other areas affected by inflammation as occurs with osteoarthritis and rheumatoid arthritis. Inhibition of COX-2 reduces the production of compounds associated with inflammation and pain. EXAMPLES: Celebrex (celecoxib) and Mobic (meloxicam)
biologics	Include a wide range of medicinal products such as vaccines, blood and blood components, and drugs made from recombinant DNA technology. EXAMPLES: Humira (adalimumab), Enbrel (etanercept), Remicade (infliximab), and Orencia (abatacept)
agents used to treat gout	Acute attacks of gout are treated with colchicine. Once the acute attack of gout has been controlled, drug therapy to control hyperuricemia can be initiated. EXAMPLES: Zyloprim (allopurinol) and probenecid
agents used to treat or prevent postmenopausal osteoporosis	
antiresorptive agents	Antiresorptive agents decrease the removal of calcium from bones. *Fosamax* reduces the activity of the cells that cause bone loss and increases the amount of bone in most patients. *Actonel* inhibits osteoclast-mediated bone resorption and modulates bone metabolism. To receive the clinical benefits of either of these drugs, the patient must be informed and follow the prescribed drug regimen. EXAMPLES: Fosamax (alendronate), Actonel (risedronate), Evista (raloxifene), Boniva (ibandronate), Reclast (zoledronate), and calcitonin
estrogen hormone therapy (EHT)	After menopause, EHT has been shown to prevent bone loss, increase bone density, and prevent bone fractures. It is useful in preventing osteoporosis in postmenopausal women. EXAMPLES: Premarin, Estrace, Estratest (oral estrogen), Estraderm, Vivelle (transdermal estrogen via skin patch) Estrogen is also available in combination with progesterone as pills and patches.
analgesics	Agents that relieve pain. They are classified as narcotic or non-narcotic.
narcotic	EXAMPLES: Demerol (meperidine HCl), morphine sulfate, Oxycontin (oxycodone HCl), and Hysingla (hydrocodone bitartrate)
non-narcotic	EXAMPLES: Tylenol (acetaminophen), aspirin, ibuprofen (Advil, Motrin, Nuprin), and Naprosyn (naproxen)

Diagnostic *and* Laboratory Tests

Test	Description
arthrography (ăr-thrŏg′ră-fē)	Diagnostic examination of a joint (usually the knee) in which air and then a radiopaque contrast medium are injected into the joint space, x-rays are taken, and internal injuries of the meniscus, cartilage, and ligaments can be seen, if present.
arthroscopy (ăr-thrŏs′kō-pē)	Process of examining and inspecting the internal structures of a joint using an arthroscope; usually done after an arthrography and before joint surgery. See Figure 5.23.

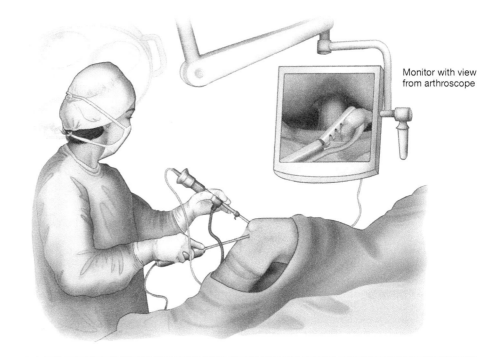

Monitor with view from arthroscope

FIGURE 5.23 Arthroscopic surgery involves the surgery of a joint with the use of a flexible arthroscope and other surgical tools. In this example, the surgeon inserts the arthroscope to evaluate the damage to the knee joint and then uses instruments to perform the necessary procedure.

computed tomography (CT) (kŏm-pū′těd tō-mŏg′ră-fē)	Advanced x-ray scanning system with a minicomputer that provides cross-section imaging. CT scans reveal both bone and soft tissue, including organs, muscles, and tumors. See Figure 5.24.

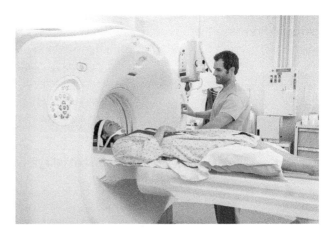

FIGURE 5.24 Technician assisting a patient undergoing a computed tomography (CT) scan.
Source: Tyler Olson/Shutterstock

Test	Description
dual-energy x-ray absorptiometry (DXA) scan (ăb-sorp″ shē-ŏm′ ĕ-trē)	Test used to measure bone mass or bone mineral density; used for diagnosing osteoporosis. The bone density of the patient is compared to the average peak bone density of young adults of the same gender and race. This score is called the *T score*, and it expresses the bone density in terms of the number of standard deviations (SDs) below peak young adult bone mass. Osteoporosis is defined as a bone density *T* score of –2.5 or below. Osteopenia (between normal and osteoporosis) is defined as a bone density *T* score between –1 and –2.5.

 fyi In women, osteoporosis is defined by the World Health Organization (WHO) as a bone mineral density –2.5 SDs below peak bone mass (compared to an average 25- to 35-year-old healthy female of the same ethnicity) as measured by a DXA scan. The standard deviation is the difference between the bone mineral density (BMD) and that of the healthy young adult. This result is the *T* score. Positive *T* scores indicate the bone is stronger than normal; negative *T* scores indicate the bone is weaker than normal. The risk for bone fracture doubles with every SD below normal. Thus, a person with a BMD of 1 SD below normal (*T* score of –1) has twice the risk for bone fracture as a person with a normal BMD. A person with a *T* score of –2 has four times the risk for bone fracture as a person with a normal BMD. People with a high risk for bone fracture can be treated with the goal of preventing future fractures. A DXA scan is recommended every 2 years after osteoporosis is diagnosed to evaluate effectiveness of treatment.

goniometry (gō″ nē-ŏm′ ĕ-trē)	Measurement of joint movements, especially range of motion (ROM) and angles via a goniometer. See Figure 5.25.

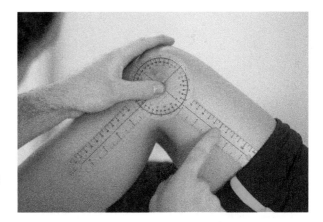

FIGURE 5.25 Physiotherapist measuring knee angle with a goniometer.
Source: ESB Professional/Shutterstock

Test	Description
magnetic resonance imaging (MRI)	Noninvasive imaging technique used to view organs, bone, and other internal body structures. The imaged body part is exposed to radio waves while in a magnetic field. The picture is produced by energy emitted from hydrogen atoms in the human body. See Figure 5.26.

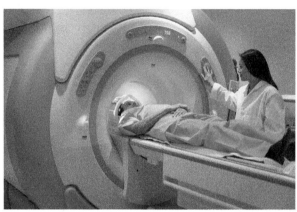

FIGURE 5.26 Technician prepares a patient to enter a magnetic resonance imaging (MRI) scanner.
Source: Image Source Trading Ltd./Shutterstock

Test	Description
photon absorptiometry (fō´ tŏn ăb-sorp˝ shē-ŏm´ ĕ-trē)	Bone scan that uses a low beam of radiation to measure bone mineral density and bone loss in the lumbar vertebrae; useful in monitoring osteoporosis.
thermography (thĕr-mŏg´ ră-fē)	Process of recording heat patterns of the body's surface; can be used to investigate the pathophysiology of rheumatoid arthritis.
x-ray	Examination of bones using an electromagnetic wave of high energy produced by the collision of a beam of electrons with a target in a vacuum tube; used to identify fractures and pathological conditions of the bones and joints such as rheumatoid arthritis, spondylitis, and tumors. See Figures 5.27 and 5.28.

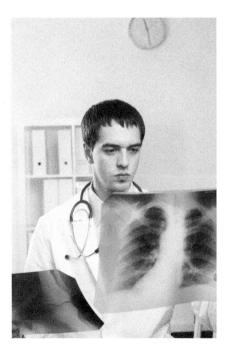

FIGURE 5.27 Radiologist examines an x-ray of the chest.
Source: adam121/Fotolia

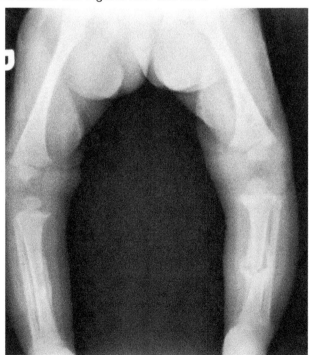

FIGURE 5.28 X-ray of a child's legs showing fractures in the right tibia and right fibula.
Source: Pearson Education, Inc.

Test	Description
alkaline phosphatase blood test (ăl´ kă-līn fŏs´ fă-tās)	Blood test to determine the level of alkaline phosphatase; increased level in osteoblastic bone tumors, rickets, osteomalacia, and during fracture healing.
antinuclear antibodies (ANA) (ăn˝ tĭ-nū´ klē-ăr ăn´ tĭ-bŏd˝ ēs)	Present in a variety of immunological diseases; positive result can indicate rheumatoid arthritis, lupus, and other autoimmune diseases.
bone mineral density (BMD) test	Test used to measure bone mass or bone mineral density. Several different machines measure bone density. Peripheral machines measure density in the finger, wrist, kneecap, shin bone, and heel. Central machines measure density in the hip, spine, and total body.
calcium (Ca) blood test	Calcium level of the blood can be increased in metastatic bone cancer, acute osteoporosis, prolonged immobilization, and during fracture healing; can be decreased in osteomalacia and rickets.
C-reactive protein (CRP) blood test (sē-rē-ăk´ tĭv prō´ tēn)	Positive result can indicate rheumatoid arthritis, acute inflammatory change, and widespread metastasis.
phosphorus (P) blood test (fŏs´ fă-rŭs)	Phosphorus level of the blood can be increased in osteoporosis and fracture healing.
serum rheumatoid factor (RF) (sēr´ ŭm roo´ mă-toyd)	Immunoglobulin present in the serum of a majority of adults with rheumatoid arthritis.
uric acid blood test (ū´ rĭk ăs´ ĭd)	Uric acid is increased in gout, arthritis, multiple myeloma, and rheumatism.

Abbreviations *and* Acronyms

Abbreviation/ Acronym	Meaning	Abbreviation/ Acronym	Meaning
ANA	antinuclear antibodies	jt	joint
BMD	bone mineral density (test)	L1	lumbar vertebra, first
C1	cervical vertebra, first	L2	lumbar vertebra, second
C2	cervical vertebra, second	L3	lumbar vertebra, third
C3	cervical vertebra, third	lig	ligament
Ca	calcium	MRI	magnetic resonance imaging
CRP	C-reactive protein blood test	NSAIDs	nonsteroidal anti-inflammatory drugs
DMARDs	disease-modifying antirheumatic drugs	OA	osteoarthritis
DXA	dual-energy x-ray absorptiometry scan	Orth, ortho	orthopedics, orthopaedics
EHT	estrogen hormone therapy	P	phosphorus
Fx	fracture	RA	rheumatoid arthritis

Abbreviation/Acronym	Meaning	Abbreviation/Acronym	Meaning
RF	rheumatoid factor	T2	thoracic vertebra, second
ROM	range of motion	T3	thoracic vertebra, third
SDs	standard deviations	TJA	total joint arthroplasty
T1	thoracic vertebra, first	Tx	traction

Study *and* Review III

Building Medical Terms

Using the following word parts, fill in the blanks to build the correct medical terms.

dactyl	-dynia	oste/o	-poiesis	-al
meta-	-oid	patell	scoli	-osis

Definition   **Medical Term**

1. Pain in the coccyx (tailbone) — coccygo _____

2. Pertaining to a finger or toe — _____ic

3. An abnormal anterior curvature of the lumbar spine — lord _____

4. Pertaining to the bones of the hand — _____carpals

5. Formation of bone marrow — myelo _____

6. Softening of bone — _____malacia

7. Pertaining to the kneecap — _____ar

8. Pertaining to the bones of the fingers and the toes — phalange _____

9. An abnormal lateral curvature of the spine — _____osis

10. Literally means resembling a sword — xiph _____

Combining Form Challenge

Using the combining forms provided, write the medical term correctly.

cost/o   chondr/o   arthr/o

dactyl/o   burs/o   carp/o

1. Surgical procedure used to repair a joint: _____plasty

2. Inflammation of a bursa: _____itis

3. Pertaining to the wrist: _____al

4. Pertaining to cartilage: _____al

5. Pertaining to the rib cartilage: _____al

6. Medical term for fingerprint: _____gram

Select the Right Term

Select the correct answer, and write it on the line provided.

1. Abnormal condition of stiffening of a joint is _____.

    acroarthritis   acromion   ankyloses   arthrocentesis

2. Surgical excision of a portion of the skull is _____.

    craniectomy   craniotomy   cranectomy   craniotomy

3. Pain in the hip is _____.

    ischial   ischialgia   ischalgia   ischial

4. Pertaining to the lower jaw is _____.

    maxillary   meniscus   mandibular   mandibular

5. Malignant tumor of the bone; cancer growing from cells of "fleshy" connective tissue is _____.

    osteocarcioma   osteosarcoma   osteogenesis   myeloma

6. Surgery performed to permanently connect two or more vertebrae in the spine is _____.

    myelitis   acroarthritis   spondylodesis   vertebral

Drug Highlights

Match the appropriate lettered description or examples of drug(s) with the class of drug.

_____	1.	disease-modifying antirheumatic drugs
_____	2.	agents used to treat gout
_____	3.	antiresorptive agents
_____	4.	nonsteroidal anti-inflammatory drugs
_____	5.	examples of COX-2 inhibitors
_____	6.	anti-inflammatory agents
_____	7.	examples of narcotic analgesics
_____	8.	biologics
_____	9.	estrogen hormone therapy
_____	10.	examples of non-narcotic analgesics

a. Tylenol (acetaminophen), aspirin, ibuprofen (Advil, Motrin, Nuprin), and Naprosyn (naproxen)

b. Celebrex (celecoxib) and Mobic (meloxicam)

c. Include a wide range of medicinal products such as vaccines, blood and blood components, and drugs made from recombinant DNA technology

d. Demerol (meperidine HCl), morphine sulfate, Oxycontin (oxycodone HCl)

e. Zyloprim (allopurinol) and probenecid

f. Introduced in early cases of rheumatoid arthritis to limit irreversible joint damage

g. Prevents bone loss, increases bone density, and prevents bone fractures in postmenopausal women

h. Used in the treatment of arthritis and related disorders

i. Relieve the swelling, tenderness, redness, and pain of inflammation; can be classified as steroidal and nonsteroidal

j. Decrease the removal of calcium from bones

Diagnostic and Laboratory Tests

Select the best answer to each multiple-choice question. Circle the letter of your choice.

1. _____ is a diagnostic examination of a joint in which air and then a radiopaque contrast medium are injected into the joint space, x-rays are taken, and internal injuries of the meniscus, cartilage, and ligaments may be seen, if present.

   a. Arthroscopy

   b. Goniometry

   c. Arthrography

   d. Thermography

2. The process of recording heat patterns of the body's surface is _____.

a. arthrography **c.** goniometry

b. arthroscopy **d.** thermography

3. _____ is increased in gout, arthritis, multiple myeloma, and rheumatism.

a. Calcium **c.** Uric acid

b. Phosphorus **d.** Alkaline phosphatase

4. The _____ level of the blood can be increased in osteoporosis and fracture healing.

a. antinuclear antibodies **c.** uric acid

b. phosphorus **d.** alkaline phosphatase

5. _____ is/are present in a variety of immunological diseases.

a. Alkaline phosphatase **c.** C-reactive protein

b. Antinuclear antibodies **d.** Uric acid

Abbreviations and Acronyms

Write the correct word, phrase, or abbreviation/acronym in the space provided.

1. antinuclear antibodies _____

2. fracture _____

3. BMD _____

4. OA _____

5. phosphorus _____

6. RA _____

7. range of motion _____

8. T1 _____

9. lig _____

10. traction _____

Practical Application

Medical Record Analysis

This exercise contains information, abbreviations/acronyms, and medical terminology from an actual medical record or case study that has been adapted for this text. The names and any personal information have been created by the author. Read and study each form or case study and then answer the questions that follow. You may refer to Appendix III, *Abbreviations, Acronyms, and Symbols*.

CLEAR SHOT IMAGING SERVICES

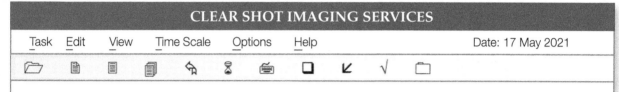

| Task | Edit | View | Time Scale | Options | Help | Date: 17 May 2021 |

Phone (123) 456-7890

NAME: BELL, CRYSTAL JANE

DATE OF BIRTH: 5/26/55

CLINICAL DATA: v49.81 POST MENO

REQUESTING PHYSICIAN: Kyle Preston, MD

EXAM CODE: XRDXA/76075

LOCATION: SHORTER MEDICAL

EXAM: XR DXA, BONE DENSITY SCAN, 03/19/2021

BONE DENSITOMETRY, 3/19/2021

ORD: 07DX00145

ORDER DATE: 03/19/2021

Routine bone densitometry of the lumbar spine and both hips was performed.

The results of the examination expressed as standard deviations (SDs) from the mean bone mineral density (BMD) are as follows:

Spine (L1–L4) *T* score	0.6 Z-score	1.7
Femoral neck *T* score	−2.3 Z-score	−0.8

Impression:

There is a discrepancy between the lumbar spine and hips due to what I believe is spondylosis. The hips are of a more accurate reading, which is consistent with osteopenia.
Follow-up in 18–24 months is recommended.

DICTATED: Lions, Daniel

TECHNOLOGIST: 303768

transcribed: rs 03/19/2021

24599

VERIFIED: Daniel Lions, MD

Medical Record Questions

Write the correct answer in the space provided.

1. What is the meaning of DXA? _____

2. The medical term *osteopenia* means _____.

3. Divide ostopenia into its component parts and define each part.

_____   _____

_____   _____

4. The results of the routine bone densitometry of the lumbar spine and both hips are expressed as _____

_____ (SDs) from the bone mineral density (_____).

5. The recommended follow-up for the next bone densitometry is _____.

MyLab Medical Terminology™

MyLab Medical Terminology is a premium online homework management system that includes a host of features to help you study. Registered users will find:

- A multitude of quizzes and activities built within the MyLab platform
- Powerful tools that track and analyze your results—allowing you to create a personalized learning experience
- Videos and audio pronunciations to help enrich your progress
- Streaming lesson presentations (guided lectures) and self-paced learning modules
- A space where you and your instructor can check your progress and manage your assignments

Muscular System

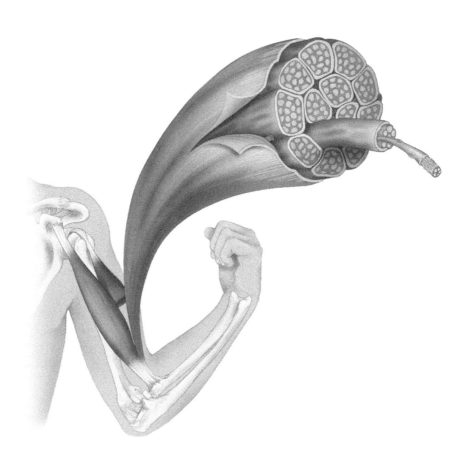

Learning Outcomes

On completion of this chapter, you will be able to:

1. Describe the muscular system.
2. Describe the three basic types of muscle tissue.
3. Explain the primary functions of muscles.
4. Analyze, build, spell, and pronounce medical words.
5. Classify the drugs highlighted in this chapter.
6. Describe diagnostic and laboratory tests related to the muscular system.
7. Identify and define selected abbreviations and acronyms.

Anatomy and Physiology

The muscular system is composed of all the **muscles** in the body and works in coordination with the skeletal and nervous systems. Muscles provide the mechanism for movement of the body and locomotion from one place to another. In addition to causing movement, muscles produce heat and help the body maintain posture and stability. There are three basic types of muscles: skeletal, smooth, and cardiac. Table 6.1 provides an at-a-glance look at the muscular system.

The muscles are the primary tissues of the system. They make up approximately 42% of a person's body weight and are composed of long, slender cells known as **fibers**. Muscle fibers are of different lengths and shapes and vary in color from white to deep red. Each muscle consists of a group of fibers held together by connective tissue and enclosed in a fibrous sheath or **fascia**. See Figure 6.1.

Each fiber within a muscle receives its own nerve impulses and has its own stored supply of glycogen, which it uses as fuel for energy. Muscles must be supplied with proper nutrition and oxygen to perform correctly; these essentials are supplied via the blood, thus blood and lymphatic vessels permeate muscle tissues.

TABLE 6.1	Muscular System at-a-Glance
Organ/Structure	**Primary Functions/Description**
Muscles	Cause movement, help to maintain posture, and produce heat
Skeletal muscles	Produce various types of body movement through contractility, extensibility, and elasticity
Smooth muscles	Produce relatively slow contraction with greater degree of extensibility in the internal organs, especially organs of the digestive, respiratory, and urinary tract, plus certain muscles of the eyes and skin, and walls of blood vessels
Cardiac muscle	Contraction of the myocardium, which is controlled by the autonomic nervous system and specialized neuromuscular tissue located within the right atrium
Tendons	Bands of connective tissue that attach muscles to bones

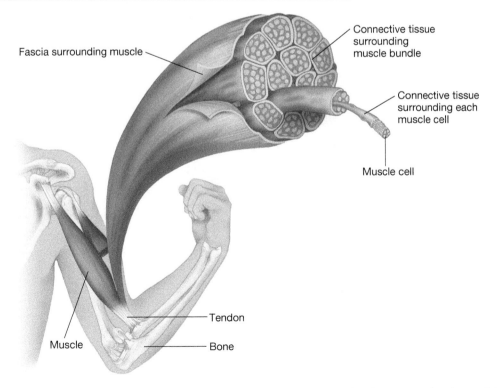

Fascia surrounding muscle

Connective tissue surrounding muscle bundle

Connective tissue surrounding each muscle cell

Muscle cell

Tendon

Muscle

Bone

FIGURE 6.1 Skeletal muscle consists of a group of fibers held together by connective tissue. It is enclosed in a fibrous sheath (fascia).

Types of Muscles

Skeletal muscle, smooth muscle, and cardiac muscle are the three basic types of muscles in the body. They are composed of different types of muscle tissue (e.g., striated or smooth) and classified according to their functions and appearance. See Figure 6.2.

Skeletal Muscle

Also known as **voluntary** or **striated muscles**, **skeletal muscles** are controlled by the conscious part of the brain and attach to the bones. These muscles have a cross-striped appearance (striated) and vary in size, shape, arrangement of fibers, and means of attachment to bones. Selected skeletal muscles are listed with their functions in Table 6.2 and are shown in Figure 6.3.

There are over 600 skeletal muscles in the body that, through contractility, extensibility, excitability, and elasticity, are responsible for the movement of the body. **Contractility** allows muscles to change shape to become shorter and thicker. With **extensibility**, living muscle cells can be stretched and extended. They become longer and thinner. In **excitability**, muscles receive and respond to stimulation. With **elasticity**, once the stretching force is removed, a living muscle cell returns to its original shape.

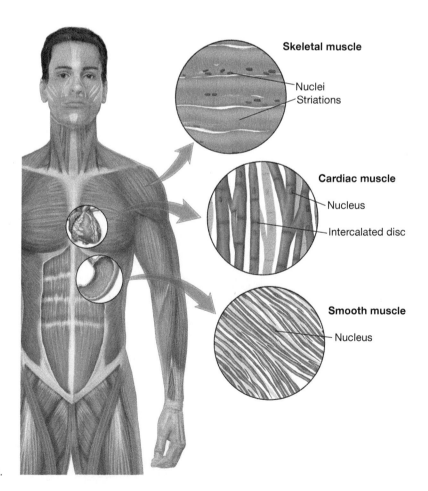

FIGURE 6.2 Types of muscle tissue.

TABLE 6.2   Selected Skeletal Muscles

Muscle	Direction	Action
Sternocleidomastoid	Anterior	Rotates and laterally flexes neck
Trapezius	Anterior/posterior	Draws head back and to the side; rotates scapula
Deltoid	Anterior/posterior	Raises and rotates arm
Rectus femoris	Anterior	Extends leg and assists flexion of thigh
Sartorius	Anterior	Flexes and rotates the thigh and leg
Tibialis anterior	Anterior	Dorsiflexes foot and increases the arch in the beginning process of walking
Pectoralis major	Anterior	Flexes, adducts, and rotates arm
Biceps brachii	Anterior	Flexes arm and forearm and supinates forearm
External oblique	Anterior	Contracts abdomen and viscera (internal organs)
Rectus abdominis	Anterior	Compresses or flattens abdomen
Gastrocnemius	Anterior/posterior	Plantar flexes foot and flexes knee
Soleus	Anterior	Plantar flexes foot
Triceps	Posterior	Extends forearm
Latissimus dorsi	Posterior	Adducts, extends, and rotates arm; used during swimming
Gluteus medius	Posterior	Abducts and rotates thigh
Gluteus maximus	Posterior	Extends and rotates thigh
Biceps femoris	Posterior	Flexes knee and rotates it outward
Semitendinosus	Posterior	Flexes and rotates leg; extends thigh
Semimembranosus	Posterior	Flexes and rotates leg; extends thigh
Achilles tendon	Posterior	Plantar (sole of the foot) flexion and extension of ankle

 fyi   The movements of a newborn are uncoordinated and random. Muscular development proceeds from head to foot and from the center of the body to the periphery. Head and neck muscles are the first ones that a baby can control. A baby can hold his or her head up before he or she can sit erect.

Muscles have three distinguishable parts: the **body** or main portion, an **origin**, and an **insertion**. The origin is the more fixed attachment of the muscle to the stationary bone and the insertion is the point of attachment of a muscle to the bone that it moves. See Figure 6.4. The means of attachment is a band of connective tissue called a **tendon**, which can vary in length from less than 1 inch to more than 1 foot. Some muscles, such as those in the abdominal region, the dorsal lumbar region, and the palmar region, form attachments using a wide, thin, sheetlike tendon known as an **aponeurosis**.

Skeletal muscles move body parts by pulling from one bone across its joint to another bone, with movement occurring at the freely movable (diarthrosis/synovial) joint. The types of body movement occurring at the freely movable joints are described in Chapter 5.

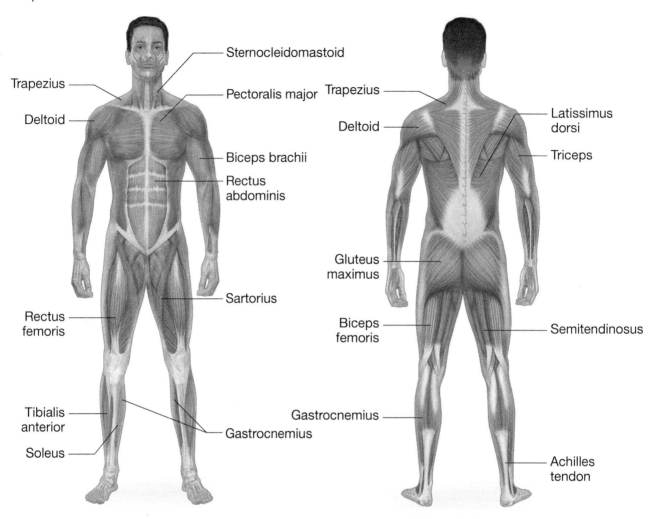

FIGURE 6.3 Selected skeletal muscles and the Achilles tendon (anterior and posterior views).

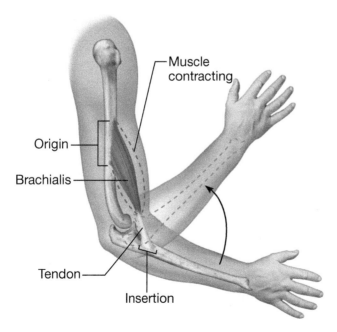

FIGURE 6.4 Muscle attachments. Origin and insertion of the brachialis muscle.
Source: MARIEB, ELAINE N.; KELLER, SUZANNE M., ESSENTIALS OF HUMAN ANATOMY & PHYSIOLOGY, 12th Ed., ©2018.
Reprinted and Electronically reproduced by permission of Pearson Education, Inc., New York, NY.

Muscles and nerves function together as a motor unit. For skeletal muscles to contract, it is necessary to have stimulation by impulses from motor nerves. Skeletal muscles perform in groups and are classified as follows:

- **Antagonist.** Muscle that counteracts the action of another muscle; when one contracts, the other relaxes
- **Prime mover** or **agonist.** Muscle that is primary in a given movement; the movement is produced by its contraction
- **Synergist.** Muscle that acts with another muscle to produce and assist movement

All movement is a result of the contraction of a prime mover (agonist) and the relaxation of the opposing muscle (antagonist). See Figure 6.5.

fyi Have you ever wondered about the bands that some football players wear around their biceps? These items are called bicep bands. They are made of a variety of materials such as nylon, cotton, and synthetic blends. Bicep bands are used to catch and absorb sweat on the arms, preventing the sweat on the shoulders and upper arms from sliding down to the forearm and hands.

Smooth Muscle

Also called *involuntary*, *visceral*, or *unstriated*, **smooth muscles** are not controlled by the conscious part of the brain. They are under the control of the autonomic nervous system and, in most cases, produce relatively slow contraction with a greater degree of extensibility. These muscles lack the cross-striped appearance of skeletal muscle and are smooth. Included in this type are the muscles of internal organs of the digestive, respiratory, and urinary tract plus certain muscles of the eyes and skin.

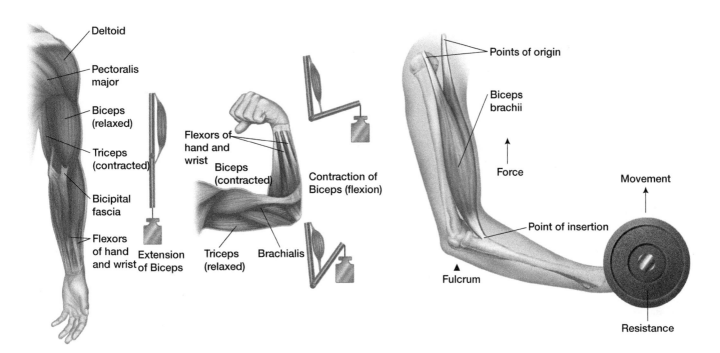

FIGURE 6.5 Coordination of antagonist muscles to perform movement.

Cardiac Muscle

The muscle of the heart, the **cardiac muscle** (**myocardium**), is *involuntary* but *striated* in appearance. It is under the control of the autonomic nervous system and has specialized neuromuscular tissue located within the right atrium. Cardiac muscle differs from the other two muscle types in that contraction can occur even without an initial nervous input. The cells that produce the stimulation for contraction without nervous input are called the **pacemaker cells**. Coordinated contraction of cardiac muscle cells in the heart propels blood from the atria and ventricles to the blood vessels of the circulatory system. Cardiac muscle cells, like all tissues in the body, rely on an ample blood supply to deliver oxygen and nutrients and to remove waste products such as carbon dioxide. The coronary arteries fulfill this function.

 In the older adult, the heart muscle becomes less able to propel the large amount of blood that is needed by the body. This makes a person feel tired more quickly and takes longer for recovery to occur.

Functions of Muscles

The following is a list of the primary functions of muscles:

1. Muscles are responsible for movement. The types of movement are locomotion where chemical energy is changed into mechanical energy, propulsion of substances through tubes as in circulation and digestion, and changes in the size of openings as in the contraction and relaxation of the iris of the eye.

2. Muscles help to maintain posture through a continual partial contraction of skeletal muscles. This process is known as **tonicity**.

3. Muscles help to produce heat through the chemical changes involved in muscular action.

 As a person grows older, the number and size of muscle fibers diminish and the water content of tendons is reduced. Decrease in handgrip strength can make performing routine activities such as opening a jar or turning a key more difficult.

Study *and* Review I

Anatomy and Physiology

Write your answers to the following questions.

1. The muscular system is made up of three types of muscle tissue. Name the three types.

a. _____   c. _____

b. _____

2. Muscles make up approximately _____ % of a person's body weight.

3. Name the two essentials that must be supplied for a muscle to perform correctly.

   a. _____   **b.** _____

4. Name the two points of attachment for a skeletal muscle.

   a. _____   **b.** _____

5. Skeletal muscle is also known as _____ or _____.

6. A wide, thin, sheetlike tendon is known as an _____.

7. Name the three distinguishable parts of a muscle.

   a. _____   **c.** _____

   b. _____

8. Define the following:

   a. Antagonist _____

   b. Prime mover _____

   c. Synergist _____

9. Smooth muscle is also called _____, _____, or
   _____.

10. Smooth muscles are found in the internal organs. Name five examples of these locations.

   a. _____   **d.** _____

   b. _____   **e.** _____

   c. _____

11. _____ is the muscle of the heart.

12. Name the three primary functions of the muscular system.

   a. _____   **c.** _____

   b. _____

ANATOMY LABELING   Identify the structures shown below by filling in the blanks.

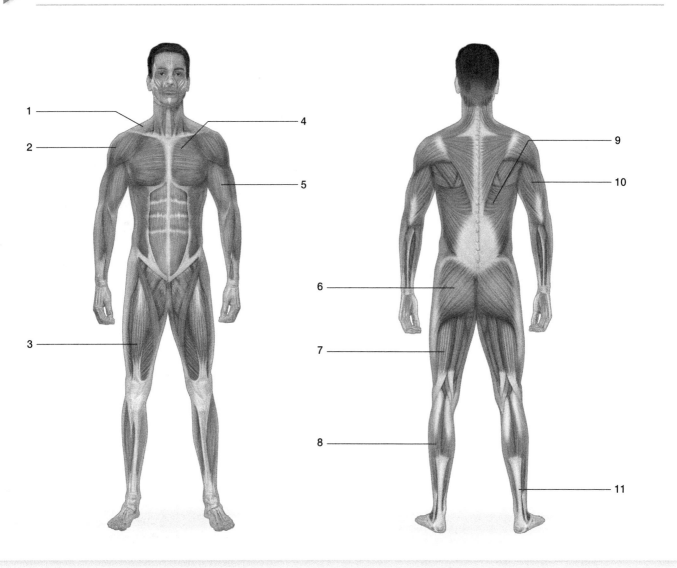

Building Your Medical Vocabulary

This section provides the foundation for learning medical terminology. Review the alphabetized list of medical terms in the following pages. Note how common prefixes and suffixes are repeatedly applied to word roots and combining forms to create different meanings. A combining form is a word root plus a vowel. The chart below lists the combining forms and word roots used in this chapter and can help to strengthen your understanding of how medical words are built and spelled.

You will find that some terms have not been divided into word parts. These are common words or specialized terms that are included to enhance your medical vocabulary.

Combining Forms

agon/o	agony, a contest	**prosth/e**	an addition
amputat/o	to cut through	**rhabd/o**	rod
brach/i, brachi/o	arm	**rheumat/o**	discharge
cleid/o	clavicle	**rotat/o**	to turn
dactyl/o	finger or toe	**sarc/o**	flesh
dermat/o	skin	**scler/o**	hardening
duct/o	to lead	**stern/o**	sternum
fasci/o	a band	**synov/o**	synovial
fibr/o	fiber	**ten/o**	tendon
is/o	equal	**therm/o**	hot, heat
mast/o	mastoid process	**ton/o**	tone, tension
metr/o	to measure	**tors/o**	twisted
muscul/o	muscle	**tort/i**	twisted
my/o(s)	muscle	**tract/o**	to draw
neur/o	nerve	**troph/o**	nourishment, development
path/o	disease	**volunt/o**	will

Word Roots

collis	neck	**relaxat**	to loosen
gravis	grave	**sert**	to gain
levat	lifter	**spastic**	convulsive
log	study		

Medical Word	Word Parts		Definition
	Part	**Meaning**	
abductor (ăb-dŭk´ tōr)	**ab-** **duct** **-or**	away from to lead a doer	Muscle that on contraction draws *away from* the middle
adductor (ă-dŭk´ tōr)	**ad-** **duct** **-or**	toward to lead a doer	Muscle that draws a part *toward* the middle

> **! ALERT!**
>
> The only difference in the terms **ab**/duct/or and **ad**/duct/or are the prefixes **ab-** (away from) and **ad-** (toward). What a difference a couple of letters can make!

amputation (ăm˝ pū-tā´ shŭn)	**amputat** **-ion**	to cut through process	Surgical or traumatic removal of a limb, part, or other appendage. See Figure 6.6.

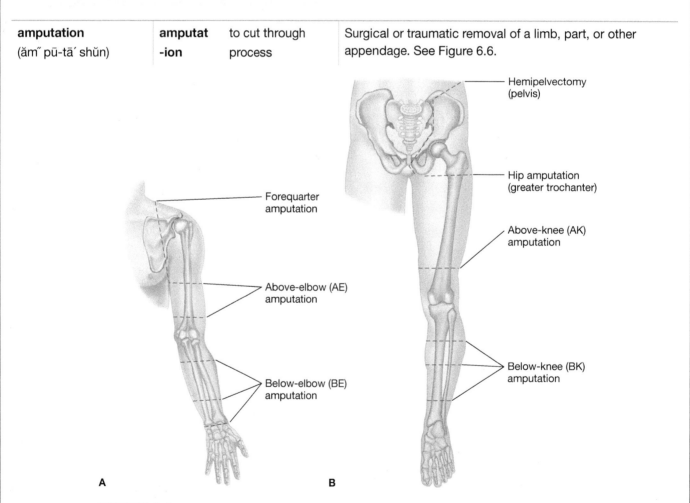

FIGURE 6.6 Common sites of amputation. **A** Upper extremities. **B** Lower extremities. The surgeon determines the level of amputation based on blood supply and tissue condition.

Medical Word	Word Parts		Definition
	Part	Meaning	
antagonist (ăn-tăg′ ō-nĭst)	ant- agon -ist	against agony, a contest agent	Muscle that counteracts the action of another muscle; when one contracts, the other relaxes (refer to Figure 6.5)
aponeurosis (ăp″ ō-nū-rō′ sĭs)			A strong, flat sheet of fibrous connective tissue that serves as a tendon to attach muscles to bone or as fascia to bind muscles together or to other tissues at their origin or insertion
ataxia (ă-tăk′ sē-ă)	a- -taxia	lack of order	Lack of muscular coordination; an inability to coordinate voluntary muscular movements that is symptomatic of some nervous disorders
atonic (ă-tŏn′ ĭk)	a- ton -ic	lack of tone, tension pertaining to	Pertaining to a lack of normal tone or tension; the lack of normal muscle tone
atrophy (ăt′ rō-fē)	a- -trophy	lack of nourishment, development	Literally means a lack of nourishment; wasting-away of muscular tissue that may be caused by lack of use or lack of nerve stimulation of the muscle. Lipoatrophy (also called lipodystrophy) is atrophy of fat tissue. This condition can occur at the site of an insulin and/or corticosteroid injection.
biceps (bī′ sĕps)	bi- -ceps	two head	Muscle with two heads or points of origin
brachialgia (brā″ kē-ăl′ jē-ă)	brach/i -algia	arm pain	Pain in the arm
bradykinesia (brăd″ ĭ-kĭ-nē′ sē-ă)	brady- -kinesia	slow motion	Slowness of motion or movement
contraction (kŏn-trăk′ shŭn)	con- tract -ion	with, together to draw process	Process of drawing-up and thickening of a muscle fiber

Medical Word	Word Parts		Definition
	Part	Meaning	
contracture (kŏn-trăk´ chūr)	con- tract -ure	with, together to draw process	A fibrosis of connective tissue in skin, fascia, muscle, or joint capsule that prevents normal mobility of the related tissue or joint. With a muscular contracture, a muscle shortens and renders the muscle resistant to the normal stretching process. For example, *Dupuytren contracture* is a thickening and tightening of subcutaneous tissue of the palm, causing the ring and little fingers to bend into the palm so that they cannot be extended. See Figure 6.7.

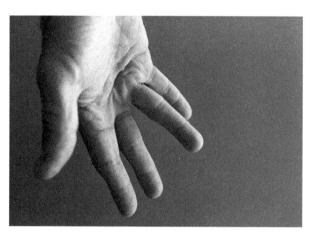

FIGURE 6.7 Dupuytren contracture.
Source: Fineart1/Shutterstock

fyi The term *fibrosis* is defined as the overgrowth, hardening, and/or scarring of various tissues and is attributed to excess deposition of extracellular matrix components including collagen. Fibrosis is the end result of chronic inflammatory reactions induced by a variety of stimuli including persistent infections, autoimmune reactions, allergic responses, chemical insults, radiation, and tissue injury.

dactylospasm (dăk´ tǐ-lō-spăzm)	dactyl/o -spasm	finger or toe tension, spasm	Medical term for cramp of a finger or toe

Medical Word	Word Parts		Definition
	Part	Meaning	
dermatomyositis (dĕr″ mă-tō-mī″ ō-sī′ tĭs)	dermat/o my/o(s) -itis	skin muscle inflammation	Acute or chronic disease with systemic pathology; inflammation of the muscles and the skin; a connective tissue disease characterized by edema, dermatitis, and inflammation of the muscles. Occurs in children and adults, and in the latter may be associated with neoplastic disease (cancer) or other disorders of connective tissue. Also referred to as *dermatopolymyositis*. See Figure 6.8.

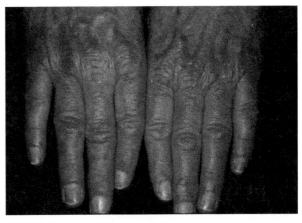

FIGURE 6.8 Dermatomyositis.
Source: Courtesy of Jason L. Smith, MD

diaphragm (dī′ ă-frăm)	dia- -phragm	through fence, partition	Partition of muscles and membranes that separates the chest cavity and the abdominal cavity. It is the major muscle of breathing. See Figure 6.9.

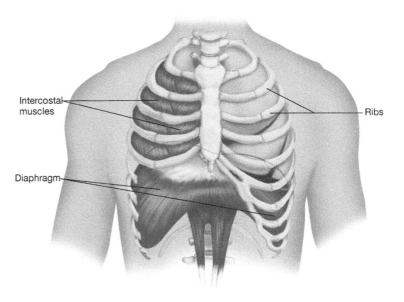

FIGURE 6.9 Diaphragm, the major muscle of breathing.

Medical Word	Word Parts		Definition
	Part	**Meaning**	
diathermy (dī´ ă-thĕr˝ mē)	**dia-**	through	Treatment using high-frequency current to produce heat within a part of the body; used to increase blood flow but should not be used in acute stage of recovery from trauma
	therm	hot, heat	
	-y	pertaining to	
dystonia (dĭs-tō´ nē-ă)	**dys-**	difficult	Condition of impaired muscle tone
	ton	tone, tension	
	-ia	condition	
dystrophin (dĭs-trōf´ ĭn)	**dys-**	difficult	Protein found in muscle cells. When the gene that is responsible for this protein is defective and sufficient dystrophin is not produced, muscle wasting occurs. For example, in *Duchenne muscular dystrophy*, this protein is absent.
	troph	nourishment, development	
	-in	substance	
dystrophy (dĭs´ trō-fē)	**dys-**	difficult	Any condition of abnormal development caused by defective nourishment, often noted by the degeneration of muscles
	-trophy	nourishment, development	
exercise			Performed activity of the muscles for improvement of health or correction of deformity

fyi Types of exercise include:

Active. Muscular contraction and relaxation by patient

Assistive. Muscular contraction and relaxation with the assistance of a therapist

Isometric. Active muscular contraction performed against stable resistance, thereby not shortening muscle length

Passive. Exercise performed by another individual without patient assistance

Range of motion (ROM). Movement of each joint through its full range of motion (FROM); used to prevent loss of mobility or to regain usage after an injury or fracture

Relief of tension. Technique used to promote relaxation of the muscles and provide relief from tension

The National Institutes of Health (NIH) recommends that adults ages 18–64 engage in regular aerobic physical activity for 2.5 hours at moderate intensity or 1.25 hours at vigorous intensity each week. Moderate activities are those during which a person could talk but not sing. Vigorous activities are those during which a person could say only a few words without stopping for breath. *Note:* According to a study by the National Cancer Institute (NCI), people who engaged in leisure-time physical activity had life expectancy gains of as much as 4.5 years.

Medical Word	Word Parts		Definition
fascia (făsh´ ē-ă)	**fasc**	a band	Thin layer of connective tissue covering, supporting, or connecting the muscles or inner organs of the body
	-ia	condition	
fasciitis (făsh˝ ē-ī´ tĭs)	**fasci**	a band	Inflammation of a fascia
	-itis	inflammation	

Medical Word	Word Parts		Definition
	Part	Meaning	
fatigue (fă-tēg′)			State of tiredness occurring in a muscle as a result of repeated contractions
fibromyalgia syndrome (FMS) (fī″ brō-mī-ăl′ jē-ă sĭn′ drōm)	**fibr/o** **my** **-algia**	fiber muscle pain	Disorder that affects the muscles and soft tissue; symptoms include chronic muscle pain (myalgia), fatigue, sleep disorders, irritable bowel syndrome, depression, and chronic headaches. Although the exact cause is still unknown, fibromyalgia is often traced to an injury or physical or emotional trauma. The American College of Rheumatology (ACR) classifies a patient with fibromyalgia if at least 11 of 18 specific areas of the body (called *trigger points*) are painful under pressure. See Figure 6.10. The location of some of these trigger points includes the inside of the elbow joint, the front of the collarbone, and the base of the skull. Treatments for fibromyalgia are geared toward improving the quality of sleep, as well as reducing pain.

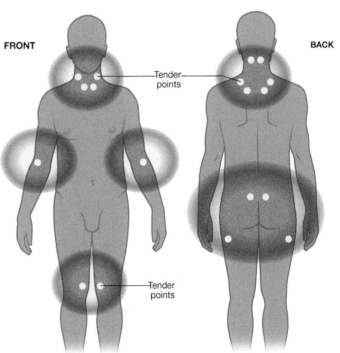

FIGURE 6.10 The 18 tender points of fibromyalgia.

Medical Word	Word Parts		Definition
fibromyitis (fī″ brō-mī-ī′ tĭs)	**fibr/o** **my** **-itis**	fiber muscle inflammation	Inflammation of muscle and fibrous tissue; also known as *fibromyositis*

Medical Word	Word Parts		Definition
	Part	**Meaning**	
First Aid Treatment—RICE (Rest Ice Compression Elevation)			**Cryotherapy** (use of cold) is the treatment of choice for soft-tissue and muscle injuries. It causes vasoconstriction of blood vessels and is effective in diminishing bleeding and edema. Ice should not be placed directly onto the skin. **Compression** by an elastic bandage is generally determined by the type of injury and physician preference. Some experts disagree on the use of elastic bandages. When used, the bandage should be 3–4 inches wide and applied firmly. Toes or fingers should be periodically checked for blue or white discoloration, indicating that the bandage is too tight. **Elevation** is used to reduce swelling. The injured part should be elevated above the level of the heart.
flaccid (flăk′ sĭd)			Lacking muscle tone; *weak, soft, flabby*
heat			Treatment using application of heat (thermotherapy) can be used 48–72 hours after the injury. Types of thermotherapy include heating pad, hot water bottle, hot packs, infrared light, and immersion of body part in warm water.
hydrotherapy (hī-drō-thĕr′ ă-pē)	hydro- -therapy	water treatment	Treatment using scientific application of water; types: hot tub, cold bath, whirlpool, and vapor bath
insertion (ĭn-sĕr′ shŭn)	in- sert -ion	into to gain process	Point of attachment of a muscle to the part that it moves
intramuscular (IM) (ĭn″ tră-mŭs′ kū-lăr)	intra- muscul -ar	within muscle pertaining to	Pertaining to within a muscle, such as an IM injection
isometric (ī″ sō-mě′ trĭk)	is/o metr -ic	equal to measure pertaining to	Literally means *pertaining to having equal measure*; increasing tension of muscle while maintaining equal length
isotonic (ī″ sō-tŏn′ ĭk)	is/o ton -ic	equal tone, tension pertaining to	Pertaining to having the same tone or tension
levator (lē-vā′ tor)	levat -or	lifter a doer	Muscle that raises or elevates a part
massage (măh-săhzh)			Kneading that applies pressure and friction to external body tissues

Medical Word	Word Parts		Definition
	Part	Meaning	
muscle spasm (mŭs′ ĕl spăzm)			Involuntary contraction of one or more muscles; usually accompanied by pain and limitation of function. A "charley horse" is a common name for a muscle spasm or cramp. Muscle spasms can occur in any muscle in the body, but often happen in the leg. When a muscle is in spasm, it contracts without your control and does not relax.
muscular dystrophy (MD) (mŭs′ kū-lăr dĭs′ trō-fē)			Refers to a group of genetic diseases characterized by progressive weakness and degeneration of the skeletal or voluntary muscles that control movement. The muscles of the heart and some other involuntary muscles are also affected in some forms of MD, and a few forms involve other organs as well.

fyi MD can affect people of all ages, with some forms apparent in infancy or childhood and others not appearing until middle age or later. Duchenne muscular dystrophy, the most common form of MD affecting children, is an X-linked disorder seen mostly in males. In this disorder, the protein dystrophin is absent from muscle cells, leading to necrosis in muscle fibers and their replacement with connective tissue and fat. Myotonic MD is the most common form affecting adults. There is no specific treatment for any of the forms of MD. Physical therapy to prevent *contractures* (a condition in which shortened muscles around joints cause abnormal and sometimes painful positioning of the joints), *orthoses* (orthopedic appliances used for support), and corrective orthopedic surgery could be needed to improve the quality of life in some cases. Some cases of MD are mild and other cases have marked progressions of muscle weakness, functional disability, and loss of ambulation. See Figure 6.11.

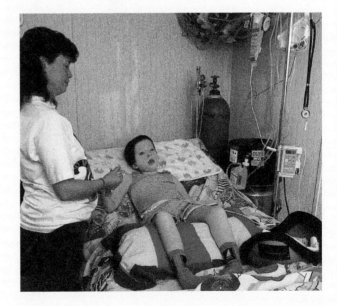

FIGURE 6.11 This young boy with muscular dystrophy needs to receive tube feedings and home nursing care. He attends school when possible and is able to use an adapted computer.
Source: Pearson Education, Inc.

fyi The **Gowers maneuver**, as seen in Figure 6.12, is the use of the upper-extremity muscles to raise oneself to a standing position. This is a good indicator of muscle weakness of the legs caused by muscular dystrophy. Early in the diagnostic process, a serum creatine kinase (CK) test, an electromyography (EMG), and a muscle biopsy are ordered.

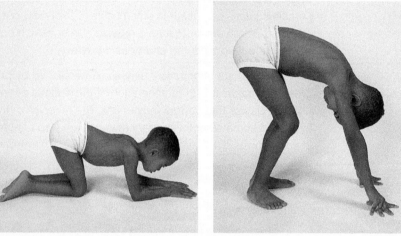

A

B

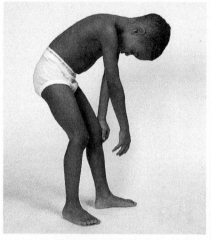

C

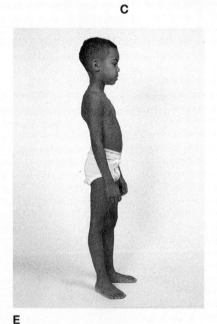

D

E

FIGURE 6.12 Because the leg muscles of children with muscular dystrophy are weak, they must perform the Gowers maneuver to rise to a standing position. **A** and **B** The child first maneuvers to a position supported by arms and legs. **C** The child next pushes off the floor and rests one hand on the knee. **D** and **E** The child then pushes himself upright.
Source: Pearson Education, Inc.

Medical Word	Word Parts		Definition
	Part	**Meaning**	
myalgia (mī-ăl´jē-ă)	**my** **-algia**	muscle pain	Pain in the muscle
myasthenia gravis (MG) (mī-ăs-thē´nē-ă gră-vĭs)	**my** **-asthenia** **gravis**	muscle weakness grave	Chronic autoimmune neuromuscular disease characterized by varying degrees of weakness of the skeletal (voluntary) muscles of the body. Its name, which is Latin and Greek in origin, literally means *grave muscle weakness*. The primary symptom is muscle weakness that increases during periods of activity and improves after periods of rest.
myoblast (mī´ō-blăst)	**my/o** **-blast**	muscle immature cell, germ cell	Embryonic cell that develops into a cell of muscle fiber
myofibroma (mī˝ō-fī-brō´mă)	**my/o** **fibr** **-oma**	muscle fiber tumor	Tumor that contains muscle and fiber
myograph (mī´ō-grăf)	**my/o** **-graph**	muscle instrument for recording	Instrument used to record muscular contractions
myokinesis (mī˝ō-kĭn-ē´sĭs)	**my/o** **-kinesis**	muscle motion	Muscular motion or activity
myoma (mī-ō´mă)	**my** **-oma**	muscle tumor	Tumor containing muscle tissue
myomalacia (mī˝ō-mă-lā´sē-ă)	**my/o** **-malacia**	muscle softening	Softening of muscle tissue
myoparesis (mī˝ō-păr´ĕ-sĭs)	**my/o** **-paresis**	muscle weakness	Weakness or slight paralysis of a muscle
myopathy (mī-ŏp´ă-thē)	**my/o** **-pathy**	muscle disease	Muscle disease
myoplasty (mī´ō-plăs˝tē)	**my/o** **-plasty**	muscle surgical repair	Surgical repair of a muscle
myorrhaphy (mī-ōr´ă-fē)	**my/o** **-rrhaphy**	muscle suture	Surgical suture of a muscle wound
myosarcoma (mī˝ō-săr-kō´mă)	**my/o** **sarc** **-oma**	muscle flesh tumor	Malignant tumor derived from muscle tissue
myosclerosis (mī˝ō-sklĕr-ō´sĭs)	**my/o** **scler** **-osis**	muscle hardening condition	Abnormal condition of hardening of muscle

Medical Word	Word Parts		Definition
	Part	Meaning	
myositis (mī″ ō-sī′ tĭs)	my/o(s) -itis	muscle inflammation	Inflammation of muscle tissue, especially skeletal muscles; may be caused by infection, trauma, or parasitic infestation
myospasm (mī′ ō-spăzm)	my/o -spasm	muscle tension, spasm	Spasmodic contraction of a muscle
myotome (mī′ ō-tōm)	my/o -tome	muscle instrument to cut	Surgical instrument used to cut muscle
myotomy (mī″ ŏt′ ō-mē)	my/o -tomy	muscle incision	Surgical incision into a muscle
neuromuscular (nū″ rō-mŭs′ kū-lăr)	neur/o muscul -ar	nerve muscle pertaining to	Pertaining to both nerves and muscles
neuromyopathic (nū″ rō-mī″ ō-păth′ ĭk)	neur/o my/o path -ic	nerve muscle disease pertaining to	Pertaining to a disease condition involving both nerves and muscles
polyplegia (pŏl″ ē-plē′ jē-ă)	poly- -plegia	many paralysis	Paralysis affecting many muscles
position			Bodily posture or attitude; the manner in which a patient's body may be arranged for examination. See Table 6.3.

TABLE 6.3 Types of Patient Positions

Position	Description
anatomic	Body erect, head facing forward, arms by the sides with palms to the front; used as a standard anatomical position of reference
dorsal recumbent	On back with lower extremities flexed and rotated outward; used in application of obstetric forceps, vaginal and rectal examination, and bimanual palpation
Fowler	Head of the bed or examining table is raised about 18 inches or 46 cm; patient is in a semi-upright sitting position (45–60 degrees) with knees either bent or straight

45° angle

Fowler position
Source: MARIEB, ELAINE N.; KELLER, SUZANNE M., ESSENTIALS OF HUMAN ANATOMY & PHYSIOLOGY, 12th Ed., ©2018. Reprinted and Electronically reproduced by permission of Pearson Education, Inc., New York, NY.

TABLE 6.3   Types of Patient Positions *(continued)*

Position	Description
knee-chest	On knees, thighs upright, head and upper part of chest resting on bed or examining table, arms crossed and above head; used in sigmoidoscopy, displacement of prolapsed uterus, rectal exams, and flushing of intestinal canal
lithotomy	On back with lower extremities flexed and both legs placed in stirrups; a gynecologic position used in vaginal examination, Pap smear, vaginal operations, and diagnosis and treatment of diseases of the urethra and bladder

Lithotomy position
Source: MARIEB, ELAINE N.; KELLER, SUZANNE M., ESSENTIALS OF HUMAN ANATOMY & PHYSIOLOGY, 12th Ed., ©2018. Reprinted and Electronically reproduced by permission of Pearson Education, Inc., New York, NY.

Position	Description
orthopneic	Sitting upright or erect; used for patients with dyspnea, shortness of breath (SOB)
prone	Lying face downward; used in examination of the back, injections, and massage

Prone position
Source: MARIEB, ELAINE N.; KELLER, SUZANNE M., ESSENTIALS OF HUMAN ANATOMY & PHYSIOLOGY, 12th Ed., ©2018. Reprinted and Electronically reproduced by permission of Pearson Education, Inc., New York, NY.

TABLE 6.3   Types of Patient Positions *(continued)*

Position	Description
Sims	Lying on left side, right knee and thigh flexed well up above left leg that is slightly flexed, left arm behind the body, and right arm forward, flexed at elbow; used in examination of rectum, sigmoidoscopy, enema, and intrauterine irrigation after labor
supine	Lying flat on back with face upward and arms at the sides; used in examining the head, neck, chest, abdomen, and extremities and in assessing vital signs

Supine position

Source: MARIEB, ELAINE N.; KELLER, SUZANNE M., ESSENTIALS OF HUMAN ANATOMY & PHYSIOLOGY, 12th Ed., ©2018. Reprinted and Electronically reproduced by permission of Pearson Education, Inc., New York, NY.

Position	Description
Trendelenburg	Body supine on a bed or examining table that is tilted at about a 45-degree angle with the head lower than the feet; used to displace abdominal organs during surgery and in treating cardiovascular shock

Trendelenburg position

Source: MARIEB, ELAINE N.; KELLER, SUZANNE M., ESSENTIALS OF HUMAN ANATOMY & PHYSIOLOGY, 12th Ed., ©2018. Reprinted and Electronically reproduced by permission of Pearson Education, Inc., New York, NY.

Medical Word	Word Parts		Definition
	Part	Meaning	
prosthesis (prŏs thē´ sĭs)	prosth/e -sis	an addition state of	Artificial device used to replace an organ or body part, such as a hand, arm, leg, or hip. See Figures 6.13 and 6.14.

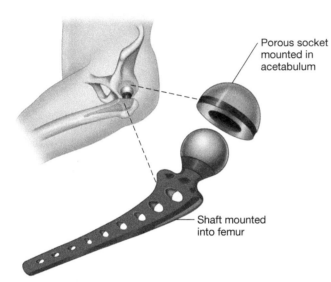

Porous socket mounted in acetabulum

Shaft mounted into femur

FIGURE 6.13 Total hip prosthesis.

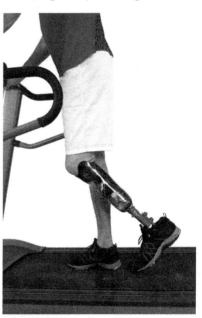

FIGURE 6.14 A man with a leg prosthesis exercising on a treadmill.
Source: Belushi/Shutterstock

Medical Word	Word Parts		Definition
quadriceps (kwŏd´ rĭ-sĕps)	quadri- -ceps	four head	Muscle that has four heads or points of origin
relaxation (rē-lăk-sā´ shŭn)	relaxat -ion	to loosen process	Process in which a muscle loosens and returns to a resting stage
rhabdomyoma (răb˝ dō-mī-ō´ mă)	rhabd/o my -oma	rod muscle tumor	Tumor of striated muscle tissue
rheumatism (roo´ mă-tĭzm)	rheumat -ism	discharge condition	General term used to describe conditions characterized by inflammation, soreness, and stiffness of muscles and pain in joints
rheumatology (roo˝ mă-tŏl´ ō-jē)	rheumat/o -logy	discharge study of	Study of rheumatic diseases
rheumatologist (roo˝ mă-tŏl´ ō-jĭst)	rheumat/o log -ist	discharge study one who specializes	One who specializes in rheumatic diseases
rigor mortis (rĭg´ ur mōr´ tĭs)			Stiffness of skeletal muscles seen in death; develops between the 4th and 24th hour after death, then ceases

Medical Word	Word Parts		Definition
	Part	**Meaning**	
rotation (rō-tā′ shŭn)	**rotat** **-ion**	to turn process	Process of moving a body part around a central axis
rotator cuff (rō-tā′ tor kŭf)			Group of muscles and their tendons that act to stabilize the shoulder

 fyi The rotator cuff is the area that enables people to reach above their heads and lift with the arms. Rotator cuff injuries and/or tears can occur as the result of years of overuse of the muscles and tendons or from a single traumatic injury. The four muscles of the rotator cuff (subscapularis, supraspinatus, infraspinatus, and teres minor), along with the teres major and the deltoid, make up the six **scapulohumeral** muscles (those that connect to the humerus and scapula and act on the glenohumeral joint) of the human body.

Medical Word	Word Parts		Definition
sarcolemma (săr″ kō-lĕm′ ă)	**sarc/o** **-lemma**	flesh sheath	Plasma membrane surrounding each striated muscle fiber
spasticity (spăs-tĭs′ ĭ-tē)	**spastic** **-ity**	convulsive condition	Condition of increased muscular tone causing stiff and awkward movements
sternocleidomastoid (stur″ nō-klī″ dō-măs′ toyd)	**stern/o** **cleid/o** **mast** **-oid**	sternum clavicle mastoid process resemble	Muscle arising from the sternum and clavicle with its insertion in the mastoid process; flexes the neck and helps with movement of the head
strain			Excessive, forcible stretching of a muscle or the musculotendinous unit
synergism (sĭn′ ĕr-jĭzm)	**syn-** **erg-** **-ism**	with, together work condition	Certain muscles working together to produce an effect greater than the sum of their individual effects
synovitis (sĭn″ ō-vī′ tĭs)	**synov** **-itis**	synovial membrane inflammation	Inflammation of a synovial membrane
tendon (tĕn′ dŭn)			Band of fibrous connective tissue serving for the attachment of muscles to bones; a giant cell tumor of a tendon sheath is a benign, small, yellow, tumor-like nodule. See Figure 6.15.

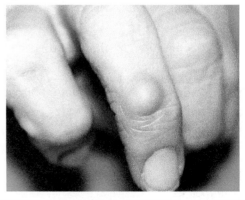

FIGURE 6.15 Giant cell tumor of tendon sheath.
Source: Courtesy of Jason L. Smith, MD

Medical Word	Word Parts		Definition
	Part	Meaning	
tenodesis (těn-ŏd´ ě-sĭs)	ten/o -desis	tendon binding	Surgical binding of a tendon
tenodynia (těn˝ ō-dĭn´ ē-ă)	ten/o -dynia	tendon pain	Pain in a tendon
tetany (tĕt´ ă-nē)			Condition characterized by cramps, convulsions, twitching of the muscles, and sharp flexion of the wrist and ankle joints; generally caused by an abnormality in calcium (Ca) metabolism
tonic (tŏn´ ĭk)	ton -ic	tone, tension pertaining to	Pertaining to tone, especially muscular tension
torsion (tor´ shŭn)	tors -ion	twisted process	Process of being twisted
torticollis (tor´ tĭ-kŏl´ ĭs)	tort/i collis	twisted neck	Stiff neck caused by spasmodic contraction of the muscles of the neck; sometimes called *wryneck*
triceps (trī´ sěps)	tri- -ceps	three head	Muscle having three heads with a single insertion
voluntary (vŏl´ ŭn-těr˝ ē)	volunt -ary	will pertaining to	Under the control of one's will

Study *and* Review II

Word Parts

Prefixes   Give the definitions of the following prefixes.

1. a- _____
2. ab- _____
3. ad- _____
4. ant- _____
5. bi- _____

6. brady- _____
7. con- _____
8. dia- _____
9. dys- _____
10. in- _____

11. intra- _____

12. hydro- _____

13. quadri- _____

14. syn- _____

15. tri- _____

Combining Forms   Give the definitions of the following combining forms.

1. agon/o _____

2. amputat/o _____

3. brach/i _____

4. cleid/o _____

5. duct/o _____

6. fasci/o _____

7. fibr/o _____

8. is/o _____

9. metr/o _____

10. muscul/o _____

11. my/o _____

12. neur/o _____

13. path/o _____

14. prosth/e _____

15. rhabd/o _____

16. rotat/o _____

17. sarc/o _____

18. synov/o _____

19. ten/o _____

20. ton/o _____

21. tors/o _____

22. troph/o _____

23. volunt/o _____

Suffixes   Give the definitions of the following suffixes.

1. -algia _____

2. -ar _____

3. -ary _____

4. -asthenia _____

5. -blast _____

6. -ceps _____

7. -desis _____

8. -dynia _____

9. -in _____

10. -therapy _____

11. -graph _____

12. -ia _____

13. -ic _____

14. -ion _____

15. -ist _____

16. -itis _____

17. -ity _____   **29.** -phragm _____

18. -kinesia _____   **30.** -plasty _____

19. -kinesis _____   **31.** -plegia _____

20. -logy _____   **32.** -rrhaphy _____

21. -ure _____   **33.** -y _____

22. -malacia _____   **34.** -spasm _____

23. -oid _____   **35.** -taxia _____

24. -oma _____   **36.** -tome _____

25. -or _____   **37.** -tomy _____

26. -osis _____   **38.** -trophy _____

27. -paresis _____   **39.** -sis _____

28. -pathy _____   **40.** -ism _____

Identifying Medical Terms

In the spaces provided, write the medical terms for the following meanings.

1. _____ Pertaining to a lack of normal tone or tension

2. _____ Slowness of motion or movement

3. _____ Medical term for cramp of a finger or toe

4. _____ Any condition of abnormal development caused by defective nourishment, often noted by the degeneration of muscles

5. _____ Pertaining to within a muscle, such as an IM injection

6. _____ Muscle that raises or elevates a part

7. _____ Chronic autoimmune neuromuscular disease characterized by varying degrees of weakness of the skeletal (voluntary) muscles of the body

8. _____ Weakness or slight paralysis of a muscle

9. _____ Surgical repair of a muscle

10. _____ Malignant tumor derived from muscle tissue

Matching

Select the appropriate lettered meaning for each of the following words.

_____ **1.** dermatomyositis

_____ **2.** fibromyalgia

_____ **3.** muscular dystrophy

_____ **4.** flaccid

_____ **5.** prosthesis

_____ **6.** rotator cuff

_____ **7.** strain

_____ **8.** tenodynia

_____ **9.** torsion

_____ **10.** voluntary

a. Group of muscles and their tendons that act to stabilize the shoulder

b. Process of being twisted

c. Pain in a tendon

d. Chronic immunological disease with systemic pathology

e. Lacking muscle tone; *weak*, *soft*, and *flabby*

f. Under the control of one's will

g. Refers to a group of genetic diseases characterized by progressive weakness and degeneration of the skeletal or voluntary muscles that control movement

h. Excessive, forcible stretching of a muscle or the musculotendinous unit

i. A chronic widespread musculoskeletal pain and fatigue disorder

j. Artificial device used to replace an organ or a body part, such as a hand, arm, leg, or hip

Medical Case Snapshots

This learning activity provides an opportunity to relate the medical terminology you are learning to sample patient case presentations. In the spaces provided, write in your answers.

Case 1

The 30-year-old female states, "I feel so tired all the time. I can't sleep at night and my muscles ache." The diagnosis is abbreviated FMS. The American College of Rheumatology classifies a patient with _____

_____ (FMS) if at least 11 of 18 trigger points are painful under pressure. This patient had 12 trigger

points, including tiredness or fatigue, and muscle pain also known as _____.

Case 2

In the middle of the night, a 51-year-old man awoke with a sudden, severe pain in his left calf muscle. He immediately flexed his left foot and began massaging his calf muscle. He felt a tight knotted area and cried out in pain. After about 3 minutes, the knot was gone, and the pain subsided. What is the medical term for this described condition?

_____   _____

Case 3

The instructor thought it would be a fun and educational experience to ask her students to stand and demonstrate the standard anatomic position. The student should stand with his or her _____ _____, head facing _____, arms by the sides with _____ to the front. (See Table 6.3.)

Drug Highlights

Classification of Drug	Description and Examples
skeletal muscle relaxants	Used to treat muscle spasms that can result from strains, sprains, spasticity, and musculoskeletal trauma or disease. Muscle spasms or "cramps" are sudden, involuntary contractions of a muscle or group of muscles. They can be caused by too much muscle strain and lead to pain. They're associated with conditions such as lower back pain, neck pain, and fibromyalgia.
	Muscle spasticity, on the other hand, is a continuous muscle spasm that causes stiffness, rigidity, or tightness that can interfere with normal walking, talking, or movement. Muscle spasticity is caused by injury to parts of the brain or spinal cord involved with movement. Conditions that can cause muscle spasticity include multiple sclerosis (MS), cerebral palsy, and amyotrophic lateral sclerosis (ALS).
	Centrally acting muscle relaxants depress the central nervous system (CNS) and can be administered orally or by injection. The patient must be informed of the sedative effect produced by these drugs. Drowsiness, dizziness, and blurred vision can diminish the patient's ability to drive a vehicle, operate equipment, or climb stairs.
	EXAMPLES: Fexnid, Flexeril (cyclobenzaprine HCl), and Robaxin (methocarbamol)
anti-inflammatory agents and analgesics	(See *Drug Highlights* in Chapter 5 for a description of anti-inflammatory agents and analgesics.)

Diagnostic *and* Laboratory Tests

Test	Description
aldolase (ALD) blood test (ăl′ dō-lāz)	Test performed on serum that measures ALD enzyme present in skeletal and heart muscle; helpful in the diagnosis of Duchenne muscular dystrophy before symptoms appear.
calcium blood test (kăl′ sē-ŭm)	Test performed on serum to determine levels of calcium, which is essential for muscular contraction, nerve transmission, and blood clotting.
creatine kinase (CK) (krē′ ă-tĭn kīn′ āz)	Blood test to determine the level of CK, which is increased in necrosis or atrophy of skeletal muscle, traumatic muscle injury, strenuous exercise, and progressive muscular dystrophy.
electromyography (EMG) (ē-lĕk″ trō-mī-ŏg′ ră-fē)	Test to measure electrical activity across muscle membranes by means of electrodes attached to a needle that is inserted into the muscle. Electrical activity can be heard over a loudspeaker, viewed on an oscilloscope, or printed on a graph (electromyogram). Abnormal results can indicate myasthenia gravis, amyotrophic lateral sclerosis, muscular dystrophy, peripheral neuropathy, and anterior poliomyelitis.
lactic dehydrogenase (LDH, LD) (lăk′ tĭk dē-hī-drŏj′ ĕ-nāz)	Blood test to determine the level of LDH enzyme, which is increased in muscular dystrophy, damage to skeletal muscles, after a pulmonary embolism, and during skeletal muscle malignancy.
muscle biopsy	Surgical removal of a small piece of muscle tissue for examination. There are two types. A *needle biopsy* involves inserting a needle into the muscle. When the needle is removed, a small piece of tissue remains in the needle. The tissue is sent to a laboratory for examination. An *open biopsy* involves making a small cut in the skin and into the muscle. The muscle tissue is then removed. A muscle biopsy may be done to identify or detect diseases of the connective tissue and blood vessels (e.g., polyarteritis nodosa); infections that affect the muscles (e.g., trichinosis or toxoplasmosis); muscular disorders such as muscular dystrophy or congenital myopathy; and metabolic defects of the muscle.
aspartate aminotransferase (AST) (ă-spăr′ tāt″ ă-mē″ nō-trăns′ fĕr-ās)	Blood test to determine the level of AST enzyme, which is increased in skeletal muscle damage and muscular dystrophy
alanine aminotransferase (ALT) (ăl′ ăh-nēn ă-mē″ nō-trăns′ fĕr-ās)	Blood test to determine the level of ALT enzyme, which is increased in skeletal muscle damage

Abbreviations *and* Acronyms

Abbreviation/ Acronym	Meaning	Abbreviation/ Acronym	Meaning
ACR	American College of Rheumatology	**ALD**	aldolase
AE	above elbow	**ALT**	alanine aminotransferase
AK	above knee	**AST**	aspartate aminotransferase

Abbreviation/ Acronym	Meaning	Abbreviation/ Acronym	Meaning
BE	below elbow	LDH, LD	lactic dehydrogenase
BK	below knee	MD	muscular dystrophy
Ca	calcium	MG	myasthenia gravis
CK	creatine kinase	MS	musculoskeletal
EMG	electromyography	NCI	National Cancer Institute
FMS	fibromyalgia syndrome	NIH	National Institutes of Health
FROM	full range of motion	ROM	range of motion
IM	intramuscular	SOB	shortness of breath

Study *and* Review III

Building Medical Terms

Using the following word parts, fill in the blanks to build the correct medical terms.

a-	poly-	ten/o	-ary	-graph
bi-	rhabd/o	-ion	-or	-lemma

Definition

1. Surgical removal of a limb, part, or other appendage

2. Lack of muscular coordination

3. Muscle with two points of origin

4. Muscle that raises or elevates a part

5. Instrument used to record muscular contractions

6. Paralysis affecting many muscles

7. Tumor of striated muscle tissue

Medical Term

1. amputat_____

2. _____taxia

3. _____ceps

4. levat_____

5. myo_____

6. _____plegia

7. _____myoma

Definition	Medical Term
8. Plasma membrane surrounding each striated muscle fiber	sarco_____
9. Pain in a tendon	_____dynia
10. Under the control of one's will	volunt_____

Combining Form Challenge

Using the combining forms provided, write the medical term correctly.

is/o	fasci/o	ten/o
my/o	dactyl/o	brach/i

1. Pain in the arm: _____algia

2. Medical term for cramp of a finger or toe: _____spasm

3. Inflammation of a fascia: _____itis

4. Literally means pertaining to having equal measure: _____metric

5. Weakness or slight paralysis of a muscle: _____paresis

6. Pain in a tendon: _____dynia

Select the Right Term

Select the correct answer, and write it on the line provided.

1. Muscle that counteracts the action of another muscle is _____.

   adductor   aponeurosis   antagonist   atrophy

2. Process of drawing-up and thickening of a muscle fiber is _____.

   bradykinesia   contraction   contracture   dystonia

3. Lacking muscle tone; weak, soft, and flabby is _____.

   isotonic   myokinesis   flaccid   relaxation

4. Surgical repair of a muscle is _____.

   myopathy   myoplasty   myorrhaphy   myotome

5. Certain muscles working together to produce an effect greater than the sum of their individual effects is
_____.

    synergism   synovitis   adductor   tetany

6. Stiff neck, sometimes called wryneck, is _____.

    triceps   torticollis   tonic   tenodesis

Drug Highlights

Write in the correct answer for each of the following questions.

1. Which type of drug classification is used to treat painful muscle spasms? _____ _____ _____

2. Muscle spasms can result from strains, _____, _____, and musculoskeletal trauma or disease.

3. Muscle "cramps" are sudden, _____ contractions of a muscle.

4. _____ _____ is a continuous muscle spasm.

5. Fexnid is an example of a skeletal _____ _____ with the generic name of _____.

6. The patient must be informed of the _____ effect produced by these drugs.

7. The patient is advised not to _____ a vehicle, _____ _____, or climb stairs.

Diagnostic and Laboratory Tests

Select the best answer to each multiple-choice question. Circle the letter of your choice.

1. Diagnostic test to help diagnose Duchenne muscular dystrophy before symptoms appear.

  a. creatine kinase   **c.** calcium blood test

  b. aldolase blood test   **d.** muscle biopsy

2. Test to measure electrical activity across muscle membranes by means of electrodes that are attached to a needle that is inserted into the muscle.

  a. muscle biopsy   **c.** creatine kinase

  b. lactic dehydrogenase   **d.** electromyography

3. Blood test to determine the level of _____ enzyme, which is increased in skeletal muscle damage and muscular dystrophy.

    a. lactic dehydrogenase   **c.** aldolase

    b. aspartate aminotransferase   **d.** creatine kinase

4. Blood test to determine the level of _____ enzyme, which is increased in skeletal muscle damage, is:

    a. lactic dehydrogenase   **c.** alanine aminotransferase

    b. aldolase   **d.** creatine kinase

5. _____ is the surgical removal of a small piece of muscle tissue for examination.

    a. Muscle biopsy   **c.** Bone biopsy

    b. Electromyography   **d.** Electrocardiography

Abbreviations and Acronyms

Write the correct word, phrase, or abbreviation/acronym in the space provided.

1. AE _____

2. AST _____

3. calcium _____

4. electromyography _____

5. FROM _____

6. MS _____

7. range of motion _____

8. MG _____

9. MD _____

10. FMS _____

Practical Application

Medical Record Analysis

This exercise contains information, abbreviations/acronyms, and medical terminology from an actual medical record or case study that has been adapted for this text. The names and any personal information have been created by the author. Read and study each form or case study and then answer the questions that follow. You may refer to Appendix III, *Abbreviations, Acronyms, and Symbols*.

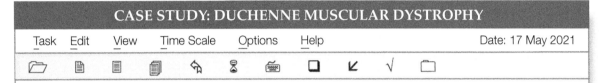

CASE STUDY: DUCHENNE MUSCULAR DYSTROPHY						
Task Edit View Time Scale Options Help					Date: 17 May 2021	

A 3-year-old male child was seen by a physician; the following is a synopsis of the visit.

Present History: The mother states that she noticed that her son has been falling a lot and seems to be very clumsy. She says that he has a waddling gait, is very slow in running and climbing, and walks on his toes. She is most concerned as she is at risk for carrying the gene that causes muscular dystrophy (MD).

Signs and Symptoms: A waddling gait, very slow in running and climbing, walks on his toes, frequent falling, clumsy.

Diagnosis: Duchenne muscular dystrophy. The diagnosis was determined by the characteristic symptoms, family history, a muscle biopsy, an electromyography (EMG), and an elevated serum creatine kinase (CK) level.

Treatment: Physical therapy, deep breathing exercises to help delay muscular weakness, supportive measures such as splints and braces to help minimize deformities and to preserve mobility. Counseling and referral services are essential. For more information and resources, the family may visit the website of the Muscular Dystrophy Association at www.mda.org.

Case Study Questions

Write the correct answer in the space provided.

1. Signs and symptoms of Duchenne muscular dystrophy include a _____ gait, frequent falls, clumsiness, slowness in running and climbing, and walking on toes.

2. The diagnosis was determined by the characteristic symptoms, family history, a muscle biopsy, an _____, and an elevated serum creatine kinase level.

3. As part of the treatment for Duchenne muscular dystrophy, the use of splints and braces help to

(a) _____ and (b) _____.

4. Define *electromyography*. _____

5. Define *muscle biopsy*. _____

MyLab Medical Terminology™

MyLab Medical Terminology is a premium online homework management system that includes a host of features to help you study. Registered users will find:

- A multitude of activities and assignments built within the MyLab platform
- Powerful tools that track and analyze your results—allowing you to create a personalized learning experience
- Videos and audio pronunciations to help enrich your progress
- Streaming lesson presentations (guided lectures) and self-paced learning modules
- A space where you and your instructor can check your progress and manage your assignments

Digestive System

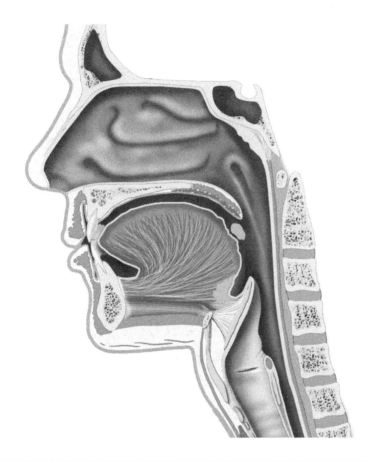

 Learning Outcomes

On completion of this chapter, you will be able to:

1. Describe the digestive system.
2. Explain the primary functions of the organs of the digestive system.
3. Describe the two sets of teeth found in humans.
4. Identify the three main portions of a tooth.
5. Discuss the accessory organs of the digestive system and state their functions.
6. Analyze, build, spell, and pronounce medical words.
7. Classify the drugs highlighted in this chapter.
8. Describe diagnostic and laboratory tests related to the digestive system.
9. Identify and define selected abbreviations and acronyms.

Anatomy and Physiology

A general description of the digestive or gastrointestinal (GI) system is that of a continuous tube beginning with the mouth and ending at the anus. This tube is known as the **alimentary canal** and/or **gastrointestinal tract**. It measures about 30 feet in adults and contains both primary and accessory organs for the conversion of food and fluids into a semiliquid that can be absorbed for the body to use. The primary organs of the digestive system are the mouth, pharynx, esophagus, stomach, small intestine, and large intestine. The accessory organs of the digestive system are the salivary glands, liver, gallbladder, and pancreas.

The three main functions of the digestive system are digestion, absorption, and elimination. **Digestion** is the process by which food is changed in the mouth, stomach, and intestines by chemical, mechanical, and enzymatic action, so that the body can absorb it. Digestion begins in the mouth, as food is broken apart by the action of the teeth, moistened and lubricated by saliva, and formed into a **bolus** (small mass of chewed food ready to be swallowed). Digestive enzymes increase chemical reactions and, in so doing, break down complex nutrients. Digestive enzymes are secreted by different exocrine glands including the salivary glands, secretory cells in the stomach, secretory cells in the pancreas, and secretory glands in the small intestine. **Absorption** is the process by which nutrient material is taken into the bloodstream or lymph and travels to all cells of the body. Valuable nutrients such as amino acids, glucose, fatty acids, and glycerol can then be utilized for energy, growth, and development of the body. **Elimination** is the process whereby the solid waste (end) products of digestion are excreted. Each of the various organs commonly associated with digestion is described in this chapter. See Table 7.1 for the digestive system at-a-glance. The organs of digestion are shown in Figure 7.1.

TABLE 7.1 Digestive System at-a-Glance

Organ/Structure	Primary Functions/Description
Mouth	Mechanically breaks food apart by the action of the teeth; moistens and lubricates food with saliva; food formed into a bolus, a soft mass of chewed food ready to be swallowed
Teeth	Used in mastication (chewing)
Salivary glands	Secrete saliva to moisten and lubricate food
Pharynx	Common passageway for both respiration and digestion; muscular constrictions move the swallowed bolus into the esophagus
Esophagus	Moves the bolus by peristalsis (wavelike contractions) down the esophagus into the stomach
Stomach	Reduces food to a digestible state; converts the food to a semiliquid state called **chyme** (mixture of partly digested food and digestive secretions)
Small intestine	Digestion and absorption take place chiefly in the small intestine; nutrients are absorbed and transferred to body cells by the circulatory system
Large intestine	Reabsorbs water from the fecal material, stores, and then eliminates waste from the body via the rectum and anus
Liver	Changes glucose to glycogen and stores it until needed; changes glycogen back to glucose; desaturates fats; assists in protein *catabolism* (the metabolic breaking-down of complex substances into more basic elements); manufactures bile, fibrinogen, prothrombin, heparin, and blood proteins; stores vitamins; produces heat; and detoxifies toxins
Gallbladder	Stores and concentrates bile that has been produced by the liver
Pancreas	Secretes pancreatic juice into the small intestine, contains cells that produce digestive enzymes, produces the hormones insulin and glucagon

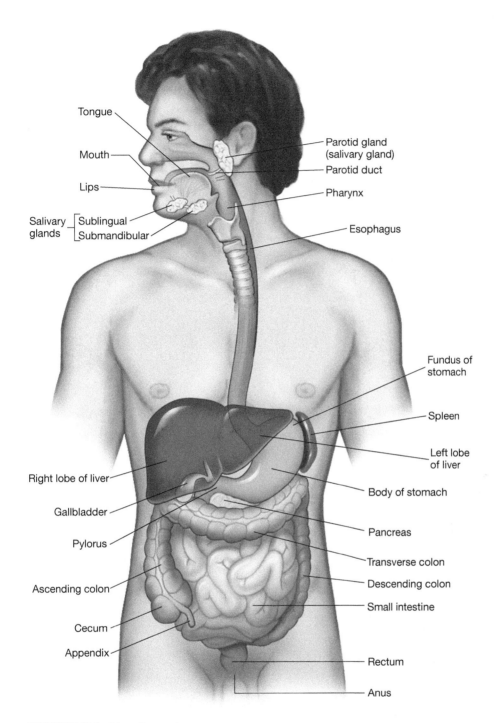

FIGURE 7.1 Digestive system.

fyi

With aging, the digestive system becomes less motile as muscle contractions become weaker. Glandular secretions decrease, thus causing a drier mouth and a lower volume of gastric juices. Nutrient absorption is mildly reduced due to **atrophy** of the mucosal lining. The teeth are mechanically worn down with age, and the gums begin to recede from the teeth. There is a loss of taste buds, and food preferences change. Gastric motor activity slows; as a result, gastric emptying is delayed and hunger contractions diminish.

Mouth

The **mouth** or *oral cavity* is formed by the hard and soft palates at the top or roof, the cheeks on the sides, the tongue at the floor, and the lips that frame the opening to the cavity. See Figure 7.2. Contained within are the teeth and salivary glands. The vestibule includes the space between the cheeks and the teeth. The **gingivae** (gums) surround the necks of the teeth. The free portion of the tongue is connected to the underlying epithelium by a thin fold of mucous membrane, the **lingual frenulum**, which prevents extreme movement of the tongue.

The **tongue** is made of skeletal muscle and is covered with mucous membrane. It manipulates food during chewing and assists in swallowing. The tongue can be divided into a blunt rear portion called the **root**, a pointed **tip**, and a central **body**. Located on the surface of the tongue are **papillae** (elevations) and **taste buds** (sweet, sour, salty, bitter, and savory).

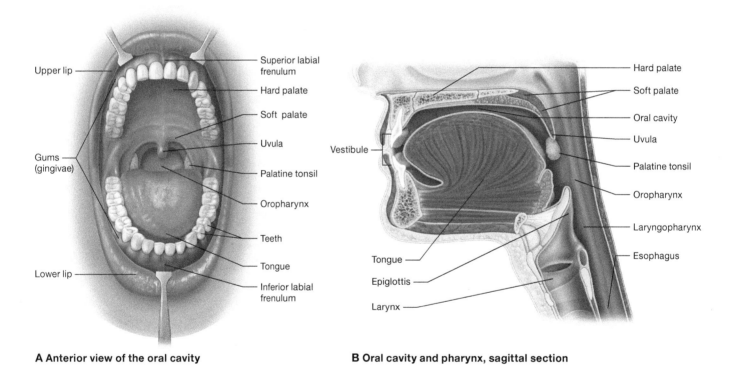

A Anterior view of the oral cavity

B Oral cavity and pharynx, sagittal section

FIGURE 7.2 Oral cavity: **A** anterior view as seen through the open mouth; **B** sagittal section of oral cavity and pharynx.
Source: AMERMAN, ERIN C., HUMAN ANATOMY & PHYSIOLOGY, 2nd Ed., ©2019. Reprinted and Electronically reproduced by permission of Pearson Education, Inc., New York, NY.

fyi

Umami (oo-mŏm' ē), or savory taste, has become one of the five basic tastes. It has been described as savoriness or deliciousness and is a characteristic of certain broths and cooked meats. People taste umami through taste receptors that typically respond to glutamate, which is widely present in meat broths and fermented products and commonly added to some foods in the form of monosodium glutamate (MSG). Because umami has its own taste receptors rather than arising out of a combination of the traditionally recognized taste receptors (sweet, sour, salty, and bitter), scientists now consider umami to be a distinct taste. Most taste buds on the tongue and other regions of the mouth can detect umami taste, irrespective of their location. The taste responsible for the sense of umami was first noted by a Japanese scientist. There is no English word that is synonymous with umami, so the term *savory* is used to designate umami.

Three pairs of salivary glands secrete saliva into the oral cavity. The posterior margin of the soft palate supports the dangling uvula and two pairs of muscular pharyngeal arches. On either side, a palatine tonsil lies between an anterior glossopalatine arch and a posterior pharyngopalatine arch. A curving line that connects the palatine arches and uvula forms the boundaries of the fauces, the passageway between the oral cavity and the pharynx. Digestion begins as food is broken apart by the action of the teeth, moistened and lubricated by saliva, and formed into a bolus. See Figure 7.3.

Teeth

Human beings are provided two sets of teeth. The 20 **deciduous teeth**, the temporary teeth of the primary dentition, include eight incisors, four canines (cuspids), and eight molars. Deciduous teeth are also referred to as *milk teeth* or *baby teeth*. There are 32 **permanent** or **secondary dentition teeth**: eight incisors, four canines, eight premolars, and 12 molars. See Figure 7.4.

The **incisors** are so named because they present a sharp cutting edge, adapted for biting into food. They form the four front teeth in each dental arch. The **canine** or **cuspid** teeth are larger and stronger than the incisors. Their roots sink deeply into the bones and cause well-marked prominences upon the surface. The **premolars** or **bicuspid** teeth are situated lateral to and behind the canine teeth. The **molar** teeth are the largest of the permanent set, and their broad crowns are adapted for grinding and pounding food. The deciduous teeth are smaller than, but generally resemble in form, the teeth that bear the same names in the permanent set.

Each tooth consists of three main portions: the **crown**, projecting above the gum; the **root**, embedded in the alveolus; and the **neck**, the constricted portion between the crown and root. On making a vertical section of a tooth, a cavity will be found in the interior of the crown and the center of each root; it opens by a minute orifice at the extremity of the latter. See Figure 7.5.

This cavity is called the **pulp cavity**, which contains the dental pulp, a loose connective tissue richly supplied with vessels and nerves that enter the cavity through the small aperture at the point of each root. The pulp cavity receives blood vessels and nerves from the **root canal**, a narrow tunnel located at the root, or base, of the tooth. Blood vessels and nerves enter the root canal through an opening called the **apical foramen** to supply the pulp cavity.

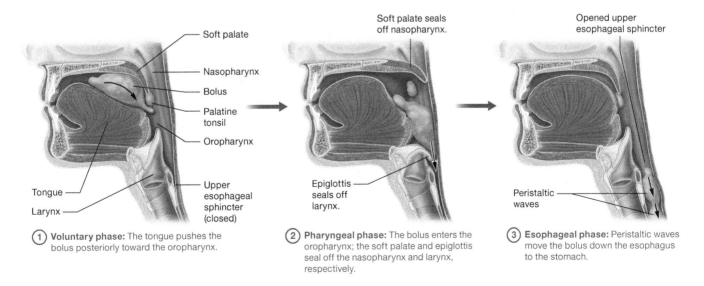

① **Voluntary phase:** The tongue pushes the bolus posteriorly toward the oropharynx.

② **Pharyngeal phase:** The bolus enters the oropharynx; the soft palate and epiglottis seal off the nasopharynx and larynx, respectively.

③ **Esophageal phase:** Peristaltic waves move the bolus down the esophagus to the stomach.

FIGURE 7.3 Movement of a bolus of food from the mouth to the esophagus. The bolus then travels to the stomach.

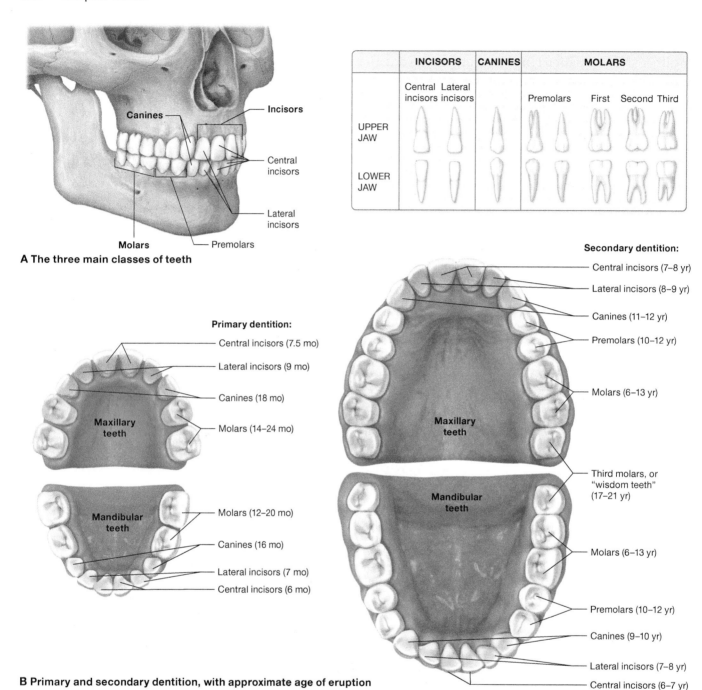

A The three main classes of teeth

	INCISORS		CANINES	MOLARS			
	Central incisors	Lateral incisors		Premolars	First	Second	Third
UPPER JAW							
LOWER JAW							

Primary dentition:
- Central incisors (7.5 mo)
- Lateral incisors (9 mo)
- Canines (18 mo)
- Molars (14–24 mo)

Maxillary teeth

Mandibular teeth
- Molars (12–20 mo)
- Canines (16 mo)
- Lateral incisors (7 mo)
- Central incisors (6 mo)

Secondary dentition:
- Central incisors (7–8 yr)
- Lateral incisors (8–9 yr)
- Canines (11–12 yr)
- Premolars (10–12 yr)
- Molars (6–13 yr)

Maxillary teeth

Mandibular teeth
- Third molars, or "wisdom teeth" (17–21 yr)
- Molars (6–13 yr)
- Premolars (10–12 yr)
- Canines (9–10 yr)
- Lateral incisors (7–8 yr)
- Central incisors (6–7 yr)

B Primary and secondary dentition, with approximate age of eruption

FIGURE 7.4 Types of teeth and the primary and secondary dentition.

Source: AMERMAN, ERIN C., HUMAN ANATOMY & PHYSIOLOGY, 2nd Ed., ©2019. Reprinted and Electronically reproduced by permission of Pearson Education, Inc., New York, NY.

The root of each tooth sits in a bony socket called an *alveolus*. Collagen fibers of the **periodontal ligament** extend from the dentin of the root to the bone of the alveolus, creating a strong articulation known as a *gomphosis*, which binds the teeth to bony sockets in the maxillary bone and mandible. A layer of **cementum** (a thin layer of bone) covers the dentin of the root, providing protection and firmly anchoring the periodontal ligament.

The solid portion of the tooth consists of the **dentin**, which forms the bulk of the tooth; the **enamel**, which covers the exposed part of the crown and is the hardest and most compact part of a tooth; and the cementum, which is deposited on the surface of the root.

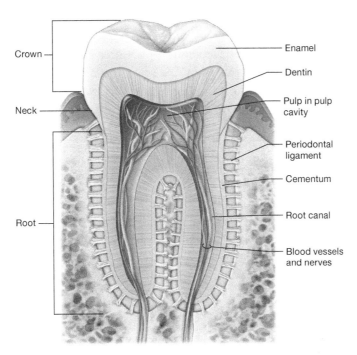

Crown

Neck

Root

Enamel

Dentin

Pulp in pulp
cavity

Periodontal
ligament

Cementum

Root canal

Blood vessels
and nerves

FIGURE 7.5 Structure of a tooth.
Source: AMERMAN, ERIN C., HUMAN ANATOMY & PHYSIOLOGY,
2nd Ed., ©2019. Reprinted and Electronically reproduced by permission
of Pearson Education, Inc., New York, NY.

The neck of the tooth marks the boundary between the root and the crown, the exposed portion of the tooth that projects above the soft tissue of the *gingiva*. A shallow groove called the **gingival sulcus** surrounds the neck of each tooth.

Pharynx

The **pharynx**, or throat, is a chamber that extends between the internal nares and the entrance to the larynx and esophagus (refer to Figures 7.1 and 7.2B). Its three subdivisions are the nasopharynx, oropharynx, and laryngopharynx. The upper portion, the **nasopharynx**, is above the soft palate. The middle portion, the **oropharynx**, lies between the palate and the hyoid bone and has an opening to the oral cavity. The lowest portion, the **laryngopharynx**, is below the hyoid bone and opens inferiorly to the larynx anteriorly and the esophagus posteriorly.

The pharynx is a common passageway for both respiration and digestion. Both the **larynx**, or voice box, and the esophagus begin in the pharynx. Food that is swallowed passes through the pharynx into the esophagus reflexively. Muscular contractions move the bolus into the esophagus and the **epiglottis** (a flap of tissue) blocks the opening of the larynx, preventing food from entering the airway leading to the trachea (windpipe).

Esophagus

The **esophagus** is a muscular tube about 10 inches long that leads from the pharynx to the stomach (refer to Figures 7.1 and 7.2B). Food and liquids pass down the esophagus and into the stomach. At the junction with the stomach is the lower esophageal sphincter (LES) or **cardiac sphincter**. This sphincter relaxes to permit passage of food and then contracts to prevent the backup of stomach contents. Food is carried along the esophagus by a series of wavelike muscular contractions called **peristalsis**.

Stomach

The **stomach** is a muscular, distensible saclike portion of the alimentary canal between the esophagus and duodenum. See Figure 7.6. The upper region of the stomach is called the *fundus,* the main portion is called the *body,* and the lower region is the *antrum.* There are folds in the mucous membrane lining the stomach called *rugae* that stretch when the stomach fills with food and contain glands that produce digestive juices.

Food and liquids pass from the esophagus into the stomach. Here food is reduced to a digestible state by mechanical churning and the release of chemicals such as hydrochloric acid, digestive hormones, and enzymes. Hydrochloric acid and gastric juices help convert food to a semiliquid state called **chyme,** which is passed at intervals through a valve called the pyloric sphincter into the small intestine. An empty stomach has a volume of about 50 mL. Typically after a meal, its capacity can expand to about 1 liter and may expand to hold as much as 4 liters.

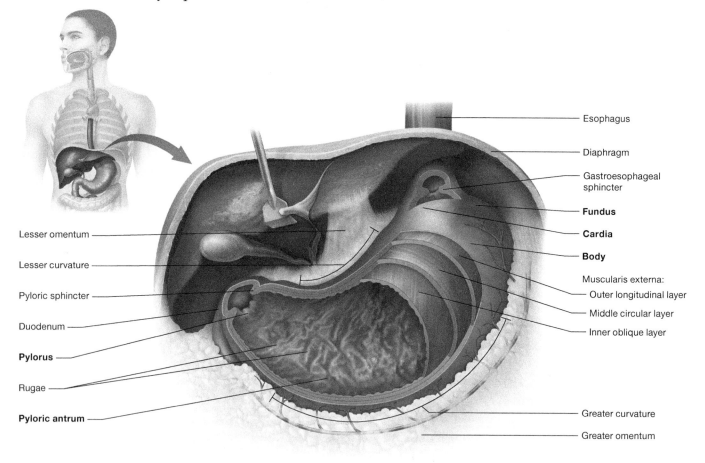

FIGURE 7.6 Regions and tissue layers of the stomach.
Source: AMERMAN, ERIN C., HUMAN ANATOMY & PHYSIOLOGY, 2nd Ed., ©2019. Reprinted and Electronically reproduced by permission of Pearson Education, Inc., New York, NY.

 fyi Have you ever experienced "hunger pains"? *Hunger* is a sensation arising from a lack of food and is characterized by a dull, aching feeling felt in the *epigastrium* (the part of the upper abdomen immediately over the stomach). Hunger pains are linked to contractions of the stomach. Hunger is the physical drive to eat, while *appetite* is the psychological drive to eat. Hunger is affected by the physiological interactions of hormones, while appetite is affected by habits, culture, taste, and other factors. A *craving* is a desire for a specific substance, such as a food, a beverage, or an addictive substance.

Small Intestine

The **small intestine** is about 21 feet long and 1 inch in diameter. It extends from the pyloric sphincter at the base of the stomach to the entrance of the large intestine. The small intestine is divided into three parts: the **duodenum**, the **jejunum**, and the **ileum**. The duodenum is the first 12 inches just beyond the stomach. The jejunum is the next 8 feet or so, and the ileum is the remaining 12 feet of the tube. See Figure 7.7.

Digestion and absorption take place chiefly in the small intestine. Chyme is received from the stomach through the pylorus and is mixed with bile from the liver and gallbladder along with pancreatic juice from the pancreas. Intestinal villi, the tiny, finger-like projections in the wall of the small intestine, increase the surface area and thus the absorptive area of the intestinal wall, providing more places for food to be absorbed. It is important that food is absorbed at a considerably fast rate so as to allow more food to be absorbed.

Digested nutrients (including sugars and amino acids) pass into the villi through diffusion. Complex proteins are broken down into simple amino acids, complicated sugars are reduced to simple sugars (glucose), and large fat molecules (triglycerides) are broken down to fatty acids and glycerol. Circulating blood then transmits these nutrients to body cells. Enzymes within the villi capillaries collect amino acids and simple sugars, which are taken up by the villi and sent into the bloodstream. Villus lacteals (lymph capillary) collect absorbed lipoproteins and are taken to the rest of the body through the lymph fluid.

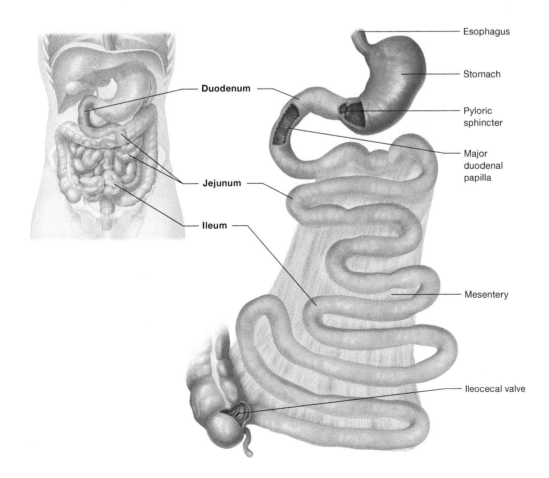

FIGURE 7.7 Small intestine.

Source: AMERMAN, ERIN C., HUMAN ANATOMY & PHYSIOLOGY, 2nd Ed., ©2019. Reprinted and Electronically reproduced by permission of Pearson Education, Inc., New York, NY.

Large Intestine

The **large intestine** is about 5 feet long and 2½ inches in diameter. It extends from the ileocecal valve at the small intestine to the anus. The large intestine is divided into the **cecum**, the **colon**, the **rectum**, and the **anal canal**. The cecum is a pouchlike structure forming the beginning of the large intestine. It is about 3 inches long and has the **appendix** attached to it. The colon makes up the bulk of the large intestine and is divided into the ascending colon, the transverse colon, the descending colon, and the sigmoid colon. See Figure 7.8. With digestion and absorption completed in the large intestine, the waste product of digestion (feces, stool) is expelled through the anus during defecation (evacuation of the bowel).

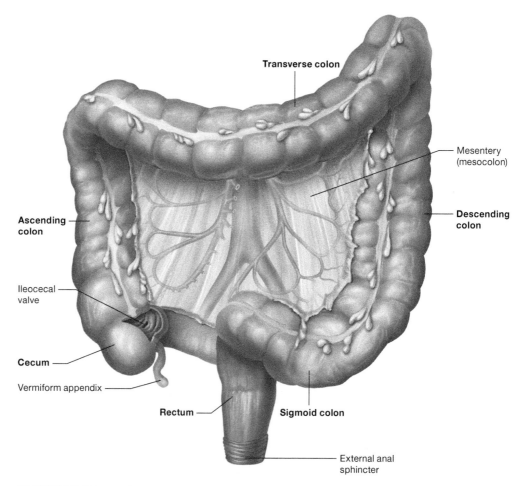

FIGURE 7.8 Large intestine.
Source: AMERMAN, ERIN C., HUMAN ANATOMY & PHYSIOLOGY, 2nd Ed., ©2019. Reprinted and Electronically reproduced by permission of Pearson Education, Inc., New York, NY.

fyi **Meconium**, the first stool, is a mixture of amniotic fluid and secretions of the intestinal glands. It is thick, sticky, and dark green in color. It is usually passed 8–24 hours following birth. The stool during the first week is loose and greenish-yellow. The stool of a breast-fed baby is bright yellow, soft, and pasty. The stool of a bottle-fed baby is more solid than that of a breast-fed baby, and the color varies from yellow to brown.

Accessory Organs

The salivary glands, liver, gallbladder, and pancreas are not actually part of the digestive tube; however, they are closely related to the digestive process.

Salivary Glands

There are three pairs of major salivary glands under and behind the jaw. These are the parotid, sublingual, and submandibular. Many other tiny salivary glands are in the lips, inside the cheeks, and throughout the mouth and throat. The **salivary glands** secrete **saliva** in response to the sight, smell, taste, or mental image of food. Human saliva is composed of 98% water, while the other 2% consists of other compounds such as electrolytes, mucus, antibacterial compounds, and various enzymes that help start the process of digestion. The various salivary glands are the **parotid**, located on either side of the face slightly below the ear; the **submandibular**, located in the floor of the mouth; and the **sublingual**, located below the tongue. All salivary glands secrete through openings (salivary ducts) into the mouth to lubricate food and begin the digestion of carbohydrates. See Figure 7.9.

Liver

The largest glandular organ in the body, the **liver** weighs about 3½ pounds and is located in the upper right part of the abdomen. See Figure 7.10. The liver plays an essential role in the normal metabolism of carbohydrates, fats, and proteins. In carbohydrate (CHO) metabolism, it changes glucose to glycogen and stores the glycogen until needed by body cells. When required, glycogen is converted back to glucose. In fat metabolism, the

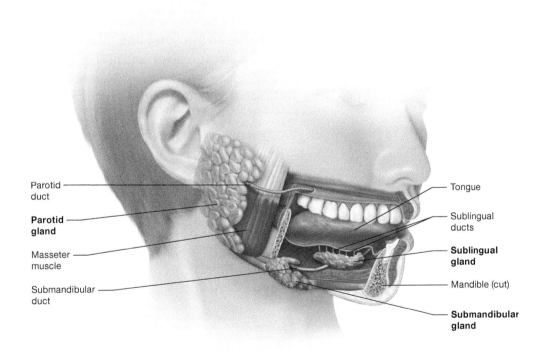

FIGURE 7.9 Anatomy of the salivary glands.

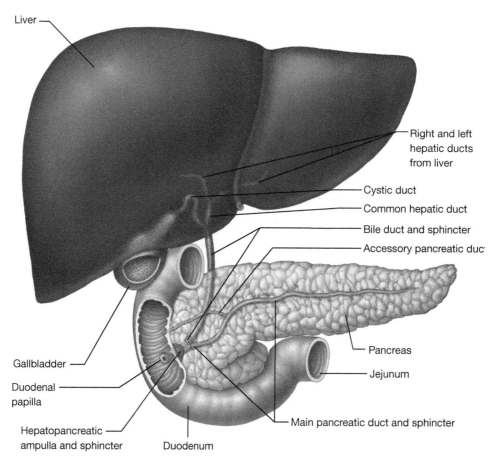

FIGURE 7.10 The liver, gallbladder, and pancreas.
Source: MARIEB, ELAINE N.; KELLER, SUZANNE M., ESSENTIALS OF HUMAN ANATOMY & PHYSIOLOGY, 12th Ed., ©2018.
Reprinted and Electronically reproduced by permission of Pearson Education, Inc., New York, NY.

liver serves as a storage place and acts to desaturate fats before releasing them into the bloodstream. In protein metabolism, the liver acts as a storage place and assists in both protein **catabolism** (metabolic breaking-down of complex substances into more basic elements) and **anabolism** (building-up of the body substances in the constructive phase of metabolism).

The liver manufactures the following important substances:

- **Bile.** Digestive juice important in fat emulsification (the breakdown of large fat globules into smaller particles)
- **Fibrinogen** and **prothrombin.** Coagulants essential for blood clotting
- **Heparin.** Anticoagulant that helps to prevent the clotting of blood
- **Blood proteins.** Albumin, gamma globulin

Additionally, the liver stores iron and vitamins B_{12}, A, D, E, and K. It also detoxifies many harmful substances (toxins) such as drugs and alcohol.

fyi Newborns produce very little saliva until they are 3 months of age and swallowing is a reflex action. The infant's stomach is small and empties rapidly. The liver of the newborn is often immature, thereby causing **jaundice.** Fat absorption is poor because of a decreased level of bile production.

Gallbladder

The **gallbladder (GB)** is a small pear-shaped sac under the liver. The gallbladder stores bile, which is produced by the liver, and then concentrates it for future use. Refer to Figures 7.1 and 7.10. Bile leaving the gallbladder is 6–10 times more concentrated as that which comes to it from the liver. Concentration is accomplished by removal of water.

Pancreas

The **pancreas** is a large, elongated gland situated behind the stomach that secretes pancreatic juice into the small intestine. Refer to Figures 7.1 and 7.10. The pancreas is 6–9 inches long and contains cells that produce digestive **enzymes**. Other specialized cells in the pancreas secrete the hormones insulin and glucagon directly into the bloodstream. The beta cells of the islets of Langerhans make and release insulin. The alpha cells of the islets of Langerhans synthesize and secrete glucagon.

GOOD TO KNOW ▶

Salmonellosis is a common bacterial infection caused by any of more than 2,000 strains of *Salmonella* bacteria. These bacteria infect the intestinal tract and occasionally the blood. Salmonellosis is typically a foodborne illness acquired from contaminated raw meat, eggs, and unpasteurized milk and cheese products, but all foods including vegetables and cereal may become contaminated. Food and food products can be contaminated by the hands of an infected food handler. *Salmonella* bacteria may also be found in the feces of some pets, especially those with diarrhea, and in the feces of reptiles. People can become infected if they do not wash their hands after contact with these pets. Symptoms typically develop between 12 and 72 hours after infection, and the illness usually lasts about 4–7 days. Most healthy individuals recover without the need for treatment. However, some cases are so severe that patients need to be hospitalized. The infection can spread from the intestines to the bloodstream and other parts of the body. These cases can become deadly if not promptly treated with antibiotics.

According to the Centers for Disease Control and Prevention, *Salmonella* bacteria causes about 1.2 million illnesses each year in the United States, with approximately 23,000 cases in which patients have to be hospitalized. Infants, older adults, and people with weakened immune systems are at an increased risk of serious complications from *Salmonella* infection. Salmonellosis is blamed for about 450 deaths in the United States each year.

Study *and* Review I

Anatomy and Physiology

Write your answers to the following questions.

1. Name the primary organs commonly associated with digestion.

a. _____   d. _____

b. _____   e. _____

c. _____   f. _____

2. Name four accessory organs of digestion.

a. _____   c. _____

b. _____   d. _____

3. State the three main functions of the digestive system.

a. _____   c. _____

b. _____

4. Define *bolus*. _____

5. Define *peristalsis*. _____

6. _____ and _____ convert the food into a semiliquid state.

7. The _____ is the first portion of the small intestine.

8. Semiliquid food is called _____.

9. The _____ transports nutrients to body cells.

10. The large intestine can be divided into four distinct sections called the _____, the _____, the _____, and the _____.

11. The _____ is the largest glandular organ in the body.

12. State the function of the gallbladder. _____

13. Name an important function of the pancreas. _____

14. State three functions of the liver.

a. _____   c. _____

b. _____

15. Where does digestion and absorption chiefly take place? _____

16. The salivary glands located in and about the mouth are called the _____, the _____, and the _____.

17. The two hormones secreted into the bloodstream by the pancreas are the _____ and _____.

ANATOMY LABELING   Identify the structures shown below by filling in the blanks.

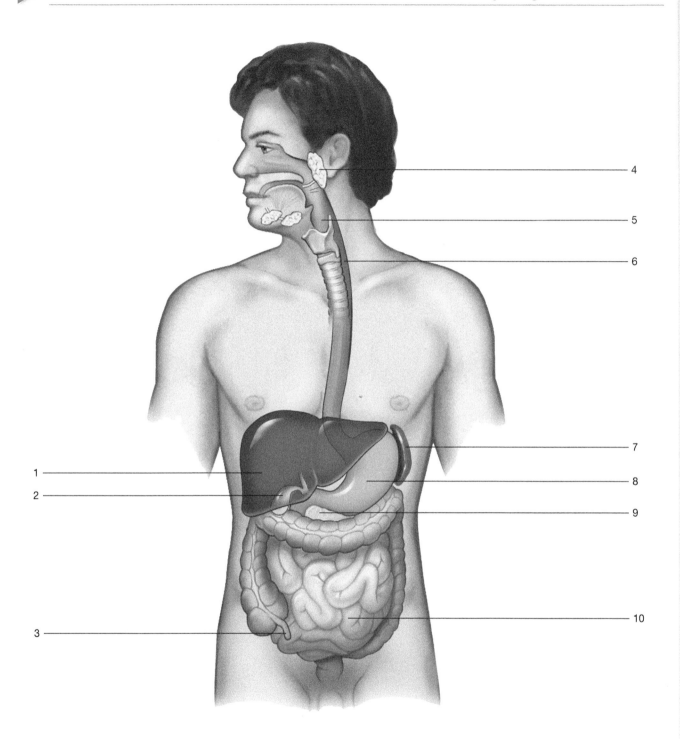

Building Your Medical Vocabulary

This section provides the foundation for learning medical terminology. Review the alphabetized list of medical terms in the following pages. Note how common prefixes and suffixes are repeatedly applied to word roots and combining forms to create different meanings. A combining form is a word root plus a vowel. The chart below lists the combining forms and word roots used in this chapter and can help to strengthen your understanding of how medical words are built and spelled.

You will find that some terms have not been divided into word parts. These are common words or specialized terms that are included to enhance your medical vocabulary.

Combining Forms

absorpt/o	to take in	**glyc/o**	sweet, sugar
aden/o	gland	**halit/o**	breath
amyl/o	starch	**hemat/o**	blood
anabol/o	building-up	**hemorrh/o**	vein liable to bleed
append/o	appendix	**hepat/o**	liver
appendic/o	appendix	**herni/o**	hernia
bil/i	gall, bile	**ile/o**	ileum
bucc/o	cheek	**labi/o**	lip
catabol/o	casting-down	**lapar/o**	abdomen
celi/o	abdomen, belly	**lingu/o**	tongue
cheil/o	lip	**mes/o**	middle
chol/e	gall, bile	**odont/o**	tooth
choledoch/o	common bile duct	**pancreat/o**	pancreas
cirrh/o	orange-yellow	**pept/o**	to digest
col/o	colon	**pharyng/e, pharyng/o**	pharynx
colon/o	colon	**pil/o**	hair
cyst/o	bladder	**prand/i**	meal
dent/o	tooth	**proct/o**	anus and rectum
diverticul/o	diverticula	**pylor/o**	pylorus, gatekeeper
duoden/o	duodenum	**rect/o**	rectum
enter/o	intestine	**sial/o**	saliva, salivary
esophage/o, esophag/o	esophagus	**sigmoid/o**	sigmoid
gastr/o	stomach	**splen/o**	spleen
gingiv/o	gums	**stomat/o**	mouth
gloss/o	tongue	**verm/i**	worm

Word Roots

constipat	to press together	**masticat**	to chew
eme	to vomit	**nid**	nest
laxat	to loosen	**paralyt**	to disable, paralysis
log	study	**volvul**	to roll

Medical Word	Word Parts		Definition
	Part	Meaning	
absorption (ăb-sōrp´ shŭn)	**absorpt** -ion	to take in process	Process by which nutrient material is transferred from the gastrointestinal tract into the bloodstream or lymph
amylase (ăm´ ĭ-lās)	**amyl** -ase	starch enzyme	Enzyme that breaks down starch. Ptyalin is a salivary amylase and amylopsin is a pancreatic amylase.
anabolism (ă-năb´ ō-lĭzm)	**anabol** -ism	building-up condition	Building-up of body substances in the constructive phase of metabolism
anorexia (ăn˝ ō-rĕk´ sē-ă)	**an-** -orexia	lack of appetite	Lack of appetite; decreased desire for food
appendectomy (ăp˝ ĕn-dĕk´ tō-mē)	**append** -ectomy	appendix surgical excision	Surgical excision of the appendix. See Figure 7.11.

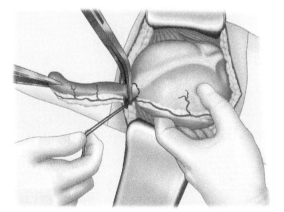

FIGURE 7.11 Appendectomy. The appendix and cecum are brought through the incision to the surface of the abdomen. The base of the appendix is clamped and ligated, and the appendix is then removed.

Medical Word	Word Parts		Definition
	Part	**Meaning**	
appendicitis (ă-pĕn″dĭ-sī′tĭs)	**appendic** **-itis**	appendix inflammation	Inflammation of the appendix. A point of tenderness in acute appendicitis is known as *McBurney point*, located on the right side of the abdomen, 1–2 inches above the anterosuperior spine of the ilium on a line between the ilium and the umbilicus. See Figure 7.12.

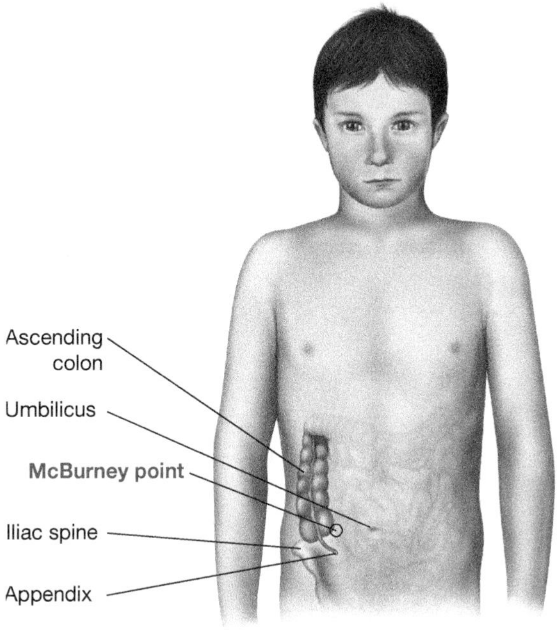

Ascending colon

Umbilicus

McBurney point

Iliac spine

Appendix

FIGURE 7.12 McBurney point is the common location of pain in children and adolescents with appendicitis.

ascites (ă-sī′tēz)			Significant accumulation of serous fluid in the peritoneal cavity
biliary (bĭl′ē-ār″ē)	**bil/i** **-ary**	gall, bile pertaining to	Pertaining to bile
bilirubin (bĭl″ĭ-roo′bĭn)			Orange-colored bile pigment produced by the separation of hemoglobin into parts that are excreted by the liver cells

Medical Word	Word Parts		Definition
	Part	Meaning	
black hairy tongue			Condition in which the tongue is covered by hairlike papillae entangled with threads produced by *Aspergillus niger* or *Candida albicans* fungi or by bacteria. This unusual condition could be caused by poor oral hygiene and/or overgrowth of fungi due to antibiotic therapy. See Figure 7.13.

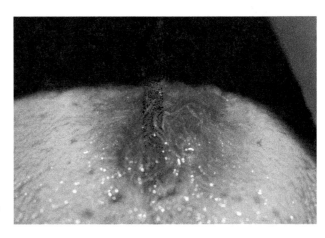

FIGURE 7.13 Black hairy tongue.
Source: Courtesy of Jason L. Smith, MD

bowel (bou´ l)			Intestine; the long tube in the body that stores and then eliminates waste out of the body
buccal (bŭk´ ăl)	bucc -al	cheek pertaining to	Literally means *pertaining to the cheek*; relating to the cheek or mouth
catabolism (kă-tăb´ ō-lĭzm)	catabol -ism	casting-down condition	Literally *a casting-down*; in metabolism a breaking-down of complex substances into more basic elements
celiac (sē´ lē-ăk)	celi -ac	abdomen, belly pertaining to	Pertaining to the abdomen

GOOD TO KNOW ▶

Celiac disease is an autoimmune disease in which an individual cannot eat food containing gluten because the person's immune system responds to gluten by damaging the small intestine. Gluten is a protein found in wheat, rye, and barley. It may also be in products like vitamins and other supplements, hair and skin products, toothpastes, and lip balm.

Celiac disease affects each person differently. Some people have no symptoms; in many people, symptoms occur in the digestive system or in other parts of the body. One person might have diarrhea and abdominal pain, while another person may be irritable or depressed. Irritability is one of the most common symptoms of celiac disease in children.

Medical Word	Word Parts		Definition
	Part	Meaning	
cheilosis (kī-lō´ sĭs)	**cheil** **-osis**	lip condition	Abnormal condition of the lip as seen in riboflavin and other B-complex deficiencies
cholecystectomy (kō˝ lē-sĭs-tĕk´ tō-mē)	**chol/e** **cyst** **-ectomy**	gall, bile bladder surgical excision	Surgical excision of the gallbladder. With laparoscopic cholecystectomy, the gallbladder is removed through a small incision near the navel. Gallstones (*cholelithiasis*) are usually present in the removed gallbladder. See Figure 7.14.

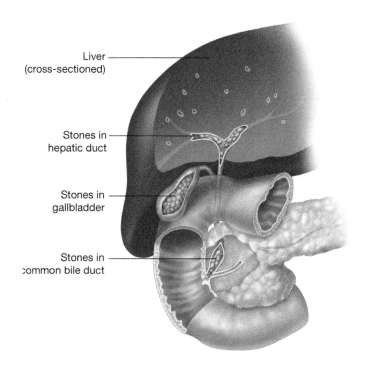

Liver
(cross-sectioned)

Stones in
hepatic duct

Stones in
gallbladder

Stones in
common bile duct

FIGURE 7.14 Gallbladder with gallstones. Note the stones in the hepatic duct, gallbladder, and common bile duct.

cholecystitis (kō˝ lē-sĭs-tī´ tĭs)	**chol/e** **cyst** **-itis**	gall, bile bladder inflammation	Inflammation of the gallbladder
choledochotomy (kō˝ lĕd-ō-kŏt´ ō-mē)	**choledoch/o** **-tomy**	common bile duct incision	Surgical incision of the common bile duct

Medical Word	Word Parts		Definition
	Part	Meaning	
cirrhosis (sĭ-rō´ sĭs)	cirrh -osis	orange- yellow condition	Chronic degenerative liver disease characterized by changes in the lobes; parenchymal cells and the lobules are infiltrated with fat. See Figure 7.15.

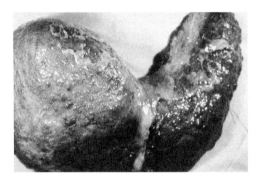

FIGURE 7.15 The liver in this photograph was from a deceased patient with an advanced state of cirrhosis.
Source: Pearson Education, Inc.

Medical Word	Word Parts		Definition
colectomy (kō-lĕk´ tō-mē)	col -ectomy	colon surgical excision	Surgical excision of part of the colon
colon cancer (kō´ lŏn kăn´ sĕr)			Malignancy of the colon; sometimes called *colorectal cancer*. See Figure 7.16.

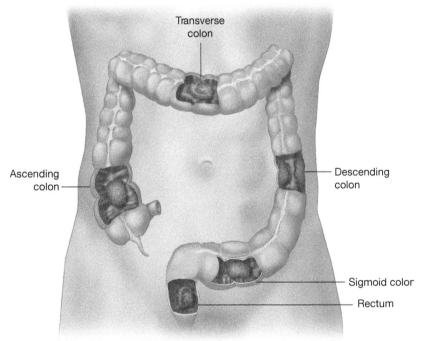

Transverse colon

Ascending colon

Descending colon

Sigmoid color

Rectum

FIGURE 7.16 Common sites of colorectal cancer.

Medical Word	Word Parts		Definition
	Part	Meaning	
colonoscope (kō-lŏn′ ō-skōp)	**colon/o** **-scope**	colon instrument for examining	Thin, lighted, flexible instrument that is used to view the interior of the colon during a colonoscopy
colonoscopy (kō-lŏn-ŏs′ kō-pē)	**colon/o** **-scopy**	colon to view, examine, visual examination	Visual examination of the colon via a colonoscope. See Figure 7.17.

! ALERT!

The combining forms **col/o** and **colon/o** mean *colon*. You can build medical words by using various suffixes such as **-ectomy**, **-ic**, **-scope**, **-scopy**, and **-stomy** to change the meaning of the word.

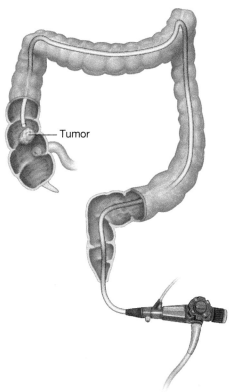

Tumor

FIGURE 7.17 Note the tumor visualized with the use of a colonoscope.

Medical Word	Word Parts		Definition
	Part	Meaning	
colostomy (kō-lŏs′ tō-mē)	col/o -stomy	colon new opening	A surgical procedure that brings one end of the large intestine out through an opening (stoma) made in the abdominal wall. Stool moving through the intestine drains through the stoma into a bag attached to the abdomen. A colostomy can be permanent or temporary. The most common types are transverse, descending, and sigmoid, so named due to the site of the disorder and the location of the stoma. See Figure 7.18 and Figure 7.19.

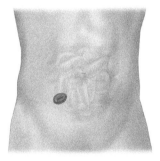 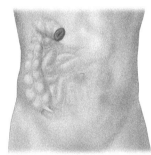 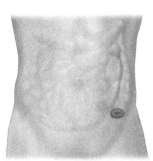

FIGURE 7.18 Alternate sites that can be used to create a new opening (-stomy) in the colon.

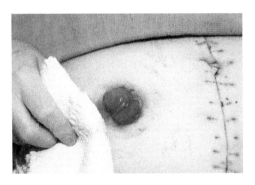

FIGURE 7.19 Patient with stoma after undergoing a colostomy.
Source: PavleMarjanovic/Shutterstock

constipation (kon″ stĭ-pā′ shŭn)	constipat -ion	to press together process	Infrequent passage of unduly hard and dry feces; *difficult defecation*

fyi Constipation is a frequent problem among older adults. It is believed that constipation is not a normal age-related change but is caused by low fluid intake, dehydration, lack of dietary fiber, inactivity, medicines, depression, and other health-related conditions. Over time, narcotic medications can slow the bowel and lead to symptoms of constipation, bloating, and nausea. This is known as **opioid-induced constipation (OIC)**.

Medical Word	Word Parts		Definition
	Part	Meaning	
Crohn disease (krōn)			Chronic autoimmune disease that can affect any part of the gastrointestinal tract but most commonly occurs in the ileum. See Figure 7.20.

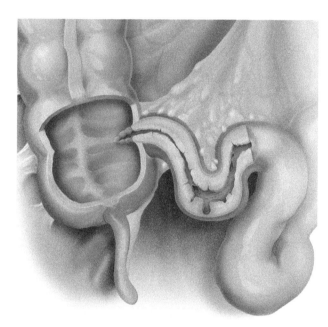

FIGURE 7.20 Note the thickening of the intestinal wall and the erosion of the inner lining of the ileum, often seen in Crohn disease.

Medical Word	Word Parts		Definition
dentalgia (dĕn-tăl′ jē-ă)	dent -algia	tooth pain, ache	Pain in a tooth; *toothache*
dentition (dĕn-tĭ′ shŭn)			Type, number, and arrangement of teeth in the dental arch
diarrhea (dī-ă-rē′ ă)	dia- -rrhea	through flow	Frequent passage of unformed watery stool

Medical Word	Word Parts		Definition
	Part	**Meaning**	
diverticulitis (dī″ věr-tĭk″ ū-lī′ tĭs)	**diverticul** **-itis**	diverticula inflammation	Inflammation of the diverticula (pouches in the walls of an organ) in the colon. Symptoms include pain, fever, chills, cramping, bloating, constipation, and diarrhea. Treatment depends on the severity of the condition. See Figure 7.21.

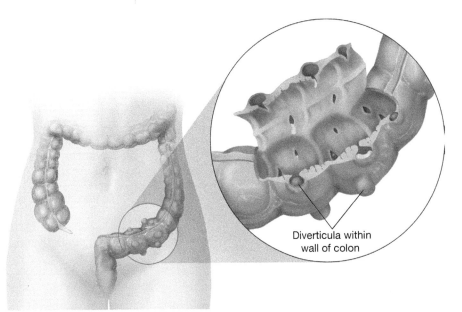

Diverticula within wall of colon

FIGURE 7.21 Diverticulitis.

duodenal (dū″ ō-dē′ năl)	**duoden** **-al**	duodenum pertaining to	Pertaining to the duodenum, the first part of the small intestine
dysentery (dĭs′ ĕn-tĕr″ ē)	**dys-** **enter** **-y**	difficult intestine pertaining to	An intestinal disease characterized by inflammation of the mucous membrane
dyspepsia (dĭs-pĕp′ sē-ă)	**dys-** **-pepsia**	difficult to digest, digestion	Difficulty in digestion; *indigestion*
dysphagia (dĭs-fā′ jē-ă)	**dys-** **-phagia**	difficult to eat, to swallow	Difficulty in swallowing
emesis (ĕm′ ĕ-sĭs)	**eme** **-sis**	to vomit condition	Vomiting
enteric (ĕn-tĕr′ ĭk)	**enter** **-ic**	small intestine pertaining to	Pertaining to the small intestine
enteritis (ĕn″ tĕr-ī′ tĭs)	**enter** **-itis**	small intestine inflammation	Inflammation of the small intestine

Medical Word	Word Parts		Definition
	Part	Meaning	
enzyme (ĕn´ zīm)			Protein substance capable of causing rapid chemical changes in other substances without being changed itself
epigastric (ĕp˝ ĭ-găs´ trĭk)	**epi-** **gastr** **-ic**	above stomach pertaining to	Pertaining to the region above the stomach
esophageal (ē-sŏf˝ ă-jē´ ăl)	**esophage** **-al**	esophagus pertaining to	Pertaining to the esophagus
feces (fē´ sēz)			Body waste discharged from the bowel by way of the anus; also called *bowel movement (BM)*, *stool*, *excreta*
flatus (flā´ tŭs)			Literally means *a blowing* in Latin; the expelling of gas from the anus. The average person passes 400–1200 mL of gas each day.
gastrectomy (găs-trĕk´ tō-mē)	**gastr** **-ectomy**	stomach surgical excision	Surgical excision of a part of or the whole stomach
gastric (găs´ trĭk)	**gastr** **-ic**	stomach pertaining to	Pertaining to the stomach
gastroenteritis (găs˝ trō-ĕn˝ tĕr-ī´ tĭs)	**gastr/o** **enter** **-itis**	stomach intestine inflammation	Inflammation of the stomach and intestine
gastroenterologist (găs˝ trō-ĕn˝ tĕr-ŏl´ ō-jĭst)	**gastr/o** **enter/o** **log** **-ist**	stomach intestine study one who specializes	Physician who specializes in the stomach and intestine
gastroenterology (găs˝ trō-ĕn˝ tĕr-ŏl´ ō-jē)	**gastr/o** **enter/o** **-logy**	stomach intestine study of	Study of the stomach and intestine
gastroesophageal (găs˝ trō-ĕ-sŏf˝ ă-jē´ al)	**gastr/o** **esophage** **-al**	stomach esophagus pertaining to	Pertaining to the stomach and esophagus

 fyi **Erosive esophagitis (EE)** is a condition in which areas of the esophageal lining are inflamed and ulcerated. The most common cause of erosive esophagitis is chronic acid reflux. **Barrett esophagus (BE)** can also develop as an advanced stage of erosive esophagitis, leading to abnormal changes in the cells of the esophagus, which puts a patient at risk for esophageal cancer.

Medical Word	Word Parts		Definition
	Part	**Meaning**	
gastroesophageal reflux disease (GERD) (găs″ trō-ĕ-sŏf″ ă-jē´ al rē´ flŭks)			Condition that occurs when the muscle between the esophagus and the stomach, the lower esophageal sphincter, is weak or relaxes inappropriately, allowing the stomach's contents to back up (*reflux*) into the esophagus. Symptoms include heartburn, belching, and regurgitation of food. See Figure 7.22.

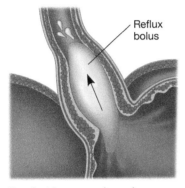

Transient lower esophageal sphincter relaxation

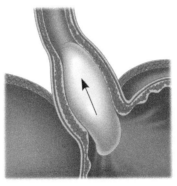

Incompetent lower esophageal sphincter

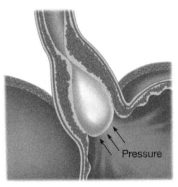

Increased intragastric pressure

FIGURE 7.22 Mechanisms of gastroesophageal reflux.

fyi Dietary and lifestyle choices may contribute to GERD. Studies show that cigarette smoking relaxes the lower esophageal sphincter (LES). Obesity and pregnancy can also cause GERD. Some doctors believe a **hiatal hernia** may weaken the lower esophageal sphincter and cause reflux.

Medical Word	Word Parts		Definition
gavage (gă-văzh´)			To feed liquid or semiliquid food via a tube (stomach or nasogastric [NG])
gingivitis (jĭn″ jĭ-vī´ tĭs)	**gingiv** **-itis**	gums inflammation	Inflammation of the gums
glossectomy (glŏs-ĕk´ tō-mē)	**gloss** **-ectomy**	tongue excision	Partial or complete surgical excision of the tongue
glycogenesis (glī″ kŏ-jĕn´ ĕ-sĭs)	**glyc/o** **-genesis**	sweet, sugar formation, produce	Formation of glycogen from glucose
halitosis (hăl″ ĭ-tō´ sĭs)	**halit** **-osis**	breath condition	Bad breath
hematemesis (hĕm″ ă-tĕm´ ĕ-sĭs)	**hemat** **-emesis**	blood vomiting	Vomiting of blood

Medical Word	Word Parts		Definition
	Part	Meaning	
hemorrhoid (hěm′ ŏ-royd)	**hemorrh** **-oid**	vein liable to bleed resemble	Mass of dilated, tortuous veins in the anorectum; can be internal or external. See Figure 7.23.

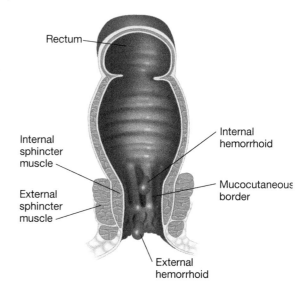

FIGURE 7.23 Location of internal and external hemorrhoids.

| **hepatitis**
(hĕp″ ă-tī′ tĭs) | **hepat**
-itis | liver
inflammation | Inflammation of the liver |

fyi Hepatitis also refers to a group of viral infections that affect the liver. The most common types in the United States are hepatitis A (HAV), hepatitis B (HBV), and hepatitis C (HCV). There are vaccines to prevent hepatitis A and B; however, there is not one for hepatitis C. The common signs and symptoms of hepatitis are malaise, anorexia, hepatomegaly, jaundice, and abdominal pain.

HAV infection is primarily transmitted by the fecal–oral route, by either person-to-person contact or consumption of contaminated food or water. HBV is transmitted by blood transfusion, sexual contact, or the use of contaminated needles or instruments. HCV is most efficiently transmitted through large or repeated percutaneous exposure to infected blood (through the sharing of equipment to inject drugs, needlestick injuries in healthcare settings, and being born to a mother who is HCV positive).

Hepatitis D (HDV), which can be acute or chronic, is uncommon in the United States. Hepatitis E (HEV) is a serious liver disease that usually results in an acute infection. While rare in the United States, hepatitis E is common in many parts of the world.

Medical Word	Word Parts		Definition
	Part	Meaning	
hernia (hĕr′ nē-ă)			Abnormal protrusion of an organ or a part of an organ through the wall of the body cavity that normally contains it. A *hiatal hernia* occurs when the upper part of the stomach moves up into the chest through a small opening in the diaphragm. An *umbilical hernia* occurs when part of the intestine protrudes through an opening in the abdominal muscles. Umbilical hernias are most common in infants, but they can affect adults as well. In an infant, an umbilical hernia may be especially evident when the infant cries, causing the baby's navel (belly button) to protrude. An *inguinal hernia* occurs when a loop of intestine enters the inguinal canal, a tubular passage through the lower layers of the abdominal wall. See Figure 7.24.

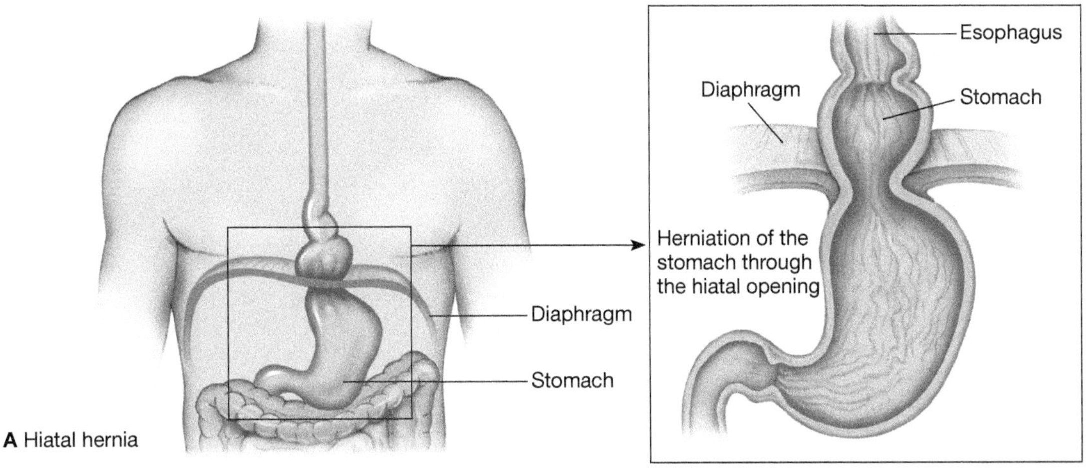

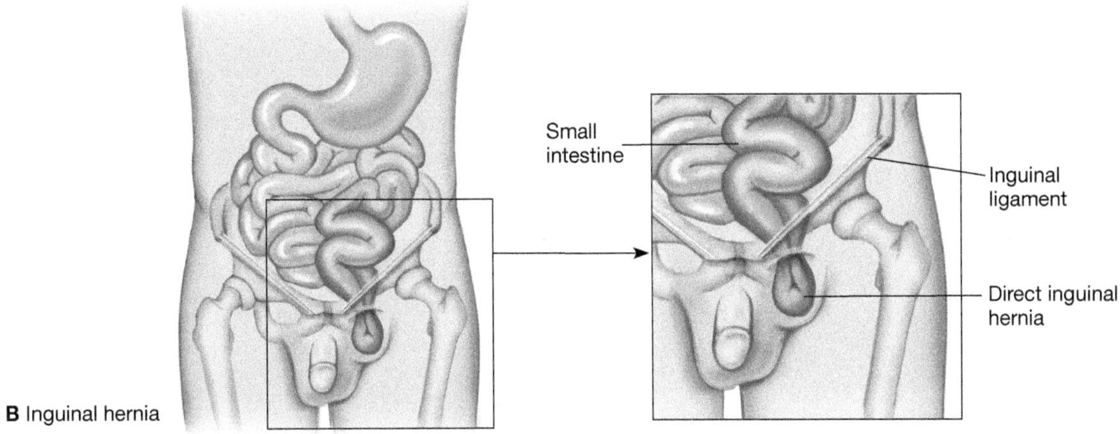

A Hiatal hernia

B Inguinal hernia

FIGURE 7.24 Hernias.

Medical Word	Word Parts		Definition
	Part	Meaning	
herniorrhaphy (hĕr″ nē-or´ ă-fē)	herni/o -rrhaphy	hernia suture	Surgical repair of a hernia
hyperemesis (hī″ pĕr-ĕm´ ĕ-sĭs)	hyper- -emesis	excessive, above vomiting	Excessive vomiting
hypogastric (hī″ pō-găs´ trĭk)	hypo- gastr -ic	deficient, below stomach pertaining to	Pertaining to below the stomach
ileostomy (ĭl″ ē-ŏs´ tō-mē)	ile/o -stomy	ileum new opening	The surgical creation of a new opening through the abdominal wall into the ileum. See Figure 7.25.

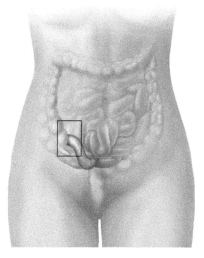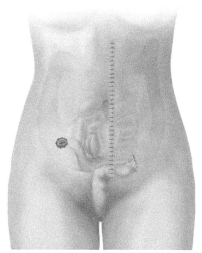

FIGURE 7.25 Ileostomy. Note that the cecum and colon have been surgically removed.

inflammatory bowel disease (IBD)		Broad term that describes conditions with chronic or recurring abnormal immune response and inflammation of the gastrointestinal tract. The two most common inflammatory bowel diseases are ulcerative colitis (UC) (inflammation of the large intestine) and Crohn disease (CD) (inflammation of any portion of the digestive tract).

 fyi The medical approach for patients with IBD is symptomatic care (relief of symptoms) and mucosal healing following a *step-up* or *stepwise* approach to medication, which means the medical regimen is escalated until a response is achieved.

Medical Word	Word Parts		Definition
	Part	Meaning	
intussusception (ĭn″ tŭ-sŭ-sĕp′ shŭn)			The slipping or telescoping of one part of an intestine into another part just below it; noted chiefly in children and occurring in the ileocecal region
irritable bowel syndrome (IBS)			Disorder that affects the muscular contractions of the colon and interferes with its normal functioning; characterized by a group of symptoms, including crampy abdominal pain, bloating, constipation, and diarrhea. *Note:* Inflammatory bowel diseases such as ulcerative colitis and Crohn disease should not be confused with IBS. Intestinal inflammation is not a symptom of IBS.
labial (lā′ bē-ăl)	labi -al	lip pertaining to	Pertaining to the lip
laparotomy (lăp″ ăr-ŏt′ ō-mē)	lapar/o -tomy	abdomen incision	Surgical incision into the abdomen
lavage (lă-văzh′)			To wash out a cavity. Gastric lavage is used to remove or dilute gastric contents in cases of acute poisoning or ingestion of a caustic substance. *Vomiting should not be induced.* A closed-system irrigation uses an ordered amount of solution until the desired results are obtained.
laxative (lăk′ să-tĭv)	laxat -ive	to loosen nature of, quality of	Substance that acts to loosen the bowel
lingual (lĭng′ gwal)	lingu -al	tongue pertaining to	Pertaining to the tongue
malabsorption (măl″ ăb-sōrp′ shŭn)	mal- absorpt -ion	bad to take in process	An inadequate absorption of nutrients from the intestinal tract
mastication (măs″ tĭ-kā′ shŭn)	masticat -ion	to chew process	Chewing; the physical breaking-up of food and mixing with saliva in the mouth
melena (mĕl′ ĕ-nă)			Black, tarry feces (stool) that has a distinctive odor and contains digested blood; usually results from bleeding in the upper GI tract; can be a sign of a peptic ulcer
mesentery (mĕs′ ĕn-tĕr″ ē)	mes enter -y	middle small intestine pertaining to	Pertaining to the peritoneal fold encircling the small intestine and connecting the intestine to the posterior abdominal wall
nausea (naw′ zē-ă)			Uncomfortable feeling of the inclination to vomit

Medical Word	Word Parts		Definition
	Part	**Meaning**	
pancreatitis (păn″ krē-ă-tī′ tĭs)	**pancreat** -itis	pancreas inflammation	Inflammation of the pancreas
paralytic ileus (păr″ ă-lĭt′ ĭk ĭl′ ē-ŭs)	**paralyt** -ic ile -us	to disable, paralysis pertaining to ileum pertaining to	Paralysis of the intestines that causes distention and symptoms of acute bowel obstruction and inactivity
peptic (pĕp′ tĭk)	**pept** -ic	to digest pertaining to	Pertaining to gastric digestion
peptic ulcer disease (PUD) (pĕp′ tĭk ŭl′ sĕr)	**pept** -ic	to digest pertaining to	Disease in which an ulcer forms in the mucosal wall of the stomach, the pylorus, the duodenum, or the esophagus. See Figure 7.26.

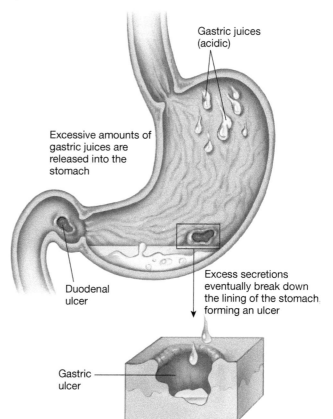

Gastric juices (acidic)

Excessive amounts of gastric juices are released into the stomach

Duodenal ulcer

Excess secretions eventually break down the lining of the stomach, forming an ulcer

Gastric ulcer

FIGURE 7.26 Peptic ulcer disease.

fyi Peptic ulcers are referred to as *gastric*, *duodenal*, or *esophageal*, depending on the location. The erosion of the mucosa that characterizes peptic ulcers is often caused by infection with a bacterium called *Helicobacter pylori (H. pylori)*. Approximately 90% of duodenal ulcers and 80% of peptic ulcers are associated with *Helicobacter pylori*. By killing the bacteria with antibiotics, it is estimated that 90% of the ulcers caused by *H. pylori* can be cured.

Medical Word	Word Parts		Definition
	Part	Meaning	
periodontal (pĕr″ ē-ō-dŏn′ tăl)	peri- odont -al	around tooth pertaining to	Pertaining to the area around a tooth
periodontal disease			Inflammation and degeneration of the gums and surrounding bone, which frequently causes loss of teeth
peristalsis (pĕr″ ĭ-stăl′ sĭs)	peri- -stalsis	around contraction	Wavelike contractions that occur involuntarily in hollow tubes of the body, especially the alimentary canal
pharyngeal (făr-ĭn′ jē-ăl)	pharyng/e -al	pharynx pertaining to	Pertaining to the pharynx
pilonidal cyst (pī″ lō-nī′ dăl sĭst)	pil/o nid -al cyst	hair nest pertaining to sac	Closed sac in the crease of the sacrococcygeal region caused by a developmental defect that permits epithelial tissue and hair to be trapped below the skin and cause pain or swelling above the area of the anus or near the tailbone
postprandial (PP) (pōst-prăn′ dē-ăl)	post- prand/i -al	after meal pertaining to	Pertaining to after a meal
probiotics			Live microorganisms that, when administered in adequate amounts, confer a health benefit on the digestive system. In the United States, probiotics are available as dietary supplements (including capsules, tablets, and powders) and in dairy foods (such as yogurts with live active cultures). The FDA has not approved any health claims for probiotics; however, they are used for a variety of gastrointestinal conditions such as infectious diarrhea, diarrhea associated with using antibiotics, irritable bowel syndrome, and inflammatory bowel disease.
proctoscope (prŏk′ tō-skōp)	proct/o -scope	anus and rectum instrument for examining	An instrument used in a medical procedure to view the interior of the rectal cavity; a short (10 in. or 25 cm long), straight, rigid, hollow metal tube, usually with a small light bulb mounted at the end

Medical Word	Word Parts		Definition
	Part	**Meaning**	
pyloric (pī-lōr´ ĭk)	**pylor**	pylorus, gatekeeper	Pertaining to the gatekeeper, the opening between the stomach and the duodenum. See Figure 7.27.
	-ic	pertaining to	

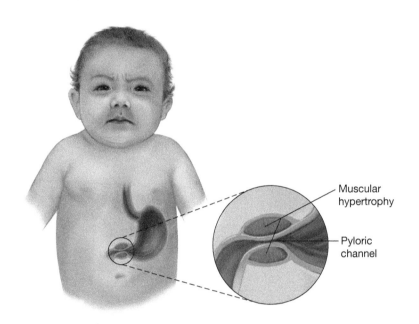

Muscular hypertrophy

Pyloric channel

FIGURE 7.27 In pyloric stenosis, shown here in an infant, the hypertrophied pyloric muscle causes symptoms of projectile vomiting and visible peristalsis.

Source: PEARSON EDUCATION; SERVICES, PEARSON; PEARSON EDUCATION, . ., NURSING: A CONCEPT-BASED APPROACH TO LEARNING, VOLUME I, 1st Ed., ©2019. Reprinted and Electronically reproduced by permission of Pearson Education, Inc., New York, NY.

Medical Word	Word Parts		Definition
rectocele (rĕk´ tō-sēl)	**rect/o** **-cele**	rectum hernia	Hernia of part of the rectum into the vagina
sialadenitis (sī´ ăl-ăd˝ ĕ-nī´ tĭs)	**sial** **aden** **-itis**	saliva gland inflammation	Inflammation of a salivary gland
sigmoidoscope (sĭg-moy´ dō-skōp)	**sigmoid/o** **-scope**	sigmoid instrument for examining	An instrument used in a medical procedure to view the interior of the sigmoid colon
splenomegaly (splē˝ nō-mĕg´ ă-lē)	**splen/o** **-megaly**	spleen enlargement, large	Enlargement of the spleen

Medical Word	Word Parts		Definition
	Part	Meaning	
stomatitis (stō″ mă-tī′ tĭs)	**stomat** **-itis**	mouth inflammation	Inflammation of the mouth
sublingual (sŭb-lĭng′ gwăl)	**sub-** **lingu** **-al**	below tongue pertaining to	Pertaining to below the tongue. See Figure 7.28.

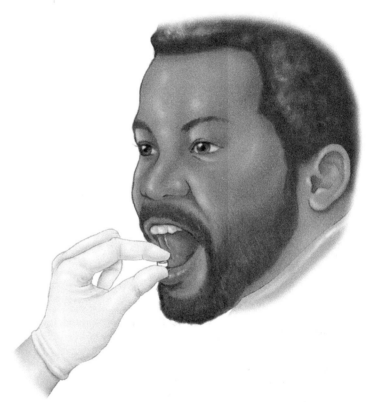

FIGURE 7.28 Sublingual drug administration.

| **ulcerative colitis (UC)**
(ŭl′ sĕr-ă-tĭv kō-lī′ tĭs) | | | Disease that causes inflammation and ulcers in the lining of the large intestine. The inflammation usually occurs in the rectum and lower part of the colon but can affect the entire colon; also called *colitis* or *proctitis*. |

Medical Word	Word Parts		Definition
	Part	Meaning	
vermiform (vĕr´ mĭ-form)	**verm/i** **-form**	worm shape	Shaped like a worm; the vermiform appendix is so named because of its wormlike shape
volvulus (vŏl´ vū-lŭs)	**volvul** **-us**	to roll pertaining to	Twisting of the bowel on itself that causes an obstruction. See Figure 7.29.

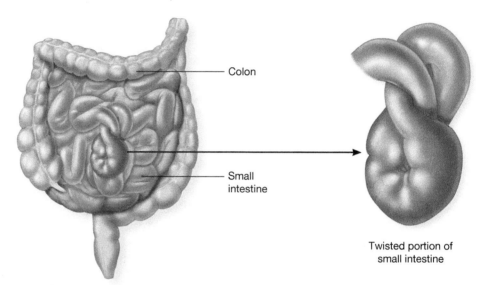

Colon

Small intestine

Twisted portion of small intestine

FIGURE 7.29 Volvulus.

vomit			To eject stomach contents through the mouth

Study *and* Review II

Word Parts

Prefixes   Give the definitions of the following prefixes.

1. an- _____

2. dys- _____

3. epi- _____

4. hyper- _____

5. hypo- _____

6. mal- _____

7. peri- _____

8. post- _____

9. dia- _____

10. sub- _____

Combining Forms   Give the definitions of the following combining forms.

1. amyl/o _____
2. append/o _____
3. bil/i _____
4. bucc/o _____
5. celi/o _____
6. chol/e _____
7. cirrh/o _____
8. colon/o _____
9. dent/o _____
10. enter/o _____
11. esophage/o _____
12. gastr/o _____

13. gingiv/o _____
14. gloss/o _____
15. hepat/o _____
16. ile/o _____
17. labi/o _____
18. lapar/o _____
19. lingu/o _____
20. odont/o _____
21. prand/i _____
22. proct/o _____
23. rect/o _____
24. stomat/o _____

Suffixes   Give the definitions of the following suffixes.

1. -ac _____
2. -al _____
3. -algia _____
4. -ary _____
5. -ase _____
6. -cele _____
7. -oid _____
8. -sis _____
9. -ectomy _____
10. -emesis _____
11. -form _____
12. -genesis _____

13. -ic _____
14. -ion _____
15. -ism _____
16. -ist _____
17. -itis _____
18. -ive _____
19. -logy _____
20. -megaly _____
21. -orexia _____
22. -osis _____
23. -rrhea _____
24. -pepsia _____

25. -us _____   **30.** -stomy _____

26. -phagia _____   **31.** -tomy _____

27. -scope _____   **32.** -y _____

28. -scopy _____   **33.** -rrhaphy _____

29. -stalsis _____

Identifying Medical Terms

In the spaces provided, write the medical terms for the following meanings.

1. _____ Enzyme that breaks down starch

2. _____ Building-up of the body substance in the constructive phase of metabolism

3. _____ Lack of appetite

4. _____ Surgical excision of the appendix

5. _____ Inflammation of the appendix

6. _____ Pertaining to bile

7. _____ Pertaining to the abdomen

8. _____ Difficulty in swallowing

9. _____ Inflammation of the liver

10. _____ Surgical repair of a hernia

Matching

Select the appropriate lettered meaning for each of the following words.

_____ **1.** cirrhosis

_____ **2.** constipation

_____ **3.** diarrhea

_____ **4.** gavage

_____ **5.** hemorrhoid

a. To wash out a cavity

b. To feed liquid or semiliquid food via a tube

c. Twisting of the bowel on itself that causes an obstruction

d. Frequent passage of unformed watery stool

e. Chronic degenerative liver disease

f. Infrequent passage of unduly hard and dry feces

_____ 6. hernia

_____ 7. hyperemesis

_____ 8. lavage

_____ 9. pilonidal cyst

_____ 10. volvulus

g. Closed sac in the crease of the sacrococcygeal region

h. Abnormal protrusion of an organ or a part of an organ through the wall of the body cavity that normally contains it

i. Mass of dilated, tortuous veins in the anorectum

j. Excessive vomiting

Medical Case Snapshots

This learning activity provides an opportunity to relate the medical terminology you are learning to sample patient case presentations. In the spaces provided, write in your answers.

Case 1

A 54-year-old male was scheduled for a routine visual examination of the colon, also known as a

_____. The exam revealed a malignancy of the colon. He was scheduled for a

_____ (a procedure to create a new opening into the colon).

Case 2

A 72-year-old male presents with symptoms of infrequent passage of hard, dry feces. A rectal exam reveals a mass of dilated, tortuous veins in the anorectum. The patient is advised that he has _____ and

_____. He is to take a laxative to loosen the bowel and is advised to increase his intake of fluids and fiber.

Case 3

A 37-year-old male complains of dull, aching pain in the stomach and back. He has "heartburn and belching."

His symptoms suggest peptic ulcer disease, which is mostly caused by _____

_____ (a bacterium). This condition can often be cured with the use of a combination of medications, including _____ (drugs that kill bacteria).

Drug Highlights

Classification of Drug	Description and Examples
antacids	Neutralize hydrochloric acid in the stomach; classified as nonsystemic and systemic.
nonsystemic	EXAMPLES: Amphojel (aluminum hydroxide), Tums (calcium carbonate), Riopan (magaldrate), and Milk of Magnesia (magnesium hydroxide)
systemic	EXAMPLE: sodium bicarbonate
antacid mixtures	Products that combine aluminum (may cause constipation) and/or calcium compounds with magnesium salts (may cause diarrhea). By combining the antacid properties of two single-entity agents, these products provide the antacid action of both yet tend to counter the adverse effects of each other. EXAMPLES: Gaviscon, Gelusil, Maalox Plus, and Mylanta
histamine H_2-receptor antagonists	Inhibit both daytime and nocturnal basal gastric acid secretion and inhibit gastric acid stimulated by food, histamines, caffeine, and insulin used in the treatment of active duodenal ulcer. EXAMPLES: Tagamet (cimetidine), Pepcid (famotidine), Axid (nizatidine), and Zantac (ranitidine)
mucosal protective medications	Medicines that protect the stomach's mucosal lining from acids but do not inhibit the release of acid. EXAMPLES: Carafate (sucralfate) and Cytotec (misoprostol)
gastric acid pump inhibitors (proton-pump inhibitors [PPIs])	Antiulcer agents that suppress gastric acid secretion by specific inhibition of the H + /K + ATPase enzyme at the secretory surface of the gastric parietal cell. Because this enzyme system is regarded as the acid (proton) pump within the gastric mucosa, gastric acid pump inhibitors are so classified because they block the final step of acid production. EXAMPLES: Prilosec (omeprazole), Aciphex (rabeprazole sodium), Prevacid (lansoprazole), Protonix (pantoprazole), and Nexium (esomeprazole magnesium)
other ulcer medications	Treatment regimen for active duodenal ulcers associated with *H. pylori* can involve a two-, three-, or four-drug program. EXAMPLES: A two-drug program—Biaxin (clarithromycin) and Prilosec (omeprazole), a three-drug program—Flagyl (metronidazole) and either tetracycline or amoxicillin and Pepto-Bismol, and a four-drug program—a proton pump inhibitor plus a single capsule containing bismuth subcitrate potassium, metronidazole, and tetracycline *Note:* For the treatment to be effective, the patient must complete the full treatment program, which usually involves taking the drugs for a total of at least 10–14 days for the two- and three-drug program and 10 days for the four-drug program.

Classification of Drug	Description and Examples
agents used for inflammatory bowel disease	Step I—Aminosalicylates (oral, enema, suppository formulations): For treating flare-ups and maintaining remission; more effective in ulcerative colitis (UC) than in Crohn disease (CD) Step IA—Antibiotics: Used sparingly in UC (limited efficacy, increased risk for antibiotic-associated pseudomembranous colitis); in CD, most commonly used for perianal disease, fistulas, intra-abdominal inflammatory masses Step II—Corticosteroids (intravenous, oral, topical, rectal): For acute disease flare-ups only Step III—Immunomodulators: Effective for steroid-sparing action in refractory disease; primary treatment for fistulas and maintenance of remission in patients intolerant of or not responsive to aminosalicylates
laxatives	Used to relieve constipation and to facilitate the passage of feces through the lower gastrointestinal tract. EXAMPLES: Dulcolax (bisacodyl), Milk of Magnesia (magnesium hydroxide), Metamucil (psyllium hydrophilic mucilloid), and Ex-Lax (phenolphthalein)
antidiarrheal agents	Used to treat diarrhea. EXAMPLES: Pepto-Bismol (bismuth subsalicylate), Kaopectate (kaolin mixture with pectin), and Imodium (loperamide HCl)
antiemetics	Prevent or arrest vomiting; also used in the treatment of vertigo, motion sickness, and nausea. EXAMPLES: Dramamine, Gravol (dimenhydrinate), Benadryl (diphenhydramine), Bonine (meclizine), and Phenergan (promethazine)
emetics	Used to induce vomiting in people who have taken an overdose of oral drugs or who have ingested certain poisons. An emetic agent should not be given to a person who is unconscious, in shock, or in a semicomatose state. Emetics are also contraindicated in individuals who have ingested strongly caustic substances, such as lye or acid, because their use could result in additional injury to the person's esophagus. Apomorphine is a powerful emetic and has been used for that effect in acute poisoning. It has also been used in the diagnosis and treatment of parkinsonism, but its adverse effects limit its use. EXAMPLE: Apokyn (apomorphine)

Diagnostic *and* Laboratory Tests

Test	Description
alcohol toxicology (ethanol and ethyl) (ăl′ kō-hŏl tŏks″ ĭ-kŏl′ ō-jē)	Test performed on blood serum or plasma to determine levels of alcohol. All 50 states and the District of Columbia have laws defining it as a crime to drive with a blood alcohol concentration (BAC) at or above 0.08%. Increased values indicate alcohol consumption that could lead to cirrhosis of the liver, gastritis, malnutrition, vitamin deficiencies, and other gastrointestinal disorders.
carcinoembryonic antigen (CEA) (kăr″ sĭn-ō-ĕm″ brē-ŏn′ ĭk ăn′ tĭ-jĕn)	Test performed on whole blood or plasma to determine the presence of CEA (antigens originally isolated from colon tumors). Increased values can indicate stomach, intestinal, rectal, and various other cancers and conditions. This test is nonspecific and must be combined with other tests for a final diagnosis. It is being used to monitor the course of cancer therapy.
cholangiography (kō-lăn″ jē-ŏg′ ră-fē)	An x-ray examination of the common bile duct, cystic duct, and hepatic ducts in which radiopaque dye is injected and then films are taken. Abnormal results can indicate obstruction, stones, and tumors.
cholecystography (kō″ lē-sĭs-tŏg′ ră-fē)	An x-ray examination of the gallbladder in which radiopaque dye is injected and then films are taken. Abnormal results can indicate cholecystitis, cholelithiasis, and tumors.
colonoscopy (kō″ lŏn-ŏs′ kō-pē)	Direct visual examination of the colon via a colonoscope; used to diagnose growths to confirm findings of other tests and to rule out or rule in colon cancer. It can also be used to remove small polyps and to collect tissue samples for analysis. See Figure 7.30. The patient is lightly sedated during the procedure. **FIGURE 7.30** Illustration of a polyp in the colon. Source: Sebastian Kaulitzki/Shutterstock
comprehensive metabolic panel (CMP)	Includes 14 tests that provide information about the current status of a patient's metabolism, including the health of the kidneys and liver, electrolyte and acid–base balance, and levels of blood glucose and blood proteins. Abnormal results, and especially combinations of abnormal results, can indicate a problem that needs to be addressed.
endoscopic retrograde cholangiopancreatography (ERCP) (ĕn″ dō-skŏp′ ĭk rĕt′ rō-grād kō-lăn″ jē-ō-păn″ krē-ă-tŏg′ ră-fē)	An x-ray examination of the biliary and pancreatic ducts by injecting a contrast medium and then films are taken. Abnormal results can indicate fibrosis, biliary or pancreatic cysts, strictures, stones, and chronic pancreatitis.

Test	Description
esophagogastroduodenos-copy (EGD) (ĕ-sŏf″ă-gō′găs″trō-doo″ŏd-ē-nos′kŏ-pē)	Endoscopic examination of the esophagus, stomach, and first part of the small intestine. During the procedure, photographs, biopsy, or brushings may be done.

fyi Esophagogastroduodenoscopy (EGD) is considered the reference method of diagnosis of peptic ulcer disease. The diagnosis of *H. pylori* can be made by several methods. The biopsy urease test is a colorimetric test based on the ability of *H. pylori* to produce urease; it provides rapid testing at the time of biopsy. Histological identification of organisms is considered the gold standard of diagnostic tests. Culture of biopsy specimens for *H. pylori*, which requires an experienced laboratory, is necessary when antimicrobial susceptibility testing is desired.

Test	Description
fiberoptic colonoscopy (fī″bĕr-ŏp′tĭk kō″lŏn-ŏs′kō-pē)	Fiberoptic colonoscopy, a direct visual examination of the colon via a flexible colonoscope; used as a diagnostic aid for removal of foreign bodies, polyps, and tissue. The patient is lightly sedated during the procedure.
gamma-glutamyltransferase (GGT) (găm′ă gloo″tăm-ĭl-trăns′fĕr-ās)	Test performed on blood serum to determine the level of GGT (enzyme found in the liver, kidney, prostate, heart, and spleen). Increased values can indicate cirrhosis, liver necrosis, hepatitis, alcoholism, neoplasms, acute pancreatitis, acute myocardial infarction, nephrosis, and acute cholecystitis.
gastric analysis (găs′trĭk ă-năl′ĭ-sĭs)	Test performed to determine quality of secretion, amount of free and combined hydrochloric acid (HCl), and absence or presence of blood, bacteria, bile, and fatty acids. Increased level of HCl can indicate peptic ulcer disease, Zollinger–Ellison syndrome (a condition caused by non-insulin-secreting pancreatic tumors, which secrete excess amounts of gastrin), and hypergastrinemia. Decreased level of HCl can indicate stomach cancer, pernicious anemia, and atrophic gastritis.
gastrointestinal (GI) series (găs″trō-ĭn-tes′tĭn″ăl)	Fluoroscopic examination of the esophagus, stomach, and small intestine in which barium is given orally and is observed as it flows through the GI system. Abnormal results can indicate esophageal varices, ulcers, gastric polyps, malabsorption syndrome, hiatal hernias, diverticula, pyloric stenosis, and foreign bodies.
hepatitis panel (hĕp″ă-tī′tĭs)	A blood test used to find markers of hepatitis infection. There are different hepatitis panels. Some tests look for proteins (antibodies) that the body makes to fight the infection. Other tests look for antigens or the genetic material (DNA or RNA) of the viruses that cause hepatitis. A common panel checks for hepatitis A IgM antibodies (HA Ab-IgM), hepatitis B surface antigen (HBsAg), hepatitis B IgM core antibody (HBcAb-IgM), and hepatitis C antibodies (HC Ab).
liver biopsy	Microscopic examination of liver tissue. Abnormal results can indicate cirrhosis, hepatitis, and tumors.
occult blood (ŏ-kŭlt′)	Test performed on feces to determine gastrointestinal bleeding that is not visible. Positive results can indicate gastritis, stomach cancer, peptic ulcer, ulcerative colitis, bowel cancer, bleeding esophageal varices, portal hypertension, pancreatitis, and diverticulitis.
ova and parasites (O&P) (ō′vă and păr′ă-sīts)	Test performed on stool to identify ova and parasites. Positive results indicate protozoa infestation.

Test	Description
stool culture	Test performed to detect and identify bacteria that cause infection of the lower digestive tract. The test distinguishes between the types of bacteria that cause disease (pathogenic) and the types that are normally found in the digestive tract (normal flora).
ultrasonography, gallbladder (ŭl-tră-sŏn-ŏg′ră-fē)	Test to visualize the gallbladder by using high-frequency sound waves. The echoes are recorded and transformed into video or photographic images. Abnormal results can indicate biliary obstruction, cholelithiasis, and acute cholecystitis.
ultrasonography, liver	Test to visualize the liver by using high-frequency sound waves. The echoes are recorded and transformed into video or photographic images. See Figure 7.31. Abnormal results can indicate hepatic tumors, cysts, abscess, and cirrhosis.

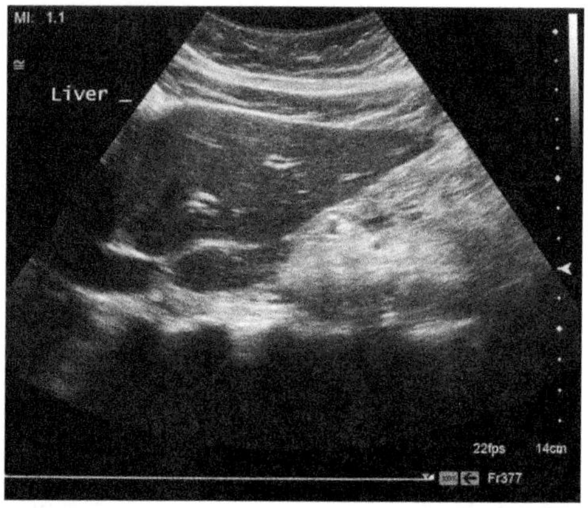

FIGURE 7.31 Ultrasound of the abdomen showing the liver.
Source: Monet_3k/Shutterstock

upper gastrointestinal (UGI) endoscopy (găs′trō-ĭn-tĕs′tĭn″ăl ĕn-dŏs′kō-pē)	Direct visual examination of the gastric mucosa via a flexible fiberoptic endoscope when gastric neoplasm is suspected. Colored photographs or motion pictures can be taken during the procedure.

Abbreviations *and* Acronyms

Abbreviation/ Acronym	Meaning	Abbreviation/ Acronym	Meaning
Ba	barium	ERCP	endoscopic retrograde cholangiopancreatography
BAC	blood alcohol concentration		
BE	Barrett esophagus	GB	gallbladder
BM	bowel movement	GERD	gastroesophageal reflux disease
CD	Crohn disease	GGT	gamma-glutamyltransferase
CEA	carcinoembryonic antigen	GI	gastrointestinal
CHO	carbohydrate	HAV	hepatitis A virus
CMP	comprehensive metabolic panel	HBsAg	hepatitis B surface antigen
EE	erosive esophagitis	HBV	hepatitis B
EGD	esophagogastroduodenoscopy	HCl	hydrochloric acid

Abbreviation/ Acronym	Meaning	Abbreviation/ Acronym	Meaning
HCV	hepatitis C virus	O&P	ova and parasites
HDV	hepatitis D virus	OIC	opioid-induced constipation
HEV	hepatitis E virus	PP	postprandial (after meals)
IBD	inflammatory bowel disease	PPIs	proton-pump inhibitors
IBS	irritable bowel syndrome	PUD	peptic ulcer disease
LES	lower esophageal sphincter	UC	ulcerative colitis
MSG	monosodium glutamate	UGI	upper gastrointestinal
NG	nasogastric (tube)		

Study *and* Review III

Building Medical Terms

Using the following word parts, fill in the blanks to build the correct medical terms.

dys-   gingiv   -al   -osis   -itis
bucc   lapar/o   -ectomy   -stomy   -cele

Definition	Medical Term
1. Surgical excision of the appendix	append_____
2. Literally means pertaining to the cheek	_____al
3. Chronic degenerative liver disease	cirrh_____
4. The creation of a new opening into the colon	colo_____
5. Inflammation of the diverticula in the colon	diverticul_____
6. Difficulty in digestion; indigestion	_____pepsia
7. Inflammation of the gums	_____itis
8. Surgical incision into the abdomen	_____tomy
9. Pertaining to the tongue	lingu_____
10. Hernia of part of the rectum into the vagina	recto_____

Combining Form Challenge

Using the combining forms provided, write the medical term correctly.

esophage/o	bil/i	hepat/o
stomat/o	absorpt/o	gloss/o

1. Process by which nutrient material is transferred from the gastrointestinal tract into the bloodstream or lymph: _____ion

2. Inflammation of the mouth: _____itis

3. Pertaining to bile: _____ary

4. Pertaining to the esophagus: _____al

5. Partial or total surgical excision of the tongue: _____ectomy

6. Inflammation of the liver: _____itis

Select the Right Term

Select the correct answer, and write it on the line provided.

1. Inflammation of the gallbladder is _____.

   choledochotomy   cholecystitis   cheilosis   appendicitis

2. Significant accumulation of fluid in the peritoneal cavity is _____.

   ascites   anabolism   cirrhosis   celiac

3. A surgical procedure that brings one end of the large intestine out through an opening (stoma) made in the abdominal wall is called a _____.

   colonoscopy   colostomy   colectomy   cholecystectomy

4. The term that means pertaining to the stomach and esophagus is _____.

   gastroenterology   gastroesophageal   gastoesophaeal   gastroenteritis

5. To feed liquid or semiliquid food via a tube is _____.

   gastric   enteric   gavage   deglutition

6. Chewing; the physical breaking-up of food and mixing with saliva is _____.

   malabsorption   mastication   lavage   gavage

Drug Highlights

Match the appropriate lettered description or examples of drug(s) with the class of drug.

_____ 1. agents used for inflammatory bowel disease

_____ 2. examples of antidiarrheal agents

_____ 3. antacids

_____ 4. antiemetics

_____ 5. histamine H2-receptor antagonists

_____ 6. examples of gastric acid pump inhibitors

_____ 7. emetics

_____ 8. laxatives

a. Neutralize hydrochloric acid in the stomach

b. Inhibit daytime and nocturnal basal gastric acid secretion and inhibit gastric acid stimulated by food, caffeine, etc.

c. Used to induce vomiting in people who have taken an overdose of oral drugs or who have ingested certain poisons

d. Prilosec (omeprazole), Aciphex (rabeprazole sodium), Prevacid (lansoprazole), Nexium (esomeprazole magnesium)

e. Pepto-Bismol (bismuth subsalicylate), Kaopectate (kaolin mixture with pectin), and Imodium (loperamide HCl)

f. Aminosalicylates, antibiotics, corticosteroids, immunomodulators

g. Used to relieve constipation and to facilitate the passage of feces through the lower gastrointestinal tract

h. Prevent or arrest vomiting

Diagnostic and Laboratory Tests

Select the best answer to each multiple-choice question. Circle the letter of your choice.

1. An x-ray examination of the common bile duct, cystic duct, and hepatic ducts.

a. cholangiography
b. cholecystography
c. cholangiopancreatography
d. ultrasonography

2. Direct visual examination of the colon via a flexible colonoscope.

a. cholangiography
b. ultrasonography
c. fiberoptic colonoscopy
d. cholecystography

3. Fluoroscopic examination of the esophagus, stomach, and small intestine.

    a. colonoscopy

    b. ultrasonography

    c. cholangiography

    d. gastrointestinal series

4. Endoscopic examination of the esophagus, stomach, and small intestine.

    a. cholangiography

    b. gastroduodenoesophagoscopy

    c. esophagogastroduodenoscopy

    d. gastric analysis

5. Test performed to determine the presence of the hepatitis B virus.

    a. occult blood test

    b. stool culture

    c. hepatitis B surface antigen

    d. ova and parasites test

Abbreviations and Acronyms

Write the correct word, phrase, or abbreviation/acronym in the space provided.

1. barium _____

2. CHO _____

3. HCV _____

4. hydrochloric acid _____

5. gallbladder _____

6. hepatitis A virus _____

7. NG _____

8. irritable bowel syndrome _____

9. postprandial (after meals) _____

10. proton-pump inhibitors _____

Practical Application

Medical Record Analysis

The Patient Referral Form is an important part of a patient's chart. As part of your learning process and in preparation for a career in a medical environment, you are to assume the role of a medical employee and use the following information—together with your own input—to complete the Patient Referral Form.

PATIENT REFERRAL FORM

Task	Edit	View	Time Scale	Options	Help	Date: 28 September 2021

Patient referred to Dalton Moss, MD, Endoscopy Center, 14 Maddox Dr., Rome, GA 30165, phone number (706) 235-3957, fax (706) 235-8877, for a screening colonoscopy on October 17, 2021, at 8:45 a.m. Advise patient to bring a driver, all current medications, driver's license, and proof of insurance.

Referring physician, Angel De'Crohn, MD, Family Practice, 1165 Berry Blvd., Rome, GA 30165, (706) 235-7765, fax (706) 235-6676.

Patient Referral Form

Our practice is affiliated with Mercy Medical Center.

Please refer this patient to Mercy Medical Center for any needed surgery or diagnostic procedures so that we can better coordinate this patient's care.

Date: 09/28/2021

Patient Name: Ralph J. Starr DOB: 2/24/57 Phone Number 123-456-7890

Appointment Date: _____ Time: _____

Referred to: _____

_____

For:

_____ Diagnostic Procedure _____

_____ Consultation

_____ Evaluate and treat, initiating appropriate diagnostic and/or therapeutic services

_____ Report test results to: _____

Reason for referral: _____

Patient Instructions: _____

_____

_____

Referring Physician's Name: _____ Date: _____

Phone #: _____ Fax #: _____

Remit the Record of this Patient's Visit to the Physician Noted Above.

For Office Use Only (appointment made at a time when the patient was not present)

Patient notified of appointment: Date: _____ Initials: _____

Unable to contact patient

Attempts to notify: Date/Time/Initials

1. _____

2. _____

3. _____

Comments: _____

Certified Letter Sent: Date: _____ Initials: _____

Referral Form Questions

Write the correct answer in the space provided.

1. Write in the Appointment Date: _____ Time: _____

2. The patient was referred to (write in name of physician, center name, and address):

_____

_____

_____

_____

3. The patient was referred for:

_____ Diagnostic Procedure

_____ Screening Colonoscopy

_____ Consultation

_____ Evaluate and treat, initiating appropriate diagnostic and/or therapeutic services

_____ Report test results to: Angel De'Crohn, MD

4. The patient was advised to: _____
_____

5. Write in the name of:

Referring Physician: _____

Date: _____

Phone #: _____

Fax #: _____

MyLab Medical Terminology™

MyLab Medical Terminology is a premium online homework management system that includes a host of features to help you study. Registered users will find:

- A multitude of quizzes and activities built within the MyLab platform
- Powerful tools that track and analyze your results—allowing you to create a personalized learning experience
- Videos and audio pronunciations to help enrich your progress
- Streaming lesson presentations (guided lectures) and self-paced learning modules
- A space where you and your instructor can check your progress and manage your assignments

8 Cardiovascular System

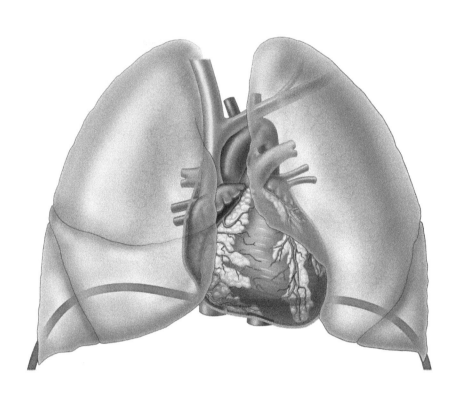

Learning Outcomes

On completion of this chapter, you will be able to:

1. State the description and primary functions of the organs/structures of the cardiovascular system.
2. Explain the circulation of blood through the chambers of the heart.
3. Identify and locate the commonly used sites for taking a pulse.
4. Explain blood pressure.
5. Analyze, build, spell, and pronounce medical words.
6. Classify the drugs highlighted in this chapter.
7. Describe diagnostic and laboratory tests related to the cardiovascular system.
8. Identify and define selected abbreviations and acronyms.

Anatomy and Physiology

The cardiovascular system includes the heart, blood, and blood vessels (arteries, veins, and capillaries). It is also called the *circulatory system* and, by the action of the heart, circulates blood to all parts of the body. This process provides the body's cells with oxygen and nutritive elements and removes waste materials and carbon dioxide. The heart, a muscular pump, is the central organ of the system. It beats approximately 100,000 times each day, pumping roughly 8,000 liters of blood, enough to fill about 8,500 quart-sized milk cartons. Arteries, veins, and capillaries comprise the network of vessels that transport blood (fluid consisting of blood cells and plasma) throughout the body. Blood flows through the heart, to the lungs, back to the heart, and on to the various body parts. Table 8.1 provides an at-a-glance look at the cardiovascular system. Figure 8.1 shows a schematic overview of the cardiovascular system.

TABLE 8.1 Cardiovascular System at-a-Glance	
Organ/Structure	**Primary Functions/Description**
Heart	The muscular pump that circulates blood through the heart, the lungs (pulmonary circulation), and the rest of the body (systemic circulation)
Arteries	Branching system of vessels that transports blood from the right and left ventricles of the heart to all body parts; transports blood away from the heart
Veins	Vessels that transport blood from peripheral tissues back to the heart
Capillaries	Microscopic blood vessels that connect arterioles with venules and facilitate passage of life-sustaining fluids containing oxygen and nutrients to cell bodies and removal of accumulated waste and carbon dioxide
Blood	Fluid consisting of formed elements (erythrocytes, thrombocytes, leukocytes) and plasma. It is a specialized bodily fluid that delivers necessary substances to the body's cells (oxygen, food, salts, hormones) and transports waste products (carbon dioxide, urea, lactic acid) away from those same cells. Blood is circulated around the body through blood vessels by the pumping action of the heart. See Chapter 9, *Blood and Lymphatic System*, for a further discussion of blood.

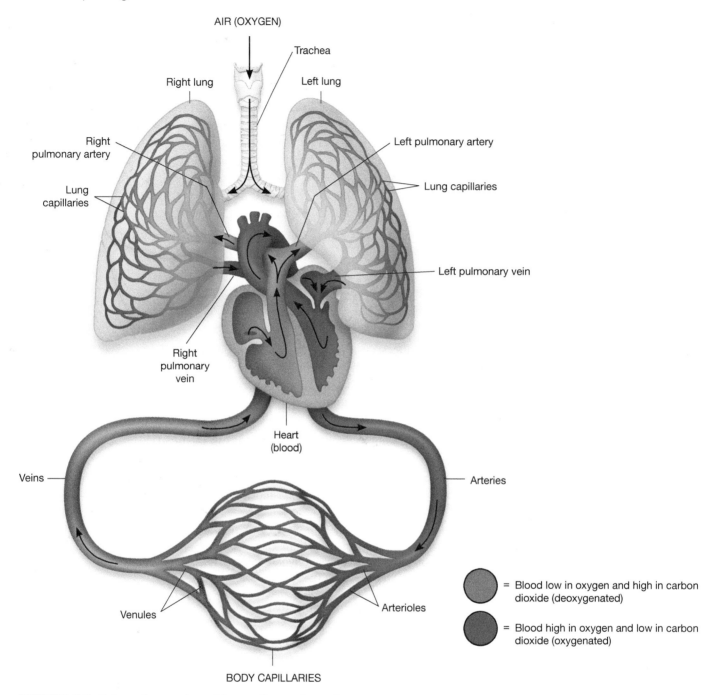

AIR (OXYGEN)

Trachea

Right lung

Left lung

Right pulmonary artery

Left pulmonary artery

Lung capillaries

Lung capillaries

Left pulmonary vein

Right pulmonary vein

Heart (blood)

Veins

Arteries

○ = Blood low in oxygen and high in carbon dioxide (deoxygenated)

● = Blood high in oxygen and low in carbon dioxide (oxygenated)

Venules

Arterioles

BODY CAPILLARIES

FIGURE 8.1 Schematic overview of the cardiovascular system.

Heart

The **heart** is the center of the cardiovascular system from which the various blood vessels originate and later return. Figure 8.2 shows the anatomy of the heart. It is slightly larger than a person's fist and weighs approximately 300 g in the average adult. It lies slightly to the left of the midline of the body, behind the sternum. See Figure 8.3.

The heart has three layers or linings:

- **Endocardium.** The inner lining of the heart.
- **Myocardium.** The muscular middle layer of the heart.
- **Pericardium.** The outer membranous sac surrounding the heart.

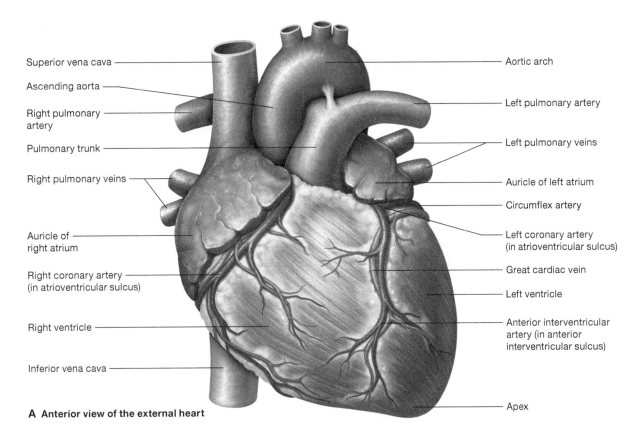

Superior vena cava

Ascending aorta

Right pulmonary artery

Pulmonary trunk

Right pulmonary veins

Auricle of right atrium

Right coronary artery (in atrioventricular sulcus)

Right ventricle

Inferior vena cava

Aortic arch

Left pulmonary artery

Left pulmonary veins

Auricle of left atrium

Circumflex artery

Left coronary artery (in atrioventricular sulcus)

Great cardiac vein

Left ventricle

Anterior interventricular artery (in anterior interventricular sulcus)

Apex

A Anterior view of the external heart

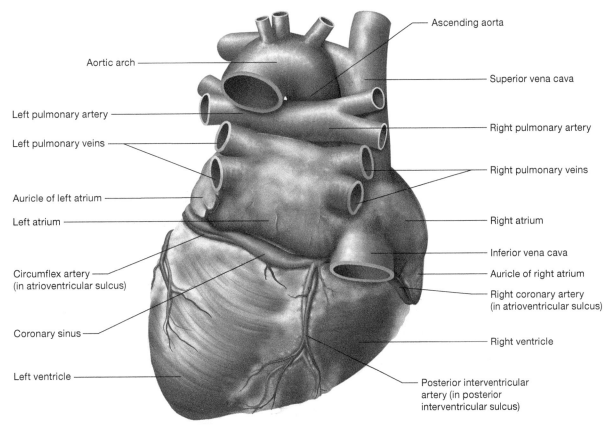

Aortic arch

Left pulmonary artery

Left pulmonary veins

Auricle of left atrium

Left atrium

Circumflex artery (in atrioventricular sulcus)

Coronary sinus

Left ventricle

Ascending aorta

Superior vena cava

Right pulmonary artery

Right pulmonary veins

Right atrium

Inferior vena cava

Auricle of right atrium

Right coronary artery (in atrioventricular sulcus)

Right ventricle

Posterior interventricular artery (in posterior interventricular sulcus)

B Posterior view of the external heart

FIGURE 8.2 External anatomy of the heart.

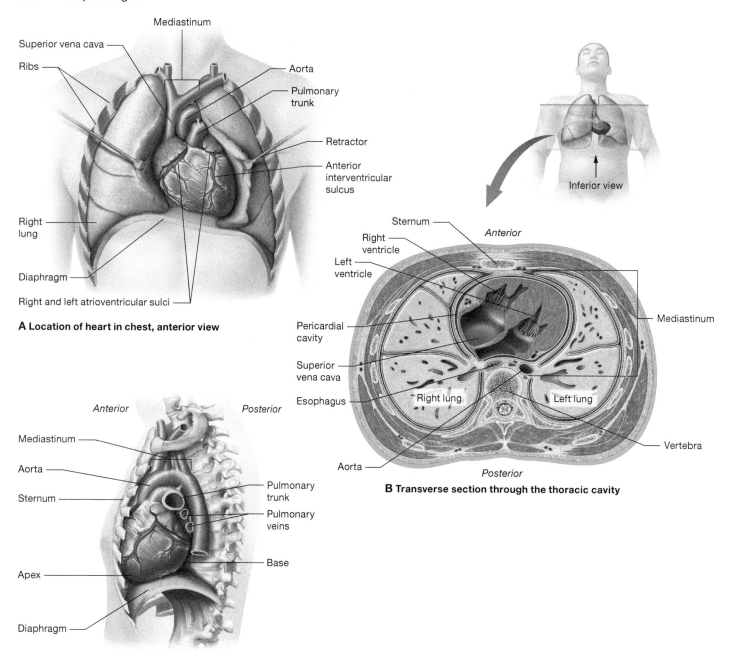

A Location of heart in chest, anterior view

B Transverse section through the thoracic cavity

C Location of heart in chest, left lateral view

FIGURE 8.3 Location of the heart in the chest cavity.

Circulation of Blood through the Chambers of the Heart

The heart is a pump and is divided into the right and left heart by a partition called the **septum**. Each side contains an upper and lower chamber. See Figure 8.4. The **atria**, or upper chambers, are separated by the interatrial septum. The **ventricles**, or lower chambers, are separated by the interventricular septum. The atria receive blood from the various parts of the body. The ventricles pump blood to body parts. Valves control the intake and outflow of blood in the heart chambers. Figure 8.5 shows the functioning of the heart valves and flow of blood through the heart.

RIGHT ATRIUM

The right upper portion of the heart is called the **right atrium (RA)**. It is a thin-walled space that receives blood from the upper and lower parts of the body (except the lungs). Two large veins, the superior vena cava and inferior vena cava, bring deoxygenated blood

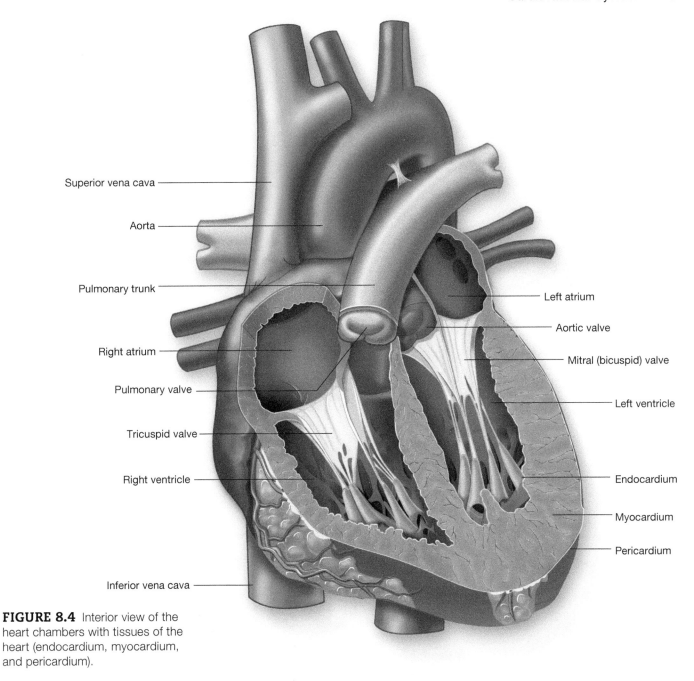

Superior vena cava
Aorta
Pulmonary trunk
Right atrium
Pulmonary valve
Tricuspid valve
Right ventricle
Inferior vena cava

Left atrium
Aortic valve
Mitral (bicuspid) valve
Left ventricle
Endocardium
Myocardium
Pericardium

FIGURE 8.4 Interior view of the heart chambers with tissues of the heart (endocardium, myocardium, and pericardium).

into the right atrium. Deoxygenated blood fills the right atrium before passing through the tricuspid (atrioventricular) valve and into the right ventricle.

RIGHT VENTRICLE

The right lower portion of the heart is called the **right ventricle (RV)**. As deoxygenated blood flows into the right atrium, it passes through the tricuspid valve and into the right ventricle, which pumps the blood up through the pulmonary valve and through the pulmonary artery to the lungs. This creates pressure, closing the right atrium and forcing open the pulmonary (semilunar) valve, sending blood into the left and right pulmonary arteries, which carry it to the lungs. The pulmonary artery is the only artery in the body that carries blood deficient in oxygen. In the lungs, the blood gives up wastes and takes on oxygen as it passes through capillary beds into veins. Oxygenated blood leaves the lungs through the left and right pulmonary veins, which carry it to the heart's left atrium. The pulmonary veins are the only veins in the body that carry oxygen-rich (oxygenated) blood.

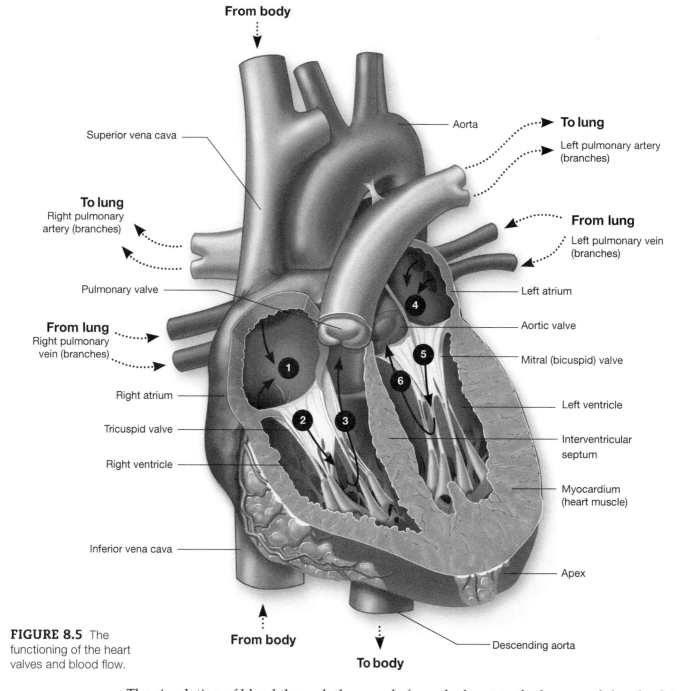

FIGURE 8.5 The functioning of the heart valves and blood flow.

The circulation of blood through the vessels from the heart to the lungs and then back to the heart again is the pulmonary circulation.

LEFT ATRIUM

The left upper portion of the heart is called the **left atrium (LA)**. It receives blood rich in oxygen as it returns from the lungs via the left and right pulmonary veins. As oxygenated blood fills the LA, it creates pressure that forces open the mitral (bicuspid) valve and allows the blood to fill the left ventricle.

LEFT VENTRICLE

The left lower portion of the heart is called the **left ventricle (LV)**. It receives blood from the left atrium through the mitral valve. When filled, the LV contracts. This creates pressure closing the mitral valve and forcing open the aortic valve. The oxygenated blood from the LV flows through the aortic valve and into a large artery known as the aorta and from there to all parts of the body via a branching system of arteries and capillaries.

fyi Pediatric cardiologists have recognized more than 50 congenital heart defects. If the left side of the heart is not completely separated from the right side, various septal defects develop. If the four chambers of the heart do not develop normally, complex anomalies form, such as tetralogy of Fallot (TOF), a congenital heart condition involving four defects: pulmonary artery stenosis, ventricular septal defect (VSD), displacement of the aorta to the right, and hypertrophy of the right ventricle.

Heart Valves

The **valves** of the heart are located at the entrance and exit of each ventricle and, as you learned in the preceding section, control the flow of blood within the heart. See Figure 8.6.

TRICUSPID VALVE

The *tricuspid* or *right atrioventricular valve* guards the opening between the right atrium and the right ventricle. In a normal state, the tricuspid valve opens to allow the flow of blood into the ventricle and then closes to prevent any backflow of blood.

PULMONARY (SEMILUNAR) VALVE

The exit point for blood leaving the right ventricle is called the *pulmonary (semilunar) valve*. Located between the right ventricle and the pulmonary artery, it allows blood to flow from the right ventricle through the pulmonary artery to the lungs.

MITRAL (BICUSPID) VALVE

The left atrioventricular valve between the left atrium and the left ventricle is called the *mitral valve (MV)* or *bicuspid valve*. It allows blood to flow to the left ventricle and closes to prevent its return to the left atrium.

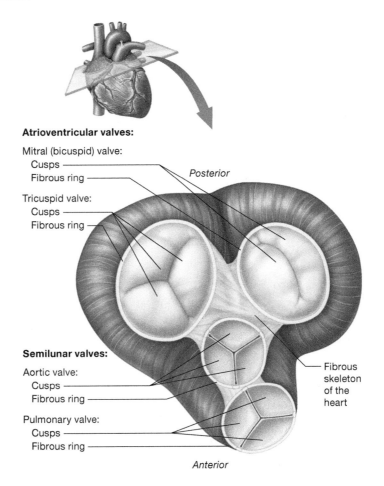

FIGURE 8.6 Valves of the heart.
Source: AMERMAN, ERIN C., HUMAN ANATOMY & PHYSIOLOGY, 2nd Ed., ©2019. Reprinted and Electronically reproduced by permission of Pearson Education, Inc., New York, NY.

AORTIC (SEMILUNAR) VALVE

Blood exits from the left ventricle through the *aortic (semilunar) valve*. Located between the left ventricle and the aorta, it allows blood to flow into the aorta and prevents its backflow to the ventricle.

Vascular System of the Heart

Due to the membranous lining of the heart (endocardium) and the thickness of the myocardium, the heart has its own vascular system to meet its high oxygen demand. The coronary arteries supply the heart with oxygen-rich blood, and the cardiac veins, draining into the coronary sinus, collect the blood (oxygen poor) and return it to the right atrium. See Figure 8.7.

Conduction System of the Heart

The autonomic nervous system controls the rate and rhythm of the **heartbeat**. It is normally generated by specialized neuromuscular tissue of the heart that is capable of causing cardiac muscle to contract rhythmically. This tissue of the heart comprises the **sinoatrial node**, the **atrioventricular node**, and the **atrioventricular bundle**. See Figure 8.8.

SINOATRIAL NODE (SA NODE)

Called the *pacemaker* of the heart, the *SA node* is located in the upper wall of the right atrium, just below the opening of the superior vena cava. It consists of a dense network of Purkinje fibers (*atypical muscle fibers*) considered to be the source of impulses initiating the heartbeat. Electrical impulses discharged by the SA node are distributed to the right and left atria and cause them to contract.

ATRIOVENTRICULAR NODE (AV NODE)

Located beneath the endocardium of the right atrium, the *AV node* transmits electrical impulses to the bundle of His (*atrioventricular bundle*).

ATRIOVENTRICULAR BUNDLE (BUNDLE OF HIS)

The *atrioventricular bundle* or *bundle of His* forms a part of the conduction system of the heart. It is a collection of heart muscle cells specialized for electrical conduction that transmits the electrical impulses from the AV node to the point of the apex of the fascicular branches.

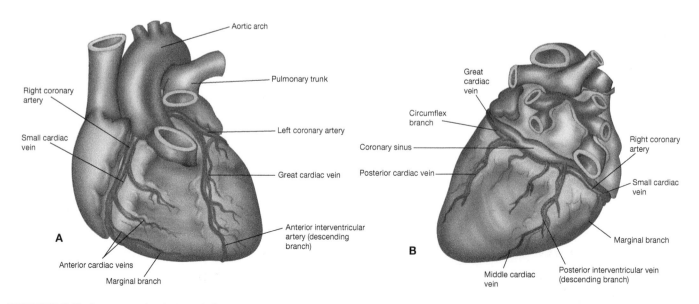

FIGURE 8.7 Coronary circulation. **A** Coronary vessels portraying the complexity and extent of the coronary circulation. **B** Coronary vessels that supply the posterior surface of the heart.

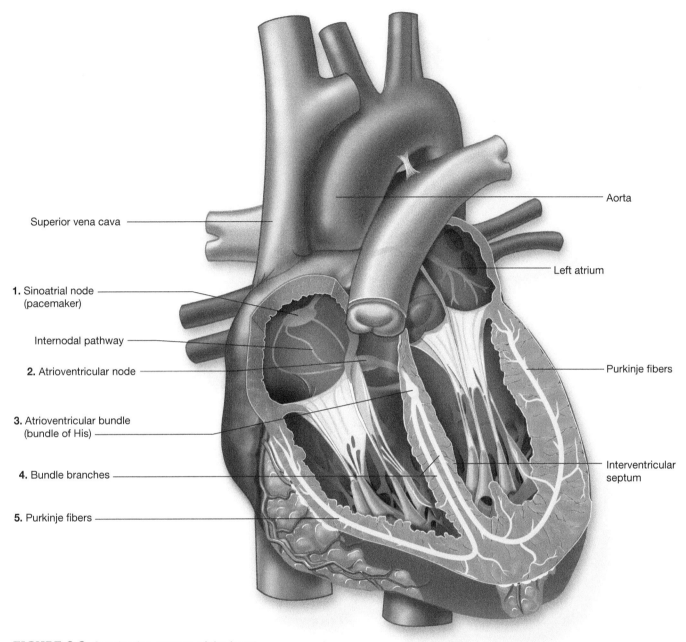

FIGURE 8.8 Conduction system of the heart.

The bundle of His branches into the two bundle branches that run along the interventricular septum. The bundles give rise to thin filaments known as *Purkinje fibers*. These fibers distribute the impulse to the ventricular muscle. Together, the bundle branches and Purkinje network comprise the ventricular conduction system.

The average adult heartbeat (*pulse*) is between 60 and 100 beats per minute. The rate of the heartbeat can be affected by emotions, smoking, disease, body size, age, stress, the environment, and many other factors.

The heart's electrical activity can be recorded by an **electrocardiogram (ECG, EKG)**, which provides valuable information in diagnosing cardiac abnormalities, such as myocardial damage and arrhythmias (see the section "Diagnostic and Laboratory Tests" and Figure 8.41).

Blood Vessels

There are three main types of blood vessels: arteries, veins, and capillaries. Blood circulates throughout the body through their pathways.

Arteries

The **arteries** constitute a branching system of vessels that transports blood away from the heart to all body parts. See Figure 8.9. In a normal state, arteries are elastic tubes that recoil and carry blood in pulsating waves. All arteries have a pulse, reflecting the rhythmical beating of the heart; however, certain points are commonly used to check the rate, rhythm, and condition of the arterial wall.

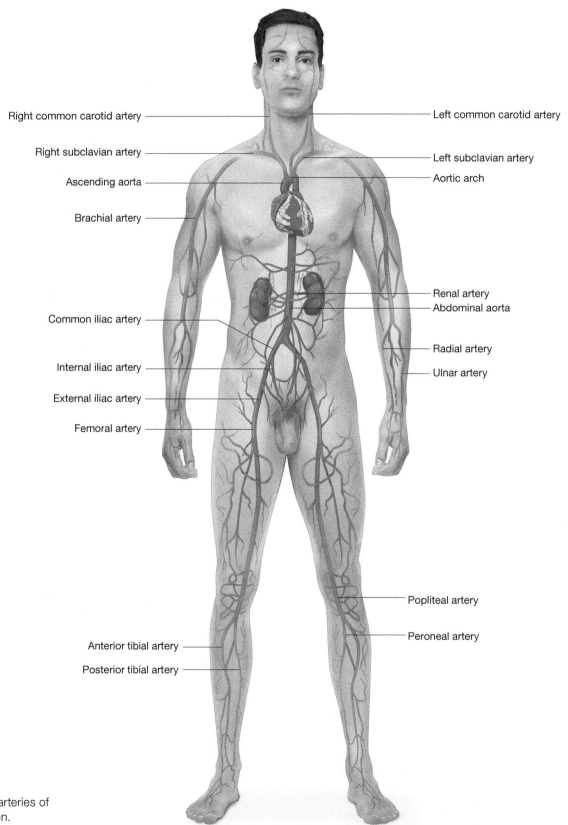

FIGURE 8.9 Major arteries of the systemic circulation.

A person's pulse can be felt in a place that allows for an artery to be compressed against a bone. The most commonly used sites for taking a pulse are the radial artery, the brachial artery, and the carotid artery. See Table 8.2 and Figure 8.10. The pulse rate can also be measured by using a stethoscope (*auscultation*) and counting the heartbeat for 1 full minute. This is known as the **apical pulse** and is taken over the heart itself. In contrast with other pulse sites, the apical pulse site is unilateral and is located at the apex of the heart or at the fifth intercostal space, just to the left of the midclavicular line. It is commonly used to check pulse rate in infants and children and when the radial pulse is difficult to palpate (to feel by touch).

Veins

Veins are the vessels that transport blood from peripheral tissues back to the heart. In a normal state, veins have thin walls and valves that prevent the backflow of blood. The great saphenous vein is an important superficial vein of the lower limb. The pulmonary veins carry oxygenated blood from the lungs to the heart. The superior and inferior venae cavae carry deoxygenated blood from the upper and lower systemic circulation. See Figure 8.11.

TABLE 8.2	**Pulse Checkpoints**
Checkpoint	**Site/Use**
Temporal	Temple area of the head. Used to control bleeding from the head and scalp and to monitor circulation.
Carotid	Neck. In an emergency (*cardiac arrest*), most readily accessible site.
Brachial	Antecubital space of the elbow. Most common site used to check blood pressure.
Radial	Radial (*thumb side*) of the wrist. Most common site for taking a pulse.
Femoral	Groin area. Monitor circulation.
Popliteal	Behind the knee. Monitor circulation.
Dorsalis pedis	Dorsal surface of the foot. Assess for peripheral artery disease (PAD).

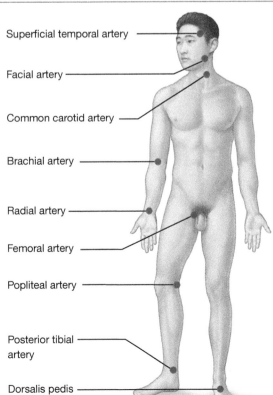

FIGURE 8.10 Primary pulse points of the body.
Source: MARIEB, ELAINE N.; KELLER, SUZANNE M., ESSENTIALS OF HUMAN ANATOMY & PHYSIOLOGY, 12th Ed., ©2018. Reprinted and Electronically reproduced by permission of Pearson Education, Inc., New York, NY.

Superficial temporal artery

Facial artery

Common carotid artery

Brachial artery

Radial artery

Femoral artery

Popliteal artery

Posterior tibial artery

Dorsalis pedis artery

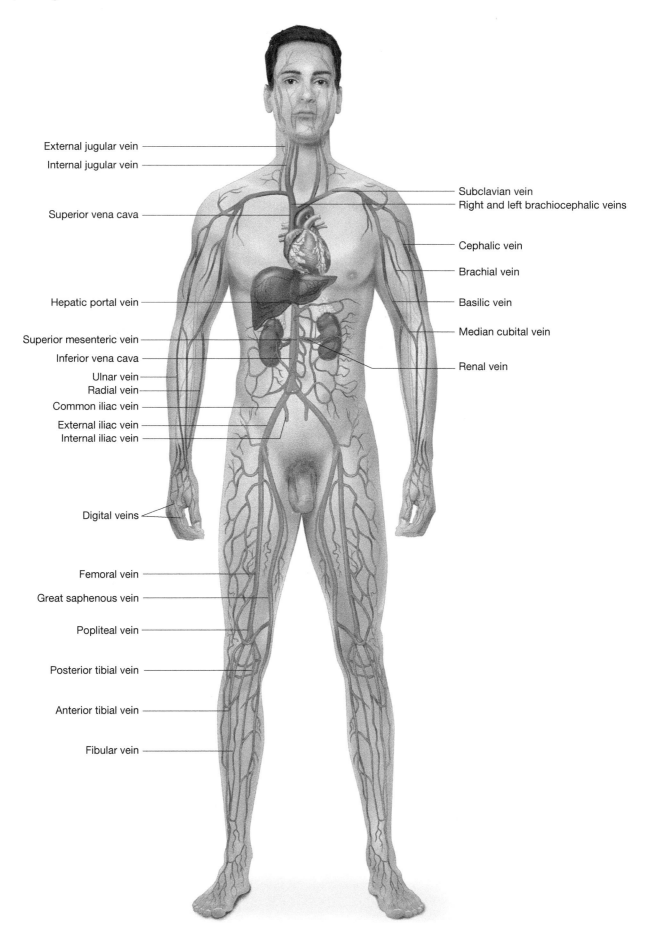

External jugular vein

Internal jugular vein

Superior vena cava

Hepatic portal vein

Superior mesenteric vein

Inferior vena cava

Ulnar vein

Radial vein

Common iliac vein

External iliac vein

Internal iliac vein

Digital veins

Femoral vein

Great saphenous vein

Popliteal vein

Posterior tibial vein

Anterior tibial vein

Fibular vein

Subclavian vein

Right and left brachiocephalic veins

Cephalic vein

Brachial vein

Basilic vein

Median cubital vein

Renal vein

FIGURE 8.11 Major veins of the systemic circulation.

Capillaries

The **capillaries** are microscopic blood vessels with single-celled walls that connect **arterioles** (*small arteries*) with **venules** (*small veins*). See Figure 8.12. Blood passing through capillaries gives up the oxygen and nutrients carried to this point by the arteries and picks up waste and carbon dioxide as it enters the veins. Veins lead away from the capillaries as tiny vessels and increase in size until they join the superior and inferior venae cavae as they return to the heart. The extremely thin walls of capillaries facilitate passage of oxygen and nutrients to cell bodies and the removal of accumulated waste and carbon dioxide.

Blood Pressure

Blood pressure (BP) is the pressure exerted by the blood on the walls of the arteries. It results from two forces. One is created by the heart as it pumps blood into the arteries and through the circulatory system. The other is the force of the arteries as they resist the blood flow. The higher (systolic) number represents the pressure while the heart contracts to pump blood to the body. The lower (diastolic) number represents the pressure when the heart relaxes between beats. Blood pressure is reported in millimeters of mercury (mmHg) and is measured with a **sphygmomanometer**. See Figure 8.13.

The systolic pressure is always stated first. For example, 116/74 (116 over 74); systolic = 116, diastolic = 74. According to the American Heart Association and the Centers for Disease Control and Prevention, blood pressure measuring 120 mmHg over 80 mmHg or less is considered optimal for adults; high blood pressure (HBP) or *hypertension* is diagnosed when blood pressure measurements are higher than 140/90. See Figure 8.14.

Pulse (P), **blood pressure (BP)**, and **respiration (R)** rates vary according to a child's age. A newborn's pulse rate is irregular and rapid, varying from 120 to 160 beats/minute. Blood pressure is low and can vary with the size of the cuff used. The average blood pressure at birth is 64/41. Respirations are approximately 40–60 per minute.

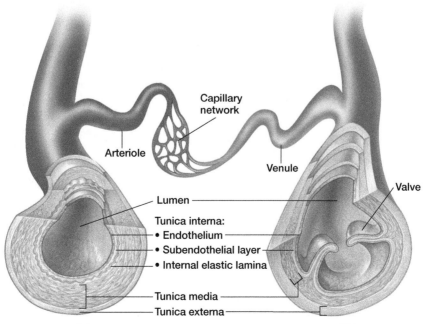

FIGURE 8.12 Capillaries.

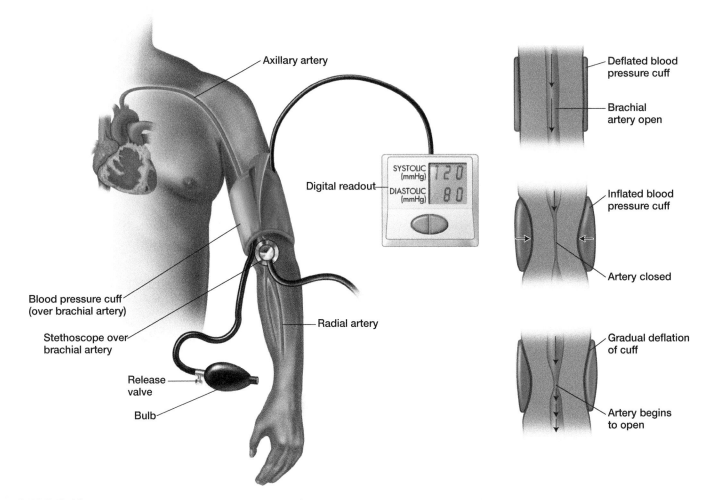

FIGURE 8.13 Blood pressure measurement using a sphygmomanometer.

BLOOD PRESSURE CLASSIFICATIONS		
Systolic Reading	*Diastolic Reading*	*Classification*
< 120 mmHg	< 80 mmHg	**Normal**
120–129 mmHg	< 80 mmHg	**Elevated**
130–139 mmHg	80–89 mmHg	**At risk for High Blood Pressure** (Prehypertension)
> 140 mmHg	> 90 mmHg	**High Blood Pressure** (Hypertension)
> 180 mmHg	> 120 mmHg	**Hypertensive Crisis** (Seek medical attention immediately)
< (less than)		
> (more than)		
mmHg (millimeters of Mercury) This measurement is used to measure pressure.		

FIGURE 8.14 Blood pressure classifications.

PULSE PRESSURE

The pulse pressure is the difference between the systolic and diastolic readings. This reading indicates the tone of the arterial walls. The normal pulse pressure is found when the systolic pressure is about 40 points higher than the diastolic reading. For example, if the blood pressure is 120/80, the pulse pressure would be 40. A pulse pressure over 50 points or under 30 points is considered abnormal.

Study *and* Review I

Anatomy and Physiology

Write your answers to the following questions.

1. The cardiovascular system includes the heart, _____ and _____.

2. Name the three layers of the heart.

   a. _____   c. _____

   b. _____

3. The heart weighs approximately _____ grams.

4. The _____ or upper chambers of the heart are separated by the

   _____ septum.

5. The _____ or lower chambers of the heart are separated by the

   _____ septum.

6. A/An _____ records the heart's electrical activity.

7. The _____ nervous system controls the heartbeat.

8. The _____ _____ is called the *pacemaker of the heart*.

9. Together, the bundle branches and _____ comprise the ventricular conduction system.

10. Name the three primary pulse points and state their locations on the body.

    a. _____ located _____

    b. _____ located _____

    c. _____ located _____

11. Define the following terms:

    a. Blood pressure _____

    b. Pulse pressure _____

12. The average adult heart is about the size of a _____ and normally beats at a pulse

    rate of _____ to _____ beats per minute.

13. A systolic pressure of _____ mmHg or higher or a diastolic pressure of

    _____ mmHg or higher is considered "hypertension stage 2" and needs to be

    monitored on a regular basis.

14. State the primary function of arteries. _____

_____

_____

15. State the primary function of veins. _____

_____

_____

▶ **ANATOMY LABELING**   Identify the structures shown below by filling in the blanks.

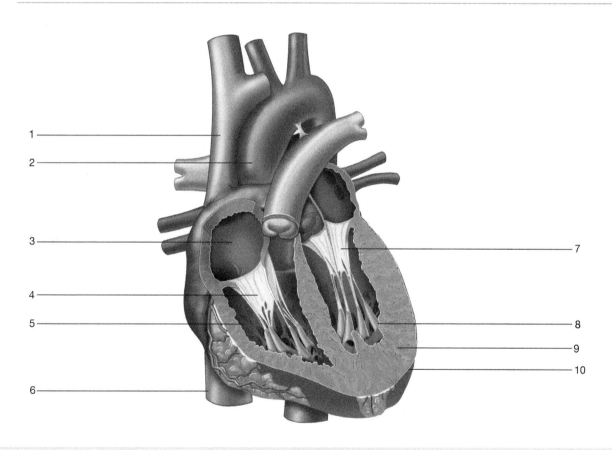

Building Your Medical Vocabulary

This section provides the foundation for learning medical terminology. Review the alphabetized list of medical terms in the following pages. Note how common prefixes and suffixes are repeatedly applied to word roots and combining forms to create different meanings. A combining form is a word root plus a vowel. The chart below lists the combining forms and word roots used in this chapter and can help to strengthen your understanding of how medical words are built and spelled.

You will find that some terms have not been divided into word parts. These are common words or specialized terms that are included to enhance your medical vocabulary.

Combining Forms

angi/o	vessel	**man/o**	thin
angin/o	to choke	**mitr/o**	mitral valve
arteri/o	artery	**my/o**	muscle
ather/o	fatty substance	**occlus/o**	to close up
atri/o	atrium	**ox/i**	oxygen
auscultat/o	listen to	**pector/o**	chest
cardi/o	heart	**phleb/o**	vein
chol/e	bile	**pulmon/o**	lung
circulat/o	circular	**rrhythm/o**	rhythm
claudicat/o	to limp	**scler/o**	hardening
corpor/o	body	**sept/o**	a partition
cyan/o	dark blue	**sin/o**	a curve
dilat/o	to widen	**sphygm/o**	pulse
dynam/o	power	**sten/o**	narrowing
embol/o	to cast, to throw	**steth/o**	chest
glyc/o	sweet, sugar	**thromb/o**	clot
hem/o	blood	**valvul/o**	valve
infarct/o	infarct (necrosis of an area)	**vas/o**	vessel
isch/o	to hold back	**vascul/o**	small vessel
lipid/o	fat	**ventricul/o**	ventricle
lun/o	moon	**vers/o**	turning

Word Roots

anastom	opening	**palpitat**	throbbing
arter	artery	**sterol**	solid (fat)
card	heart	**strict**	to draw, to bind
fibrillat	fibrils (small fibers)	**tel**	end
log	study	**tens**	pressure
oxy	sour, sharp, acid	**ton**	tone

Medical Word	Word Parts		Definition
	Part	Meaning	
anastomosis (ă-năs″ tō-mō´ sĭs)	**anastom** **-osis**	opening condition	Connection of two things that are normally diverging, which can occur naturally in the body; however, in medicine an anastomosis typically refers to a surgical connection between blood vessels or the joining of one hollow or tubular organ to another
aneurysm (ăn´ ū-rĭzm)			Abnormal widening or ballooning of a portion of an artery due to weakness in the wall of the blood vessel. See Figure 8.15.

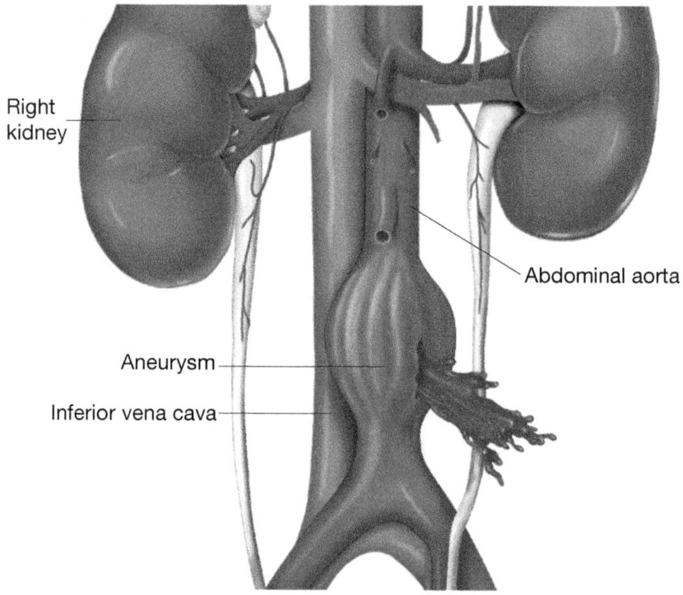

FIGURE 8.15 Ruptured abdominal aortic aneurysm.

Medical Word	Word Parts		Definition
angina pectoris (ăn´ jĭ-nă pĕk´ tōr″ ĭs)	**angin (a)** **pector** **-is**	to choke chest pertaining to	Chest pain that occurs when diseased blood vessels restrict blood flow to the heart. It is the most common symptom of coronary artery disease (CAD) and is often referred to as *angina*. The pain can radiate to the neck, jaw, or left arm. It is often described as a crushing, burning, or squeezing sensation. Patients with CAD can present with stable angina pectoris, unstable angina pectoris, or a myocardial infarction (MI), a heart attack.

Medical Word	Word Parts		Definition
	Part	**Meaning**	
angioma (ăn″ jē-ō′ mă)	**angi** **-oma**	vessel tumor	Tumor of a blood vessel. See Figure 8.16.

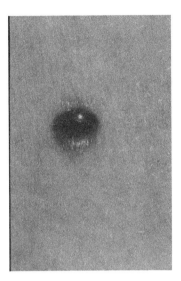

FIGURE 8.16 Infarction angioma.
Source: Courtesy of Jason L. Smith, MD

Medical Word	Word Parts		Definition
angioplasty (ăn′ jē-ō-plăs″ tē)	**angi/o** **-plasty**	vessel surgical repair	Surgical repair of a blood vessel(s) or a nonsurgical technique for treating diseased arteries by temporarily inflating a tiny balloon inside an artery
angiostenosis (ăn″ jē-ō-stĕ-nō′ sĭs)	**angi/o** **sten** **-osis**	vessel narrowing condition	Pathological condition of the narrowing of a blood vessel
arrhythmia (ă-rĭth′ mē-ă)	**a-** **rrhythm** **-ia**	lack of rhythm condition	Irregularity or loss of rhythm of the heartbeat; also called *dysrhythmia*. *Note:* The prefix **dys-** means *difficult*.

fyi A *cardiac ablation* is a procedure that can correct heart rhythm problems (arrhythmias). It is used to scar small areas of the heart that may be involved in the arrhythmia. There are two methods. *Radiofrequency ablation* uses heat energy to eliminate the difficult area. *Cryoablation* uses very cold temperatures. During the procedure, small electrodes are placed inside the heart to measure the heart's electrical activity. When the source of the arrhythmia is found, the tissue causing the difficulty is destroyed.

Medical Word	Word Parts		Definition
arterial (ăr-tē′ rē-ăl)	**arter/i** **-al**	artery pertaining to	Pertaining to an artery

Medical Word	Word Parts		Definition
	Part	**Meaning**	
arteriosclerosis (ăr-tē″ rē-ō-sklĕ-rō′ sĭs)	**arteri/o** **scler** **-osis**	artery hardening condition	Pathological condition of hardening of arteries. Arteriosclerotic heart disease (ASHD) is hardening of the coronary arteries.

 fyi In some older adults, the heart must work harder to pump blood because of hardening of the arteries (*arteriosclerosis*) and a buildup of fatty plaques (cholesterol deposits and triglycerides) in the arterial walls (*atherosclerosis*). Arteries can gradually become stiff and lose their elastic recoil. The aorta and arteries supplying the heart and brain are generally affected first. **Arteriosclerotic heart disease (ASHD)** occurs when the arterial vessels are marked by thickening, hardening, and loss of elasticity in the arterial walls. Reduced blood flow, elevated blood lipids, and defective endothelial repair that can be seen in aging accelerate the course of cardiovascular disease.

| **arteritis** (ăr″ tĕ-rī′ tĭs) | **arter** **-itis** | artery inflammation | Inflammation of an artery. See Figure 8.17. |

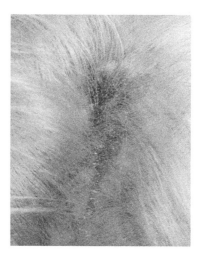

FIGURE 8.17 Temporal arteritis.
Source: Courtesy of Jason L. Smith, MD

Medical Word	Word Parts		Definition
	Part	**Meaning**	
artificial pacemaker			Electronic device that stimulates impulse initiation within the heart. It is a small, battery-operated device that helps the heart beat in a regular rhythm. See Figure 8.18.

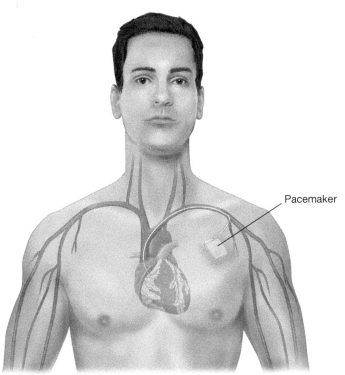

Pacemaker

FIGURE 8.18 A permanent epicardial pacemaker. The pulse generator can be placed in subcutaneous pockets in the subclavian or abdominal regions.

Medical Word	Word Parts		Definition
atheroma (ăth″ĕr-ō′ mă)	**ather** **-oma**	fatty substance tumor	Tumor of an artery containing a fatty substance
atherosclerosis (ăth″ĕr-ō-sklĕ-rō′ sĭs)	**ather/o** **scler** **-osis**	fatty substance hardening condition	Pathological condition of the arteries characterized by the buildup of fatty substances (cholesterol deposits and triglycerides) and hardening of the walls. Refer to Figures 8.22 and 8.23.

Medical Word	Word Parts		Definition
	Part	Meaning	
auscultation (aws″ kŭl-tā´ shŭn)	auscultat -ion	listen to process	Method of physical assessment using a stethoscope to listen to sounds within the chest, abdomen (Abd, abd), and other parts of the body. See Figure 8.19.

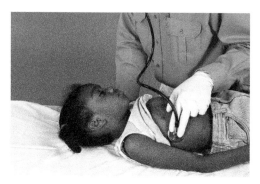

FIGURE 8.19 During auscultation, sounds can be heard via a stethoscope.
Source: Pearson Education, Inc.

Medical Word	Word Parts		Definition
automated external defibrillator (AED) (aw´ tō-māt-ĕd eks-tĕr´ năl dē-fĭb´ rĭ-lā-tor)			Portable automatic device used to restore normal heart rhythm to patients in cardiac arrest. An AED is applied outside the body. It automatically analyzes the patient's heart rhythm and advises the rescuer whether a shock is needed to restore a normal heartbeat. If the patient's heart resumes beating normally, the heart has been defibrillated.
bicuspid (bī-kŭs´ pĭd)	bi- -cuspid	two point	Valve with two cusps; pertaining to the mitral valve
bradycardia (brăd″ ĭ-kăr´ dē-ă)	brady- card -ia	slow heart condition	Abnormally slow heartbeat defined as fewer than 60 beats per minute
bruit (broot)			Pathological noise; a sound of venous or arterial origin heard on auscultation
cardiac (kăr´ dē-ăk)	cardi -ac	heart pertaining to	Pertaining to the heart
cardiac arrest			Loss of effective heart function, which results in cessation of functional circulation. Sudden cardiac arrest (SCA) results in sudden death.
cardiologist (kăr-dē-ŏl´ ō-jĭst)	cardi/o log -ist	heart study one who specializes	Physician who specializes in the study of the heart
cardiology (kăr´ dē-ŏl´ ō-jē)	cardi/o -logy	heart study of	Literally means *study of the heart*

Medical Word	Word Parts		Definition
	Part	**Meaning**	
cardiomegaly (kăr″ dē-ō-mĕg′ ă-lē)	**cardi/o** **-megaly**	heart enlargement, large	Enlargement of the heart
cardiometabolic syndrome (CMS) (kăr″ dē-ō-mĕt″ ă-bŏl′ ĭk sĭn′ drōm)			A combination of metabolic dysfunctions mainly characterized by insulin resistance, impaired glucose tolerance, *dyslipidemia* (abnormally elevated cholesterol or fats in the blood), hypertension, and *central adiposity* (accumulation of fat around the abdominal area)

G**OO**D TO KNOW ▶

CMS consists of maladies of the cardiovascular, renal, metabolic, and prothrombotic systems plus inflammatory abnormalities. It was recognized in 2017 as a disease entity by the American Society of Endocrinology, the National Cholesterol Education Program, and the World Health Organization. The cardiovascular and metabolic derangements in CMS individually and interdependently lead to a substantial increase in cardiovascular disease (CVD) morbidity and mortality, making CMS an established and strong risk factor for premature and severe CVD and stroke.

In the U.S. adult population, hypertension (HTN) affects approximately 29%, overweight/obesity affects about 66%, diabetes affects almost 10%, and chronic kidney disease (CKD) affects 14%, with CMS affecting 35–40%. All of these factors lead to increasing rates of cardiovascular disease and stroke.

Established and evolving treatment strategies including moderate physical activity, weight reduction, rigorous blood pressure control, correction of dyslipidemia, and glycemic control have proven beneficial in reversing the abnormal responses of CMS and decreasing CVD risk.

cardiomyopathy (CMP) (kăr″ dē-ō-mī-ŏp′ ă-thē)	**cardi/o** **my/o** **-pathy**	heart muscle disease	Disease of the heart muscle that leads to generalized deterioration of the muscle and its pumping ability. It can be caused by multiple factors, including viral infections. See Figure 8.20.

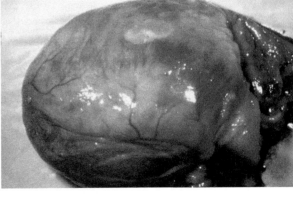

FIGURE 8.20 An enlarged heart showing the results of cardiomyopathy.
Source: Pearson Education, Inc.

Medical Word	Word Parts		Definition
	Part	Meaning	
cardiopulmonary (kăr″ dē-ō-pŭl′ mō-nĕr-ē)	cardi/o pulmon -ary	heart lung pertaining to	Pertaining to the heart and lungs (H&L)
cardiotonic (kăr″ dē-ō-tŏn′ ĭk)	cardi/o ton -ic	heart tone pertaining to	A class of medication that is used to increase the tone (pumping strength) of the heart
cardiovascular (CV) (kăr″ dē-ō-văs′ kū-lăr)	cardi/o vascul -ar	heart small vessel pertaining to	Pertaining to the heart and small blood vessels
cardioversion (kăr′ dē-ō-vĕr″ zhŭn)	cardi/o vers -ion	heart turning process	Medical procedure used to treat cardiac arrhythmias. An electrical shock is delivered to the heart to restore its normal rhythm. The electrical energy can be delivered externally through electrodes placed on the chest or directly to the heart by placing paddles on the heart during an open chest surgery.

! ALERT!

The combining form **cardi/o** means *heart*. By adding various suffixes, you can build medical words. How many terms can you build?

cholesterol (chol) (kō-lĕs′ tĕr-ŏl)	chol/e sterol	bile solid (fat)	A normal, soft, waxy substance found among the lipids (fats) in the bloodstream and all body cells. It is the building block of steroid hormones, but it is dangerous when it builds up on arterial walls and can contribute to the risk of coronary heart disease.

fyi There is evidence that cholesterol can begin clogging the arteries during childhood, leading to atherosclerosis and heart disease later in life. The American Heart Association recommends children and teenagers with high cholesterol take steps to bring it down, as should adults. Ideally, total cholesterol should be below 170 mg/dL in people ages 2–19, and below 200 mg/dL in adults over age 20.

circulation (sĭr″ kū-lā′ shŭn)	circulat -ion	circular process	The moving of the blood in the veins and arteries throughout the body
claudication (klaw-dĭ-kā′ shŭn)	claudicat -ion	to limp process	Literally means *process of lameness or limping*. It is a dull, cramping pain in the hips, thighs, calves, or buttocks caused by an inadequate supply of oxygen to the muscles, due to narrowed arteries. It is one of the symptoms in peripheral artery disease (PAD).

Medical Word	Word Parts		Definition
	Part	Meaning	
constriction (kŏn-strĭk´ shŭn)	con- strict -ion	together, with to draw, to bind process	Process of drawing together, as in the narrowing of a vessel
coronary artery bypass graft (CABG) (kor´ ŏ-nĕr-ē ăr´ tĕr-ē bī´ păs grăft)			Surgical procedure to assist blood flow to the myocardium by using a section of a saphenous vein or internal mammary artery to bypass or reroute blood around an obstructed or occluded coronary artery, thus improving blood flow and oxygen to the heart. See Figure 8.21.

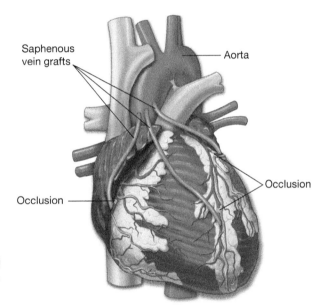

FIGURE 8.21 A coronary artery bypass graft (CABG) is a procedure to bypass a blocked coronary artery. The procedure involves isolating the blocked coronary artery and grafting a vessel to bypass it. The graft vessel is usually a portion of the saphenous vein of the leg or the internal mammary artery. It is grafted with very fine sutures.

 fyi Cardiopulmonary bypass with a pump oxygenator (heart–lung machine) is used for most coronary artery bypass graft operations. Another option is *off-pump coronary bypass (OPCAB)* surgery. During this surgery, the heart continues beating while the bypass graft is sewn in place. In some patients, OPCAB may reduce intraoperative bleeding (and the need for blood transfusion), renal complications, and postoperative neurological deficits (problems after surgery). Increasing blood flow to the heart muscle can relieve chest pain and reduce the risk of heart attack. A patient may undergo several bypass grafts, depending on how many coronary arteries are blocked.

Medical Word	Word Parts		Definition
	Part	Meaning	
coronary artery disease (CAD)			Most common form of heart disease; it is a progressive disease that increases the risk of myocardial infarction (heart attack) and sudden death.
			CAD usually results from the buildup of fatty material and plaque in the coronary arteries (atherosclerosis). As the coronary arteries narrow, the flow of blood to the heart can slow or stop. Blockage can occur in one or many coronary arteries. See Figures 8.22 and 8.23.

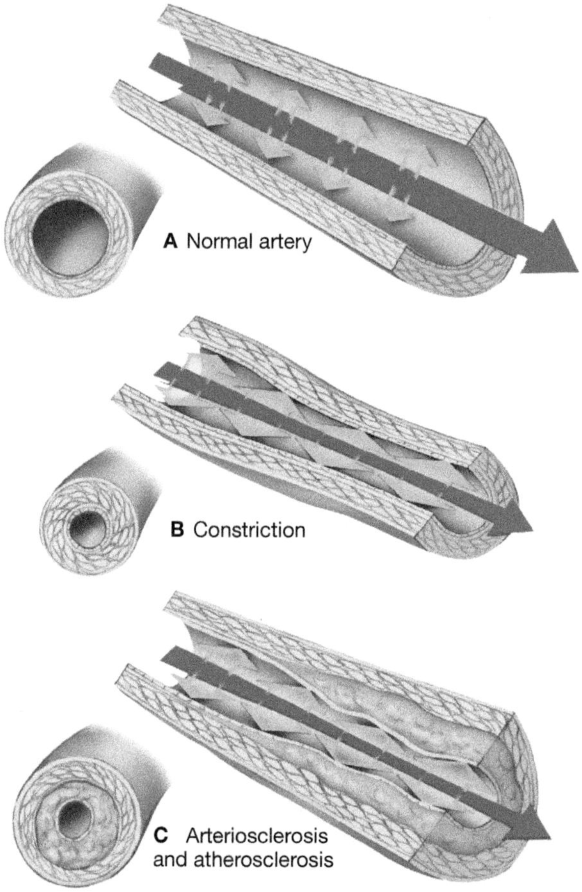

A Normal artery

B Constriction

C Arteriosclerosis and atherosclerosis

FIGURE 8.22 Blood vessels: **A** normal artery, **B** constriction, and **C** arteriosclerosis and atherosclerosis.

Medical Word	Word Parts		Definition
	Part	Meaning	

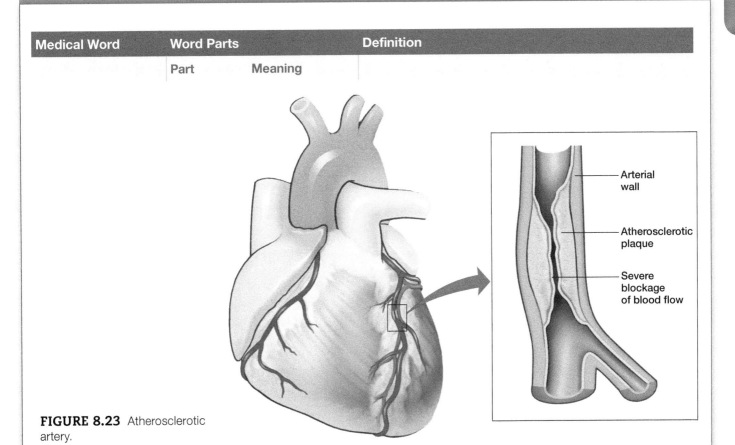

FIGURE 8.23 Atherosclerotic artery.

 Acute coronary syndrome is a name given to three types of coronary artery disease that are associated with sudden rupture of plaque inside a coronary artery:

- *Unstable angina* occurs when the pattern of chest pain changes abruptly.
- *Non-ST-segment elevation myocardial infarction (NSTEMI)* (a type of heart attack).
- *ST-segment elevation myocardial infarction (STEMI)* (a type of heart attack). The coronary artery is completely blocked off by a blood clot. Changes can be noted on the ECG as well as in blood levels of key chemical markers.

The type of acute coronary syndrome is determined by the location of the blockage, the length of time blood flow is blocked, and the amount of damage that occurs. These life-threatening conditions require immediate emergency medical care.

Medical Word	Word Parts		Definition
cyanosis (sī-ă-nō´ sĭs)	cyan	dark blue	Abnormal condition of the skin and mucous membranes caused by oxygen deficiency in the blood. The skin, fingernails, and mucous membranes can appear slightly blue or gray.
	-osis	condition	

Medical Word	Word Parts		Definition
	Part	Meaning	
defibrillator (dē-fĭb′ rĭ-lā″ tor)			Medical device used to restore a normal heart rhythm by delivering an electric shock; also called a *cardioverter*. See Figure 8.24.

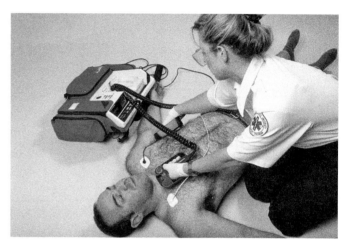

FIGURE 8.24 Defibrillator (cardioverter).
Source: Pearson Education, Inc.

Medical Word	Word Parts		Definition
diastole (dī-ăs′ tō-lē)			Relaxation phase of the heart cycle during which the heart muscle relaxes and the heart chambers fill with blood
dysrhythmia (dĭs-rĭth′ mē-ă)	**dys-** **rhythm** **-ia**	difficult, abnormal rhythm condition	Abnormality of the rhythm or rate of the heartbeat. It is caused by a disturbance of the normal electrical activity within the heart and can be divided into two main groups: *tachycardias* and *bradycardias*. Dysrhythmia is also referred to as *arrhythmia*.
embolism (ĕm′ bō-lĭzm)	**embol** **-ism**	to cast, to throw condition	Pathological condition caused by obstruction of a blood vessel by foreign substances or a blood clot
endarterectomy (ĕn″ dăr-tĕr-ĕk′ tō-mē)	**end-** **arter** **-ectomy**	within artery surgical excision	Surgical excision of the inner lining of an artery
endocarditis (ĕn″ dō-kăr-dī′ tĭs)	**endo-** **card** **-itis**	within heart inflammation	Inflammation of the endocardium (inner lining of the heart), usually involving the heart valves. It typically occurs when microorganisms, especially bacteria from another part of the body such as the gums/teeth, spread through the bloodstream and attach to damaged areas of the heart. Treatments for endocarditis include antibiotics and, in severe cases, surgery. See Figure 8.25.

Medical Word	Word Parts		Definition
	Part	Meaning	

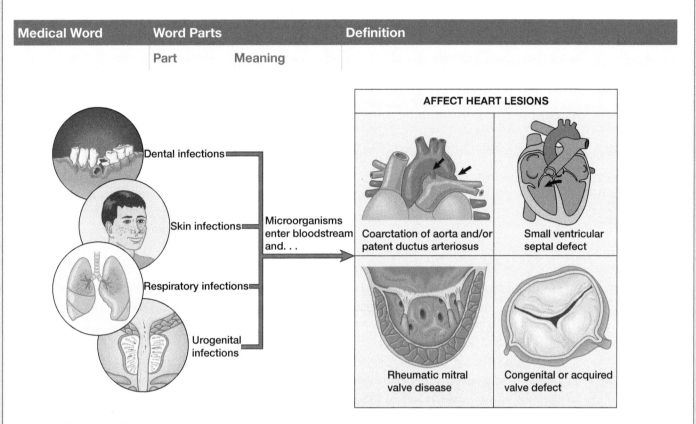

FIGURE 8.25 How microorganisms enter bloodstream and affect heart lesions, which could result in bacterial endocarditis.

Medical Word	Word Parts		Definition
	Part	Meaning	
extracorporeal circulation (ECC) (ĕks″ tră-kor-por´ ē-ăl)	**extra-** **corpor** -eal **circulat** -ion	outside body pertaining to circular process	Pertaining to the circulation of the blood outside the body via a heart–lung machine or in hemodialysis
fibrillation (fĭ″ brĭl-ā´ shŭn)	**fibrillat** -ion	fibrils (small fibers) process	Quivering or spontaneous contraction of individual muscle fibers; an abnormal bioelectric potential occurring in neuropathies and myopathies; disorganized pathological rhythm that can lead to death if not immediately corrected

 fyi   **Atrial fibrillation (AF, AFib)** is an irregular and often rapid heart rate that can increase the risk of stroke, heart failure, and other heart-related complications. It occurs when rapid, disorganized electrical signals cause the heart's two upper chambers (atria) to *fibrillate* (contract very fast and irregularly). Blood pools in the atria and it is not pumped completely into the heart's two lower chambers (ventricles). As a result, the heart's upper and lower chambers don't work together as they should. Symptoms often include heart palpitations, shortness of breath, and weakness. Episodes of atrial fibrillation can come and go, or one may develop atrial fibrillation that doesn't go away and may require treatment. Although atrial fibrillation itself usually isn't life-threatening, it is a serious medical condition that sometimes requires emergency treatment.

Medical Word	Word Parts		Definition
	Part	Meaning	
flutter			Pathological rapid heart rate that may cause cardiac output (CO) to be decreased. With atrial flutter, the heartbeat is 200–400 beats per minute. With ventricular flutter, the heartbeat is 250 beats or more per minute. On an EKG recording, a flutter will demonstrate a "sawtooth" appearance.
heart failure (HF)			Pathological condition in which the heart loses its ability to pump blood efficiently. Left-sided heart failure is commonly called *congestive heart failure (CHF)*.

fyi

Heart failure is one of the most common types of cardiovascular disease seen in the older adult. It can involve the heart's left side, right side, or both sides. Left-sided failure leads to a backup of blood, which causes a buildup of fluid in the lungs, or **pulmonary edema**, which causes **dyspnea** and shortness of breath (SOB). Left-sided heart failure is commonly called **congestive heart failure (CHF)**. There are two types of left-sided heart failure. Drug treatments are different for the two types.

- *Systolic failure:* The left ventricle loses its ability to contract normally. The heart can't pump with enough force to push enough blood into circulation.
- *Diastolic failure* (also called *diastolic dysfunction*)**:** The left ventricle loses its ability to relax normally (because the muscle has become stiff). The heart can't properly fill with blood during the resting period between each beat.

Right-sided or right-ventricular (RV) heart failure usually occurs as a result of left-sided failure. When the left ventricle fails, increased fluid pressure is, in effect, transferred back through the lungs, ultimately damaging the heart's right side. Right-sided failure is a result of a buildup of blood flowing into the right side of the heart, which can lead to enlargement of the liver, distention of the neck veins, and edema of the ankles. See Figure 8.26 for the multisystem effects of heart failure.

A normal heart pumps a little more than half the heart's blood volume with each beat. **Ejection fraction (EF)** is the percentage of blood that is pumped (ejected) out of the ventricles with each contraction of the heart. It should be measured initially with the first diagnosis of a heart condition, and again as needed, based on changes in the patient's condition. **Left-ventricular ejection fraction (LVEF)** is the measurement of how much blood is being pumped out of the left ventricle of the heart with each contraction. **Right-ventricular ejection fraction (RVEF)** is the measurement of how much blood is being pumped out of the right side of the heart to the lungs for oxygen.

EF Measurement: What It Means

55–70%	Normal
40–55%	Below normal
Less than 40%	May confirm diagnosis of heart failure
Less than 35%	Patient may be at risk of life-threatening irregular heartbeats

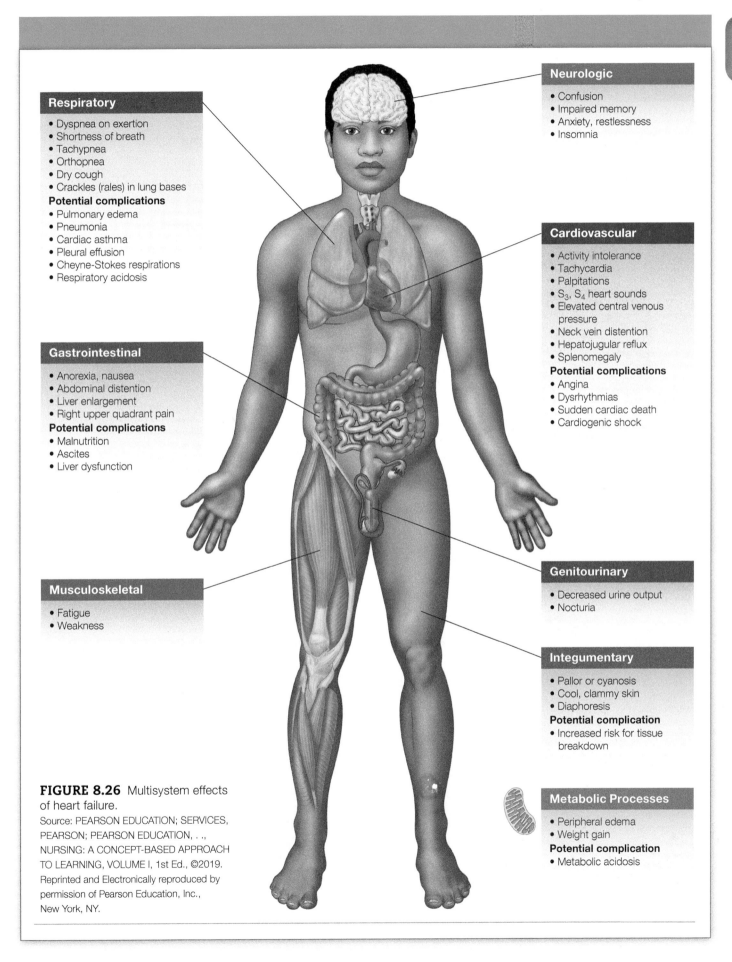

Neurologic
- Confusion
- Impaired memory
- Anxiety, restlessness
- Insomnia

Respiratory
- Dyspnea on exertion
- Shortness of breath
- Tachypnea
- Orthopnea
- Dry cough
- Crackles (rales) in lung bases

Potential complications
- Pulmonary edema
- Pneumonia
- Cardiac asthma
- Pleural effusion
- Cheyne-Stokes respirations
- Respiratory acidosis

Cardiovascular
- Activity intolerance
- Tachycardia
- Palpitations
- S_3, S_4 heart sounds
- Elevated central venous pressure
- Neck vein distention
- Hepatojugular reflux
- Splenomegaly

Potential complications
- Angina
- Dysrhythmias
- Sudden cardiac death
- Cardiogenic shock

Gastrointestinal
- Anorexia, nausea
- Abdominal distention
- Liver enlargement
- Right upper quadrant pain

Potential complications
- Malnutrition
- Ascites
- Liver dysfunction

Genitourinary
- Decreased urine output
- Nocturia

Integumentary
- Pallor or cyanosis
- Cool, clammy skin
- Diaphoresis

Potential complication
- Increased risk for tissue breakdown

Musculoskeletal
- Fatigue
- Weakness

Metabolic Processes
- Peripheral edema
- Weight gain

Potential complication
- Metabolic acidosis

FIGURE 8.26 Multisystem effects of heart failure.
Source: PEARSON EDUCATION; SERVICES, PEARSON; PEARSON EDUCATION, . ., NURSING: A CONCEPT-BASED APPROACH TO LEARNING, VOLUME I, 1st Ed., ©2019. Reprinted and Electronically reproduced by permission of Pearson Education, Inc., New York, NY.

Medical Word	Word Parts		Definition
	Part	Meaning	
heart–lung transplant			Surgical procedure of transferring the heart and lungs from a donor to a patient
heart transplant			Surgical procedure of transferring the heart from a donor to a patient
hemangioma (hē-măn″ jē-ō′ mă)	**hem**	blood	Benign tumor of a blood vessel. See Figures 8.27 and 8.28.
	angi	vessel	
	-oma	tumor	

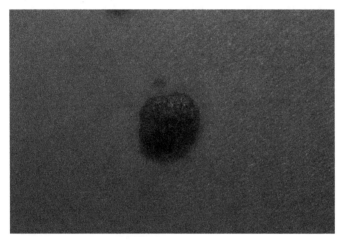

FIGURE 8.27 Hemangioma.
Source: Courtesy of Jason L. Smith, MD

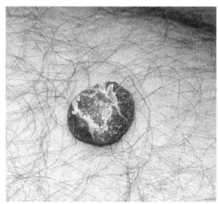

FIGURE 8.28 Sclerosing hemangioma.
Source: Courtesy of Jason L. Smith, MD

Medical Word	Word Parts		Definition
hemodynamic (hē″ mō-dī-năm′ ĭk)	**hem/o**	blood	The dynamic study of the heart's function and movement of the blood and pressure
	dynam	power	
	-ic	pertaining to	
hyperlipidemia (hī″ pĕr-lĭp″ ĭ-dē′ mē-ă)	**hyper-**	excessive	Abnormally high levels of lipids (fatty substances) in the blood. Lipids include sterols (cholesterol and cholesterol esters), free fatty acids (FFA), triglycerides (glycerol esters of FFA), and phospholipids (phosphoric acid esters of lipid substances).
	lipid	fat	
	-emia	blood condition	
hypertension (HTN) (hī″ pĕr-tĕn′ shŭn)	**hyper-**	excessive, above	A condition in which the force of blood flowing through the blood vessels is consistently too high; commonly called *high blood pressure (HBP)*. Hypertension often has no symptoms and is frequently called the *silent killer* because, if left untreated, it can lead to kidney failure, stroke, heart attack, peripheral artery disease, and eye damage. Various factors can contribute to developing hypertension, and it is important to know these factors. See Table 8.3.
	tens	pressure	
	-ion	process	

Medical Word	Word Parts		Definition
	Part	Meaning	

TABLE 8.3 Factors Contributing to Hypertension

Factors That One Can Control

Smoking	Avoid the use of tobacco products
Overweight	Maintain a proper weight for age and body size
Lack of exercise	Exercise regularly
Stress	Learn to manage stress
Alcohol	Limit intake of alcohol

Factors That One Cannot Control

Heredity	Family history of high blood pressure, heart attack, stroke, or diabetes
Race	Incidence of hypertension increases among African Americans
Gender	Chance of developing hypertension increases for males
Age	Likelihood of hypertension increases with age

Medical Word	Part	Meaning	Definition
hypotension (hī″ pō-těn′ shŭn)	**hypo-** **tens** **-ion**	deficient, below pressure process	Low blood pressure
infarction (ĭn-fărk′ shŭn)	**infarct** **-ion**	infarct (necrosis of an area) process	Process of development of an infarct, which is death of tissue resulting from obstruction of blood flow
ischemia (ĭs-kē′ mē-ă)	**isch** **-emia**	to hold back blood condition	Condition in which there is a lack of oxygen due to decreased blood supply to a part of the body caused by constriction or obstruction of a blood vessel

fyi *Ischemic heart disease*, also called *coronary artery disease* or *coronary heart disease*, is a term given to heart problems caused by narrowed coronary arteries. When arteries are narrowed, less blood and oxygen reach the heart muscle. Ischemia often causes chest pain or discomfort (angina pectoris). *Silent ischemia* is a term given to ischemia without chest pain and a person may experience a heart attack with no prior warning. People who have had previous heart attacks or those with diabetes are especially at risk for developing silent ischemia.

Medical Word	Word Parts		Definition
	Part	Meaning	
lipoprotein (lĭp″ ō-prō′ tēn)			Fat (lipid) and protein molecules that are bound together. They are classified as **VLDL**—very-low-density lipoproteins; **LDL**—low-density lipoproteins; and **HDL**—high-density lipoproteins. High levels of VLDL and LDL are associated with cholesterol and triglyceride deposits in arteries, which could lead to coronary heart disease, hypertension, and atherosclerosis. See *lipid profile* in the section "Diagnostic and Laboratory Tests."
mitral stenosis (MS) (mī′ trăl stĕ-nō′ sĭs)	**mitr** **-al** **sten** **-osis**	mitral valve pertaining to narrowing condition	Pathological condition of narrowing of the mitral valve (bicuspid valve) orifice
mitral valve prolapse (MVP) (mī′ trăl vălv prō-lăps′)			Pathological condition that occurs when the leaflets of the mitral valve (bicuspid valve) between the left atrium and left ventricle bulge into the atrium and permit backflow of blood into the atrium. The condition is often associated with progressive mitral regurgitation (blood flows back into the left atrium instead of moving forward into the left ventricle).
murmur (mŭr′ mŭr)			An abnormal sound ranging from soft and blowing to loud and booming heard on auscultation of the heart and adjacent large blood vessels. Murmurs range from very faint to very loud. They sometimes sound like a whooshing or swishing noise. Normal heartbeats make a "lub-DUPP" or "lub-DUB" sound. This is the sound of the heart valves closing as blood moves through the heart. Most abnormal murmurs in children are due to congenital heart defects. In adults, abnormal murmurs are most often due to heart valve problems caused by infection, disease, or aging.
myocardial (mī″ ō-kăr′ dē-ăl)	**my/o** **cardi** **-al**	muscle heart pertaining to	Pertaining to the heart muscle (myocardium)

Medical Word	Word Parts		Definition
	Part	**Meaning**	
myocardial infarction (MI) (mī″ ō-kăr′ dē-ăl ĭn-fărk′ shŭn)	**my/o**	muscle	Occurs when a focal area of the heart muscle dies or is permanently damaged because of an inadequate supply of oxygen to that area; also known as a *heart attack*. The most common symptom of a heart attack is *angina*, which is chest pain often described as a feeling of crushing pressure, fullness, heaviness, or aching in the center of the chest. Many times people try to ignore the symptoms or say that "it's just indigestion." It is imperative to seek medical help immediately. Calling 911 is almost always the fastest way to get lifesaving treatment.
	cardi	heart	
	-al	pertaining to	
	infarct	infarct (necrosis of an area)	
	-ion	process	

fyi *Broken heart syndrome* is a term used to describe a type of heart problem that is often brought on by grief or emotional stress. It is a real medical condition with symptoms similar to a heart attack. Traumatic events can trigger the sympathetic nervous system, the "fight-or-flight" mechanism, and the sudden flood of chemicals, including adrenaline, can stun the heart muscle, leaving it temporarily unable to pump properly. Although symptoms may be similar, it is not the same as a heart attack.

Medical Word	Word Parts		Definition
myocarditis (mī″ ō-kăr-dī′ tĭs)	**my/o**	muscle	Inflammation of the heart muscle that is usually caused by viral, bacterial, or fungal infections that reach the heart
	card	heart	
	-itis	inflammation	
occlusion (ŏ-kloo′ zhŭn)	**occlus**	to close up	A blockage in a vessel, canal, or passage of the body
	-ion	process	
oximetry (ŏk-sĭm′ ĕ-trē)	**ox/i**	oxygen	Process of measuring the oxygen saturation of blood. A photoelectric medical device (oximeter) measures oxygen saturation of the blood by recording the amount of light transmitted or reflected by deoxygenated versus oxygenated hemoglobin (Hgb). A *pulse oximetry* is a noninvasive method of indicating the arterial oxygen saturation of functional hemoglobin. See Figure 8.29.
	-metry	measurement	

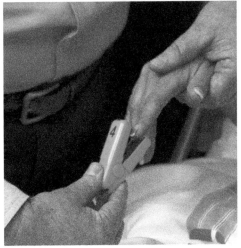

FIGURE 8.29 Pulse oximetry with the sensor probe applied securely, flush with skin, making sure that both sensor probes are aligned directly opposite each other.
Source: Pearson Education, Inc.

Medical Word	Word Parts		Definition
	Part	**Meaning**	
oxygen (O₂) (ŏk′ sĭ-jĕn)	**oxy**	sour, sharp, acid	Colorless, odorless, tasteless gas essential to respiration in animals
	-gen	formation, produce	
palpitation (păl-pĭ-tā′ shŭn)	**palpitat**	throbbing	An abnormal rapid throbbing or fluttering of the heart that is perceptible to the patient and may be felt by the physician during a physical exam
	-ion	process	
percutaneous transluminal coronary angioplasty (PTCA) (pĕr″ kū-tā′ nē-ŭs trăns-lū′ mĭ-năl kor′ ŏ-nĕr-ē ăn′ jē-ō-plăs″ tē)			Use of a balloon-tipped catheter to compress fatty plaques against an artery wall. When successful, the plaques remain compressed, which permits more blood to flow through the artery, therefore providing more oxygen to relieve the symptoms of coronary heart disease. See Figure 8.30.

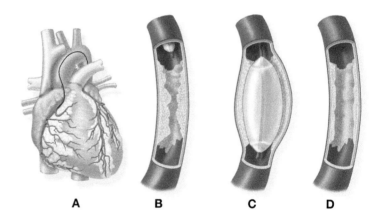

FIGURE 8.30 Balloon angioplasty. **A** The balloon catheter is threaded into the affected coronary artery. **B** The balloon is positioned across the area of obstruction. **C** The balloon is then inflated, flattening the plaque against the arterial wall. **D** Plaque remains flattened after balloon catheter is removed.

A   **B**   **C**   **D**

Medical Word	Word Parts		Definition
pericardial (pĕr″ ĭ-kăr′ dē-ăl)	**peri-**	around	Pertaining to the pericardium, the sac surrounding the heart
	cardi	heart	
	-al	pertaining to	

Medical Word	Word Parts		Definition
	Part	Meaning	
pericardiocentesis (pĕr″ĭ-kăr″ dē-ō-sĕn-tē′ sĭs)	peri- cardi/o -centesis	around heart surgical puncture	Surgical procedure to remove fluid from the pericardial sac for therapeutic or diagnostic purposes. See Figure 8.31.

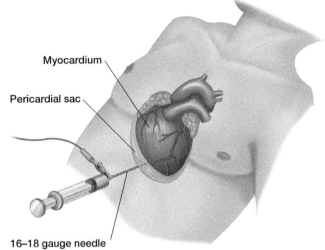

Myocardium

Pericardial sac

FIGURE 8.31 Pericardiocentesis.   16–18 gauge needle

pericarditis (pĕr″ĭ-kăr″ dī′ tĭs)	peri- card -itis	around heart inflammation	Inflammation of the pericardium (outer membranous sac surrounding the heart)
peripheral artery disease (PAD) (pĕ-rĭf′ ĕ-răl ăr′ tĕr-ē)			Pathological condition in which fatty deposits build up in the inner linings of the artery walls. These blockages restrict blood circulation, mainly in arteries leading to the kidneys, stomach, arms, legs, and feet. In its early stages, a common symptom is cramping or fatigue in the legs and buttocks during activity. Such cramping subsides when the person stands still. This is called *intermittent claudication*. If left untreated, PAD can progress to *critical limb ischemia (CLI)*, which occurs when the oxygenated blood being delivered to the leg is not adequate to keep the tissue alive.
phlebitis (flĕ-bī′ tĭs)	phleb -itis	vein inflammation	Literally means *inflammation of a vein*. There will be redness (erythema), swelling (edema), and pain or burning along the length of the affected vein.

Medical Word	Word Parts		Definition
	Part	**Meaning**	
phlebotomy (flĕ-bŏt´ ō-mē)	**phleb/o** **-tomy**	vein incision	Medical term used to describe the puncture of a vein to withdraw blood for analysis
Raynaud phenomenon (rā-nō´ fĕ-nŏm´ ĕ-nŏn)			Disorder that affects the blood vessels in the fingers and toes; it is characterized by intermittent attacks that cause the blood vessels in the digits to constrict. The cause is believed to be the result of vasospasms that decrease blood supply to the respective regions. Emotional stress and cold are classic triggers of the phenomenon, and discoloration follows a characteristic pattern in time: white, blue, and red. See Figure 8.32.

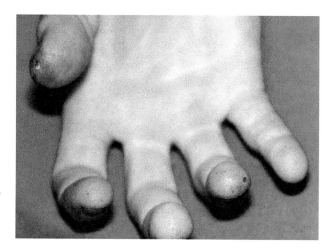

FIGURE 8.32 Raynaud phenomenon. Note the discoloration in the thumb and fingers.
Source: Courtesy of Jason L. Smith, MD

Medical Word	Word Parts		Definition
rheumatic heart disease (roo-măt´ ĭk)			Pathological condition in which permanent damage to heart valves is a result of a prior episode of rheumatic fever. The heart valve is damaged by a disease process that generally originates with a strep throat caused by streptococcus A bacteria.
semilunar (sĕm˝ ē-lū´ năr)	**semi-** **lun** **-ar**	half moon pertaining to	Valves of the aorta and pulmonary artery; shaped like a crescent (half-moon)
septum (sĕp´ tŭm)	**sept** **-um**	a partition tissue, structure	Wall or partition that divides or separates a body space or cavity
shock			A life-threatening condition that occurs when the body is not getting enough blood flow. This can damage multiple organs. Shock requires immediate medical treatment and can get worse very rapidly. In cardiogenic shock, there is failure to maintain the blood supply to the circulatory system and tissues because of inadequate cardiac output. See Figure 8.33.

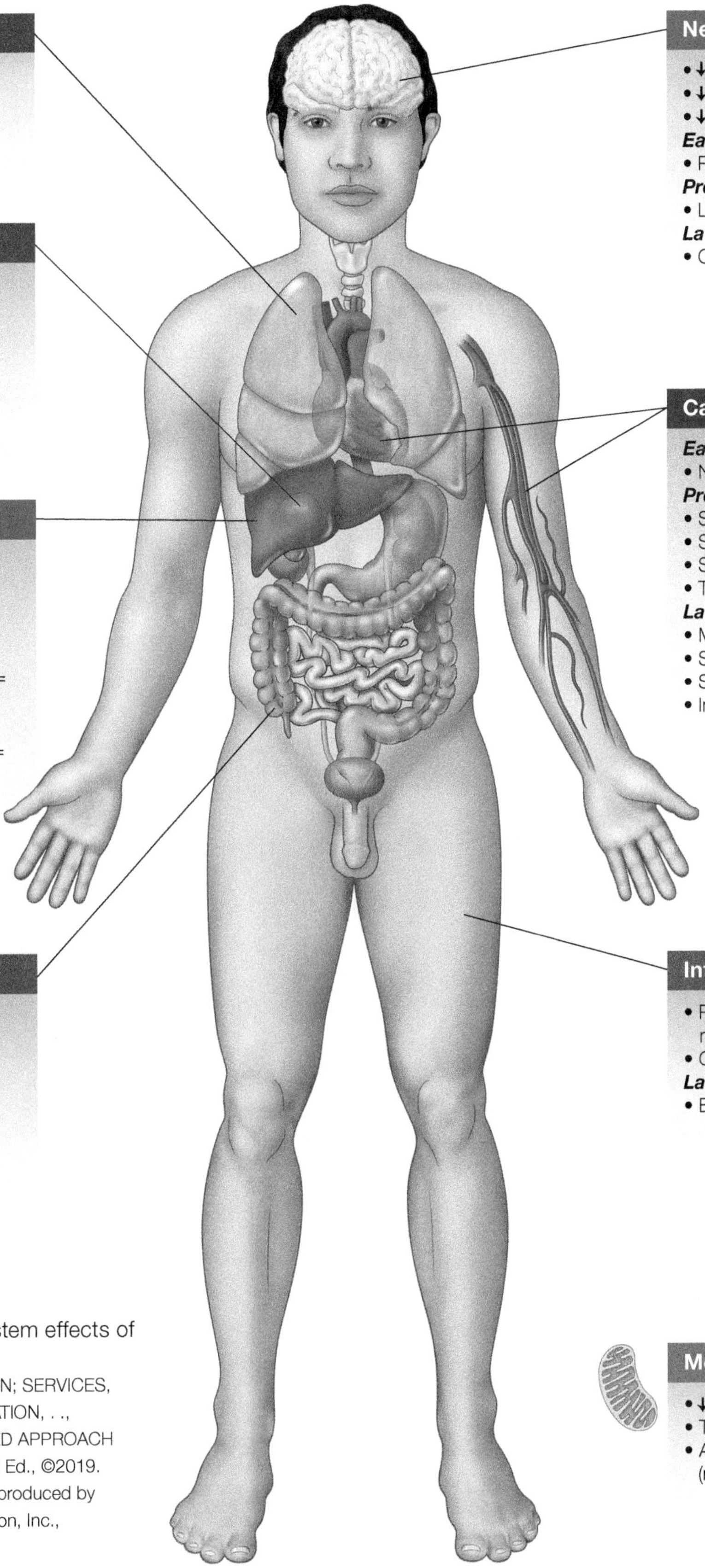

Respiratory

- ↑ respiratory rate
- Respiratory acidosis

Potential complication
- ARDS

Urinary

- ↓ renal perfusion
- ↓ GFR

Late
- Oliguria

Potential complications
- Acute tubular necrosis
- Kidney failure

Hepatic

Early
- ↑ glucose production

Progressive
- ↓ glucose production = hypoglycemia
- ↓ lactic acid conversion = metabolic acidosis

Potential complication
- Destroyed Kupffer cells = systemic bacterial infections

Gastrointestinal

Early
- ↓ GI motility

Late
- Paralytic ileus
- Ulceration of GI mucosa

Potential complication
- Bowel necrosis

Neurologic

- ↓ cognition
- ↓ sympathetic activity
- ↓ consciousness

Early
- Restlessness, apathy

Progressive
- Lethargy

Late
- Coma

Cardiovascular

Early
- No change

Progressive
- Slightly ↑BP
- Slowly ↑HR
- Sinus tachycardia
- Thready pulse

Late
- MAP <60 mmHg
- Steadily ↓BP
- Steadily ↓CO
- Imperceptible pulses

Integumentary

- Pallor (skin, lips, oral mucosa, nail beds, conjunctiva)
- Cool, moist skin

Late
- Edema

Metabolic Processes

- ↓ temperature
- Thirst
- Acidosis (metabolic and respiratory)

FIGURE 8.33 Multisystem effects of shock.

Source: PEARSON EDUCATION; SERVICES, PEARSON; PEARSON EDUCATION, . ., NURSING: A CONCEPT-BASED APPROACH TO LEARNING, VOLUME I, 1st Ed., ©2019. Reprinted and Electronically reproduced by permission of Pearson Education, Inc., New York, NY.

Medical Word	Word Parts		Definition
	Part	Meaning	
sinoatrial (SA) (sīn″ ō-ā′ trē-ăl)	sin/o atri -al	a curve atrium pertaining to	Pertaining to the sinus venosus and the atrium
sphygmomanometer (sfĭg″ mō-măn-ŏm′ ĕt-ĕr)	sphygm/o man/o -meter	pulse thin instrument to measure	Medical instrument used to measure the arterial blood pressure. Refer to Figure 8.13.
spider veins			Dilated blood vessels, typically found in the legs, that radiate from a central point; also called *telangiectasia* (refer to Figure 4.46 in Chapter 4)
stent			Medical device made of expandable, metal mesh that is placed (by using a balloon catheter) at the site of a narrowing artery. The stent is then expanded and left in place to keep the artery open. See Figure 8.34.

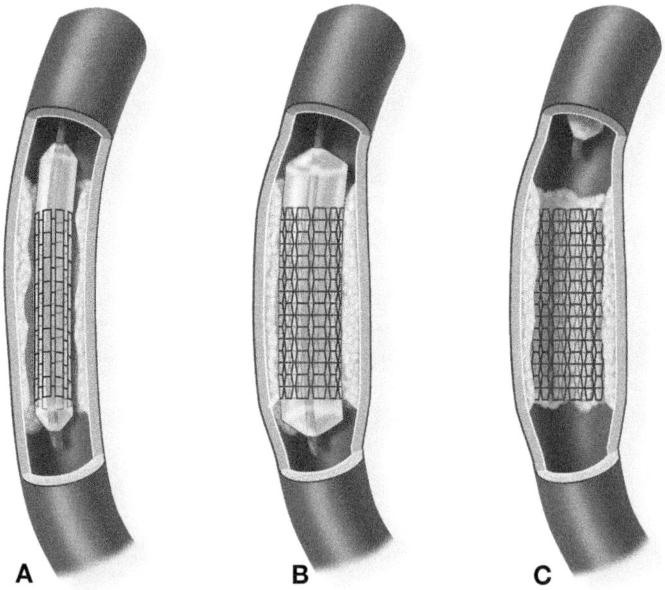

FIGURE 8.34 Placement of a stent. **A** The stainless steel stent is fitted over a balloon-tipped catheter. **B** The stent is positioned along the blockage and expanded. **C** The balloon is deflated and removed, leaving the stent in place.

Medical Word	Word Parts		Definition
stethoscope (stĕth′ ō-skōp)	steth/o -scope	chest instrument for examining	Medical instrument used to listen to the normal and pathological sounds of the heart, lungs, and other internal organs
systole (sĭs′ tō-lē)			Contractive phase of the heart cycle during which blood is forced into the systemic circulation via the aorta and the pulmonary circulation via the pulmonary artery

Medical Word	Word Parts		Definition
	Part	**Meaning**	
tachycardia (tăk″ĭ-kăr′ dē-ă)	**tachy-** **card** **-ia**	rapid heart condition	Rapid heartbeat that is over 100 beats per minute
telangiectasis (tĕl-ăn″ jē-ĕk′ tă-sĭs)	**tel** **angi** **-ectasis**	end vessel dilatation	Vascular lesion formed by dilatation of a group of small blood vessels; can appear as a birthmark or be caused by long-term exposure to the sun. See Figure 8.35.

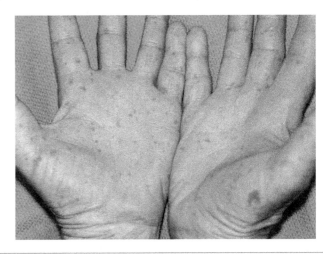

FIGURE 8.35 Telangiectasis.
Source: Courtesy of Jason L. Smith, MD

thrombophlebitis (thrŏm″ bō-flĕ-bī′ tĭs)	**thromb/o** **phleb** **-itis**	clot vein inflammation	Inflammation of a vein associated with the formation of a *thrombus* (blood clot). If the clot breaks off and travels to the lungs, it poses a potentially life-threatening condition called *pulmonary embolism (PE)*. See Figure 8.36.

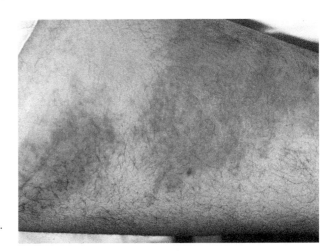

FIGURE 8.36 Thrombophlebitis.
Source: Courtesy of Jason L. Smith, MD

Medical Word	Word Parts		Definition
	Part	**Meaning**	
thrombosis	**thromb**	clot	A blood clot within the vascular system; *stationary blood*
(thrŏm-bō´ sĭs)	**-osis**	condition	*clot*. See Figure 8.37.

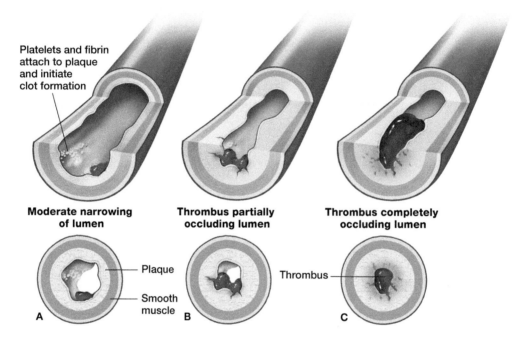

Platelets and fibrin attach to plaque and initiate clot formation

Moderate narrowing of lumen

Thrombus partially occluding lumen

Thrombus completely occluding lumen

Plaque

Smooth muscle

Thrombus

A B C

FIGURE 8.37 Thrombus formation in an atherosclerotic vessel depicting **A** the initial clot formation and **B** and **C** the varying degrees of occlusion.

Medical Word	Word Parts		Definition
tricuspid	**tri-**	three	Valve with three cusps; pertaining to the tricuspid valve
(trī-kŭs´ pĭd)	**-cuspid**	a point	
triglyceride	**tri-**	three	Pertaining to an organic compound consisting of three
(trī-glĭs´ ĕr-īd)	**glyc**	sweet, sugar	molecules of fatty acids
	-er	relating to	
	-ide	having a particular quality	
valve replacement surgery			Surgical replacement of diseased heart valve with an artificial one. There are two types of artificial valves: a mechanical heart valve is made of artificial materials and can usually last a lifetime; a biological heart valve is made from heart valves taken from animals or human cadavers and can wear out over time.
valvuloplasty	**valvul/o**	valve	Surgical repair of a cardiac valve
(văl´ vū-lō-plăs˝ tē)	**-plasty**	surgical repair	

Medical Word	Word Parts		Definition
	Part	**Meaning**	
varicose veins (văr´ ĭ-kōs)			Swollen, dilated, and knotted veins that usually occur in the lower leg(s). They result from a stagnated or sluggish flow of blood in combination with defective valves and weakened walls of the veins. See Figures 8.38 and 8.39.

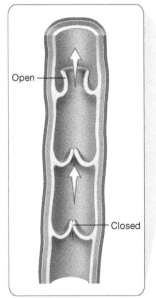
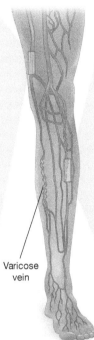
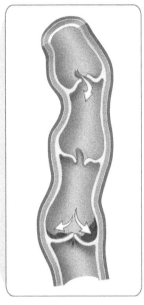
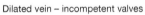

Open — Closed

Varicose vein

Normal vein – competent valves

Dilated vein – incompetent valves

FIGURE 8.38 Development of varicose veins.

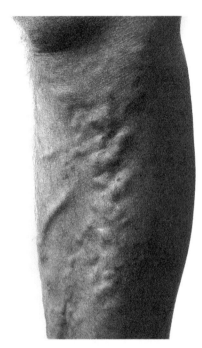

FIGURE 8.39 Varicose veins.
Source: Audie/Shutterstock

Medical Word	Word Parts		Definition
	Part	**Meaning**	
vasoconstrictive (vā˝ zō-kŏn-strĭk´ tĭv)	**vas/o** **con-** **strict** **-ive**	vessel together to draw, to bind nature of, quality of	Causing constriction of the blood vessels
vasodilator (vā˝ zō-dī-lā´ tor)	**vas/o** **dilat** **-or**	vessel to widen one who, a doer	Medicine that acts directly on smooth muscle cells within blood vessels to make them widen (dilate)
vasospasm (vā´ zō-spăzm)	**vas/o** **-spasm**	vessel contraction, spasm	Spasm of a blood vessel
venipuncture (vĕn´ ĭ-pŭnk˝ chūr)			Puncture of a vein for the removal of blood for analysis
ventricular (vĕn-trĭk´ ū-lăr)	**ventricul** **-ar**	ventricle pertaining to	Pertaining to a cardiac ventricle

Study *and* Review II

Word Parts

Prefixes   Give the definitions of the following prefixes.

1. a- _____
2. bi- _____
3. brady- _____
4. con- _____
5. end- _____
6. endo- _____
7. extra- _____

8. hyper- _____
9. hypo- _____
10. peri- _____
11. dys- _____
12. semi- _____
13. tachy- _____
14. tri- _____

Combining Forms   Give the definitions of the following combining forms.

1. angi/o _____
2. arteri/o _____
3. ather/o _____
4. cardi/o _____
5. cyan/o _____
6. dilat/o _____
7. embol/o _____
8. hem/o _____
9. isch/o _____
10. lipid/o _____
11. lun/o _____

12. man/o _____
13. mitr/o _____
14. occlus/o _____
15. ox/i _____
16. phleb/o _____
17. scler/o _____
18. sin/o _____
19. steth/o _____
20. thromb/o _____
21. vas/o _____

Suffixes   Give the definitions of the following suffixes.

1. -ac _____
2. -al _____

3. -ar, -ary _____
4. -centesis _____

5. -metry _____

6. -ectasis _____

7. -ectomy _____

8. -emia _____

9. -er _____

10. -gen _____

11. -graphy _____

12. -ia _____

13. -ic _____

14. -ide _____

15. -ion _____

16. -ism _____

17. -ist _____

18. -itis _____

19. -ive _____

20. -logy _____

21. -malacia _____

22. -megaly _____

23. -meter _____

24. -oma _____

25. -or _____

26. -osis _____

27. -pathy _____

28. -plasty _____

29. -scope _____

30. -spasm _____

31. -tomy _____

32. –um _____

Identifying Medical Terms

In the spaces provided, write the medical terms for the following meanings.

1. _____ Tumor of a blood vessel

2. _____ Surgical repair of a blood vessel(s)

3. _____ Pathological condition of narrowing of a blood vessel

4. _____ Irregularity or loss (lack of) rhythm of the heartbeat

5. _____ Inflammation of an artery

6. _____ Valve with two cusps; pertaining to the mitral valve

7. _____ Physician who specializes in the study of the heart

8. _____ Enlargement of the heart

9. _____ Pertaining to the heart and lungs

10. _____ Process of drawing together as in the narrowing of a vessel

Matching

Select the appropriate lettered meaning for each of the following words.

_____ **1.** cholesterol

_____ **2.** claudication

_____ **3.** dysrhythmia

_____ **4.** diastole

_____ **5.** fibrillation

_____ **6.** lipoprotein

_____ **7.** cardioversion

_____ **8.** palpitation

_____ **9.** percutaneous transluminal coronary angioplasty

_____ **10.** systole

a. Medical procedure used to treat cardiac arrhythmias

b. Quivering of muscle fiber

c. Fat and protein molecules that are bound together

d. A normal, soft, waxy substance found among the lipids (fats) in the bloodstream and all body cells

e. Literally means *process of lameness, limping*

f. An abnormality of the rhythm or rate of the heartbeat

g. Relaxation phase of the heart cycle

h. Contraction phase of the heart cycle

i. An abnormal rapid throbbing or fluttering of the heart

j. Use of a balloon-tipped catheter to compress fatty plaques against an artery wall

Medical Case Snapshots

This learning activity provides an opportunity to relate the medical terminology you are learning to sample patient case presentations. In the spaces provided, write in your answers.

Case 1

A 45-year-old male describes experiencing a "squeezing" sensation in his chest during a workout session. This condition, described as _____ _____, occurs when diseased blood vessels restrict blood flow to the heart, causing chest pain that can radiate to the _____ and _____, or to the left arm.

Case 2

A 72-year-old male is diagnosed with arteriosclerotic heart disease (ASHD). Upon _____ (assessment using a stethoscope to listen to sounds), Dr. Chung hears a bruit or sound of arterial origin. Two conditions often associated with ASHD are _____ (hardening of the arteries) and _____ (buildup of fatty substances with subsequent hardening of the arterial walls).

Case 3

The patient is a 62-year-old male experiencing _____ _____ (chest pain). He states that the pain radiates to his neck, jaw, and left arm. An ultrafast CT scan was ordered. After the results of this test were studied, a _____ _____ bypass graft was discussed with the patient and his wife.

Drug Highlights

Classification of Drug	Description and Examples
digitalis drugs	Strengthen the heart muscle, increase the force and velocity of myocardial systolic contraction, slow the heart rate, and decrease conduction velocity through the atrioventricular (AV) node. These drugs are used in the treatment of congestive heart failure, atrial fibrillation, atrial flutter, and paroxysmal atrial tachycardia (PAT). An overdosage of digitalis can cause toxicity. The most common early symptoms of digitalis toxicity are anorexia, nausea and vomiting, and arrhythmias. EXAMPLE: Lanoxin (digoxin)
antiarrhythmic agents	Used in the treatment of cardiac arrhythmias (irregular heart rhythms). EXAMPLES: flecainide acetate, Inderal (propranolol HCl), Calan (verapamil), and Pacerone (amiodarone)
vasopressors	Cause contraction of the muscles associated with capillaries and arteries, thereby narrowing the space through which the blood circulates. This narrowing results in an elevation of blood pressure. Vasopressors are useful in the treatment of patients suffering from shock. EXAMPLES: Levophed (norepinephrine bitartrate) and dopamine HCl
vasodilators	Cause relaxation of blood vessels and lower blood pressure. Coronary vasodilators are used for the treatment of angina pectoris. EXAMPLES: isosorbide dinitrate and nitroglycerin

Classification of Drug	Description and Examples
antihypertensive agents	Used in the treatment of hypertension. EXAMPLES: Catapres (clonidine HCl), Lopressor (metoprolol tartrate), captopril, and Toprol–XL (metoprolol succinate)

fyi

There is increasing evidence for the beneficial effects of renin angiotensin aldosterone systems (RAAS) inhibition on metabolic signaling, cardiovascular disease (CVD), and chronic kidney disease (CKD) in patients with insulin resistance or overt type 2 diabetes mellitus (T2DM).

ACE inhibitors and ANG-II receptor blockers (ARBs) have been studied extensively in hypertension (HTN), congestive heart failure (CHF), coronary artery disease (CAD), and CKD and are recommended to prevent CVD and nephropathy in patients with T2DM.

Pharmacologic blockade of RAAS not only improves blood pressure but also has a beneficial impact on inflammation, oxidative stress, insulin sensitivity, and glucose homeostasis. Several strategies are available for RAAS blockade, including ACE inhibitors, ARBs, and mineralocorticoid receptor antagonists (MRAs), which have been proven in clinical trials to result in improved CVD and CKD outcomes.

- ACE inhibitors, a class of drugs developed from snake venom, prevent the formation of a hormone, angiotensin II, that acts on the central nervous system to regulate renal sympathetic nerve activity, renal function, and, therefore, blood pressure. Ace inhibitors cause the blood vessels to relax and widen, allowing blood to flow more easily through the vessels, and blood pressure goes down.
- Angiotensin-receptor blockers (ARBs) block the angiotensin receptors on the cells of blood vessels and the proximal tubule, preventing vasoconstriction and reabsorption of sodium ions and water. This action shields blood vessels from angiotensin II and the vessels become wider, blood flows more easily, and blood pressure goes down.
- Mineralocorticoid receptor antagonists (MRAs), also called *aldosterone antagonists*, block the effects of aldosterone on the distal tubule and decrease reabsorption of sodium ions and water. This action causes diuresis and acts as a diuretic. Aldosterone is a mineralocorticoid hormone synthesized by the adrenal glands that has several regulatory functions to help the body maintain normal volume status and electrolyte balance.

New research in these areas will allow for a better understanding of the relationship between HTN, insulin resistance, and activation of RAAS, which could result in newer alternatives for more comprehensive management of HTN in the setting of cardiometabolic syndrome (CMS).

antihyperlipidemic agents	Used to lower abnormally high blood levels of fatty substances (lipids) when other treatment regimens fail. EXAMPLES: Lopid (gemfibrozil), Lipitor (atorvastatin calcium), Pravachol (pravastatin), Zocor (simvastatin), Crestor (rosuvastatin calcium), Vytorin (ezetimibe/simvastatin), Zetia (ezetimibe), niacin, and lovastatin
antiplatelet drugs	Help reduce the occurrence of and death from vascular events such as heart attacks and strokes. *Aspirin* is considered to be the reference standard antiplatelet drug and is recommended by the American Heart Association for use in patients with a wide range of cardiovascular disease. Aspirin helps keep platelets from sticking together to form clots. *Plavix (clopidogrel)* is approved by the Food and Drug Administration for many of the same indications as aspirin. It is recommended for patients for whom aspirin fails to achieve a therapeutic benefit.

Classification of Drug	Description and Examples
anticoagulants	Act to prevent blood clots from forming. They are known as "blood thinners" and are used in primary and secondary prevention of deep vein thrombosis (DVT), pulmonary embolism (PE), myocardial infarctions (MI), and cerebrovascular accidents (CVAs; strokes). EXAMPLES: Coumadin (warfarin sodium), heparin, Xarelto (rivaroxaban), and Pradaxa (diabigatran etexilate)
thrombolytic agents	Act to dissolve an existing thrombus when administered soon after its occurrence. They are often referred to as *tissue plasminogen activators* (tPA, TPA) and can reduce the chance of dying after a myocardial infarction by 50%. Unless contraindicated, the drug should be administered within 6 hours of the onset of chest pain. In some hospitals, the time period for administering thrombolytic agents has been extended to 12 and 24 hours. These agents dissolve the clot, reopen the artery, restore blood flow to the heart, and prevent further damage to the myocardium. Bleeding is the most common and potentially serious complication encountered during thrombolytic therapy. Thrombolytic agents are also used in ischemic strokes, DVT, and PE to clear a blocked artery and avoid permanent damage to the perfused tissue. *Note:* Thrombolytic therapy in hemorrhagic strokes is contraindicated because its use would prolong bleeding into the intracranial space and cause further damage. EXAMPLE: Activase (alteplase)

Diagnostic *and* Laboratory Tests

Test	Description
angiocardiography (ACG) (ăn″ jē-ō-kăr″ dē-ŏg′ ră-fē)	Video x-ray technique used to follow the passage of blood through the heart and great vessels after an intravenous (IV) injection of a radiopaque contrast substance; used to evaluate patient for cardiovascular (CV) surgery
angiography (ăn″ jē-ŏg′ ră-fē)	A minimally invasive medical test that helps physicians diagnose and treat medical conditions by using x-ray recording (-*graphy*) of a blood vessel after the injection of a radiopaque substance. Used to determine the patency of the blood vessels, organ, or tissue being studied.

Test	Description
cardiac catheterization (heart cath) (kăr′ dē-ăk kăth″ ĕ-tĕr-ĭ-zā′ shŭn)	Medical procedure used to diagnose heart disorders. A tiny catheter is inserted into an artery in the arm or leg of the patient and is fed through this artery to the heart. Dye is then pumped through the catheter, enabling the physician to locate by x-ray any blockages in the arteries supplying the heart. See Figure 8.40.

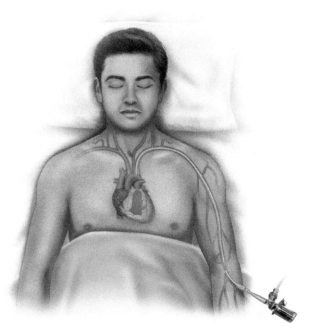

FIGURE 8.40 Cardiac catheterization.

Test	Description
cardiac enzymes (kar′ dē-ăk ĕn′ zīmz) - alanine aminotransferase (ALT) - aspartate aminotransferase (AST) - creatine kinase (CK) - creatine kinase isoenzymes	Blood tests performed to determine cardiac damage in an acute myocardial infarction (AMI). Levels begin to rise 6–10 hours after an AMI and peak at 24–48 hours. Used to detect area of damage. Level may be five to eight times normal. Used to indicate area of damage; CK-MB heart muscle, CK-MM skeletal muscle, and CK-BB brain
cardiac troponin (kăr′ dē-ăk trō′ pŏ-nĭn)	Blood test performed to determine heart muscle injury (microinfarction) not detected by cardiac enzyme tests. Troponin T and troponin I proteins control the interactions between actin and myosin, which contract or squeeze the heart muscle. Normally the level of these cardiac proteins in the blood is very low. It increases substantially within several hours (on average 4–6 hours) of muscle damage, so elevated levels can indicate a heart attack, even a mild one. It peaks at 10–24 hours and can be detected for up to 10–14 days.
cholesterol (chol) (kō-lĕs′ tĕr-ŏl)	Blood test to determine the level of cholesterol in the serum. Elevated levels can indicate an increased risk of coronary heart disease. Any level more than 200 mg/dL is considered too high for heart health.
computed tomography (CT)	Sometimes referred to as a **CAT scan** (computerized axial tomography), this test combines an advanced x-ray scanning system with a powerful minicomputer and has vastly improved imaging quality while making it possible to view parts of the body and abnormalities not previously open to radiography.

Test	Description
echocardiography (ECHO) (ĕk″ ō-kăr″ dē-ŏg′ ră-fē)	Medical procedure using sonographic sound to analyze the size, shape, and movement of structures inside the heart. Usually two echoes are taken: one of the heart at rest and another of the heart under stress. Comparison of the two images helps pinpoint abnormal valves or areas that are not receiving enough blood.
electrocardiogram (ECG, EKG) (ē-lĕk″ trō-kăr′ dē-ō-grăm)	A test that checks for problems with the electrical activity of the heart, an ECG shows the heart's electrical activity recorded as line tracings on paper or displayed on a screen. The spikes and dips in the tracings are called *waves*. A standard electrocardiograph has 12 leads with 10 electrodes placed on the patient's arms and legs and six positions on the chest, which record electrical activity of different parts of the heart. An ECG provides valuable information in diagnosing cardiac abnormalities, such as myocardial damage and arrhythmias. See Figure 8.41.

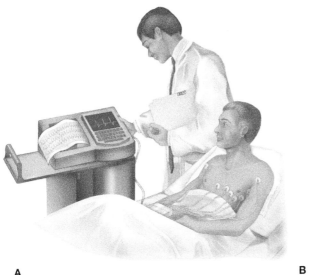

A

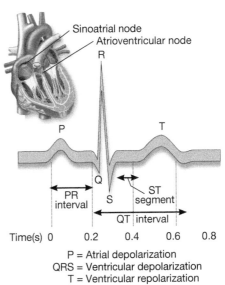

B

P = Atrial depolarization
QRS = Ventricular depolarization
T = Ventricular repolarization

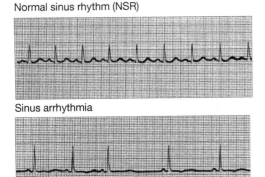

C

FIGURE 8.41 Electrocardiography is a commonly used procedure in which the electrical events associated with the beating of the heart are evaluated. **A** Skin electrodes are applied to the chest wall and send electrical signals to a computer that interprets the signals into graph form. **B** Illustration of the electrical events of the heart and a normal ECG/EKG. **C** An electrocardiogram is useful in identifying arrhythmias, as shown here.

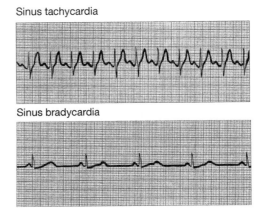

Test	Description
electrophysiology study (EPS) (intracardiac) (ē-lĕk″ trō-fĭz″ ē-ŏl′ ō-jē ĭn″ tră-kăr′ dē-ăk)	Invasive cardiac procedure that involves the placement of catheter-guided electrodes within the heart to evaluate and map the electrical conduction of cardiac arrhythmias.
Holter monitor (hōl′ tĕr mŏn′ ĭ-tŏr)	Portable medical device attached to the patient that is used to record a patient's continuous ECG for 24 hours.
lactate dehydrogenase (LD or LDH) (lăk′ tāt dē-hī-drŏj′ ĕ-nās)	Intracellular enzyme present in nearly all metabolizing cells, with the highest concentrations in the heart, skeletal muscles, red blood cells (RBCs), liver, kidney, lung, and brain. When LDH leaks from cardiac cells into the bloodstream, it can be detected and is a good indicator of tissue damage. A high serum level occurs 12–24 hours after cardiac injury.
lipid profile (lĭp′ ĭd)	Series of blood tests including cholesterol, high-density lipoproteins, low-density lipoproteins, and triglycerides. Used to determine levels of lipids and to assess risk factors of coronary heart disease.

 fyi

A fasting lipoprotein profile measures the different forms of cholesterol that are circulating in the blood after one avoids eating for 9–12 hours. The evaluations below are for adults.

LDL Cholesterol

Below 100	Optimal
100–129	Near optimal
130–159	Borderline high
160–189	High
Above 190	Very high

HDL Cholesterol

Above 60	Optimal
Below 40	Low for men
Below 50	Low for women

Total Cholesterol (LDL and HDL)

Below 200	Optimal
200–239	Borderline
Above 240	High

Triglycerides

Below 150	Optimal
150–199	Borderline high
Above 200	High

Test	Description
magnetic resonance imaging (MRI) (măg-nĕt′ ĭk rĕz′ ŏ-năns)	Medical imaging technique that uses a magnet that sets the nuclei of atoms in the heart cells vibrating. The oscillating atoms emit radio signals, which are converted by a computer into either still or moving three-dimensional images. The scan can reveal plaque-filled coronary arteries and the layer of fat that envelops most hearts. MRI is also an ideal method for scanning children with congenital heart problems. Patients with pacemakers, stents, or other metal implants cannot have MRI. An MRI scan cannot pick up calcium deposits that could signal narrowed vessels.
positron emission tomography (PET)	Nuclear medicine imaging technique that helps physicians see how the organs and tissues inside the body are functioning. The test involves injecting a very small dose of a radioactive chemical, called a *radiotracer*, into the vein of the patient's arm. The tracer travels through the body and is absorbed by the organs and tissues being studied. The PET scan detects and records the energy given off by the tracer substance and, with the use of a computer, this energy is converted into three-dimensional pictures. A physician can then look at cross-sectional images of the body organ from any angle in order to detect functional problems. Commonly called a **PET scan**.

Test	Description
stress test	A screening test used in evaluating cardiovascular fitness, also called *exercise test*, *exercise stress test*, or *treadmill test*. The ECG is monitored while the patient is subjected to increasing levels of work using a treadmill or ergometer. It is a common test for diagnosing coronary artery disease, especially in patients who have symptoms of heart disease. The test helps doctors assess blood flow through coronary arteries in response to exercise, usually walking, at varied speeds and for various lengths of time on a treadmill. A stress test can include the use of electrocardiography, echocardiography, and injected radioactive substances.
thallium-201 stress test (thăl′ ē-ŭm)	An x-ray study that follows the path of radioactive thallium carried by the blood into the heart muscle. Damaged or dead muscle can be defined, as can the extent of narrowing in an artery.
triglycerides (trī-glĭs′ ĕr-īds)	Blood test to determine the level of triglycerides in the blood. Elevated levels (more than 200 mg/dL) can indicate an increased potential risk of coronary heart disease and diabetes mellitus.
ultrafast CT scan	Ultrafast CT can take multiple images of the heart within the time of a single heartbeat, thus providing much more detail about the heart's function and structures while greatly decreasing the amount of time required for a study. It can detect very small amounts of calcium within the heart and the coronary arteries. This calcium has been shown to indicate that lesions, which can eventually block off one or more coronary arteries and cause chest pain or even a heart attack, are in the beginning stages of formation. Thus, many physicians are using ultrafast CT scanning as a means to diagnose early coronary artery disease in certain people, especially those who have no symptoms of the disease.
ultrasonography (ŭl″ tră-sŏn-ŏg′ ră-fē)	Test used to visualize an organ or tissue by using high-frequency sound waves; can be used as a screening test or as a diagnostic tool to determine abnormalities of the aorta, arteries, veins, and the heart.

Abbreviations *and* Acronyms

Abbreviation/ Acronym	Meaning	Abbreviation/ Acronym	Meaning
Abd, abd	abdomen	**AV**	atrioventricular
ACE	angiotensin-converting enzyme	**BP**	blood pressure
ACG	angiocardiography	**CABG**	coronary artery bypass graft
AED	automated external defibrillator	**CAD**	coronary artery disease
AF or AFib	atrial fibrillation	**CHD**	coronary heart disease
AMI	acute myocardial infarction	**CHF**	congestive heart failure
ARBs	ANG-II receptor blockers	**Chol**	cholesterol
ASHD	arteriosclerotic heart disease	**CK**	creatine kinase
AST	aspartate aminotransferase	**CKD**	chronic kidney disease

Abbreviation/ Acronym	Meaning	Abbreviation/ Acronym	Meaning
CLI	critical limb ischemia	MRAs	mineralocorticoid receptor antagonists
CMP	cardiomyopathy	MRI	magnetic resonance imaging
CMS	cardiometabolic syndrome	MS	mitral stenosis
CO	cardiac output	MV	mitral valve
CT	computed tomography	MVP	mitral valve prolapse
CTA	clear to auscultation	NSTEMI	non-ST-segment elevation myocardial infarction
CV	cardiovascular		
CVA	cerebrovascular accident (stroke)	O_2	oxygen
CVD	cardiovascular disease	OPCAB	off-pump coronary artery bypass surgery
DVT	deep vein thrombosis		
ECC	extracorporeal circulation	P	pulse
ECG, EKG	electrocardiogram	PAD	peripheral artery disease
ECHO	echocardiography	PAT	paroxysmal atrial tachycardia
EF	ejection fraction	PE	pulmonary embolism
EPS	electrophysiology study (intracardiac)	PET	positron emission tomography
FDA	Food and Drug Administration	PTCA	percutaneous transluminal coronary angioplasty
FFA	free fatty acids		
heart cath	cardiac catheterization	R	respiration
HBP	high blood pressure	RA	right atrium
HDL	high-density lipoprotein	RAAS	renin angiotensin aldosterone systems
HF	heart failure	RBCs	red blood cells
Hg	mercury	RV	right ventricle
Hgb	hemoglobin	RVEF	right-ventricular ejection fraction
H&L	heart and lungs	SA	sinoatrial (node)
HTN	hypertension	SCA	sudden cardiac arrest
IV	intravenous	SCD	sudden cardiac death
LA	left atrium	SOB	shortness of breath
LD, LDH	lactate dehydrogenase	STEMI	ST-segment elevation myocardial infarction
LDL	low-density lipoprotein		
LV	left ventricle	T2DM	type 2 diabetes mellitus
LVEF	left-ventricular ejection fraction	TOF	tetralogy of Fallot
MI	myocardial infarction	tPA, TPA	tissue plasminogen activator
mmHg	millimeters of Mercury	VLDL	very-low-density lipoprotein
		VSD	ventricular septal defect

Study *and* Review III

Building Medical Terms

Using the following word parts, fill in the blanks to build the correct medical terms.

bi-	sept	veni	-gen	-plasty
occlus	steth/o	-ion	-cuspid	

Definition   **Medical Term**

1. Valve with two cusps; pertaining to the mitral valve   _____cuspid

2. Literally means *process of lameness or limping*   claudicat_____

3. A blockage in a vessel, canal, or passage of the body   _____ion

4. Colorless, odorless, tasteless gas essential to respiration   oxy_____

5. An abnormal rapid throbbing or fluttering of the heart   palpitat_____

6. Wall or partition that divides a body space or cavity   _____um

7. Medical instrument used to listen to sounds of the heart   _____scope

8. Valve with three cusps   tri_____

9. Surgical repair of a cardiac valve   valvulo_____

10. Puncture of a vein for the removal of blood for analysis   _____puncture

Combining Form Challenge

Using the combining forms provided, write the medical term correctly.

angi/o	ather/o	cyan/o
arteri/o	cardi/o	phleb/o

1. Surgical repair of a blood vessel: _____plasty

2. Pertaining to an artery: _____al

3. Tumor of an artery containing a fatty substance: _____oma

4. Enlargement of the heart: _____megaly

5. When the skin, fingernails, and mucous membranes appear slightly blue: _____osis

6. Literally means *inflammation of a vein*: _____itis

Select the Right Term

Select the correct answer, and write it on the line provided.

1. Abnormally slow heartbeat defined as fewer than 60 beats per minute is _____.

   bruit   cardioversion   bradycardia   tachycardia

2. Abnormally high levels of lipids in the blood is _____.

   hyperlipidemia   hyperlipdemia   hypolipidemia   hypolipdemia

3. Pertaining to the sac surrounding the heart is _____.

   pericardial   pericardiocentesis   pericarditis   phlebitis

4. Valves of the aorta and pulmonary artery; shaped like a crescent is _____.

   sinoatrial   tricuspid   bicuspid   semilunar

5. Pertains to an organic compound consisting of three molecules of fatty acids is _____.

   tricuspid   triglyceride   systole   triglyeride

6. Condition in which there is a lack of oxygen due to decreased blood supply to a part of the body caused by constriction or obstruction of a blood vessel is _____.

   infarction   murmur   ischemia   occlusion

Drug Highlights

Match the appropriate lettered description or examples of drug(s) with the class of drug.

_____ **1.** antiarrhythmic agents

_____ **2.** antihypertensive agents

_____ **3.** thrombolytic agents

_____ **4.** anticoagulants

_____ **5.** antihyperlipidemic agents

_____ **6.** examples of antiplatelet drugs

_____ **7.** vasodilators

_____ **8.** vasopressors

_____ **9.** digitalis drugs

a. Aspirin and Plavix (clopidogrel)

b. Act to prevent blood clots from forming

c. Cause relaxation of blood vessels and lower blood pressure

d. Used to lower abnormally high blood levels of fatty substances (lipids)

e. Used in the treatment of hypertension

f. Cause an elevation of blood pressure, which is useful in the treatment of patients suffering from shock.

g. Used in the treatment of irregular heart rhythms

h. Strengthen the heart muscle, increase the force and velocity of myocardial systolic contraction, slow the heart rate, and decrease conduction velocity through the atrioventricular (AV) node

i. Also called tissue plasminogen activators (tPA, TPA), they can reduce the chance of dying after a myocardial infarction by 50%

Diagnostic and Laboratory Tests

Select the best answer to each multiple-choice question. Circle the letter of your choice.

1. An intracardiac procedure that maps the electrical conduction of cardiac arrhythmias.

a. Electrocardiogram

b. Electrocardiomyogram

c. Electrophysiology

d. Cardiac catheterization

2. Blood tests performed to determine cardiac damage in an acute myocardial infarction.

a. cardiac enzymes

b. high-density lipoproteins

c. triglycerides

d. low-density lipoproteins

3. Method of recording a patient's ECG for 24 hours.

a. stress test

b. Holter monitor

c. ultrasonography

d. angiography

4. Test used to visualize an organ or tissue by using high-frequency sound waves.

    a. electrophysiology   **c.** ultrasonography

    b. stress test   **d.** cholesterol

5. An x-ray recording of a blood vessel after the injection of a radiopaque contrast medium.

    a. ultrasonography   **c.** stress test

    b. angiography   **d.** cardiac catheterization

Abbreviations and Acronyms

Write the correct word, phrase, or abbreviation/acronym in the space provided.

1. acute myocardial infarction _____

2. atrioventricular _____

3. BP _____

4. CAD _____

5. deep vein thrombosis _____

6. ECG, EKG _____

7. HDL _____

8. heart and lungs _____

9. MI _____

10. tPA, TPA _____

Practical Application

SOAP: Chart Note Analysis

This exercise will make you aware of the information, abbreviations/acronyms, and medical terminology typically found in a cardiology patient's chart. Refer to Appendix III, *Abbreviations, Acronyms, and Symbols*.

Read the chart note and answer the questions that follow.

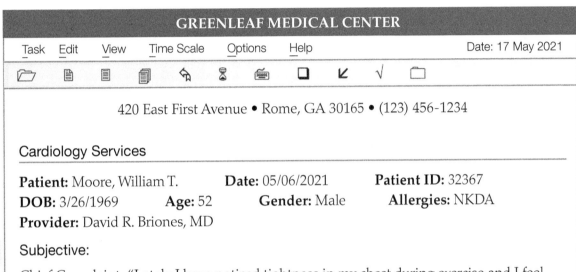

GREENLEAF MEDICAL CENTER

| Task | Edit | View | Time Scale | Options | Help | Date: 17 May 2021 |

420 East First Avenue • Rome, GA 30165 • (123) 456-1234

Cardiology Services

Patient: Moore, William T.   **Date:** 05/06/2021   **Patient ID:** 32367
DOB: 3/26/1969   **Age:** 52   **Gender:** Male   **Allergies:** NKDA
Provider: David R. Briones, MD

S

Subjective:

Chief Complaint: "Lately I have noticed tightness in my chest during exercise and I feel out of breath. I am real anxious and worried about myself."

52 y/o Caucasian male describes experiencing "tightness" in his chest during a workout session. Noted patient clenching his fist while describing dyspnea (shortness of breath) and how anxious he felt. He denies nausea, vomiting, or radiating pain to his left arm or jaw. The uncomfortable sensation "just went away" after he stopped exercising. He states that he has no prior history of cardiac disease.

O

Objective:

Vital Signs: T: 98.4 F; **P:** 84; **R:** 20; **BP:** 138/90

Ht: 5′ 11″

Wt: 196 lb

General Appearance: Well-developed and muscular. No obvious signs of physical distress noted such as edema, pallor, or diaphoresis. Overall health appears WNL.

Heart: Rate at 84 beats per minute, rhythm regular, no extra sounds, no murmurs.

Lungs: CTA

Abd: Bowel sounds all four quadrants, no masses or tenderness.

MS: Joints and muscles symmetric; no swelling, masses, or deformity; normal spinal curvature. No tenderness to palpation of joints. Full ROM, movement smooth, no crepitant (crackling) sound heard, no tenderness. Muscle strength: able to maintain flexion against resistance and without tenderness.

A Assessment:

Chest pain (angina pectoris)

P Plan:

1. Schedule patient for an EKG and blood enzyme studies ASAP.

2. Start patient on nitroglycerin (coronary vasodilator) sublingual tablets 0.4 mg prn for chest pain. Instruct patient to seek medical attention immediately if pain is not relieved by nitroglycerin tablets, taken one every 5 minutes over a 15-minute period.

3. To return in 2 weeks for follow-up.

4. Discuss family cardiac history as related to HTN, obesity, diabetes, coronary artery disease, and sudden death of any family member occurring at a young age.

5. Educate patient that angina pectoris occurs due to myocardial ischemia that results when cardiac workload and myocardial oxygen demand exceed the ability of the coronary arteries to supply oxygenated blood. This commonly occurs during exercise or other activity.

Chart Note Questions

Write the correct answer in the space provided.

1. Signs and symptoms of angina pectoris include tightness in the chest, apprehension, and shortness of breath, which is also called _____.

2. A complete physical, an EKG, and _____ _____ studies are important in determining the diagnosis of angina pectoris.

3. Myocardial ischemia is a result of the body's inability to supply _____ blood.

4. EKG is an abbreviation for _____.

5. Nitroglycerin is a coronary _____used to treat angina pectoris.

MyLab Medical Terminology™

MyLab Medical Terminology is a premium online homework management system that includes a host of features to help you study. Registered users will find:

- A multitude of quizzes and activities built within the MyLab platform

- Powerful tools that track and analyze your results—allowing you to create a personalized learning experience

- Videos and audio pronunciations to help enrich your progress

- Streaming lesson presentations (guided lectures) and self-paced learning modules

- A space where you and your instructor can check your progress and manage your assignments

Blood and Lymphatic System

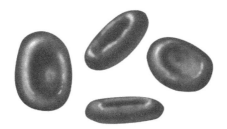

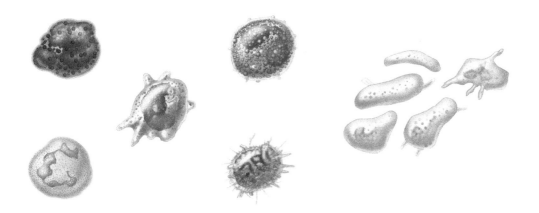

⌄ Learning Outcomes

On completion of this chapter, you will be able to:

1. State the description and primary functions of the organs/structures of the blood and lymphatic system.
2. Name the four blood types and their significance in blood typing and blood transfusion.
3. Describe and give the functions of the accessory organs of the lymphatic system.
4. Describe the immune system's response to foreign substances and the means by which it protects the body.
5. Analyze, build, spell, and pronounce medical words.
6. Classify the drugs highlighted in this chapter.
7. Describe diagnostic and laboratory tests related to blood and the lymphatic system.
8. Identify and define selected abbreviations and acronyms.

Anatomy and Physiology

Blood and lymph are two of the body's main fluids and they travel through two separate but interconnected vessel systems. Blood is circulated by the action of the heart, through the circulatory system consisting largely of arteries, veins, and capillaries. Lymph does not actually circulate. It is propelled in one direction, away from its source, through larger lymph vessels, to drain into large veins of the circulatory system located in the upper chest. Numerous valves within the lymph vessels permit one-directional flow, opening and closing as a consequence of pressure caused by the contracting action of muscles on the vessels squeezing the fluid forward.

Table 9.1 provides an at-a-glance look at the blood and lymphatic system.

TABLE 9.1	Blood and Lymphatic System at-a-Glance
Organ/Structure	**Primary Functions/Description**
Blood	Fluid consisting of formed elements (erythrocytes, thrombocytes, leukocytes) and plasma. It is a specialized bodily fluid that delivers necessary substances—such as oxygen (O_2), nutrients, hormones, and salts—to the body's cells and transports waste products—such as carbon dioxide, urea, and lactic acid—away from those same cells. Blood is circulated around the body through blood vessels by the pumping action of the heart.
Lymphatic system	Vessel system composed of lymphatic capillaries, lymphatic vessels, lymphatic ducts, and lymph nodes that transport lymph from the tissue to the blood. The three main functions of the lymphatic system are: 1. Transport proteins and fluids, lost by capillary seepage, back to the bloodstream 2. Protect the body against pathogens (microorganisms or substances capable of producing disease) by phagocytosis and immune response 3. Serve as a pathway for the absorption of fats from the small intestine into the bloodstream
Spleen	Acts as a filter for blood; recycles old erythrocytes (red blood cells); stores platelets and white blood cells; helps fight certain kinds of bacteria, especially those that cause pneumonia and meningitis
Tonsils	Trap germs (bacteria and viruses) that are breathed in; produce antibodies that can help to kill germs and may help to prevent throat and lung infections
Thymus	Plays essential role in the formation of antibodies and the development of the immune response in the newborn; manufactures infection-fighting T cells and helps distinguish normal T cells from those that attack the body's own tissue.

Blood

Blood is a fluid that circulates through the heart, arteries, veins, and capillaries. It consists of formed elements and plasma, both of which are continuously produced by the body for the purpose of transporting respiratory gases (*oxygen* and *carbon dioxide*), chemical substances (*nutrients, hormones*), and cells that act to protect the body from foreign substances. The blood volume within an individual depends on body weight. An individual weighing 154 lb (70 kg) has a blood volume of about 5 quarts (qt) or 4.7 liters (L).

Formed Elements

The formed elements in blood are the erythrocytes (red blood cells), thrombocytes (platelets), and leukocytes (white blood cells). See Table 9.2. Formed elements constitute

TABLE 9.2 Types of Blood Cells and Functions	
Blood Cell	**Function**
Erythrocyte (red blood cell)	Transports oxygen and carbon dioxide
Thrombocyte (platelet)	Responsible for blood clotting
Leukocyte (white blood cell)	Provides body's main defense against invasion of pathogens
Neutrophil	Protects against infection, especially by bacteria; is readily attracted to foreign antigens and destroys them by phagocytosis (engulfing and eating of particulate substances)
Eosinophil	Destroys parasitic organisms; plays a key role in allergic reactions
Basophil	Plays a role in releasing histamine and other chemicals that act on blood vessels; essential to nonspecific immune response to inflammation
Monocyte	Provides one of the first lines of defense in the inflammatory process, phagocytosis
Lymphocyte	Acts to recognize antigens, produce antibodies, and destroy foreign invaders

about 45% of the total volume of blood. Together, the plasma and formed elements constitute whole blood. These components can be separated for analysis and clinical purposes. See Figure 9.1.

 fyi In the embryo, plasma and blood cells are formed around the second week of life. At approximately the fifth week of development, blood formation occurs in the liver and later in the spleen, thymus, lymphatic system, and bone marrow. At 16 weeks, the fetus is 11.6 cm (4.6 in.) from the crown (or top) of the head to the rump (or bottom) and weighs 100 g (3.5 oz). The fetal **liver** is the chief producer of red blood cells, and the gallbladder secretes **bile**. At 16 weeks, blood vessels are visible through the now-transparent skin. Fetal circulation provides oxygenation and nutrition to the fetus and disposes of carbon dioxide and other waste products.

ERYTHROCYTES

Erythrocytes are commonly called *red blood cells (RBCs)*. Mature RBCs are flexible biconcave disks that lack nuclei. They transport oxygen (most of which is bound to hemoglobin contained in the cell) and carbon dioxide to and from the tissues of the body. There are approximately 5 million erythrocytes per cubic millimeter of blood, and they have a lifespan of 80–120 days. Erythrocytes are formed in the red bone marrow. Refer to Figure 9.1.

THROMBOCYTES

Thrombocytes, commonly called *platelets,* are small disk-shaped cell fragments without a nucleus. Refer to Figure 9.1. They play an important role in the clotting process by releasing *thrombokinase,* which, in the presence of calcium, reacts with *prothrombin* to form *thrombin*. Thrombin (a blood enzyme) converts fibrinogen (a blood protein) into fibrin, an insoluble protein that forms an intricate network of minute threadlike structures called fibrils and causes the blood plasma to coagulate. The blood cells and plasma are enmeshed in the network of fibrils to form the clot.

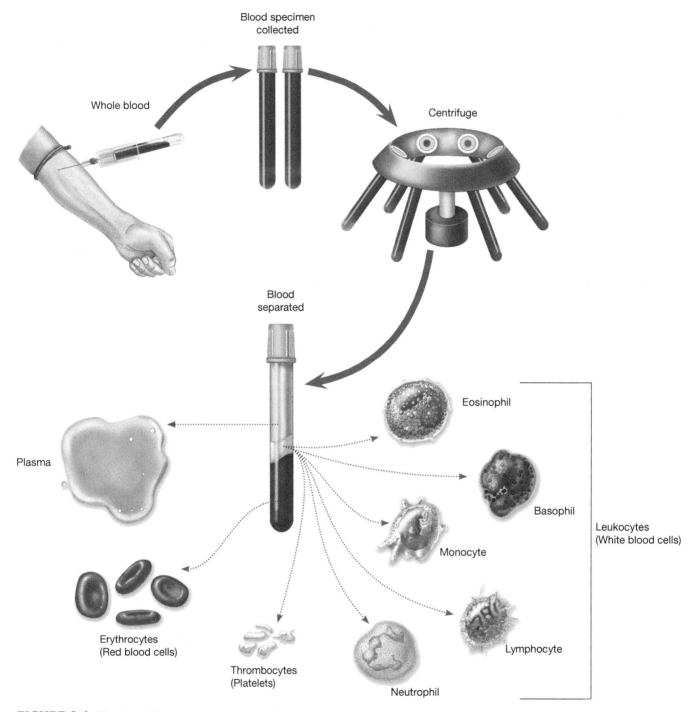

FIGURE 9.1 Blood and its components.

Coagulation is a complex process by which blood forms clots. See Figure 9.2. It is an important part of hemostasis (the cessation of blood loss from a damaged vessel), wherein a damaged blood vessel wall is covered by a platelet and fibrin-containing clot to stop bleeding and begin repair of the damaged vessel. Disorders of coagulation can lead to an increased risk of bleeding (hemorrhage) or clotting (thrombosis).

Coagulation begins almost instantly after an injury to the blood vessel has damaged the endothelium (lining of the vessel). Exposure of the blood to proteins such as tissue factor initiates changes to blood platelets and the plasma protein fibrinogen, a clotting factor. Platelets immediately form a plug at the site of injury; this is called *primary hemostasis*. *Secondary hemostasis* occurs simultaneously: Proteins in the blood plasma, called *coagulation factors* or *clotting factors*, respond in a complex cascade to form fibrin strands,

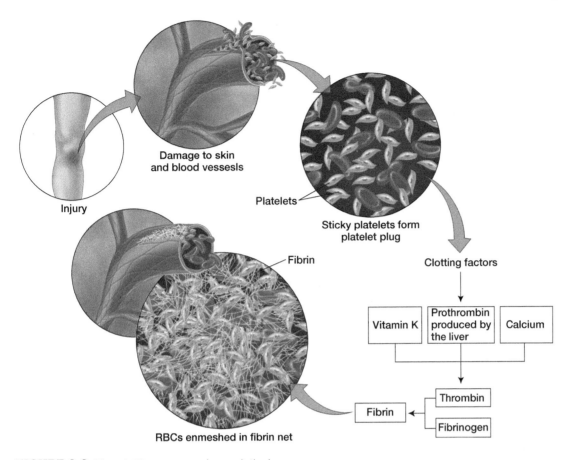

FIGURE 9.2 The clotting process (coagulation).

which strengthen the platelet plug. This complex process involves several substances—vitamin K, prothrombin, calcium, thrombin, and fibrinogen—that all aid in forming fibrin.

There are approximately 150,000–400,000 thrombocytes per cubic millimeter of blood. Thrombocytes are fragments of certain giant cells called *megakaryocytes*, which are formed in the red bone marrow.

LEUKOCYTES

Leukocytes, commonly called *white blood cells (WBCs)*, are sphere-shaped cells containing nuclei of varying shapes and sizes. Refer to Figure 9.1. Leukocytes are the body's main defense against the invasion of pathogens. In a normal body state, when pathogens enter the tissue, the leukocytes leave the blood vessels through their walls and move in an amoeba-like motion to the area of infection, where they ingest and destroy the invader. There are approximately 8,000 leukocytes per cubic millimeter of blood. The five types of leukocytes are *neutrophils* (**neutr/o** [*neither*]), *eosinophils* (**eos, eosin/o** [*rose-colored*]), *basophils* (**bas/o** [*base*]), *lymphocytes* (**lymph/o** [*lymph*]), and *monocytes* (**mono-** [*one*]).

Neutrophils, eosinophils, basophils, and monocytes contribute to the body's nonspecific defenses. These immune defenses are activated by a variety of stimuli. Neutrophils aid in the fight against bacterial infection. Lymphocytes are responsible for specific defenses against invading pathogens or foreign proteins. Monocytes are the largest of the leukocytes and fight off bacteria, viruses, and fungi.

Blood Groups

A number of human blood systems are determined by a series of two or more genes closely linked on a single autosomal chromosome. The **ABO** system, which was discovered in 1901 by Karl Landsteiner, is of great significance in blood typing and blood transfusion.

The four blood types identified in this system are types A, B, AB, and O. The differences in human blood are due to the presence or absence of certain protein molecules called *antigens* and *antibodies*. The antigens are located on the surface of the red blood cells, and the antibodies are in the blood plasma. Individuals have different types and combinations of these molecules. Individuals in the A group have the A antigen on the surface of their red blood cells and anti-B antibody in the blood plasma; B group has the B antigen and the anti-A antibody; AB group has both A and B antigens and no anti-A or anti-B antibodies; and group O has neither A or B antigens but has both anti-A and anti-B antibodies. Type AB blood is the universal donor of plasma and the universal recipient of cells, and type O is the universal donor of cells only. See Table 9.3.

Rh Factor

The presence of a substance called an **agglutinogen** in the red blood cells is responsible for what is known as the **Rh factor**. It was first discovered in the blood of the rhesus monkey, from which the factor gets its name. About 85% of the population have the Rh factor and are called *Rh positive*. The other 15% lack the Rh factor and are designated *Rh negative*. More than 20 genetically determined blood group systems are known today, but the ABO and Rh systems are the most important ones used for blood transfusions.

For a blood transfusion to be safe and successful, ABO and Rh blood groups of the donor and the recipient must be compatible. If they are not, the red blood cells from the donated blood can agglutinate and cause clogging of blood vessels and slow and/or stop the circulation of blood to various parts of the body. The agglutinated red blood cells can also hemolyze (dissolve or be destroyed) and their contents leak out in the body. This can be very dangerous, even life-threatening, to the patient. Before blood can be administered to a patient, a type and cross-match must be performed. This means mixing the donor cells with the recipient's serum and watching for agglutination. If none occurs, the blood is considered compatible. Even though the blood is checked for compatibility, blood transfusion reactions can still occur and usually involve fever and chills. These reactions typically begin during the first 15 minutes of the transfusion. Refer to Table 9.3 for blood group compatibilities.

Plasma

The fluid part of the blood is called **plasma**. Clear and somewhat straw-colored, it comprises about 55% of the total volume of blood and is composed of water (91%) and chemical compounds (9%). Plasma is the fluid part of the circulation medium of blood cells, providing nutritive substances to various body structures and removing waste products of metabolism from body structures. There are four major plasma proteins: **albumin**, **globulin**, **fibrinogen**, and **prothrombin**.

TABLE 9.3	Blood Groups and Compatibilities				
Type	Antigen	Plasma Antibody	Percentage/ Population	Compatible Donor Blood Groups	Incompatible Donor Blood Groups
A	A	Anti-B	41%	A, O	B, AB
B	B	Anti-A	10%	B, O	A, AB
AB	Both A and B	No anti-A or anti-B	4%	A, B, AB, O	None
O	No A and B	Both anti-A and anti-B	45%	O	A, B, AB

Study *and* Review I

Anatomy and Physiology—Blood

Write your answers to the following questions.

1. Blood is a fluid that _____ through the heart, arteries, veins, and capillaries.

2. What are the three formed elements in blood? Write in their medical names.

   a. _____   c. _____

   b. _____

3. Red blood cells (RBCs) transport _____ and carbon dioxide.

4. Thrombocytes play an important role in the _____ process.

5. _____ is a complex process by which blood forms clots.

6. _____ are the body's main defense against the invasion of pathogens (pertaining to producing disease).

7. Blood types A, B, AB, and O are identified in the _____ system.

8. The factor first discovered in the rhesus monkey is named the _____ factor.

9. The fluid part of the blood is called _____.

10. There are four major proteins of the answer to question 9. List these proteins.

    a. _____   c. _____

    b. _____   d. _____

Matching

Select the correct lettered function for each blood cell type.

_____ 1. erythrocyte

_____ 2. thrombocyte

_____ 3. leukocyte

_____ 4. neutrophil

_____ 5. eosinophil

_____ 6. basophil

_____ 7. monocyte

_____ 8. lymphocyte

a. Destroys parasitic organisms; plays a key role in allergic reactions

b. Provides one of the first lines of defense in the inflammatory process, phagocytosis

c. Provides body's main defense against invasion of pathogens

d. Responsible for blood clotting

e. Protects against infection, especially by bacteria

f. Transports oxygen and carbon dioxide

g. Acts to recognize antigens, produce antibodies, and destroy foreign invaders

h. Plays a role in releasing histamine and other chemicals that act on blood vessels; essential to nonspecific immune response to inflammation

Lymphatic System

The **lymphatic system** is a vessel system apart from, but connected to, the circulatory system. See Figure 9.3. The lymphatic system is composed of *lymphatic capillaries, lymphatic vessels, lymphatic ducts,* and *lymph nodes.* The system conveys lymph from the tissues to the blood.

The three main functions of the lymphatic system are:

1. Transport proteins and fluids, lost by capillary seepage, back to the bloodstream
2. Protect the body against pathogens (microorganisms or substances capable of producing disease) by phagocytosis and immune response
3. Serve as a pathway for the absorption of fats from the small intestine into the bloodstream

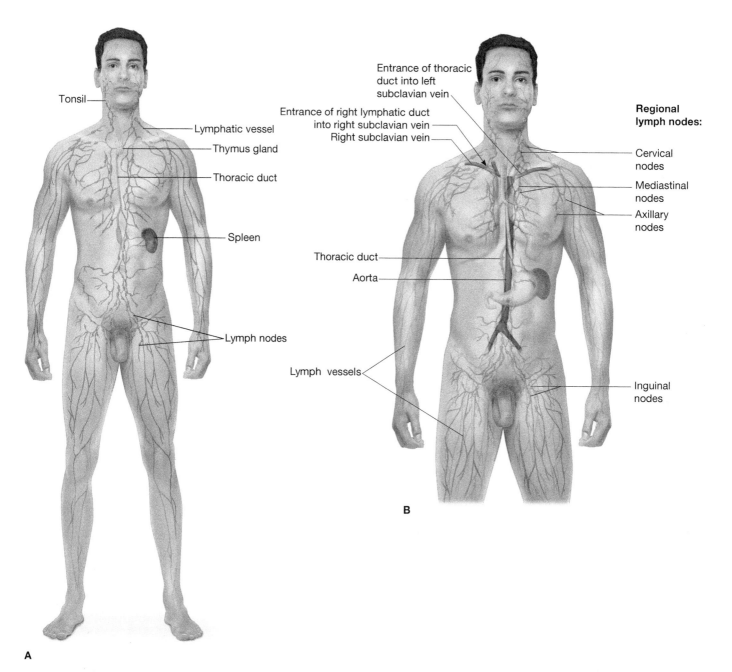

FIGURE 9.3 Lymphatic system. **A** Lymphatic vessels, major lymph nodes, and lymphatic organs. **B** Areas of lymph node concentration. The direction of lymph flow is toward the heart.

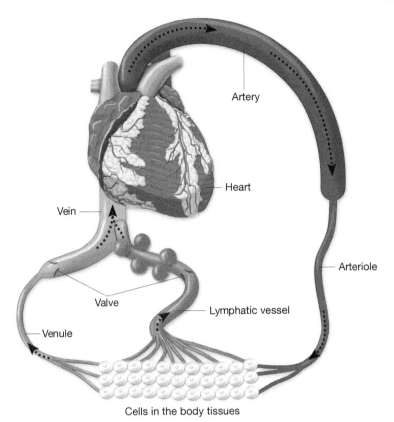

FIGURE 9.4 Lymphatic vessels pick up excess tissue fluid, purify it in the lymph nodes, and then return it to the circulatory system.

Lymph is a clear, colorless, alkaline fluid (about 95% water) found in the lymphatic vessels. It is fluid derived from body tissues. Lymph contains white blood cells and circulates throughout the lymphatic system, returning to the venous bloodstream through the thoracic duct. See Figure 9.4. The principal component of lymph is fluid from plasma that has seeped out of capillary walls into spaces among the body tissues. Lymph contains proteins (serum albumin, serum globulin, serum fibrinogen), salts, organic substances (urea, creatinine, neutral fats, glucose), and water. Cells present are principally lymphocytes, formed in the lymph nodes and other lymphatic tissues. See Figure 9.5. Lymph from the intestines contains fats and other substances absorbed from the intestines.

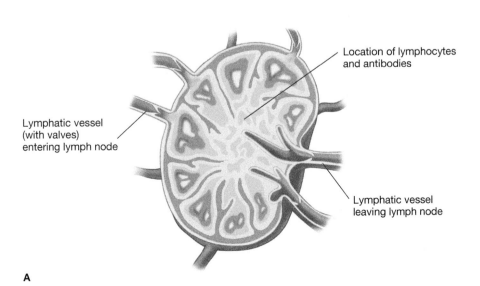

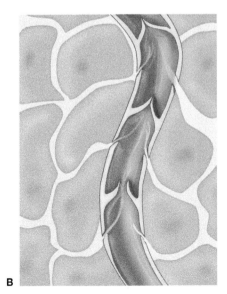

A

B

FIGURE 9.5 A Structure of a lymph node. **B** Lymphatic vessel showing valves within tissue cells.

The lymphatic system can be broadly divided into the conducting system and the lymphoid tissue. The conducting system carries the lymph and consists of tubular vessels that include the lymph capillaries, the lymph vessels, and the right and left thoracic ducts. The lymphoid tissue is primarily involved in immune responses and consists of lymphocytes and other white blood cells enmeshed in connective tissue through which the lymph passes. Regions of the lymphoid tissue that are densely packed with lymphocytes are known as *lymphoid follicles*. Lymphoid tissue can either be structurally well organized as lymph nodes or may consist of loosely organized lymphoid follicles known as mucosa-associated lymphoid tissue (MALT). These tissues are associated with mucosal surfaces of almost any organ, but especially those of the digestive, genitourinary, and respiratory tracts, which are constantly exposed to a wide variety of potentially harmful microorganisms and therefore require their own system of antigen capture and presentation to lymphocytes. For example, Peyer patches, which are mucosa-associated lymphoid tissues of the small intestine, plays a role in immunologic response by efficiently trapping antigens for exposure to T cells and B cells and destroying harmful bacteria.

The thymus and the bone marrow constitute the primary lymphoid tissues involved in the production and early selection of lymphocytes. Secondary lymphoid tissue provides the environment for the foreign or altered native molecules (antigens) to interact with the lymphocytes. Lymphocytes are concentrated in the lymph nodes, and the lymphoid follicles in the tonsils and spleen.

Accessory Organs

The accessory organs of the lymphatic system include the spleen, the tonsils, and the thymus. Refer to Figure 9.3 and Table 9.1.

Spleen

The **spleen** is a soft, dark red oval body lying in the upper left quadrant of the abdomen. It is the major site of erythrocyte destruction (old erythrocytes over 80–120 days). It serves as a reservoir for blood. The spleen plays an essential role in the immune response and acts as a filter, removing microorganisms from the blood.

Tonsils

The **tonsils** are lymphoid masses located in depressions of the mucous membranes of the face and pharynx. They consist of the *palatine tonsils, pharyngeal tonsils (adenoids),* and the *lingual tonsils*. The tonsils trap bacteria and viruses and produce antibodies that help to kill germs and may help to prevent throat and lung infections. See Figure 9.6.

Thymus

The **thymus** is considered to be one of the endocrine glands, but because of its function and appearance, it is a part of the lymphoid system. Located in the mediastinal cavity, the thymus plays an essential role in the formation of antibodies and the development of the immune response in the newborn. It manufactures infection-fighting **T cells** and helps distinguish normal T cells from those that attack the body's own tissue. T cells are important in the body's cellular immune response.

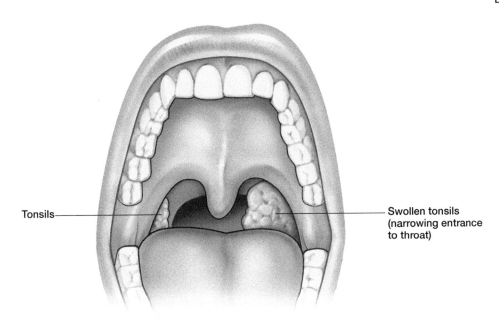

Tonsils

Swollen tonsils
(narrowing entrance
to throat)

FIGURE 9.6 Tonsils—normal and enlarged.

fyi The **thymus gland** plays an important role in the development of the immune response in the newborn. At birth, the average weight of the thymus is 10–15 g. It attains a weight of 28 g (1 oz) at puberty, after which it begins to undergo involution, which replaces the thymus with adipose and connective tissue.

Immune System

The **immune system** is part of the defense mechanism of the body. It consists of the tissues, organs, and physiological processes used by the body to identify and protect against abnormal cells, foreign substances, and foreign tissue cells that may have been transplanted into the body. Many of these tissues and organs are part of the lymphatic system.

Fortunately, the average, healthy human body is equipped with natural defenses that assist it in fighting off disease and cancer. These natural defenses are intact skin, the cleansing action of the body's secretions (such as tears, mucus), white blood cells, body chemicals (such as hormones, enzymes), and antibodies. As long as the immune system is intact and functioning properly, it can defend the body against invading foreign substances and cancer.

Immunity is the state of being immune to or protected from a disease, especially an infectious disease. This state is usually induced by having been exposed to the antigenic marker of an organism that invades the body or by having been immunized with a vaccine capable of stimulating production of specific antibodies.

Passive immunity is acquired through transfer of antibodies or activated T cells from an immune host and is short lived, usually lasting only a few months; whereas **active immunity** is induced in the host itself by an antigen and lasts much longer, sometimes lifelong. **Humoral immunity** is the aspect of immunity that is mediated by secreted antibodies, whereas the protection provided by **cell-mediated immunity** involves T lymphocytes alone.

GOOD TO KNOW

Did you know that vaccines can help protect you and your community? This concept is called *herd immunity* or *community immunity*. Microorganisms can travel quickly through a community and make a large number of people sick. If enough people get sick, it can lead to an outbreak of disease or even an epidemic. But when enough people are vaccinated against a certain disease, the germs can't travel as easily from person to person—and the entire community is less likely to get the disease. This means that even people who don't get vaccinated (such as people with serious allergies or weakened immune systems) will have some protection from getting sick. And if a person does get sick, there's less chance of an outbreak because it's harder for the disease to spread. Eventually, the disease becomes rare—and sometimes, it's wiped out altogether.

If vaccines have wiped out some diseases in the United States, can we stop getting vaccinated for them? No. Many vaccine-preventable diseases that we don't often see in the United States still make people sick in other countries. So it's possible for travelers to bring these diseases to the United States, where they could then spread. If we stop getting vaccinated, we won't be protected from these diseases—herd/community immunity protects us only if enough people continue to get vaccinated.

Immune Response

The **immune response** is the reaction of the body to foreign substances and the means by which it protects the body. See Figure 9.7. It is a complex function; the following sections provide an overview of how the immune response works.

The immune response can be described as humoral (pertaining to body fluids) immunity or antibody-mediated immunity and cellular immunity or cell-mediated immunity.

HUMORAL OR ANTIBODY-MEDIATED IMMUNITY

Humoral immunity, also called *antibody-mediated immunity*, involves the production of plasma lymphocytes (B cells) in response to antigen exposure with subsequent formation of antibodies. Humoral immunity is a major defense against bacterial infections. An antigen is any substance to which the immune system can respond. For example, it may be a foreign substance from the environment such as chemicals, bacteria, viruses, or pollen. If the immune system encounters an antigen that is not found on the body's own cells, it will launch an attack against that antigen.

The Immunue System		
Innate (nonspecific) defense mechanisms		**Adaptive (specific) defense mechanisms**
First line of defense	Second line of defense	Third line of defense
• Skin • Mucous membranes • Secretions of skin and mucous membranes	• Phagocytic cells • Natural killer cells • Antimicrobial proteins • The inflammatory response • Fever	• Lymphocytes • Antibodies • Macrophages and other antigen-presenting cells

FIGURE 9.7 An overview of the body's defenses.

Source: MARIEB, ELAINE N.; KELLER, SUZANNE M., ESSENTIALS OF HUMAN ANATOMY & PHYSIOLOGY, 12th Ed., ©2018. Reprinted and Electronically reproduced by permission of Pearson Education, Inc., New York, NY.

TABLE 9.4 Different Classes of Antibodies

Antibody	Functions
IgG	Crosses placenta to provide passive immunity for the fetus and newborn; opsonizes (coats) microorganisms to enhance phagocytosis; activates *complement system* (a group of proteins in the blood) Components of complement are labeled C1–C9. Complement acts by directly killing organisms; by opsonizing an antigen; and by stimulating inflammation and the B cell–mediated immune response
IgM	Activates complement; is first antibody produced in response to bacterial and viral infections
IgA	Protects epithelial surfaces; activates complement; is passed to breastfeeding newborn via the colostrum (first milk after birth)
IgE	Responds to allergic reactions and some parasitic infections; triggers mast cells to release histamine, serotonin, kinins, slow-reacting substance of anaphylaxis, and the neutrophil factor, mediators that produce allergic skin reaction, asthma, and hay fever
IgD	Helps regulate B-cell function

Antibodies are developed in response to a specific antigen. An antibody is also referred to as an *immunoglobulin*; it is a complex glycoprotein produced by B lymphocytes in response to the presence of an antigen. Antibodies neutralize or destroy antigens. See Table 9.4 for the functions of the five classes of antibodies: IgG, IgM, IgA, IgE, and IgD.

CELLULAR OR CELL-MEDIATED IMMUNITY

Cellular immunity or *cell-mediated immunity* involves the production of lymphocytes (T cells) of the helper type and T cells of the natural killer (NK) type that are capable of attacking foreign cells, normal cells infected with viruses, and cancer cells.

Four general phases are associated with the body's immune response to a foreign substance:

1. The first phase recognizes the foreign substance or the invader (enemy).

2. The second phase activates the body's defenses by producing more white blood cells that are designed to seek and destroy the invader(s), especially the macrophages that eat and engulf the foreign substances, and lymphocytes, B cells, and T cells. See Table 9.5.

   - T cells of the helper type identify the enemy and rush to the spleen and lymph nodes, where they stimulate the production of other cells to aid in the fight against the foreign substance.

   - T cells of the natural killer (NK) type are large granular lymphocytes that also specialize in killing cells of the body that have been invaded by foreign substances and fighting cells that have turned cancerous.

   - B cells reside in the spleen or lymph nodes and produce antibodies for specific antigens.

TABLE 9.5 Functions of Lymphocytes

Type of Cell	Functions
T cells (thymus-dependent)	Provide cellular immunity
B cells (bone marrow–derived)	Provide humoral immunity
NK cells (natural killer)	Attack foreign cells, normal cells infected with viruses, and cancer cells

3. The third phase is the attack phase during which the preceding defenders of the body produce antibodies and/or seek out to kill and/or remove the foreign invader. They do this by phagocytosis in which the macrophages squeeze out between the cells in the capillaries and crawl into the tissue to the site of the infection. Here they surround and eat the foreign substances that caused the infection. Other white blood cells respond to infection by producing antibodies, which are released into the blood-stream and carried to the site of the infection where they surround and immobilize the invaders. Later, the phagocytes can eat both antibody and invader.

4. The fourth phase is the slowdown phase in which the number of defenders returns to normal, following victory over the foreign invader.

fyi The immune response declines with age, limiting the body's ability to identify and fight foreign substances such as bacteria and viruses. With aging comes the loss of the thymus cortex, which leads to a reduced production of T lymphocytes, including T cells, natural killer cells, and B lymphocytes. Frequency and severity of infections generally increase in older adults because of a decreased ability of the immune system to respond adequately to invading microorganisms.

Study *and* Review II

Anatomy and Physiology—Lymphatic and Immune Systems

Write your answer to the following questions.

1. The lymphatic system is composed of lymphatic capillaries, lymphatic vessels, lymphatic ducts, and lymphatic glands. True or false? _____

2. The lymphatic system transports proteins, carbohydrates, and fluids back to the bloodstream. True or false? _____

3. _____ is a clear, colorless, alkaline fluid found in the lymphatic system.

4. What is the acronym for the loosely organized lymphoid follicles known as the mucosa-associated lymphoid tissue? _____

5. In which three tracts of the body would mucosa-associated lymphoid tissue be found?

   a. _____   c. _____

   b. _____

6. Where are Peyer patches located in the body? _____

7. Peyer patches play a role in immunologic response by trapping _____ for exposure to T cells and B cells and destroying harmful bacteria.

8. List the three accessory organs of the lymphatic system

a. _____   c. _____

b. _____

9. The _____ filter bacteria and aid in the formation of white blood cells.

10. The _____ plays an essential role in the formation of antibodies in the newborn.

Matching

Select the correct lettered meaning for each of the numbered medical terms.

_____ **1.** immune system

_____ **2.** immunity

_____ **3.** immune response

_____ **4.** humoral immunity

_____ **5.** antigen

_____ **6.** antibodies

_____ **7.** cellular immunity

_____ **8.** T cells

_____ **9.** B cells

_____ **10.** NK cells

a. Any substance to which the immune system can respond, such as a foreign substance, chemicals, bacteria, viruses, or pollen

b. Cell-mediated immunity that involves the production of lymphocytes (T cells) and natural killer (NK) cells

c. Provide humoral immunity

d. The state of being immune to or protected from a disease

e. Attack foreign cells, normal cells infected with viruses, and cancer cells

f. Part of the defense mechanism of the body

g. Provide cellular immunity

h. A complex glycoprotein produced by B lymphocytes in response to the presence of an antigen

i. The production of plasma lymphocytes (B cells) in response to antigen exposure with subsequent formation of antibodies

j. Reaction of the body to foreign substances and the means by which it protects the body

▶ **ANATOMY LABELING**   Identify the structures shown below by filling in the blanks.

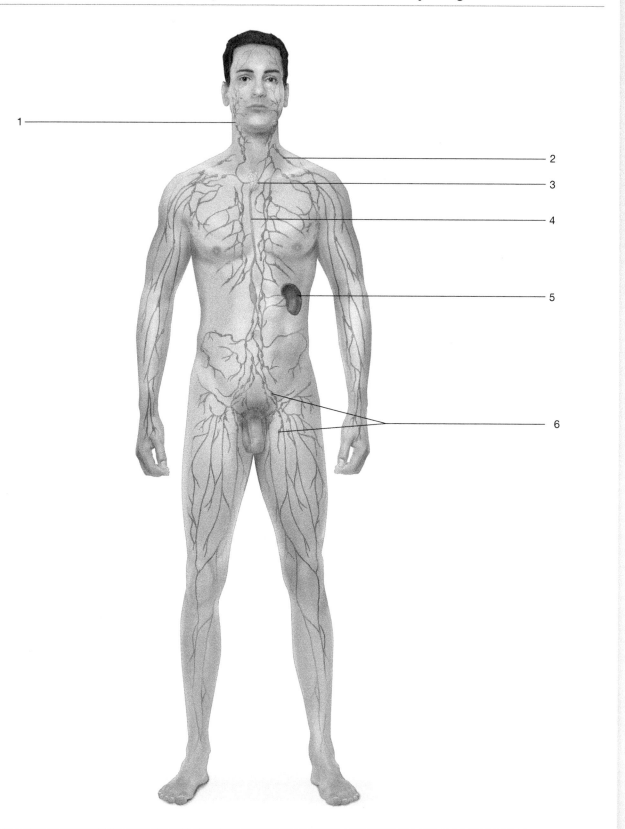

1 _____

2 _____

3 _____

4 _____

5 _____

6 _____

Building Your Medical Vocabulary

This section provides the foundation for learning medical terminology. Review the alphabetized list of medical terms in the following pages. Note how common prefixes and suffixes are repeatedly applied to word roots and combining forms to create different meanings. A combining form is a word root plus a vowel. The chart below lists the combining forms and word roots used in this chapter and can help to strengthen your understanding of how medical words are built and spelled.

You will find that some terms have not been divided into word parts. These are common words or specialized terms that are included to enhance your medical vocabulary.

Combining Forms

aden/o	gland	leuk/o	white
all/o	other	lipid/o	fat
anis/o	unequal	lymph/o	lymph
calc/o	lime, calcium	macr/o	large
coagul/o	clots, to clot	phag/o	eat, engulf
cyt/o	cell	plasm/o	plasma
erythr/o	red	reticul/o	net
fibr/o	fiber, fibrous tissue	septic/o	putrefying
fibrin/o	fiber	sider/o	iron
fus/o	to pour	splen/o	spleen
globul/o	globe	thromb/o	clot
glyc/o	sweet, sugar	thym/o	thymus
granul/o	little grain, granular	tonsill/o	tonsil
hem/o	blood	vas/o	vessel
hemat/o	blood	vascul/o	small vessel
immun/o	immunity		

Word Roots

agglutinat	clumping	plast	developing
creatin	creatine	poiet	formation
log	study	thalass	sea
nucle	kernel, nucleus		

Medical Word	Word Parts		Definition
	Part	Meaning	
acquired immunodeficiency syndrome (AIDS) (ă-kwīrd ĭm″ ū-nō dĕ-fĭsh´ ĕn-sē)			AIDS is a disease caused by the human immunodeficiency virus (HIV), which is transmitted through sexual contact, exposure to infected blood or blood components, and perinatally from mother to newborn. The HIV virus invades the T cells of the helper-type lymphocytes and, as the disease progresses, the body's immune system becomes unable to function properly. See Figure 9.8. The patient becomes severely weakened and potentially fatal infections can occur. *Pneumocystis jiroveci* pneumonia (PJP) and Kaposi sarcoma (KS) account for many of the deaths of patients with AIDS.

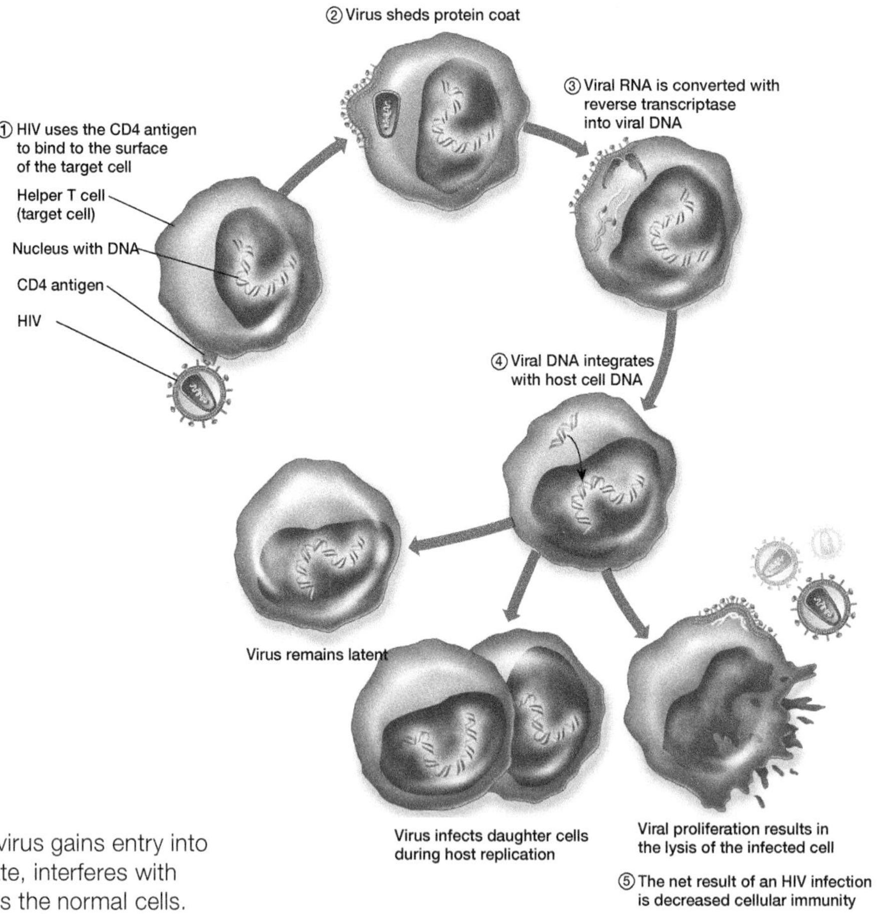

FIGURE 9.8 Human immunodeficiency virus gains entry into helper T cells, uses the cell DNA to replicate, interferes with normal function of the T cells, and destroys the normal cells.

Medical Word	Word Parts		Definition
	Part	Meaning	

Medical Word	Part	Meaning	Definition
agglutination (ă-gloo″ tĭ-nā′ shŭn)	**agglutinat** **-ion**	clumping process	Process of clumping together, as of blood cells that are incompatible
albumin (ăl-bū′ mĭn)			One of a group of simple proteins found in blood plasma and serum
allergy (ăl′ ĕr-jē)	**all** **-ergy**	other work	An individual hypersensitivity to a substance that is usually harmless. **Allergic rhinitis** is commonly known as *hay fever*. It is typically caused by the pollens of certain seasonal plants and occurs in people who are allergic to these substances. Symptoms include coughing, headache, sneezing, and itchy nose, mouth, and eyes. See Figure 9.9. This same reaction occurs with allergy to mold, animal dander, dust, and similar inhaled allergens.

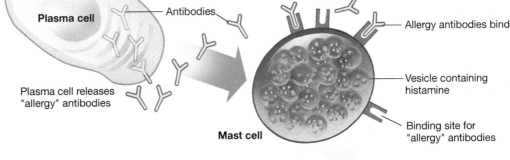

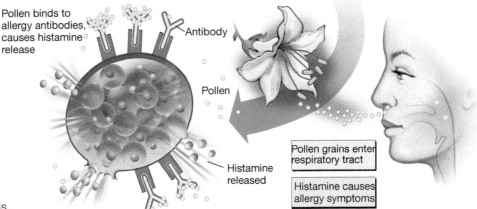

FIGURE 9.9 Allergic rhinitis.

Medical Word	Word Parts		Definition
	Part	Meaning	
anaphylaxis (ăn″ă-fĭ-lăk′sĭs)	ana- -phylaxis	up protection	Unusual or exaggerated allergic reaction to foreign proteins or other substances. It can occur suddenly, be life-threatening, and affect the whole body. During an anaphylactic allergic reaction, tissues in different parts of the body release histamine and other substances. This causes constriction of the airways, resulting in wheezing, difficulty breathing, and gastrointestinal symptoms such as abdominal pain, cramps, vomiting, and diarrhea. See Figure 9.10.

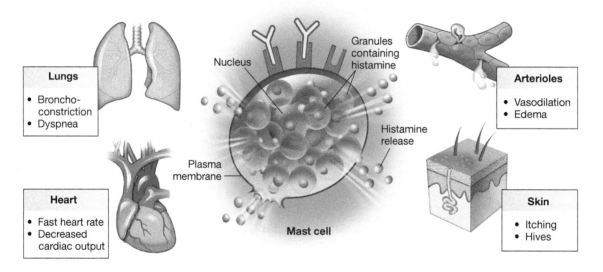

Lungs
- Broncho-constriction
- Dyspnea

Heart
- Fast heart rate
- Decreased cardiac output

Nucleus

Granules containing histamine

Histamine release

Plasma membrane

Mast cell

Arterioles
- Vasodilation
- Edema

Skin
- Itching
- Hives

FIGURE 9.10 Symptoms of anaphylaxis.

fyi
Anaphylaxis is an emergency condition that requires immediate professional medical attention. Shock can occur as a result of lowered blood pressure and blood volume. Hives and angioedema (hives on the lips, eyelids, throat, and/or tongue) often occur, and angioedema could be severe enough to cause obstruction of the airway. Prolonged anaphylaxis can cause heart arrhythmias.

Medical Word	Word Parts		Definition
anemia (ă-nē′mē-ă)	an- -emia	lack of blood condition	Condition in which there is a reduction in the number of circulating red blood cells, the amount of the hemoglobin, or the volume of packed red cells (hematocrit). A normal red blood cell is biconcave with no nucleus and transports oxygen and carbon dioxide. Refer to Figure 9.1. Symptoms of anemia are due to tissue **hypoxia**, or lack of oxygen. General symptoms include pallor, fatigue, dizziness, headaches, decreased exercise tolerance, tachycardia, and shortness of breath (SOB). There are many types of anemia, including hemolytic, pernicious, sickle cell disease (see Figure 9.11), and thalassemia.

Hemoglobin S and Red Blood Cell Sickling

Sickle cell anemia is caused by an inherited autosomal recessive defect in Hb synthesis. Sickle cell hemoglobin (HbS) differs from normal hemoglobin only in the substitution of the amino acid valine for glutamine in both beta chains of the hemoglobin molecule.

When HbS is oxygenated, it has the same globular shape as normal hemoglobin. However, when HbS loses its oxygen, it becomes insoluble in intra-cellular fluid and crystallizes into rodlike structures. Clusters of rods form polymers (long chains)

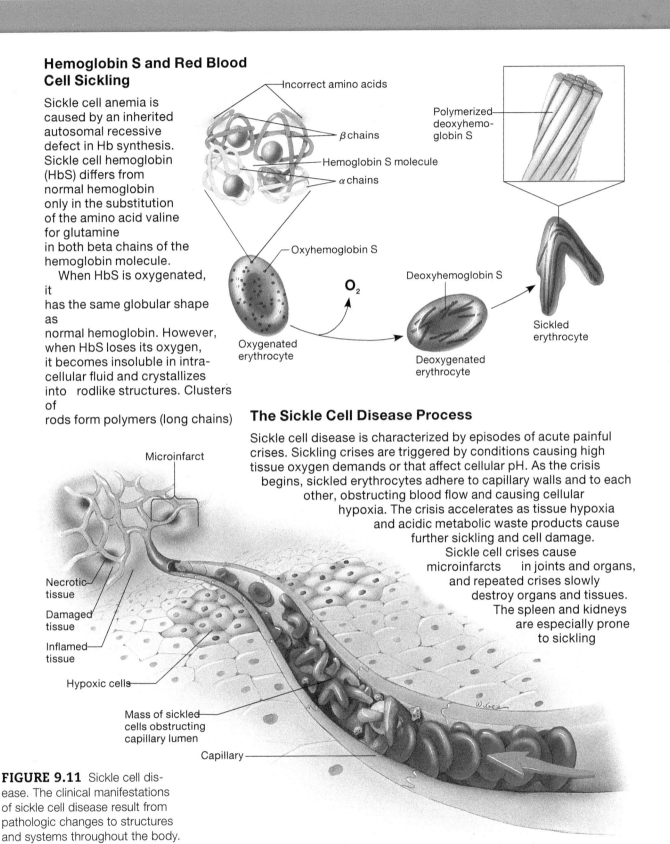

Incorrect amino acids

β chains

Hemoglobin S molecule

α chains

Polymerized deoxyhemo-globin S

Oxyhemoglobin S

Oxygenated erythrocyte

O₂

Deoxyhemoglobin S

Deoxygenated erythrocyte

Sickled erythrocyte

The Sickle Cell Disease Process

Sickle cell disease is characterized by episodes of acute painful crises. Sickling crises are triggered by conditions causing high tissue oxygen demands or that affect cellular pH. As the crisis begins, sickled erythrocytes adhere to capillary walls and to each other, obstructing blood flow and causing cellular hypoxia. The crisis accelerates as tissue hypoxia and acidic metabolic waste products cause further sickling and cell damage. Sickle cell crises cause microinfarcts in joints and organs, and repeated crises slowly destroy organs and tissues. The spleen and kidneys are especially prone to sickling

Microinfarct

Necrotic tissue

Damaged tissue

Inflamed tissue

Hypoxic cells

Mass of sickled cells obstructing capillary lumen

Capillary

FIGURE 9.11 Sickle cell disease. The clinical manifestations of sickle cell disease result from pathologic changes to structures and systems throughout the body.

Medical Word	Word Parts		Definition
	Part	**Meaning**	
anisocytosis (ăn-ī″ sō-sī-tō´ sĭs)	**anis/o** **cyt** **-osis**	unequal cell condition	Condition in which the erythrocytes are unequal in size and shape
antibody (ăn´ tĭ-bŏd″ ē)	**anti-** **-body**	against body	Protein substance produced in the body in response to an invading foreign substance (antigen)
anticoagulant (ăn″ tĭ-kō-ăg´ ū-lănt)	**anti-** **coagul** **-ant**	against clots forming	Substance that works against the formation of blood clots; a class of medication used in certain patients to prevent blood from clotting; a chemical compound used in medical equipment, such as test tubes, blood transfusion bags, and renal dialysis equipment. See "Drug Highlights" for more information.
antigen (ăn´ tĭ-jĕn)	**anti-** **-gen**	against formation, produce	Invading foreign substance that induces the formation of antibodies
autoimmune disease (aw″ tō-ĭm-mūn´)			Condition in which the body's immune system becomes defective and produces antibodies against itself. Hemolytic anemia, rheumatoid arthritis, myasthenia gravis, and scleroderma are considered to be autoimmune diseases.

 fyi The incidence of autoimmune diseases increases with age, most likely due to a decreased ability of antibodies to differentiate between self and nonself. Failure of the immune response system to recognize mutant, or abnormal, cells could be the reason for the high incidence of cancer associated with increasing age.

Medical Word	Word Parts		Definition
autotransfusion (aw″ tō-trăns-fū´ zhŭn)	**auto-** **trans-** **fus** **-ion**	self across to pour process	Process of infusing a patient's own blood. Methods used include *harvesting* the blood 1–3 weeks before elective surgery; *salvaging* intraoperative blood; and *collecting* blood from trauma or selected surgical patients for infusion within 4 hours.
coagulable (kō-ăg´ ū-lă-bl)	**coagul** **-able**	to clot capable	Capable of forming a clot
corpuscle (kŏr´ pŭs-ĕl)			Blood cell
creatinemia (krē″ ă-tĭn-ē´ mē-ă)	**creatin** **-emia**	creatine blood condition	Excess of creatine (nitrogenous compound produced by metabolic processes) in the blood
embolus (ĕm´ bō-lŭs)			Particle or mass (most likely a blood clot) that travels through the bloodstream. It can lodge in a blood vessel, producing blockage and causing organ damage. *Emboli* (plural form) can be solid, liquid, or gaseous.

Medical Word	Word Parts		Definition
	Part	Meaning	
erythroblast (ĕ-rĭth′ rō-blăst)	erythr/o -blast	red immature cell, germ cell	Immature red blood cell that is found only in bone marrow and still contains a nucleus

> **! ALERT!**
>
> **Check-It-Out!** How many words can you build using the combining form **erythr/o**?

erythrocyte (ĕ-rĭth′ rō-sīt)	erythr/o -cyte	red cell	Mature red blood cell, which does not contain a nucleus
erythrocytosis (ĕ-rĭth″ rō-sī-tō′ sĭs)	erythr/o cyt -osis	red cell condition	Abnormal condition in which there is an increase in production of red blood cells
erythropoiesis (ĕ-rĭth″ rō-poy-ē′ sĭs)	erythr/o -poiesis	red formation	Formation of red blood cells
erythropoietin (ĕ-rĭth″ rō-poy′ ĕ-tĭn)	erythr/o poiet -in	red formation substance	Hormone that stimulates the production of red blood cells
extravasation (ĕks-trăv″ ă-sā′ shŭn)	extra- vas -at(e) -ion	beyond vessel action process	Process by which fluids and/or intravenous (IV) medications can escape from the blood vessel into surrounding tissue
fibrin (fī′ brĭn)	fibr -in	fiber substance	Insoluble protein formed from fibrinogen by the action of thrombin in the blood-clotting process
fibrinogen (fī-brĭn′ ō-jĕn)	fibrin/o -gen	fiber formation, produce	Blood protein converted to fibrin by the action of thrombin in the blood-clotting process
globulin (glŏb′ ū-lĭn)	globul -in	globe substance	Plasma protein found in body fluids and cells
granulocyte (grăn′ ū-lō-sīt″)	granul/o -cyte	little grain, granular cell	Granular leukocyte (white blood cell containing granules); a polymorphonuclear white blood cell (includes neutrophils, eosinophils, or basophils)
hematologist (hē″ mă-tŏl′ ō-jĭst)	hemat/o log -ist	blood study one who specializes	Literally means *one who specializes in the study of the blood*; physician who specializes in the diagnosis and treatment of blood diseases

Medical Word	Word Parts		Definition
	Part	**Meaning**	
hematology (hē″ mă-tŏl′ ō-jē)	**hemat/o** **-logy**	blood study of	Literally means *study of the blood*
hematoma (hē″ mă-tō′ mă)	**hemat** **-oma**	blood tumor, mass, fluid collection	Collection of blood that has escaped from a blood vessel into the surrounding tissues; results from trauma or incomplete hemostasis after surgery. See Figure 9.12.

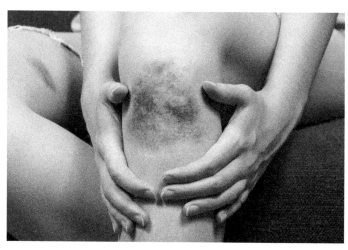

FIGURE 9.12 Hematoma.
Source: Aleksey Boyko/Shutterstock

hemochromatosis (hē″ mō-krō″ mă-tō′ sĭs)	**hem/o** **chromat** **-osis**	blood color condition	Genetic condition in which iron is not metabolized properly and accumulates in body tissues. The skin has a bronze hue, the liver becomes enlarged, and diabetes and cardiac failure can occur.

! ALERT!

Check-It-Out! How many words can you build using the combining form **hem/o**?

hemoglobin (Hb, Hgb, HGB) (hē′ mō-glō″ bĭn)	**hem/o** **-globin**	blood protein	A protein inside red blood cells that carries oxygen from the lungs to tissues and organs in the body and carries carbon dioxide back to the lungs
hemolysis (hē-mŏl′ ĭ-sĭs)	**hem/o** **-lysis**	blood destruction	Destruction of red blood cells
hemophilia (hē″ mō-fĭl′ ē-ă)	**hem/o** **-phil** **-ia**	blood attraction condition	Hereditary blood condition characterized by prolonged coagulation and tendency to bleed
hemorrhage (hĕm′ ĕ-rĭj)	**hem/o** **-rrhage**	blood bursting forth	Literally means *bursting forth of blood*; bleeding

Medical Word	Word Parts		Definition
	Part	**Meaning**	
hemostasis (hē″ mō-stā′ sĭs)	**hem/o** **-stasis**	blood control, stop	Control or stopping of bleeding. See Figure 9.13.

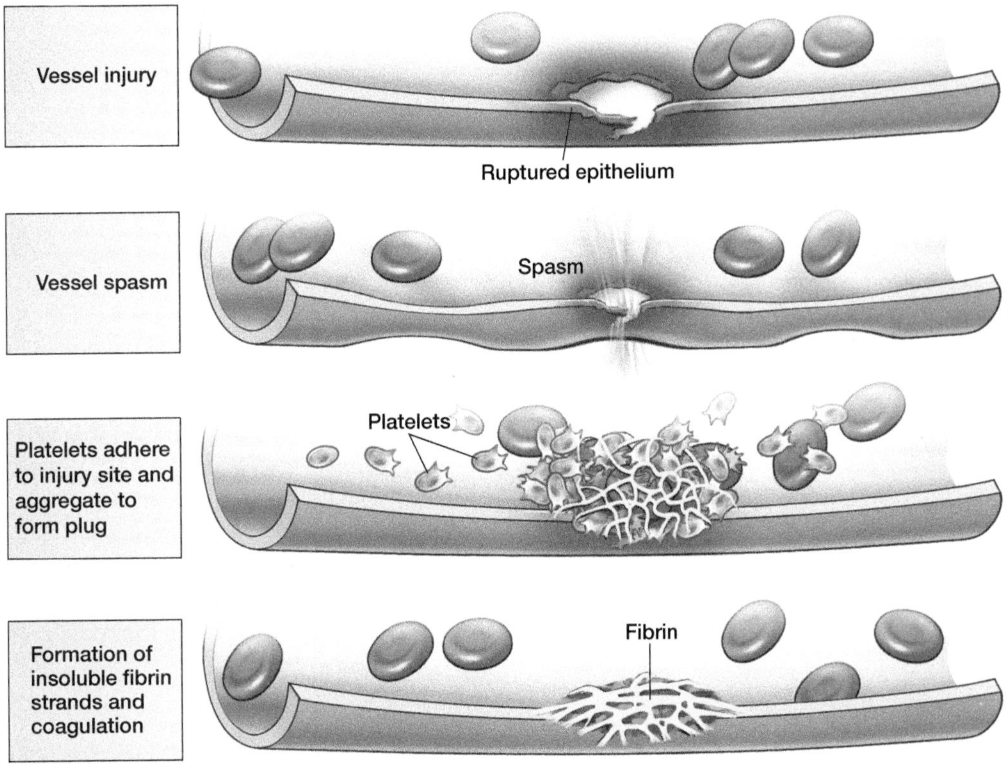

FIGURE 9.13 Basic steps in hemostasis.

heparin (hĕp′ ă-rĭn)			Natural substance found in the liver, lungs, and other body tissues that inhibits blood clotting (anticoagulant). As a drug, heparin is used during certain types of surgery and in the treatment of deep vein thrombosis or pulmonary infarction. It can be administered by either subcutaneous or intravenous injection.
hypercalcemia (hī″ pĕr-kăl-sē′ mē-ă)	**hyper-** **calc** **-emia**	excessive calcium blood condition	Pathological condition of excessive amounts of calcium in the blood
hyperglycemia (hī″ pĕr-glī-sē′ mē-ă)	**hyper-** **glyc** **-emia**	excessive sweet, sugar blood condition	Pathological condition of excessive amounts of sugar in the blood

Medical Word	Word Parts		Definition
	Part	Meaning	
hyperlipidemia (hī″ pĕr-lĭp-ĭd-ē′ mē-ă)	**hyper-** **lipid** **-emia**	excessive fat blood condition	Pathological condition of excessive amounts of lipids (fat) in the blood
hypoglycemia (hī″ pō-glī-sē′ mē-ă)	**hypo-** **glyc** **-emia**	deficient sweet, sugar blood condition	Condition of deficient amounts of sugar in the blood; low blood sugar

> **! ALERT!**
>
> It is important to know the difference between **hyper-** (*excessive*) and **hypo-**, **hyp-** (*deficient*). They are the opposite of one another.

Medical Word	Word Parts		Definition
hypoxia (hī″ pŏks′ ē-ă)	**hyp-** **-oxia**	deficient oxygen	Deficient amount of oxygen in the blood, cells, and tissues
immunoglobulin (Ig) (ĭm″ ū-nō-glŏb′ ū-lĭn)	**immun/o** **globul** **-in**	immunity globe substance	Blood protein capable of acting as an antibody. The five major types are IgA, IgD, IgE, IgG, and IgM.
Kaposi sarcoma (KS) (kăp′ ō-sē săr-kō′ mă)			Malignant neoplasm that causes violaceous (violet-colored) vascular lesions and general lymphadenopathy (diseased lymph nodes); it is the most common AIDS-related tumor. See Figure 9.14.

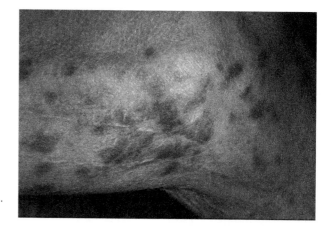

FIGURE 9.14 Kaposi sarcoma.
Source: Courtesy of Jason L. Smith, MD

Medical Word	Word Parts		Definition
leukapheresis (loo″ kă-fĕ-rē′ sĭs)	**leuk** **-apheresis**	white removal	Separation of white blood cells from the blood, which is then transfused back into the patient

Medical Word	Word Parts		Definition
	Part	Meaning	
leukemia (loo-kē′ mē-ă)	leuk -emia	white blood condition	Cancer of the white blood cells. The bone marrow produces abnormal white blood cells and these cells crowd out healthy blood cells, making it difficult for blood to do its work. Leukemia is classified by the type of white blood cell that is affected (myeloid or lymphoid) and how rapidly it progresses (chronic or acute).

 fyi Leukemia can develop slowly or quickly. Chronic lymphocytic leukemia (CLL) and chronic myeloid leukemia (CML) grow slowly. In acute lymphocytic leukemia (ALL) and acute myeloid leukemia (AML), the white blood cells increase rapidly. Adults may develop either type; children with leukemia most often have an acute type. Treatments may include chemotherapy, radiation, and stem cell transplantation.

Medical Word	Word Parts		Definition
leukocytopenia (loo″ kō-sī″ tō-pē′ nē-ă)	leuk/o cyt/o -penia	white cell lack of	Abnormal decrease of white blood cells; literally means *lack of white blood cells*
lymphadenitis (lĭm-făd″ ĕn-ī′ tĭs)	lymph aden -itis	lymph gland inflammation	Inflammation of the lymph glands
lymphedema (lĭmf-ĕ-dē′ mă)	lymph -edema	lymph swelling	Abnormal accumulation of lymph in the interstitial spaces. See Figure 9.15.

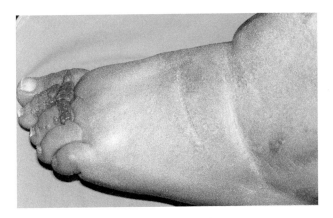

FIGURE 9.15 Chronic lymphedema.
Source: Courtesy of Jason L. Smith, MD

 fyi Vascularized lymph node transfer (VLNT) is a microsurgical procedure that involves transferring lymph nodes from the groin to the area under the arm. VLNT may be appropriate for women who have experienced complications during breast cancer surgery. Patients with leg lymphedema may require this procedure at the levels of the knee and groin. Patients with profound soft-tissue deformities may require excision (removal) of excess skin and then liposuction of the extremity in a staged fashion.

Medical Word	Word Parts		Definition
	Part	Meaning	
lymphoma (lĭm-fō´ mă)	lymph -oma	lymph tumor, mass, fluid collection	Lymphoid neoplasm, usually malignant. See Figure 9.16. Lymphomas are identified as Hodgkin disease or non-Hodgkin lymphomas. Radiation therapy is the primary treatment for early-stage Hodgkin disease.

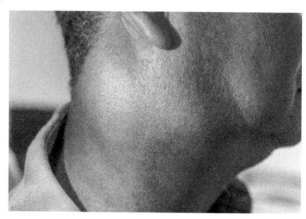

FIGURE 9.16 Lymphoid neoplasm (cancer). Lateral view of enlarged lymph nodes and submandibular gland on right side of patient's neck.
Source: Karan Bunjean/Shutterstock

Medical Word	Word Parts		Definition
lymphostasis (lĭm fŏs´ tă-sĭs)	lymph/o -stasis	lymph control, stop	Control or stopping of the flow of lymph
macrocytosis (măk˝ rō-sī-tō´ sĭs)	macr/o cyt -osis	large cell condition	Condition in which erythrocytes are larger than normal
mononucleosis (mŏn˝ ō-nū˝ klē-ō´ sĭs)	mono- nucle -osis	one kernel, nucleus condition	Infectious disease, often called *mono* or *kissing disease*, that occurs most often in teens and young adults; caused by the Epstein-Barr virus and spread through saliva. See Figure 9.17.

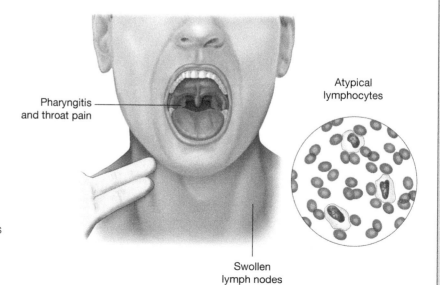

Pharyngitis and throat pain

Atypical lymphocytes

Swollen lymph nodes

FIGURE 9.17 Mononucleosis is caused by the Epstein-Barr virus. Symptoms of the infectious disease are swollen palatine tonsils (pharyngitis), swollen cervical lymph nodes (lymphadenopathy), high fever, and a blood sample that shows atypical lymphocytes.

Medical Word	Word Parts		Definition
	Part	Meaning	
opportunistic infection (ŏp″ ŏr-too-nĭs′ tĭk)			An infection that occurs more frequently or is more severe in people with weakened immune systems, such as people with HIV or people receiving chemotherapy, than in people with healthy immune systems. People with AIDS are very vulnerable to these types of infections.
pancytopenia (păn″ sī-tō-pē′ nē-ă)	pan-	all	Literally means *lack of the cellular elements of the blood*
	cyt/o	cell	
	-penia	lack of	
phagocytosis (făg″ ō-sī-tō′ sĭs)	phag/o	eat, engulf	Engulfing and eating of particulate substances such as bacteria, protozoa, cells and cell debris, dust particles, and colloids by phagocytes (leukocytes or macrophages).
	cyt	cell	
	-osis	condition	
plasmapheresis (plăz″ mă-fĕr-ē′ sĭs)	plasm	plasma	Removal of blood from the body and centrifuging it to separate the plasma from the blood and infusing the cellular elements back into the patient
	-apheresis	removal	
Pneumocystis jiroveci pneumonia (PJP)			Pneumonia resulting from infection with *Pneumocystis jiroveci*; frequently seen in the immunologically compromised, such as persons with AIDS, steroid-treated individuals, older adults, or premature or debilitated babies during their first 3 months. Patients may be only slightly febrile (or even afebrile), but are likely to be extremely weak, dyspneic, and cyanotic.
polycythemia (pŏl″ ē-sī-thē′ mē-ă)	poly-	many	Increased number of red blood cells
	cyt	cell	
	hem	blood	
	-ia	condition	
prothrombin (prō-thrŏm′ bĭn)	pro-	before	Chemical substance that interacts with calcium salts to produce thrombin
	thromb	clot	
	-in	substance	
reticulocyte (rĕ-tĭk′ ū-lō-sīt)	reticul/o	net	Red blood cell containing a network of granules; the last immature stage of a red blood cell
	-cyte	cell	

Medical Word	Word Parts		Definition
	Part	Meaning	
retrovirus (rĕt″ rō-vī′ rŭs)			Virus that contains a unique enzyme called *reverse transcriptase* that allows it to replicate within new host cells. HIV is a retrovirus; once it enters the cell, it can replicate and kill the cells, some lymphocytes directly, and disrupt the functioning of the remaining CD4 cells.

 fyi Although the HIV virus can remain inactive in infected cells for years, antibodies are produced to its proteins, a process known as **seroconversion**. These antibodies are usually detectable 6 weeks to 6 months after the initial infection. Helper T or CD4 cells are the primary cells infected by HIV; these cells are involved in cellular immunity and the body's immune response in fighting off infection and disease. The loss of these CD4 cells leads to immunodeficiencies and developing opportunistic infections. A normal CD4 lymphocyte count is 500–1,600 cells/mm3. It is not uncommon for an HIV-infected person's count to be 180 cells/mm3.

Medical Word	Word Parts		Definition
septicemia (sĕp″ tĭ-sē′ mē-ă)	septic -emia	putrefying blood condition	Pathological condition in which bacteria are present in the blood; also known as *sepsis*
serum (sēr′ ŭm)			Blood serum is the clear, thin, and sticky fluid part of the blood that remains after blood clots; any clear watery fluid that has been separated from its more solid elements, such as the exudates from a blister
sideropenia (sĭd″ ĕr-ō-pē′ nē-ă)	sider/o -penia	iron lack of	Lack of iron in the blood
splenomegaly (splē″ nō-mĕg′ ă-lē)	splen/o -megaly	spleen enlargement	Abnormal enlargement of the spleen
stem cell			A bone marrow cell that gives rise to different types of blood cells

 fyi Myelodysplastic syndromes are a group of diseases of the blood and bone marrow in which the bone marrow does not make enough healthy blood cells, thus the blood stem cells do not mature into healthy red blood cells, white blood cells, or platelets. The immature blood cells, called *blasts*, do not function normally and either die in the bone marrow or soon after they enter the blood. This leaves less room for healthy white blood cells, red blood cells, and platelets to form in the bone marrow. When there are fewer blood cells, infection, anemia, or easy bleeding may occur. Myelodysplastic syndromes often do not cause early symptoms and are sometimes found during a routine blood test. Other conditions may cause similar symptoms, such as:

- Shortness of breath
- Weakness or feeling tired
- Having skin that is paler than usual
- Easy bruising or bleeding
- Petechiae (flat, pinpoint spots under the skin caused by bleeding)
- Fever or frequent infections

Medical Word	Word Parts		Definition
	Part	Meaning	
thalassemia (thăl-ă-sē′ mē-ă)	thalass -emia	sea blood condition	Hereditary anemia occurring in populations bordering the Mediterranean Sea and in Southeast Asia. It is a blood disorder in which the body makes an abnormal form of hemoglobin. The disorder results in large numbers of red blood cells being destroyed, which leads to anemia.
thrombectomy (thrŏm-bĕk′ tō-mē)	thromb -ectomy	clot surgical excision	Surgical excision of a blood clot
thrombin (thrŏm′ bĭn)	thromb -in	clot substance	Blood enzyme that converts fibrinogen into fibrin
thromboplastin (thrŏm″ bō-plăs′ tĭn)	thromb/o plast -in	clot developing substance	Essential factor in the production of thrombin and blood clotting
thrombosis (thrŏm-bō′ sĭs)	thromb -osis	clot condition	Formation, development, or existence of a blood clot (thrombus) within the vascular system. In venous thrombosis (thrombophlebitis), a thrombus forms on the wall of a vein, accompanied by inflammation and obstructed blood flow. Thrombi can form in either superficial or deep veins. Deep vein thrombosis (DVT) is generally a complication after hospitalization, surgery, or immobilization. See Figure 9.18.

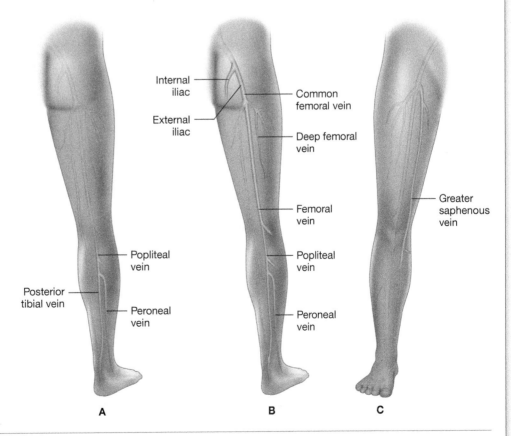

FIGURE 9.18 Common locations of venous thrombosis. **A** The most common sites of deep vein thrombosis. **B** DVT extending from the calf to the iliac veins. **C** Superficial venous thrombosis.

Internal iliac
External iliac
Common femoral vein
Deep femoral vein
Femoral vein
Popliteal vein
Peroneal vein
Greater saphenous vein
Popliteal vein
Posterior tibial vein
Peroneal vein

A

B

C

Medical Word	Word Parts		Definition
	Part	Meaning	
thymoma (thī-mō´ mă)	thym -oma	thymus tumor, mass	Tumor of the thymus
tonsillectomy (tŏn˝ sĭl-ek´ tō-mē)	tonsill -ectomy	tonsil surgical excision	Surgical excision of the tonsils

> **! ALERT!**
>
> The root *tonsill* has two *l*'s for tonsil. This is to form the correct spelling of the word *tonsillectomy* or other such words that relate to the tonsil.

Medical Word	Word Parts		Definition
transfusion (trăns-fū´ zhŭn)	trans- fus -ion	across to pour process	Process by which blood is transferred from one individual to the vein of a recipient
vasculitis (văs˝ kū-lī´ tĭs)	vascul -itis	small vessel inflammation	Inflammation of the blood vessels that can affect arteries, veins, and capillaries; also known as *angiitis*. See Figure 9.19.

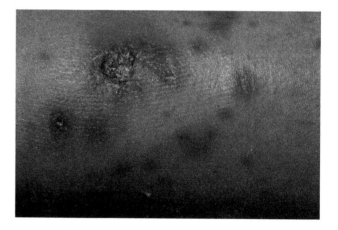

FIGURE 9.19 Vasculitis.
Source: Courtesy of Jason L. Smith, MD

GOOD TO KNOW ▶

The cause of vasculitis is often unknown, but it occurs when the body's immune system attacks the blood vessel cells by mistake. This causes changes in the blood vessel walls, including thickening, weakening, narrowing, or scarring. These changes can restrict blood flow, resulting in tissue and organ (such as skin) damage. Possible triggers for this immune system reaction include infections (such as hepatitis B and hepatitis C), blood cancers, and immune system diseases (such as rheumatoid arthritis, lupus, and scleroderma). Symptoms can vary, but usually include fever, swelling, headache, general aches and pains, and fatigue.

Study *and* Review III

Word Parts

Prefixes Give the definitions of the following prefixes.

1. an- _____
2. anti- _____
3. auto- _____
4. ana- _____
5. extra- _____
6. hyper- _____
7. hypo- _____

8. mono- _____
9. pan- _____
10. poly- _____
11. pro- _____
12. trans- _____
13. hyp- _____

Combining Forms Give the definitions of the following combining forms.

1. aden/o _____
2. anis/o _____
3. coagul/o _____
4. cyt/o _____
5. erythr/o _____
6. glyc/o _____
7. hemat/o _____
8. hem/o _____
9. immun/o _____

10. leuk/o _____
11. lymph/o _____
12. macr/o _____
13. plasm/o _____
14. septic/o _____
15. sider/o _____
16. splen/o _____
17. thym/o _____
18. vascul/o _____

Suffixes Give the definitions of the following suffixes.

1. -able _____
2. -ant _____
3. -apheresis _____

4. -blast _____
5. -body _____
6. -edema _____

7. -cyte _____

8. -ectomy _____

9. -emia _____

10. -ergy _____

11. -gen _____

12. -phylaxis _____

13. -globin _____

14. -in _____

15. -ion _____

16. -ist _____

17. -itis _____

18. -logy _____

19. -lysis _____

20. -megaly _____

21. -oma _____

22. -osis _____

23. -penia _____

24. -phil _____

25. -poiesis _____

26. -rrhage _____

27. -stasis _____

28. -ia _____

29. -oxia _____

Identifying Medical Terms

In the spaces provided, write the medical terms for the following meanings.

1. _____ Process of clumping together, as of blood cells that are incompatible

2. _____ An individual hypersensitivity to a substance that is usually harmless

3. _____ Protein substance produced in the body in response to an invading foreign substance

4. _____ Substance that works against the formation of blood clots

5. _____ Invading foreign substance that induces the formation of antibodies

6. _____ Process of infusing a patient's own blood

7. _____ Capable of forming a clot

8. _____ Excess of creatine in the blood

9. _____ Blood clot carried in the bloodstream

10. _____ Granular leukocyte

Matching

Select the appropriate lettered meaning for each of the following words.

_____ 1. autotransfusion

_____ 2. erythrocyte

_____ 3. erythropoietin

_____ 4. extravasation

_____ 5. hemorrhage

_____ 6. immunoglobulin

_____ 7. hemochromatosis

_____ 8. septicemia

_____ 9. stem cell

_____ 10. thrombectomy

a. Pathological condition in which bacteria are present in the blood

b. Genetic condition in which iron is not metabolized properly and accumulates in body tissues

c. Blood protein capable of acting as an antibody

d. Mature red blood cell that does not contain a nucleus

e. Hormone that stimulates the production of red blood cells

f. Literally means bursting-forth of blood; bleeding

g. Process by which fluids and/or medications escape from the blood vessel into surrounding tissue

h. Process of infusing a patient's own blood

i. Surgical excision of a blood clot

j. Bone marrow cell that gives rise to different types of blood cells

Medical Case Snapshots

This learning activity provides an opportunity to relate the medical terminology you are learning to sample patient case presentations. In the spaces provided, write in your answers.

Case 1

A 52-year-old female states, "It was months after the death of my husband when I began dating a younger man. We became sexually involved. I am so afraid. Bill has just told me that he is HIV positive and could have AIDS." AIDS is a disease caused by the _____ _____ virus, which invades the _____ lymphocytes.

Case 2

A 15-year-old female complains of being tired, experiencing dizziness, headaches, fast heartbeat, and shortness of breath (_____). A possible diagnosis is anemia. The symptoms of anemia are due to a deficient amount of oxygen in the blood known as _____. Bloodwork is ordered and the patient is to return in 2 weeks.

Case 3

Two weeks after the initial exam, the 15-year-old female was seen by Dr. Mann. The diagnosis of anemia was confirmed. With anemia, special attention is given to the amount of _____ (or iron-containing pigment of red blood cells) and the percentage of solid components compared to the liquid components of blood called _____. The patient was prescribed an antianemic agent that is used to treat iron-deficiency anemia.

Drug Highlights

Classification of Drug	Description and Examples
anticoagulants	Used in inhibiting or preventing a blood clot formation. Hemorrhage can occur at almost any site in patients on anticoagulant therapy. EXAMPLES: heparin sodium, Coumadin (warfarin sodium), and Lovenox (enoxaparin)
hemostatic agents	Used to control bleeding; can be administered systemically or topically. EXAMPLES: Amicar (aminocaproic acid) and vitamin K
antianemic agents (*irons*)	Used to treat iron-deficiency anemia. Oral iron preparations interfere with the absorption of oral tetracycline antibiotics. These products should not be taken within 2 hours of each other. EXAMPLES: Oral iron supplements (ferrous sulfate); prescription IV medications INFeD (iron dextran) and Venofer (iron sucrose)
antiviral agents	Main form of treatment of AIDS, antiviral therapy suppresses the replication of the HIV virus. This treatment involves a combination of several antiretroviral agents, called *highly active antiretroviral therapy (HAART),* and has been very effective in reducing the number of HIV particles in the bloodstream (as measured by a blood test called the *viral load*). This can help the immune system recover and improve the T-cell count. The FDA has approved an antiretroviral agent, Truvada (emtricitabine and tenofovir disoproxil fumarate), for *pre-exposure prophylaxis (PrEP).* The purpose of this drug is to protect uninfected people from HIV
epoetin alfa (*EPO, Procrit*)	Genetically engineered hemopoietin that stimulates the production of red blood cells. It is a recombinant version of erythropoietin and is indicated for treating anemia in patients with chronic renal failure and HIV-infected patients taking zidovudine.
other agents	Agents used in treating folic-acid deficiency include folic acid capsules, tablets, pills, tonic, powder, or drops. Agents used in treating vitamin B_{12} deficiency include vitamin B_{12} (cyanocobalamin) injection.

Diagnostic *and* Laboratory Tests

Test	Description
antinuclear antibodies (ANA) (ăn″ tĭ-nū′ klē-ăr ăn′ tĭ-bŏd″ ēs)	Blood test to identify antigen–antibody reactions. ANA antibodies are present in a number of autoimmune diseases (e.g., lupus).
blood typing (ABO groups and Rh factor)	Blood test to determine an individual's blood type (A, B, AB, and O) and Rh factor (can be negative [Rh−] or positive [Rh+]). See Figure 9.20.

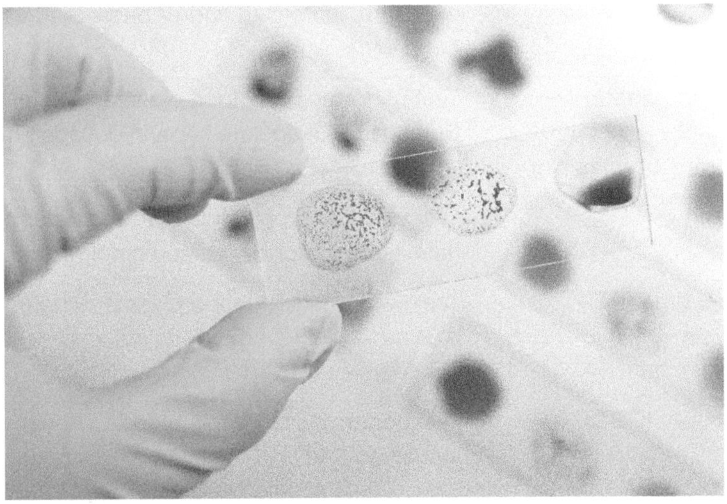

FIGURE 9.20 Blood group testing.
Source: Jarun Ontakrai/123RF

Test	Description
bone marrow aspiration (ăs-pĭ-rā′ shŭn)	Removal of bone marrow for examination; can be performed to determine aplastic anemia, leukemia, certain cancers, and polycythemia.
CD4 cell count	Most widely used serum blood test to monitor the progress of AIDS. CD4 count of less than 200/mm3 confirms AIDS diagnosis. CD4 is a protein on the surface of cells that normally helps the body's immune system fight disease. The HIV attaches itself to the protein to attack white blood cells (WBCs), causing a failure of the patient's defense system.
complete blood count (CBC)	Blood test that includes a hematocrit, hemoglobin, red and white blood cell count, and differential; usually part of a complete physical examination.
enzyme-linked immunosorbent assay (ELISA) (ĕn′ zīm-linkt ĭm″ ū-nō-sŏr′-bĕnt ă-sā)	Test performed on blood or urine and used for measuring the amount of a particular protein or substance such as infectious agents, allergens, hormones, or drugs in these bodily fluids. The test relies on the interaction between antigens and antibodies of the immune system. The latest generation of ELISA tests is 99.5% sensitive to HIV and is the most widely used screening test for HIV. Occasionally, the ELISA test will be positive for a patient without symptoms of AIDS from a low-risk group. Because this result is likely to be a false positive, the ELISA must be repeated *on the same sample of the patient's blood* by an HIV differentiation assay to confirm HIV infection.
erythrocyte sedimentation rate (ESR, sed rate) (ĕ-rĭth′ rō-sīt sĕd″ ĭ-mĕn-tā′ shŭn)	Blood test to determine the rate at which red blood cells settle in a long, narrow tube. The distance the RBCs settle in 1 hour is the rate. Higher or lower rate can indicate certain disease conditions.

Test	Description
hematocrit (Hct, HCT) (hē-măt′ ō-krĭt)	Blood test performed on whole blood to determine the percentage of red blood cells in the total blood volume. The percentage varies with age and gender: men range from 40–54%; women, 37–47%; children, 35–49%; newborns, 49–54%.
hemoglobin (Hb, Hgb, HGB) (hē′ mō-glō″ bĭn)	Blood test to measure the level of protein in red blood cells. A low count may indicate anemia; a high count may indicate polycythemia.
immunoglobulins (Ig) (ĭm″ ū-nō-glŏb′ ū-lĭns)	Serum blood test to determine the presence of IgA, IgD, IgE, IgG, and/or IgM. Lymphocytes and plasma cells produce immunoglobulins in response to antigen exposure. Increased and/or decreased values can indicate certain disease conditions.
partial thromboplastin time (PTT) (păr′ shăl thrŏm″ bō-plăs′ tĭn)	Test performed on blood plasma to determine how long it takes for fibrin clots to form; used to regulate heparin dosage and to detect clotting disorders.
platelet count (plāt′ lĕt)	Test performed on whole blood to determine the number of thrombocytes present. Increased and/or decreased amounts can indicate certain disease conditions.
prothrombin time (PT) (prō-thrŏm′ bĭn)	Test performed on blood plasma to determine the time needed for oxalated plasma to clot; used to regulate anticoagulant drug therapy and to detect clotting disorders.
red blood count (RBC)	Test performed on whole blood to determine the number of erythrocytes present. Increased and/or decreased amounts can indicate certain disease conditions.
viral load	Blood test that measures the amount of HIV in the blood. Results can range from 50 to more than 1 million copies per milliliter (mL) of blood. Two tests that are used to measure viral load are bDNA and PCR.
white blood count (WBC)	Blood test to determine the number of leukocytes present. Increased level indicates infection and/or inflammation and leukemia. Decreased level indicates aplastic anemia, pernicious anemia, and malaria.

Abbreviations *and* Acronyms

Abbreviation/ Acronym	Meaning	Abbreviation/ Acronym	Meaning
ABO	blood groups	**CML**	chronic myeloid leukemia
AIDS	acquired immunodeficiency syndrome	**diff**	differential count
ALL	acute lymphocytic leukemia	**DVT**	deep vein thrombosis
AML	acute myeloid leukemia	**ELISA**	enzyme-linked immunosorbent assay
ANA	antinuclear antibodies	**eos, eosin**	eosinophil
CBC	complete blood count	**ESR, sed rate**	erythrocyte sedimentation rate
CLL	chronic lymphocytic leukemia	**HAART**	highly active antiretroviral therapy
		Hb, Hgb, HGB	hemoglobin

Abbreviation/ Acronym	Meaning	Abbreviation/ Acronym	Meaning
Hct, HCT	hematocrit	PJP	*Pneumocystis jiroveci* pneumonia
HIV	human immunodeficiency virus	PrEP	pre-exposure prophylaxis
Ig	immunoglobulin	PT	prothrombin time
IV	intravenous	PTT	partial thromboplastin time
KS	Kaposi sarcoma	RBC	red blood cell (count)
lymphs	lymphocytes	Rh	Rhesus (factor)
MALT	mucosa-associated lymphoid tissue	SOB	shortness of breath
mL, ml	milliliter	VLNT	vascularized lymph node transfer
NK	natural killer (cells)	WBC	white blood cell (count)

Study *and* Review IV

Building Medical Terms

Using the following word parts, fill in the blanks to build the correct medical terms.

mono-	hem/o	sider/o	-in	-emia
erythr/o	lymph	thromb	-cyte	-megaly

Definition

1. Formation of red blood cells

2. Plasma protein found in body fluids and cells

3. Destruction of red blood cells

4. Red blood cell containing a network of granules

5. Lymphoid neoplasm, usually malignant

6. Red blood cell

7. Condition in which bacteria are present in the blood

8. Lack of iron in the blood

9. Abnormal enlargement of the spleen

10. Formation of a blood clot within the vascular system

Medical Term

1. _____poiesis

2. globul_____

3. _____lysis

4. reticulo_____

5. _____oma

6. _____cyte

7. septic_____

8. _____penia

9. spleno_____

10. _____osis

Combining Form Challenge

Using the combining forms provided, write the medical term correctly.

hem/o   erythr/o   leuk/o
coagul/o   hemat/o   lymph/o

1. Destruction of red blood cells: _____ lysis

2. Capable of forming a clot: _____able

3. Immature red blood cell that is found only in bone marrow: _____blast

4. Literally means *study of the blood*: _____logy

5. Disease of the blood characterized by overproduction of leukocytes: _____emia

6. Abnormal accumulation of lymph in the interstitial spaces: _____edema

Select the Right Term

Select the correct answer, and write it on the line provided.

1. An individual hypersensitivity to a substance that is usually harmless is _____.

anaphylaxis   anemia   AIDS   allergy

2. Protein substance produced in the body in response to an invading foreign substance is

_____.

antigen   antibody   albumin   fibrinogen

3. Hereditary blood disease characterized by prolonged coagulation and tendency to bleed is

_____.

hemophilia   hemolysis   hemorrhage   hemochromatosis

4. Hereditary anemia occurring in populations bordering the Mediterranean Sea and in Southeast Asia is

_____.

hemolytic   pernicious   thalassemia   sickle cell

5. A particle or mass (most likely a blood clot) that travels through the bloodstream is called a(n)

_____.

thrombus   coagulable   extravasation   embolus

6. Essential factor in the production of thrombin and blood clotting is _____.

thrombin   thromboplastin   thrombocyte   prothrombin

Drug Highlights

Match the appropriate lettered description or examples of drug(s) with the class of drug.

_____ 1. antianemic agents

_____ 2. anticoagulants

_____ 3. hemostatic agents

_____ 4. epoetin alfa (*EPO, Procrit*)

_____ 5. examples of antianemic agents

_____ 6. examples of anticoagulants

_____ 7. examples of hemostatic agents

a. Used to control bleeding

b. Used to treat iron-deficiency anemia

c. Used in inhibiting or preventing a blood clot formation

d. Amicar (aminocaproic acid), vitamin K

e. Heparin sodium, Coumadin (warfarin sodium), Lovenox (enoxaparin)

f. Oral iron supplements (ferrous sulfate); prescription IV medications INFeD (iron dextran), Venofer (iron sucrose)

g. Indicated for treating anemia in patients with chronic renal failure and HIV-infected patients taking zidovudine

Diagnostic and Laboratory Tests

Select the best answer to each multiple-choice question. Circle the letter of your choice.

1. Blood test to identify antigen–antibody reactions.

    a. erythrocyte sedimentation rate

    b. hematocrit

    c. immunoglobulins

    d. antinuclear antibodies

2. Blood test that includes a hematocrit, hemoglobin, red and white blood cell count, and differential.

    a. blood typing

    b. sedimentation rate

    c. CBC

    d. Hb, Hgb

3. Blood test performed on whole blood to determine the percentage of red blood cells in the total blood volume.

    a. RBC

    b. WBC

    c. Hct

    d. PTT

4. Blood test to determine the number of leukocytes present.

    a. RBC

    b. WBC

    c. Hct

    d. PTT

5. Most widely used screening test for HIV.

    a. ELISA

    b. viral load

    c. ESR

    d. PTT

Abbreviations and Acronyms

Place the correct word, phrase, or abbreviation/acronym in the space provided.

1. acquired immunodeficiency syndrome _____

2. acute lymphocytic leukemia _____

3. CML _____

4. hemoglobin _____

5. Hct _____

6. human immunodeficiency virus _____

7. PJP _____

8. PT _____

9. RBC _____

10. DVT _____

Practical Application

Medical Record Analysis

This exercise contains information, abbreviations/acronyms, and medical terminology from an actual medical record or case study that has been adapted for this text. The names and any personal information have been created by the author. Read and study each form or case study and then answer the questions that follow. You may refer to Appendix III, *Abbreviations, Acronyms, and Symbols*.

HARBIN CLINIC HEMATOLOGY

Task	Edit	View	Time Scale	Options	Help				Date: 17 May 2021

2324 Shorter Avenue
Rome, GA 30165
(706) 555-1234

Patient: Sanchez, Carlos
    100 Main Street
    Cedar Bluff, AL 35959

Age/DOB: 49 yrs 19 Feb. 1972
Home: (256) 123-4567

Results
Lab Accession #: 0010871292009
Ordering Provider: Mann, Keith
Performing Location: Main Harbin Clinic

Collected: 4/20/21 10:38:00 AM
Resulted: 4/21/21 10:20:00 AM
Verified By: Mann, Keith
Auto Verify: N
Stage: Final

CBC with Auto Differential Count (diff)

Test	Result	Units	Flag	Reference Range
WBC	7.9	× 10³/µL		4.8–10.8
RBC	4.44	× 10³/µL	L	4.6–6.13
HGB	14.4	g/dL		14.1–18.1
HCT	41.9	%	L	43.5–53.7
MCV	94.0	fL		80.0–99.0
MCH	35.4	Pg	H	26.0–34.0
MCHC	34.3	g/dL		33.0–37.0
RDW	12.6	%		11.6–14.8
PLATELETS	248	× 10³/µL		130–400
MPV	8.8	fL		7.4–10.4
NEUT%	56.3	%		37.0–80.0

CBC with Auto Differential Count (diff) *(continued)*

Test	Result	Units	Flag	Reference Range
LYMPH%	32.4	%		10.0–50.0
MONO%	8.2	%		0.1–10.0
EOS%	1.6	%		0.1–6.0
BASO%	1.5	%		0.0–3.0
NEUT#	4.5	× 103/μL		2.9–6.2
LYMPH#	2.6	× 103/μL		0.8–3.9
MONO#	0.7	× 103/μL		0.0–1.2
EOS#	0.1	× 103/μL		0.0–0.6
BASO#	0.1	× 103/μL		0.1–0.3

Medical Record Exercise

Select the appropriate lettered function/description for each of the following abbreviations or word.

_____ 1. WBCs

_____ 2. RBCs

_____ 3. HGB

_____ 4. platelets

_____ 5. HCT

a. Determine amount of iron-containing pigment in blood

b. Play an important role in the clotting process

c. Percentage of RBCs in total blood volume

d. Transport oxygen and carbon dioxide to and from the tissues of the body

e. Body's main defense against the invasion of pathogens

MyLab Medical Terminology™

MyLab Medical Terminology is a premium online homework management system that includes a host of features to help you study. Registered users will find:

- A multitude of quizzes and activities built within the MyLab platform
- Powerful tools that track and analyze your results—allowing you to create a personalized learning experience
- Videos and audio pronunciations to help enrich your progress
- Streaming lesson presentations (guided lectures) and self-paced learning modules
- A space where you and your instructor can check your progress and manage your assignments

Respiratory System

Learning Outcomes

On completion of this chapter, you will be able to:

1. Name the organs of the respiratory system.
2. Identify the primary functions of the organs of the respiratory system.
3. Define terms that physiologists and respiratory specialists use to describe the volume of air exchanged in breathing.
4. Analyze, build, spell, and pronounce medical words.
5. Classify the drugs highlighted in this chapter.
6. Describe diagnostic and laboratory tests related to the respiratory system.
7. Identify and define selected abbreviations and acronyms.

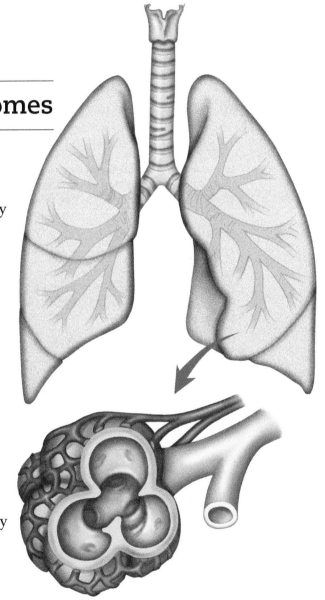

Anatomy and Physiology

The respiratory system consists of the nose, pharynx, larynx, trachea, bronchi, and lungs. Its primary function is to *supply* oxygen (O_2) for individual tissue cells to use and to *take away* their gaseous waste product, carbon dioxide (CO_2). This process is accomplished through the act of **respiration (R)**, which consists of external and internal processes. **External respiration** is the process by which the lungs are ventilated and oxygen and carbon dioxide are *exchanged* between the air in the lungs and the blood within capillaries of the alveoli. **Internal respiration** is the process by which oxygen and carbon dioxide are exchanged between the blood in tissue capillaries and the cells of the body. Table 10.1 provides an at-a-glance look at the respiratory system. See Figure 10.1.

TABLE 10.1   Respiratory System at-a-Glance

Organ/Structure	Primary Functions/Description
Nose	Serves as an air passageway; warms and moistens inhaled air; its cilia and mucous membrane trap dust, pollen, bacteria, and other foreign matter; contains special smell receptor cells (nerve cells), which assist in distinguishing various smells; contributes to phonation and the quality of voice
Pharynx	Serves as a passageway for air and for food; contributes to phonation as a chamber where the sound is able to resonate
Larynx	Produces vocal sounds. High notes are formed by short, tense vocal cords. Low notes are produced by long, relaxed vocal cords. The nose, mouth, pharynx, and bony sinuses aid in phonation and the tone that is produced to give each person a distinctive sound.
Trachea	Provides an open passageway for air to and from the lungs
Bronchi	Provide a passageway for air to and from the lungs

> **! ALERT!**
>
> Did you know that *bronchi* is the plural form of bronchus?

Lungs	Bring air into contact with blood so that oxygen and carbon dioxide can be exchanged in the *alveoli*

> **! ALERT!**
>
> Did you know that *alveoli* is the plural form of alveolus?

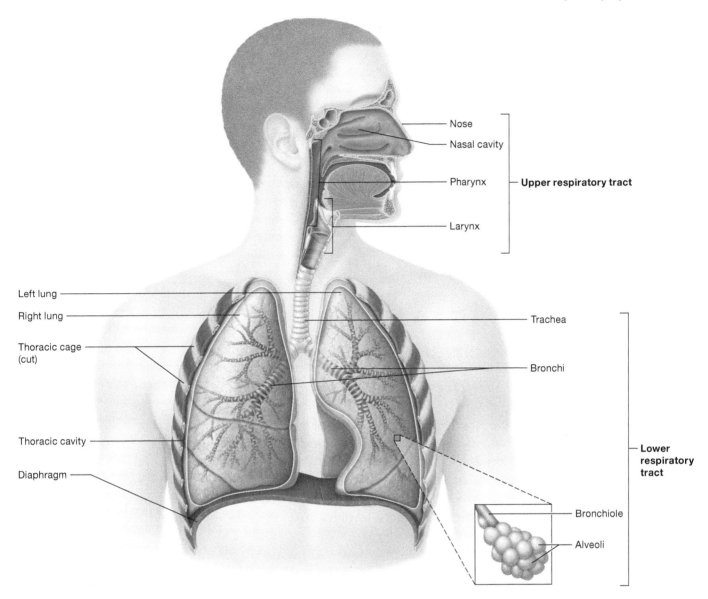

FIGURE 10.1 The respiratory system: nasal cavity, pharynx, larynx, trachea, bronchi, and lungs with expanded view of the bronchiole and alveoli.

Source: AMERMAN, ERIN C., HUMAN ANATOMY & PHYSIOLOGY, 2nd Ed., ©2019. Reprinted and Electronically reproduced by permission of Pearson Education, Inc., New York, NY.

Nose

The **nose** consists of an external and internal portion. The *external portion* is a triangle of cartilage and bone that is covered with skin and lined with mucous membrane. The external entrance of the nose is known as the **nostrils** or **anterior nares**. The *internal portion* of the nose is divided into two chambers by a partition, the **septum**, separating it into a right and a left cavity. These cavities are divided into three air passages: the *superior*, *middle*, and *inferior conchae*. These passages lead to the pharynx and are connected with the paranasal sinuses by openings, with the ears by the eustachian tube and with the region of the eyes by the nasolacrimal ducts. See Figure 10.2.

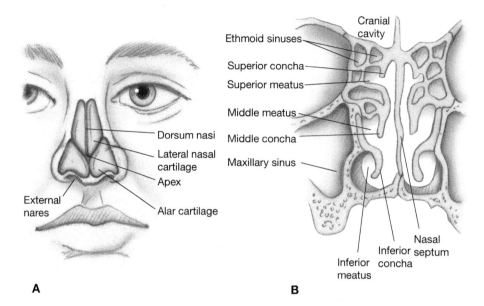

FIGURE 10.2 Nose and nasal cavity: **A** nasal cartilages and external structure; **B** meatus and positions of the entrance to the ethmoid and maxillary sinuses.
Source: MARIEB, ELAINE N.; KELLER, SUZANNE M., ESSENTIALS OF HUMAN ANATOMY & PHYSIOLOGY, 12th Ed., ©2018. Reprinted and Electronically reproduced by permission of Pearson Education, Inc., New York, NY.

The nose is lined with mucous membrane and plays an important role in the sense of smell. Smell receptor cells are located in the upper part of the nasal cavity. These cells are special nerve cells that have **cilia** (hairlike processes). The cilia of each cell are sensitive to different chemicals and, when stimulated, create a nerve impulse that is sent to the nerve cells of the olfactory bulb, which lies inside the skull just above the nose. The olfactory nerves carry the nerve impulse from the olfactory bulb directly to the brain, where it is perceived as a smell.

The nasal mucosa produces about 946 mL or 1 qt of mucus per day. Four pairs of paranasal sinuses drain into the nose. These are the *frontal, maxillary, ethmoidal,* and *sphenoidal* sinuses. See Figure 10.3. The *palatine bones* and *maxillae* separate the nasal cavities from the mouth cavity.

Cleft palate is a condition in which the two plates of the skull that form the hard palate (roof of the mouth) are not completely joined. In most cases, cleft lip, often called harelip, is also present. Cleft palate or lip occurs in about one in 700 infants born in the United States and can range from a small notch in the lip to a groove that runs into the roof of the mouth and nose. This can affect the way the child's face looks. It can also lead to problems with eating, talking, and ear infections. Treatment is usually surgery to close the lip (*cheiloplasty*) and palate (*palatoplasty*). Doctors often do this surgery in several stages. Usually the first surgery is during the baby's first year. With treatment, most children with cleft lip or palate do well.

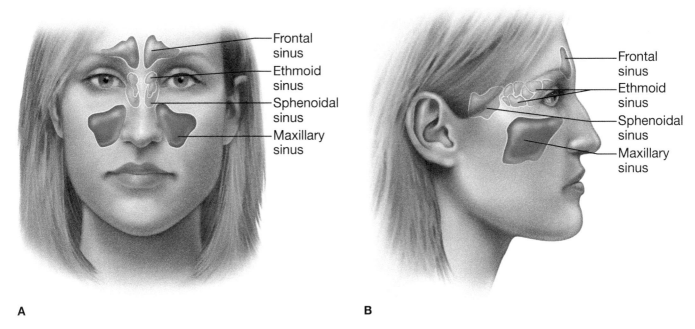

Frontal sinus

Ethmoid sinus

Sphenoidal sinus

Maxillary sinus

Frontal sinus

Ethmoid sinus

Sphenoidal sinus

Maxillary sinus

A   **B**

FIGURE 10.3 Paranasal sinuses. **A** Anterior view. **B** Medial view.

Source: AMERMAN, ERIN C., HUMAN ANATOMY & PHYSIOLOGY, 2nd Ed., ©2019. Reprinted and Electronically reproduced by permission of Pearson Education, Inc., New York, NY.

Pharynx

The **pharynx** is a musculomembranous tube about 5 inches long that extends from the base of the skull, lies anterior to the cervical vertebrae, and becomes continuous with the esophagus. It is divided into three portions: the *nasopharynx* located behind the nose, the *oropharynx* located behind the mouth, and the *laryngopharynx* located behind the larynx. Seven openings are found in the pharynx: two openings from the eustachian tubes, two openings from the posterior nares into the nasopharynx, the fauces or opening from the mouth into the oropharynx, and the openings from the larynx and the esophagus into the laryngopharynx. See Figure 10.4. Associated with the pharynx are three pairs of lymphoid tissues, which are the **tonsils**. The nasopharynx contains the *adenoids* or *pharyngeal* tonsils. The oropharynx contains the *faucial* or *palatine* tonsils and the *lingual* tonsils. The tonsils are accessory organs of the lymphatic system and aid in filtering bacteria and other foreign substances from the circulating lymph in the head and neck region.

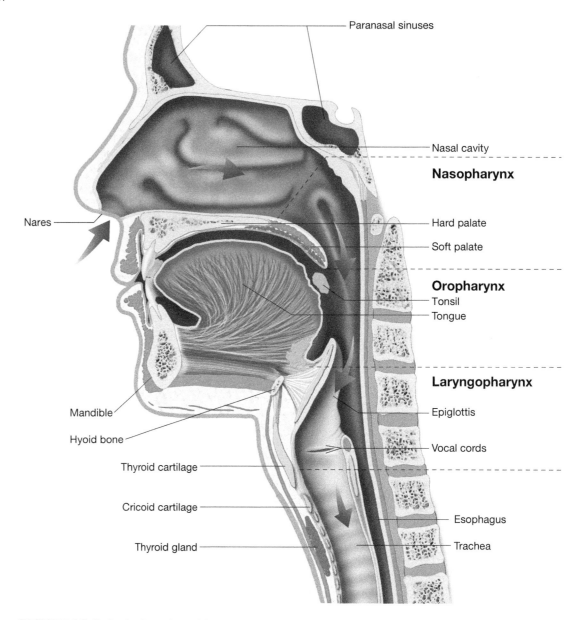

FIGURE 10.4 Sagittal section of the nasal cavity and pharynx.

Source: AMERMAN, ERIN C., HUMAN ANATOMY & PHYSIOLOGY, 2nd Ed., ©2019. Reprinted and Electronically reproduced by permission of Pearson Education, Inc., New York, NY.

Larynx

The **larynx** or *voice box* is a structure made of muscle and cartilage and lined with mucous membrane. It is the enlarged upper end of the trachea below the root of the tongue and hyoid bone. Refer to Figure 10.1.

The cavity of the larynx contains a pair of *ventricular folds* (false vocal cords) and a pair of vocal folds or true vocal cords. The cavity is divided into three regions: vestibule, ventricle, and entrance to the glottis. The **glottis** is a narrow slit at the opening between the true vocal folds.

Cartilages of the Larynx

The larynx is composed of nine cartilages bound together by muscles and ligaments. See Figure 10.5. The three unpaired cartilages, each of which is described in the following sections, are the *thyroid*, *epiglottis*, and *cricoid*, and the three paired cartilages are the *arytenoid*, *cuneiform*, and *corniculate*.

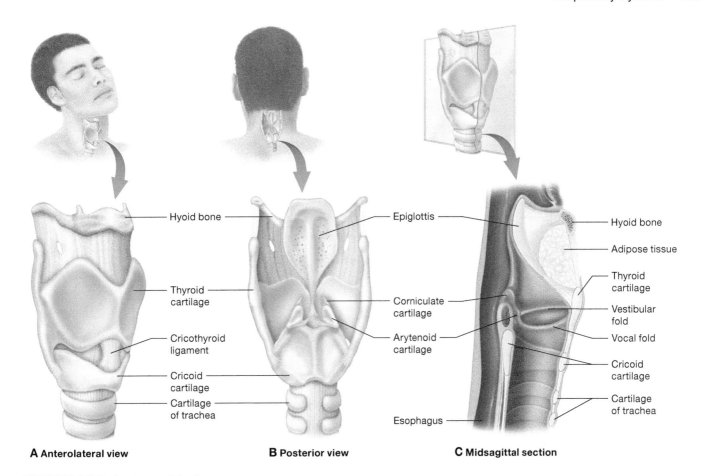

FIGURE 10.5 Anatomy of the larynx.

THYROID CARTILAGE

The **thyroid cartilage** is the largest cartilage in the larynx and forms the structure commonly called the *Adam's apple* (Figure 10.5). This structure is usually larger and more prominent in men than in women and contributes to the deeper male voice.

EPIGLOTTIS

The **epiglottis** covers the entrance of the larynx (Figure 10.5). During swallowing, it acts as a lid to prevent aspiration of food or liquid into the trachea. When the epiglottis fails to cover the entrance to the larynx, food or liquid intended for the esophagus can enter the trachea, causing irritation, coughing, or choking.

CRICOID CARTILAGE

The **cricoid cartilage** is the lowermost cartilage of the larynx (Figure 10.5). It is shaped like a signet ring with the broad portion being posterior and the anterior portion forming the arch and resembling the ring's band.

In the older adult, atrophy of the pharynx and larynx muscle can occur, causing a slackening of the vocal cords and a loss of elasticity of the laryngeal muscles and cartilages. These changes can cause a "gravelly," softer voice with a rise in pitch, making communication more difficult, especially if there is impaired hearing.

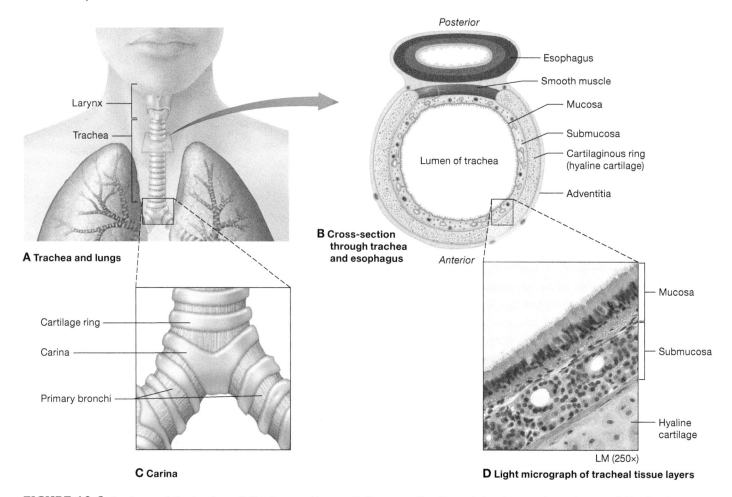

FIGURE 10.6 Anatomy of the trachea. **A** Trachea and lungs. **B** Cross-section through trachea and esophagus. **C** Tracheal carina, a ridge of cartilage at the base of the trachea that separates the openings of the right and left main bronchi. **D** Tracheal tissue layers.

Trachea

The **trachea** or *windpipe* is a semi-cylindrical cartilaginous tube that is the air passageway extending from the pharynx and larynx to the bronchi. It is about 1 inch wide and 4½ inches (11.4 cm) long. It is composed of smooth muscle that is reinforced at the front and sides by C-shaped rings of cartilage. The mucous membrane lining the trachea contains cilia, which sweep foreign matter out of the passageway. The trachea provides an open passageway for air to and from the lungs. See Figure 10.6.

Bronchi

The **bronchi** are the two main branches of the trachea, which provide the passageway for air to the lungs. Refer to Figure 10.1. The trachea divides into the **right bronchus** and the **left bronchus**. The right bronchus is larger and extends down in a more vertical direction than the left bronchus. When a foreign body is inhaled or aspirated, it more frequently lodges in the right bronchus or enters the right lung. Each bronchus enters the lung at a depression, the **hilum**. The bronchi then subdivide into the bronchial tree composed of smaller bronchi, bronchioles, and alveolar ducts. The bronchial tree terminates in the *alveoli*, which are tiny air sacs supporting a network of capillaries from pulmonary blood vessels. See Figure 10.7. The function of the bronchi is to provide an open passageway for air to and from the lungs.

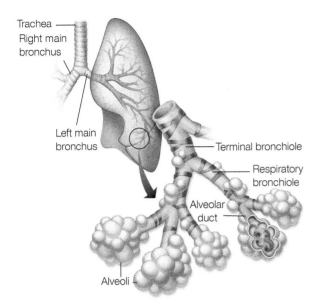

FIGURE 10.7 Respiratory bronchioles, alveolar ducts, and alveoli.
Source: PEARSON EDUCATION; SERVICES, PEARSON; PEARSON EDUCATION, . ., NURSING: A CONCEPT-BASED APPROACH TO LEARNING, VOLUME I, 1st Ed., ©2019. Reprinted and Electronically reproduced by permission of Pearson Education, Inc., New York, NY.

Lungs

The two **lungs** are conical-shaped spongy organs of respiration. They lie on both sides of the heart within the pleural cavity of the thorax. They occupy a large portion of the thoracic cavity and are enclosed in the **pleura**, a serous membrane composed of several layers. The pleural cavity is a space between the parietal and visceral pleura and contains a serous fluid that lubricates and prevents friction caused by the rubbing-together of the two layers. The thoracic cavity is separated from the abdominal cavity by a musculomembranous wall, the **diaphragm**. The central portion of the thoracic cavity, between the lungs, is a space called the **mediastinum**, containing the heart and other structures. See Figure 10.8.

fyi With advancing age, the respiratory system is vulnerable to injuries caused by infections, environmental pollutants, and allergic reactions. The number of cilia declines as one grows older. At the same time, the number of mucus-producing cells may increase, resulting in mucus clogging the airways.

Total lung capacity is relatively constant across the lifespan but vital capacity (volume of air that can be exhaled after a maximal inspiration) decreases because the residual volume increases (amount of air remaining in the lungs after maximal expiration).

The lungs consist of elastic tissue filled with interlacing networks of tubes and sacs that carry air and with blood vessels carrying blood. The broad inferior surface of the lung is the **base**, which rests on the diaphragm, while the **apex**, or pointed upper margin, rises from 2.5 to 5.0 cm above the sternal end of the first rib. The lungs are divided into **lobes**, with the right lung having three lobes and the left lung having two lobes. The left lung is slightly smaller than the right lung and has an indentation, the **cardiac depression**, which allows room for the normal placement of the heart. In an average adult male, the right lung weighs approximately 445 g (1 lb) and the left about 395 g. In an average adult male, the total lung capacity (TLC) is 3.6–9.4 L, whereas in an average adult female it is 2.5–6.9 L. A **lobule** is a primary subdivision of a lobe. In the lungs, it is a physiological unit of the lung consisting of a respiratory bronchiole and its branches

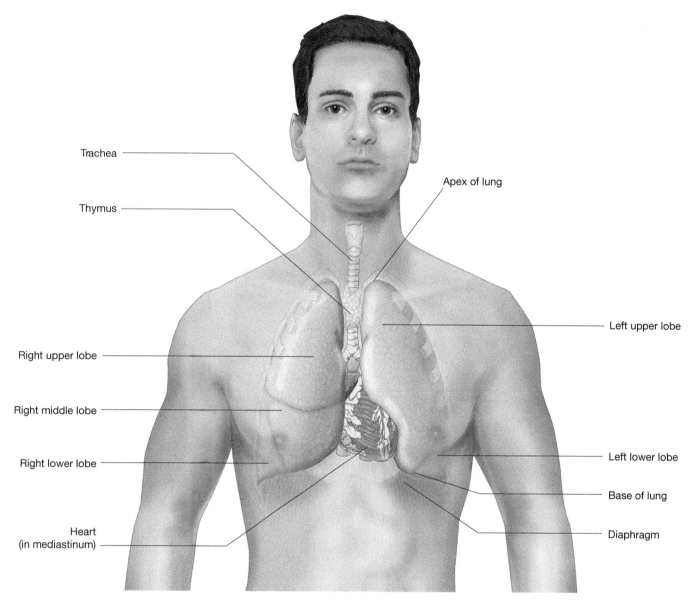

FIGURE 10.8 Position of the lungs and other thoracic organs.

(alveolar ducts, alveolar sacs, and alveoli). The lungs contain around 300 million **alveoli**, which are the air sacs where the exchange of oxygen and carbon dioxide takes place. The main function of the lungs is to bring air into contact with blood so that oxygen and carbon dioxide can be exchanged in the alveoli.

 fyi At 12 weeks' gestation, the lungs of the fetus have a definite shape. At 20 weeks, the cellular structure of the alveoli is complete; the fetus is able to suck its thumb and swallow amniotic fluid. At 24 weeks, the nostrils open and respiratory movements occur. At 26–32 weeks, **surfactant** (a substance formed in the lung that regulates the amount of surface tension of the fluid lining the alveoli) is produced. In preterm infants, the lack of surfactant contributes to *neonatal respiratory distress syndrome (NRDS)*, previously called hyaline membrane disease (HMD). It is also called infant respiratory distress syndrome (IRDS) or respiratory distress syndrome (RDS) of the newborn.

During fetal life, gaseous exchange occurs at the placental interface. The lungs do not function until birth.

Respiration

Breathing is normally an involuntary activity, meaning that it occurs without any conscious effort. The *medulla oblongata* and the *pons*, two of the structures of the brainstem, regulate and control respiration. Respiratory control centers in the brain regulate and control the rate, rhythm, and depth of respiration. Receptors in large arteries in the thorax (chest) and neck send the respiratory centers of the brain information about the blood level of oxygen, and receptors in the brain send information about the level of carbon dioxide. The respiratory rate is normally controlled by the level of carbon dioxide in the blood. When the carbon dioxide level is increased, breathing is more rapid because of the need to expel the excess. When the carbon dioxide level decreases, the respiratory rate decreases. See Figure 10.9.

Evaluation of an individual's response to changes occurring within the body can be measured by taking the vital signs: temperature, pulse, respiration, and blood pressure. The variations of certain vital signs signify a typical disease process and its stages of development. For example, in a patient who has pneumonia (inflammation of the lungs caused by bacteria, viruses, fungi, or chemical irritants), the temperature can be elevated to 101°F–106°F, and pulse and respiration can increase to almost twice their normal rates. Normally, when the temperature falls, the patient will perspire profusely and the pulse and respiration will begin to return to normal rates. You will note that not all patients will follow this sequence of events, but will need an additional intervention in care/treatment.

Individuals of different ages breathe at different respiratory rates. The following are normal resting respiratory rates for different age groups:

Newborn	30–60 per minute
1–3 years	20–30 per minute
11–14 years	12–20 per minute
Adult	16–20 per minute

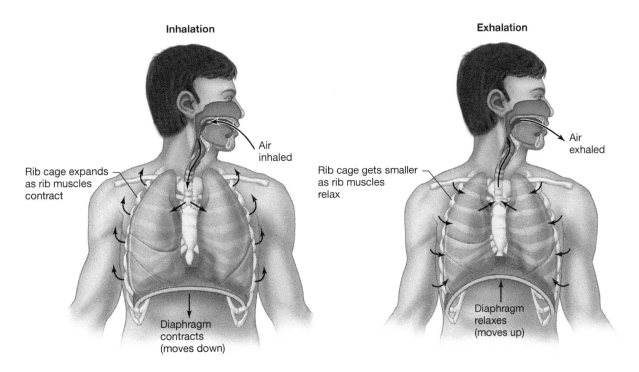

Inhalation

Air inhaled

Rib cage expands as rib muscles contract

Diaphragm contracts (moves down)

Exhalation

Air exhaled

Rib cage gets smaller as rib muscles relax

Diaphragm relaxes (moves up)

FIGURE 10.9 The process of respiration.

Volume

The following terms are used by physiologists and respiratory specialists to describe the volume of air exchanged in breathing. Read and study these terms to enhance your medical vocabulary.

Tidal volume (TV). Amount of air in a single inspiration and expiration. In the average adult male, about 500 mL of air enters the respiratory tract during normal quiet breathing.

Expiratory reserve volume (ERV). Amount of air that can be forcibly expired after a normal quiet respiration. This is also called the *supplemental air* and measures approximately 1000–1200 mL.

Inspiratory reserve volume (IRV). Amount of air that can be forcibly inspired over and above a normal inspiration and measures approximately 3000 mL.

Residual volume (RV). Amount of air remaining in the lungs after maximal expiration, about 1500 mL.

Vital capacity (VC). Volume of air that can be exhaled after a maximal inspiration.

Functional residual capacity (FRC). Volume of air that remains in the lungs at the end of a normal expiration.

Total lung capacity (TLC). Maximal volume of air in the lungs after a maximal inspiration.

Study *and* Review I

Anatomy and Physiology

Write your answers to the following questions.

1. List the organs of the respiratory system.

   a. _____   d. _____

   b. _____   e. _____

   c. _____   f. _____

2. State the primary function of the respiratory system.

   _____

   _____

3. Define *external respiration.* _____

4. Define *internal respiration.* _____

5. List the five functions of the nose.

a. _____   d. _____

b. _____   e. _____

c. _____

6. List the three functions of the pharynx.

a. _____   c. _____

b. _____

7. State the function of the epiglottis. _____

8. Define *glottis*. _____

9. State the function of the larynx. _____

10. State the function of the trachea. _____

11. State the function of the bronchi. _____

12. Give a brief description of the lungs. _____

13. Define *pleura*. _____

14. The thoracic cavity is separated from the abdominal cavity by a musculomembranous wall commonly known as the _____.

15. The central portion of the thoracic cavity between the lungs is a space called the _____.

16. The right lung has _____ lobes and the left lung has _____ lobes.

17. The air cells of the lungs are the _____.

18. State the main function of the lungs. _____

19. The vital signs, which are essential elements for determining an individual's state of health, are _____, _____, _____, and _____.

20. Define the following terms:

a. *Tidal volume* _____

b. *Residual volume* _____

c. *Vital capacity* _____

21. The _____ _____ and the

_____ of the central nervous system regulate and control respiration.

22. The normal resting respiratory rate for a newborn is _____ to

_____ breaths per minute.

23. The normal resting respiratory rate for an adult is _____ to

_____ breaths per minute.

▶ **ANATOMY LABELING**   Identify the structures shown below by filling in the blanks.

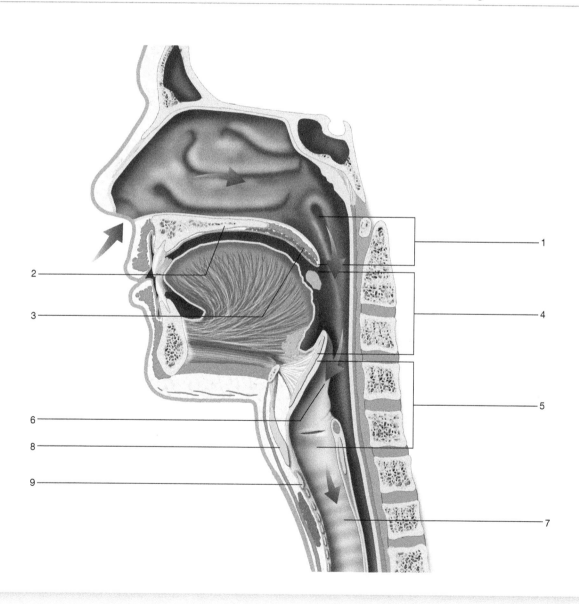

Building Your Medical Vocabulary

This section provides the foundation for learning medical terminology. Review the alphabetized list of medical terms in the following pages. Note how common prefixes and suffixes are repeatedly applied to word roots and combining forms to create different meanings. A combining form is a word root plus a vowel. The chart below lists the combining forms and word roots used in this chapter and can help to strengthen your understanding of how medical words are built and spelled.

You will find that some terms have not been divided into word parts. These are common words or specialized terms that are included to enhance your medical vocabulary.

Combining Forms

alveol/o	small, hollow air sac	**pector/o**	chest
anthrac/o	coal	**pharyng/o**	pharynx, throat
aspirat/o	to draw in	**phon/o**	voice, sound
atel/o	imperfect	**pleur/o**	pleura
bronch/o	bronchus	**pneum/o**	air
bronchi/o	bronchus	**pneumon/o**	lung
bronchiol/o	bronchiole	**pulmon/o**	lung
coni/o	dust	**py/o**	pus
cyan/o	dark blue	**respirat/o**	breathing
cyst/o	sac	**rhin/o**	nose
fibr/o	fiber	**rhonch/o**	snore
halat/o	breathe	**sarc/o**	flesh
hem/o	blood	**spir/o**	breathe
laryng/o	larynx, voice box	**thorac/o**	chest
lob/o	lobe	**tonsill/o**	tonsil
nas/o	nose	**trache/o**	trachea
olfact/o	smell	**tubercul/o**	a little swelling, nodule
orth/o	straight	**ventilat/o**	to air
ox/o	oxygen	**vir/o**	virus (poison)
palat/o	palate		

Word Roots

log	study	**sphyxis, sphyx**	pulse
sinus	curve, hollow		

Medical Word	Word Parts		Definition
	Part	Meaning	
alveolus (ăl-vē´ ō-lŭs)	alveol	small, hollow air sac	Pertaining to a small air sac in the lungs
	-us	pertaining to	

 Acute respiratory distress syndrome (ARDS) is a rapidly progressive disease occurring in critically ill patients. The main complication in ARDS is that fluid leaks into the lungs, making breathing difficult or impossible, and leads to *hypoxemia* (abnormally low level of oxygen in the blood). When the body can't carry out the work of breathing and has a low oxygen level, it causes respiratory failure. In order to improve the amount of oxygen and reduce the work of breathing, most patients with ARDS are placed on a ventilator.

Medical Word	Word Parts		Definition
anthracosis (ăn˝ thră-kō´ sĭs)	anthrac	coal	Lung condition caused by inhalation of coal dust and silica; also called *black lung*
	-osis	condition	
apnea (ăp´ nē-ă)	a-	lack of	Temporary cessation of breathing. **Sleep apnea** is a temporary cessation of breathing during sleep. To be so classified, the apnea must last for at least 10 seconds and occur 30 or more times during a 7-hour period of sleep. Sleep apnea is classified according to the mechanisms involved. **Obstructive apnea** is caused by obstruction to the upper airway. **Central apnea** is marked by absence of respiratory muscle activity.
	-pnea	breathing	
asphyxia (ăs-fĭk´ sĭ-ă)	a-	lack of	Emergency condition in which there is a depletion of oxygen in the blood with an increase of carbon dioxide in the blood and tissues; symptoms include dyspnea, cyanosis, tachycardia, impairment of senses, and, in extreme cases, convulsions, unconsciousness, and death. Some of the more common causes include drowning, electrical shock, aspiration of vomitus, lodging of a foreign body in the respiratory tract, inhalation of toxic gas or smoke, and poisoning. Artificial ventilation and oxygen should be administered as quickly as possible.
	sphyx	pulse	
	-ia	condition	
aspiration (ăs˝ pĭ-rā´ shŭn)	aspirat	to draw in	The act of drawing in or out by suction using a device such as a syringe or needle; the process of drawing foreign bodies—such as food, liquid, or other substances—into the nose, throat, or lungs on inspiration
	-ion	process	

Medical Word	Word Parts		Definition
	Part	Meaning	
asthma (ăz′ mă)			Disease of the bronchi characterized by wheezing, dyspnea, and a feeling of constriction in the chest. See Figure 10.10. Inflammation of the airways causes airflow into and out of the lungs to be restricted. During an asthma attack, the muscles of the bronchial tree constrict and the linings of the air passages swell, reducing airflow and producing the characteristic wheezing sound. See Figure 10.11.

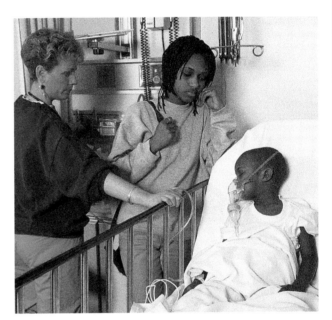

FIGURE 10.10 Acute exacerbations of asthma can require management in the emergency department. The child is placed in a sitting position to facilitate respiratory effort.
Source: Pearson Education, Inc.

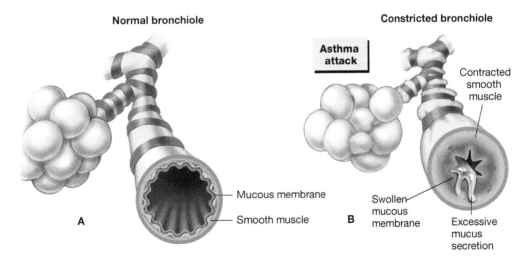

Normal bronchiole

Constricted bronchiole

Asthma attack

Mucous membrane

Smooth muscle

A

Contracted smooth muscle

Swollen mucous membrane

B

Excessive mucus secretion

FIGURE 10.11 Changes in bronchioles during an asthma attack: **A** normal bronchiole and **B** in asthma attack.

fyi In asthma-prone individuals, symptoms can be triggered by inhaled allergens, such as pet dander, dust mites, cockroach allergens, molds, or pollens. A variety of other situations can also trigger symptoms, including respiratory infections, exercise, cold air, tobacco smoke and other pollutants, stress, and food or drug allergies. Figure 10.12, from the American Lung Association, shows what can trigger an asthmatic episode.

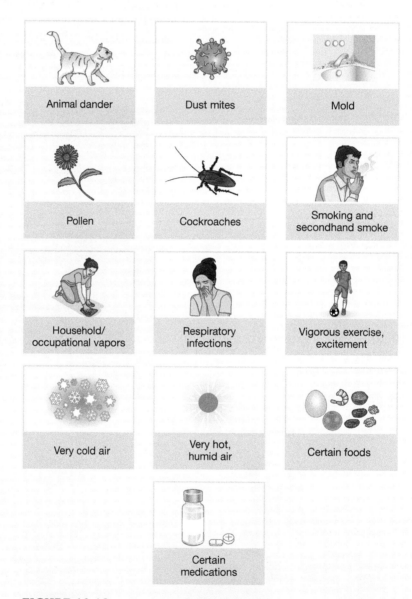

FIGURE 10.12 Asthma triggers abound.

Source: Reprinted with permission © 2006 American Lung Association. For more information about the American Lung Association or to support the work it does, visit www.lung.org.

Medical Word	Word Parts		Definition
	Part	Meaning	
atelectasis (ăt″ĕ-lĕk′tă-sĭs)	atel -ectasis	imperfect dilation, expansion	A disorder characterized by the collapse of part of or the entire lung or failure of the lung to expand (inflate) completely. This may be caused by a blocked airway, a tumor, general anesthesia, pneumonia or other lung infections, lung disease, or long-term bed rest with shallow breathing. Also called *collapsed lung*.
bronchiectasis (brŏng″kē-ĕk′tă-sĭs)	bronchi -ectasis	bronchus dilation, expansion	Chronic dilation of a bronchus or bronchi, with a secondary infection that usually involves the lower portion of a lung
bronchiolitis (brŏng″kē-ō-lī′tĭs)	bronchiol -itis	bronchiole inflammation	Inflammation of the bronchioles
bronchitis (brŏng-kī′tĭs)	bronch -itis	bronchus inflammation	Inflammation of the bronchi
bronchoscope (brŏng′kō-skōp)	bronch/o -scope	bronchus instrument for examining	Medical instrument used to visually examine the bronchi. In a bronchoscopy procedure, the larynx, trachea, and bronchi are examined by a flexible bronchoscope. See Figure 10.13.

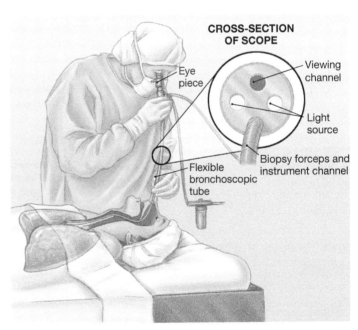

FIGURE 10.13 Use of a bronchoscope during a bronchoscopy to visualize the bronchus.

| carbon dioxide (CO₂) (kăr′bŏn dī-ŏk′sīd) | | | Colorless, odorless gas produced by the oxidation of carbon; it is a waste gas from metabolism that needs to be exhaled |

Medical Word	Word Parts		Definition
	Part	Meaning	
Cheyne–Stokes respiration (chān′–stōks′ rĕs″ pĭr-ā′ shŭn)			Rhythmic cycle of breathing with a gradual increase in respiration followed by apnea (which may last from 10 to 60 seconds), then a repeat of the same cycle
cough (kawf)			Sudden, forceful expulsion of air from the lungs; an essential protective response that clears irritants, secretions, or foreign objects from the trachea, bronchi, and/or lungs
croup (kroop)			Acute respiratory disease (ARD) characterized by obstruction of the larynx, a barking cough, dyspnea, hoarseness, and stridor (high-pitched noisy breathing). See Figure 10.14.

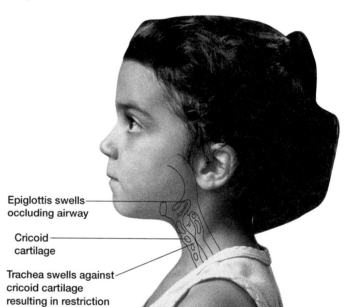

Epiglottis swells occluding airway

Cricoid cartilage

Trachea swells against cricoid cartilage resulting in restriction

FIGURE 10.14 Two important changes occur in the upper airway in croup: The epiglottis swells, thereby occluding the airway, and the trachea swells against the cricoid cartilage, causing restriction.

Source: Pearson Education, Inc.

Medical Word	Word Parts		Definition
cyanosis (sī″ ăn-ō′ sĭs)	**cyan**	dark blue	Abnormal condition of the skin and mucous membrane caused by oxygen deficiency in the blood. The skin, fingernails, and mucous membranes can appear slightly bluish or grayish.
	-osis	condition	

Medical Word	Word Parts		Definition
	Part	Meaning	
cystic fibrosis (CF) (sĭs´ tĭk fī-brō´ sĭs)	cyst -ic fibr -osis	sac pertaining to fiber condition	Inherited disease that affects the entire body, causing progressive disability and often early death. The name *cystic fibrosis* refers to the characteristic scarring (fibrosis) and cyst formation within the pancreas. Cystic fibrosis may be diagnosed by many different categories of testing, including newborn screening, sweat testing, or genetic testing. The gene responsible for this condition has been identified, and persons carrying the gene can be determined through genetic testing. See Figure 10.15.

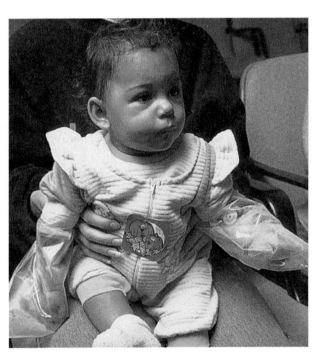

FIGURE 10.15 Evaluation of a child for cystic fibrosis with a sweat chloride test. Sweat is being collected under the wrappings for later analysis of the amount of sodium and chloride.
Source: Pearson Education, Inc.

dysphonia (dĭs-fō´ nē-ă)	dys- phon -ia	difficult voice condition	Condition of difficulty in speaking; also called *hoarseness*
dyspnea (dĭsp-nē´ ă)	dys- -pnea	difficult breathing	Literally means *difficulty in breathing*

Medical Word	Word Parts		Definition
	Part	Meaning	
emphysema (ĕm″ fĭ-sē′ mă)			Chronic pulmonary disease in which the alveoli become distended and the alveolar walls become damaged or destroyed, making it difficult to exhale air from the lungs. It is included in a group of diseases (chronic bronchitis, emphysema) called *chronic obstructive pulmonary disease*, or *COPD*. The primary cause of emphysema is cigarette smoking. See Figure 10.16.

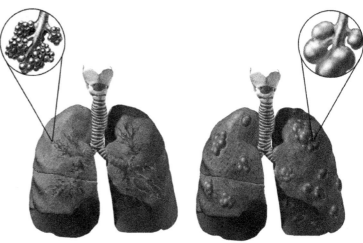

FIGURE 10.16 Normal lung and one with emphysema.

Normal lung   Emphysema

Medical Word	Word Parts		Definition
empyema (ĕm″ pī-ē′ mă)			Pus in a body cavity, especially the pleural cavity
endotracheal (ET) (ĕn″ dō-trā′ kē-ăl)	endo- trache -al	within trachea pertaining to	Within the trachea. An endotracheal tube is used in general anesthesia, intensive care, and emergency medicine for airway management and mechanical ventilation and as an alternative route for the administration of medicines when an intravenous (IV) infusion line cannot be established.
epistaxis (ĕp″ ĭ-stăk′ sĭs)	epi- -staxis	upon dripping	Nosebleed; usually results from traumatic or spontaneous rupture of blood vessels in the mucous membranes of the nose
eupnea (ūp-nē′ ă)	eu- -pnea	good, normal breathing	Good or normal breathing
exhalation (ĕks″ hă-lā′ shŭn)	ex- halat -ion	out breathe process	Process of breathing out
expectoration (ĕk-spĕk″ tō-rā′ shŭn)	ex- pector(at) -ion	out chest process	Process of coughing up and spitting out material (sputum) from the lungs, bronchi, and trachea

Medical Word	Word Parts		Definition
	Part	Meaning	
Heimlich maneuver (hīm′ lĭk mă-noo′ ver)			A first aid technique used to force an upper airway obstruction (usually a bolus of food) out of the trachea; also called *abdominal thrusts*. See Figure 10.17.

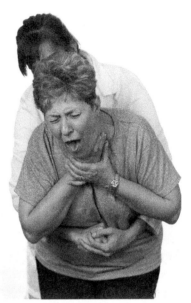

FIGURE 10.17 Administration of abdominal thrusts (the Heimlich maneuver) on a choking person.
Source: aceshot1/Shutterstock

Medical Word	Word Parts		Definition
hemoptysis (hē-mŏp′ tĭ-sĭs)	hem/o -ptysis	blood to spit	Coughing-up of blood or blood-stained mucus from the respiratory tract; literally a spitting-up of blood
hyperpnea (hī″ pĕrp-nē′ ă)	hyper- -pnea	excessive breathing	Abnormally deep and rapid breathing
hyperventilation (hī″ pĕr-vĕn″ tĭ-lā′ shŭn)	hyper- ventilat -ion	excessive to air process	Process of excessive ventilating, thereby increasing the air in the lungs beyond the normal limit
hypoxemia (hī-pŏks′ ēm-ēă)	hyp- ox -emia	deficient oxygen blood condition	Deficient amount of oxygen in the blood
influenza (ĭn″ floo-ĕn′ ză)			Acute, contagious respiratory infection caused by a virus. Onset is usually sudden, and symptoms are fever, chills, headache, myalgia, cough, and sore throat.
inhalation (ĭn″ hă-lā′ shŭn)	in- halat -ion	in breathe process	Process of breathing in
laryngeal (lă-rĭn′ jē-ăl)	laryng -eal	larynx, voice box pertaining to	Pertaining to the larynx (voice box)

Medical Word	Word Parts		Definition
	Part	Meaning	
laryngitis (lăr″ĭn-jī′tĭs)	**laryng** **-itis**	larynx, voice box inflammation	Inflammation of the larynx (voice box). See Figure 10.18.

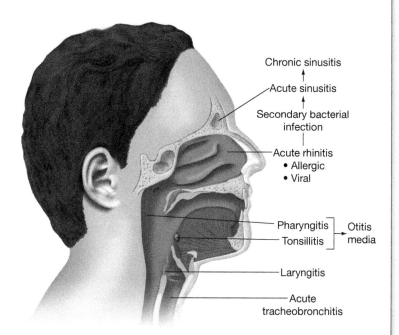

FIGURE 10.18 Paranasal sinuses are part of the upper respiratory system. From here, infections can spread via the nasopharynx to the middle ear or bronchi. Note locations of laryngitis, pharyngitis, sinusitis, and tonsillitis.

Chronic sinusitis
Acute sinusitis
Secondary bacterial infection
Acute rhinitis
• Allergic
• Viral
Pharyngitis
Tonsillitis
Otitis media
Laryngitis
Acute tracheobronchitis

Medical Word	Word Parts		Definition
laryngoscope (lă-ring′gō-skōp)	**laryng/o** **-scope**	larynx, voice box instrument for examining	Medical instrument used to visually examine the larynx (voice box). The procedure using a laryngoscope is known as *laryngoscopy*.
Legionnaires disease (lē-jŏn-ārz′)			Severe pulmonary pneumonia caused by a bacterium called *Legionella pneumophila*

GOOD TO KNOW ▶

Legionella pneumophila is commonly found in the environment, particularly in freshwater, groundwater, and soil. According to the Centers for Disease and Prevention (CDC), people can get Legionnaires' disease when they breathe in mist (small droplets of water in the air) containing the bacteria. One example might be from breathing in droplets sprayed from a hot tub or spa that has not been properly cleaned and disinfected. Outbreaks are most commonly associated with buildings or structures that have complex water systems, like hotels, hospitals, long-term care facilities, and cruise ships. Within these structures, the bacterium can become a health concern when it grows and spreads in human-made water systems, like hot tubs, cooling towers, hot water tanks, large plumbing systems, and decorative fountains. Most healthy people do not become infected with *Legionella* bacteria after exposure.

Medical Word	Word Parts		Definition
	Part	Meaning	
lobectomy (lō-běk′ tō-mē)	lob -ectomy	lobe surgical excision	Surgical excision of a lobe of any organ or gland, such as the lung

 fyi The choice for patients with lung cancer is usually a lobectomy, but in some patients with early-stage non-small-cell lung cancer (NSCLC), a *segmentectomy* (surgical removal of a segment) or segment resection of a lung may be an option. In this surgical procedure, part of one of the lobes of the lung is excised. If the cancer is advanced or metastatic (pertaining to the process whereby cancer cells spread from a primary site to distant secondary sites elsewhere in the body), then segmentectomy is not recommended.

Sleeve lobectomy is a procedure in which the involved lobe and part of the mainstem bronchus is removed. The remaining lobe is reimplanted on the mainstem bronchus. This procedure is indicated for central tumors of the lung as an alternative to pneumonectomy and/or for NSCLC.

lung cancer		A cancer that begins in the lungs (bronchi, bronchioles, and/or alveoli) and most often occurs in people who smoke, who are exposed to secondhand smoke, or to particular toxins. It is the highest cancer killer in the United States of both women and men. See Figure 10.19. Symptoms include persistent cough, chest pain, dyspnea, weight loss, and blood-streaked sputum. The deep, rattling sound of "smoker's cough" is caused by the adverse effects of chemicals, irritants, and smoke leading to the destruction of cilia of the airways. The good news for people who *stop* smoking is that cilia can regrow.

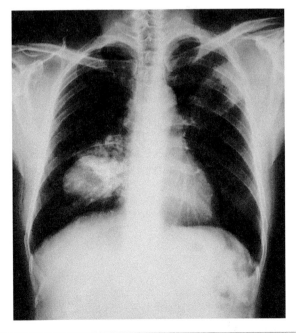

FIGURE 10.19 Chest radiograph showing large tumor in right lung.
Source: Suttha Burawonk/Shutterstock

Medical Word	Word Parts		Definition
	Part	Meaning	
mesothelioma (mĕs″ ō-thē″ lē-ō′ mă)			Malignant tumor of the mesothelium (serous membrane of the pleura) found most often in people who smoke or people with a history of exposure to asbestos
nasopharyngitis (nā″ zō-făr′ ĭn-jī′ tĭs)	nas/o pharyng -itis	nose pharynx, throat inflammation	Inflammation of the nose and pharynx (throat)
olfaction (ŏl-făk′ shŭn)	olfact -ion	smell process	Process of smelling
orthopnea (or″ thŏp′ nē-ă)	orth/o -pnea	straight breathing	Inability to breathe unless in an upright or straight position
palatopharyngoplasty (păl″ ăt-ō-făr″ ĭn′ gō-plăs″ tē)	palat/o pharyng/o -plasty	palate pharynx, throat surgical repair	Type of surgery that relieves snoring and sleep apnea by removing the uvula and the tonsils and reshaping the lining at the back of the throat to enlarge the air passageway
pertussis (pĕr-tŭs′ ĭs)			Acute, infectious disease caused by the bacterium *Bordetella pertussis*; characterized by a peculiar paroxysmal cough ending in a "crowing" or "whooping" sound; also called *whooping cough*

GOOD TO KNOW ▶

Pertussis, a serious disease that can affect people of all ages, can be deadly for babies less than a year old. This disease is on the rise in the United States and more cases are being reported to the CDC. Approximately half of the people with pertussis are not up to date with all recommended immunizations and some families have been identified as not vaccinating their children at all.

According to the CDC, the only prevention against pertussis disease is the DTaP (diphtheria, tetanus, and pertussis) vaccine for children younger than 7 years of age or the Tdap vaccine (tetanus, diphtheria, and pertussis), which is a booster immunization given to those older than 11 years of age. All family members should be up to date on all CDC Advisory Committee of Immunization Practices (ACIP) and American Academy of Pediatrics (AAP)–recommended vaccines. Pregnant women should be vaccinated with Tdap during each pregnancy as a way to protect newborns and infants.

pharyngitis (făr″ ĭn-jī′ tĭs)	pharyng -itis	pharynx, throat inflammation	Inflammation of the pharynx (throat). Refer to Figure 10.18.
pleurisy (ploo′ rĭs-ē)			Inflammation of the pleura caused by injury, infection, or a tumor. The inflamed pleural layers rub against each other every time the lungs expand to breathe in air, which can cause sharp pain with breathing (also called *pleuritic chest pain*).
pleuritis (ploo-rī′ tĭs)	pleur -itis	pleura inflammation	Inflammation of the pleura

Medical Word	Word Parts		Definition
	Part	Meaning	
pleurodynia (ploo″ rō-dĭn′ ē-ă)	**pleur/o** **-dynia**	pleura pain	Pain in the pleura
pneumoconiosis (noo″ mō-kō″ nē-ō′ sĭs)	**pneum/o** **coni** **-osis**	air dust condition	Abnormal condition of the lung caused by the inhalation of dust particles such as coal dust (*anthracosis*), stone dust (*chalicosis*), iron dust (*siderosis*), asbestos (*asbestosis*), and quartz (*silica*) dust (*silicosis*)
pneumonectomy (noo″ mŏ-nĕk′ tŏ-mē)	**pneumon** **-ectomy**	lung surgical excision	Surgical excision of the left or right lung
pneumonia (noo-mōn′ yă)	**pneumon** **-ia**	lung condition	Inflammation of the lung caused by bacteria, viruses, fungi, or chemical irritants. See Figure 10.20.

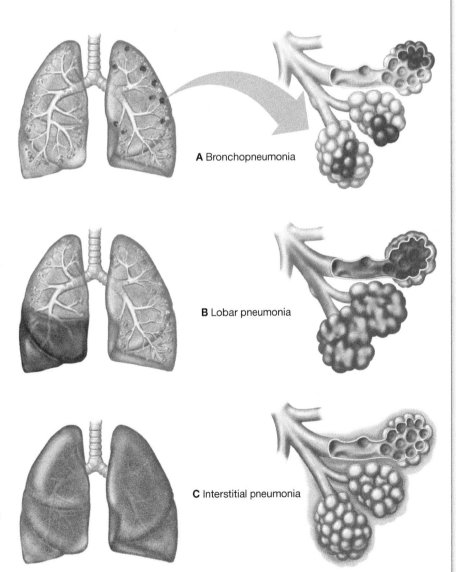

A Bronchopneumonia

B Lobar pneumonia

C Interstitial pneumonia

FIGURE 10.20 A Bronchopneumonia with localized pattern. **B** Lobar pneumonia with a diffuse pattern within the lung lobe. **C** Interstitial pneumonia is typically diffuse and bilateral.

Medical Word	Word Parts		Definition
	Part	**Meaning**	

GO👀D TO KNOW ▶

Pneumococcal disease is common in young children, but older adults with the disease are at greatest risk of serious illness and death because the immune system weakens as the body ages and cannot fight off infections as well. Older adults are also more likely to be suffering from other illnesses that make their body more susceptible to infection.

There are two kinds of vaccines that help prevent pneumococcal disease: (1) pneumococcal conjugate vaccine (PCV13 or Prevnar 1) protects against 13 of the most common bacteria that cause pneumonia and

(2) pneumococcal polysaccharide vaccine (PPSV23 or Pneumovax23) protects against an additional 23 types of pneumonia bacteria.

Symptoms of pneumococcal disease include a cough with greenish mucus or puslike sputum, chills, fever, fatigue, chest pain, and muscle aches. Initial diagnosis is made through auscultation of the chest with a stethoscope (refer to Figure 1.11 in Chapter 1). In patients with pneumonia, rales and other abnormal breathing sounds can be heard. Tests that are used to confirm the diagnosis include a chest x-ray (CXR) and a sputum culture.

Medical Word	Word Parts		Definition
pneumonitis (noo″ mō-nīt′ ĭs)	**pneumon** **-itis**	lung inflammation	Inflammation of the lung
pneumothorax (noo″ mŏ-thōr′ aks)	**pneum/o** **-thorax**	air chest	A pathological condition in which there is a collection of air between the chest wall and lungs, causing the lung to collapse. It may occur spontaneously or after physical trauma to the chest or as a complication of medical treatment. See Figure 10.21.

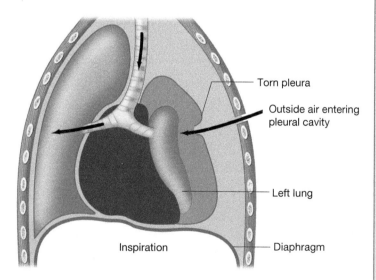

FIGURE 10.21 Pneumothorax.

Medical Word	Word Parts		Definition
pulmonologist (pŭl-mŏ-nŏl′ ŏ-jĭst)	**pulmon/o** **log** **-ist**	lung study one who specializes	Physician who specializes in the diagnosis and treatment of pulmonary diseases

Medical Word	Word Parts		Definition
	Part	**Meaning**	
pulmonology (pŭl-mŏ-nŏl´ ŏ-jē)	**pulmon/o** **-logy**	lung study of	The study of pulmonary diseases
pyothorax (pī˝ ō-thō´ răks)	**py/o** **-thorax**	pus chest	Pus in the chest cavity
rale (rāl)			Abnormal sound heard on auscultation of the chest; a crackling, rattling, or bubbling sound
respirator (rĕs´ pĭ-rā˝ tor)	**respirat** **-or**	breathing a doer	Medical device used to assist in breathing; type of machine used for prolonged artificial respiration
respiratory distress syndrome (RDS) (rĕs´ pĭ-ră-tō˝ rē)			Condition that can occur in a premature newborn in which the lungs are not matured to the point of manufacturing lecithin, a pulmonary surfactant, resulting in collapse of the alveoli, which leads to cyanosis and *hypoxia* (low levels of oxygen in body tissues); previously called *hyaline membrane disease (HMD)*
respiratory syncytial virus (RSV) infection (sĭn-sĭ´ shăl)			Most common cause of bronchiolitis and pneumonia among infants and children under 2 years of age. Illness begins with fever, runny nose, cough, and sometimes wheezing. Most children recover from illness in 8–15 days. It is contagious and spreads through the respiratory secretions of infected persons or contact with contaminated surfaces or objects.
rhinoplasty (rī´ nō-plăs˝ tē)	**rhin/o** **-plasty**	nose surgical repair	Surgical repair of the nose
rhinorrhea (rī´ nō-rē´ ă)	**rhin/o** **-rrhea**	nose flow, discharge	Discharge from the nose
rhinovirus (rī´ nō-vī´ rŭs)	**rhin/o** **vir** **-us**	nose virus pertaining to	One of a subgroup of viruses that causes the common cold (*coryza*) in humans
rhonchus (rŏng´ kŭs)	**rhonch** **-us**	snore pertaining to	Rale or rattling sound in the throat or bronchial tubes caused by a partial obstruction
sarcoidosis (sar˝ koyd-ō´ sĭs)	**sarc** **-oid** **-osis**	flesh resemble condition	Chronic granulomatous condition that can involve almost any organ system of the body, usually the lungs, causing dyspnea on exertion
severe acute respiratory syndrome (SARS)			Contagious viral respiratory infection that was first described in 2003; serious form of pneumonia resulting in acute respiratory distress and sometimes death
sinusitis (sī˝ nŭs-ī´ tĭs)	**sinus** **-itis**	curve, hollow inflammation	Inflammation of a sinus. Refer to Figure 10.18.

Medical Word	Word Parts		Definition
	Part	**Meaning**	
spirometer (spī-rŏm´ĕt-ĕr)	**spir/o** **-meter**	breathe instrument to measure	Medical instrument used to measure lung volume during inspiration and expiration; in incentive spirometry, a portable spirometer may be used by a patient for deep breathing exercises. See Figure 10.22.

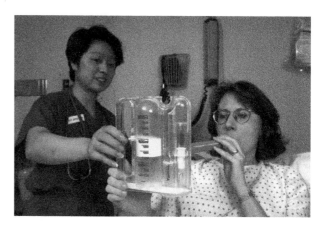

FIGURE 10.22 A portable spirometer used by a patient for deep breathing exercises.
Source: Pearson Education, Inc.

Medical Word	Word Parts		Definition
sputum (spū´ tŭm)			Substance coughed up from the lungs; can be watery, thick, purulent, clear, or bloody and can contain microorganisms
stridor (strī´ dōr)			High-pitched sound caused by partial obstruction of the air passageway
tachypnea (tăk˝ ĭp-nē´ ă)	**tachy-** **-pnea**	rapid breathing	Rapid breathing
thoracocentesis (thō˝ ră-kō-sĕn-tē´ sĭs)	**thorac/o** **-centesis**	chest surgical puncture	Surgical puncture of the chest wall for removal of fluid; also called *thoracentesis*. Can be used in pleurisy to remove excess fluid that has accumulated in the chest cavity. See Figure 10.23.

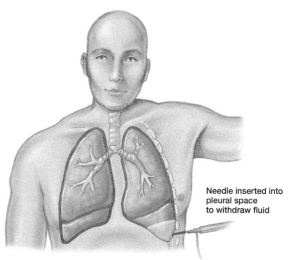

Needle inserted into pleural space to withdraw fluid

FIGURE 10.23 Thoracocentesis (also called thoracentesis).

Medical Word	Word Parts		Definition
	Part	Meaning	
thoracoplasty (thō´ ră-kō-plăs˝ tē)	**thorac/o** -**plasty**	chest surgical repair	Surgical repair of the chest wall
thoracotomy (thō˝ răk-ŏt´ ō-mē)	**thorac/o** -**tomy**	chest incision	Incision into the chest wall
tonsillitis (tŏn˝ sĭl-ī´ tĭs)	**tonsill** -**itis**	tonsil inflammation	Inflammation of the tonsils. Refer to Figure 10.18.
tracheal (trā´ kē-ăl)	**trache** -**al**	trachea, windpipe pertaining to	Pertaining to the trachea (windpipe)
tracheostomy (trā˝ kē-ŏs´ tō-mē)	**trache/o** -**stomy**	trachea, windpipe new opening	New opening into the trachea (windpipe). See Figure 10.24.

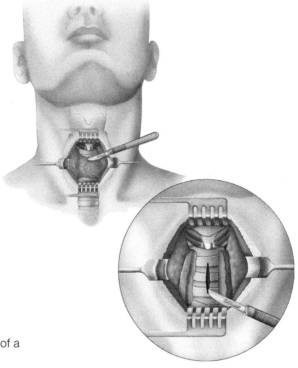

FIGURE 10.24 Tracheostomy. The surgical creation of a new opening into the trachea.

tracheotomy (trā˝ kē-ŏt´ ō-mē)	**trache/o** -**tomy**	trachea, windpipe incision	Incision into the trachea (windpipe)

Medical Word	Word Parts		Definition
	Part	Meaning	
tuberculosis (TB) (too-bĕr′ kyŭ-lō′ sĭs)	**tubercul**	a little swelling, nodule	Infectious disease caused by the tubercle bacillus *Mycobacterium tuberculosis*, which can form tubercles (soft nodules of necrosis) in the lungs and other infected parts of the body. TB can be diagnosed with a positive sputum culture, positive blood and/or skin tests, and x-rays.
	-osis	condition	

GOOD TO KNOW ▶

Mycobacterium tuberculosis usually attacks the lungs, but can attack any part of the body, such as the kidney, spine, and brain. Not everyone infected with TB bacteria becomes sick. As a result, two TB-related conditions exist: latent TB infection (LTBI) and TB disease. If not treated properly, TB disease can be fatal. Active TB may be cured by taking several medicines for a long period of time.

TB spreads through the air when a person with TB of the lungs or throat coughs, sneezes, or talks. A person who has been exposed should see a physician for testing. People with weak immune systems are more likely to get TB after exposure. Symptoms of TB in the lungs can include a bad cough that lasts 3 weeks or longer, coughing up blood-tinged mucus, night sweats, anorexia, fatigue, and weight loss.

Medical Word	Word Parts		Definition
ventilator (vent′ ĭ-lāt″ ŏr)	**ventilat**	to air	A machine that supports breathing; ventilators are used to breathe for individuals who are unable to breathe on their own; also called *respirator* or *breathing machine*
	-or	a doer	
wheeze (hwēz)			A high-pitched whistling sound caused by constriction of the air passageway associated with an asthma attack or airway obstruction

Study *and* Review II

Word Parts

Prefixes Give the definitions of the following prefixes.

1. a- _____

2. epi- _____

3. dys- _____

4. endo- _____

5. eu- _____

6. ex- _____

7. hyp- _____   **9.** in- _____

8. hyper- _____   **10.** tachy- _____

Combining Forms   Give the definitions of the following combining forms.

1. alveol/o _____   **12.** pharyng/o _____

2. anthrac/o _____   **13.** pleur/o _____

3. atel/o _____   **14.** pneum/o _____

4. bronch/o _____   **15.** py/o _____

5. coni/o _____   **16.** rhin/o _____

6. halat/o _____   **17.** rhonch/o _____

7. laryng/o _____   **18.** spir/o _____

8. nas/o _____   **19.** thorac/o _____

9. olfact/o _____   **20.** tonsill/o _____

10. orth/o _____   **21.** trache/o _____

11. pector/o _____   **22.** tubercul/o _____

Suffixes   Give the definitions of the following suffixes.

1. -al _____   **12.** -oma _____

2. -centesis _____   **13.** -staxis _____

3. -dynia _____   **14.** –plasty _____

4. -ectasis _____   **15.** -or _____

5. -ectomy _____   **16.** -pnea _____

6. -ic _____   **17.** -ptysis _____

7. -ia _____   **18.** -rrhea _____

8. -ion _____   **19.** -scope _____

9. -itis _____   **20.** -stomy _____

10. -meter _____   **21.** -tomy _____

11. -osis _____   **22.** -us _____

Identifying Medical Terms

In the spaces provided, write the medical terms for the following meanings.

1. _____ Pertaining to a small air sac in the lungs

2. _____ Chronic dilation of a bronchus or bronchi

3. _____ Inflammation of the bronchi

4. _____ Condition of difficulty in speaking

5. _____ Good or normal breathing

6. _____ Spitting up blood

7. _____ Process of breathing in

8. _____ Inflammation of the larynx

9. _____ A collection of air between the chest wall and lungs

10. _____ Surgical repair of the nose

Matching

Select the appropriate lettered meaning for each of the following words.

_____ 1. cough

_____ 2. cystic fibrosis

_____ 3. influenza

_____ 4. inhalation

_____ 5. olfaction

_____ 6. pleurodynia

_____ 7. rhinovirus

_____ 8. sputum

_____ 9. tachypnea

_____ 10. thoracocentesis

a. Substance coughed up from the lungs

b. Pain in the pleura

c. Process of smelling

d. One of a subgroup of viruses that causes the common cold in humans

e. Rapid breathing

f. Process of breathing in

g. Surgical puncture of the chest wall for removal of fluid

h. Sudden, forceful expulsion of air from the lungs

i. Inherited disease that affects the pancreas, respiratory system, and sweat glands

j. Acute, contagious respiratory infection caused by a virus

Medical Case Snapshots

This learning activity provides an opportunity to relate the medical terminology you are learning to sample patient case presentations. In the spaces provided, write in your answers.

Case 1

A 7-year-old male is seen in the emergency room with wheezing, dyspnea, and a feeling of constriction in the chest. He is experiencing an acute exacerbation of _____. The ER personnel find that he has an inability to breathe unless he is upright. This condition is called _____ and he is placed in a sitting position.

Case 2

A 58-year-old male presents with _____ (difficulty in breathing), _____ _____ _____ (abbreviated SOB), fatigue, and wheezing. A smoker for 40 years, he has had bronchitis several times during the past 5 years. With the use of a _____ (instrument for measuring lung volume), it was determined that he had emphysema or COPD, an abbreviation for _____ _____ _____ _____.

Case 3

A 28-year-old male returns to the clinic for a follow-up visit after being diagnosed with _____ (an infectious disease caused by the tubercle bacillus). The lab performs a _____ culture (to determine the presence of pathogenic microorganisms).

Drug Highlights

Classification of Drug	Description and Examples
antihistamines	Act to counter the effects of histamine by blocking histamine 1 (H1) receptors. They are used to treat allergy symptoms, prevent or control motion sickness, and in combination with cold remedies to decrease mucus secretion and produce bedtime sedation. See Figure 10.25. EXAMPLES: Benadryl (diphenhydramine HCl), Dimetane (brompheniramine maleate), Allegra (fexofenadine), Claritin (loratadine), and Zyrtec (cetirizine)

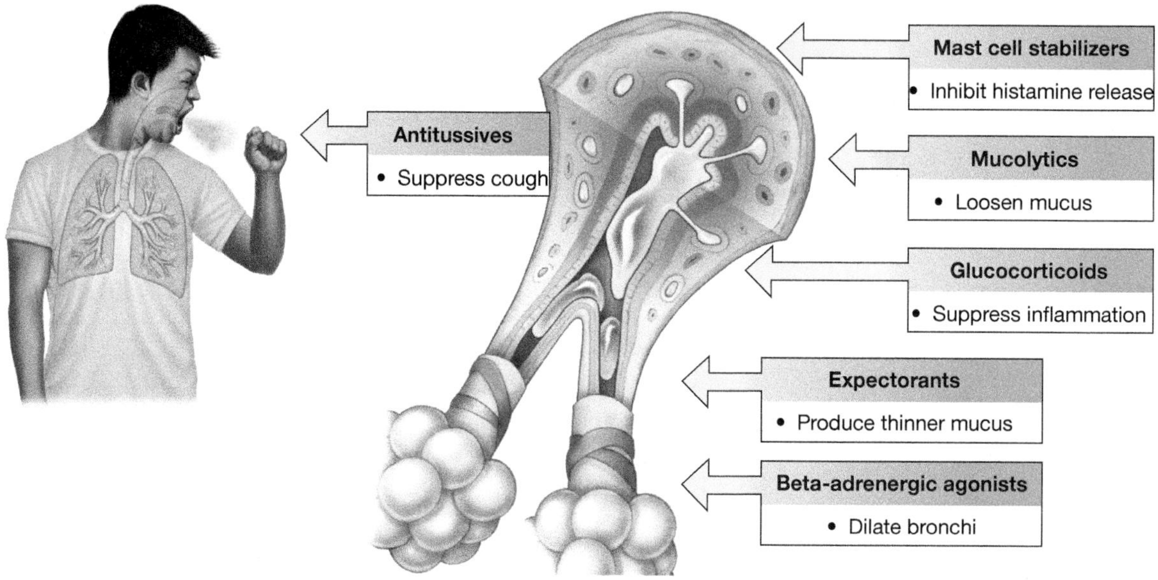

FIGURE 10.25 Drugs used to treat respiratory disorders.

decongestants	These agents are used for the temporary relief of nasal congestion associated with the common cold, hay fever, other upper respiratory allergies, and sinusitis. Refer to Figure 10.25. EXAMPLES: Sudafed (pseudoephedrine HCl) and Afrin (oxymetazoline HCl) *Note:* Sudafed is not available as an over-the-counter drug, and it can be obtained only under pharmacy supervision because it contains ingredients that can be used to make the illegal drug methamphetamine, commonly called crystal meth.
antitussives	Can be classified as non-narcotic and narcotic. Refer to Figure 10.25.
non-narcotic agents	Anesthetize the stretch receptors located in the respiratory passages, lungs, and pleura by dampening their activity and thereby reducing the cough reflex at its source. EXAMPLES: Tessalon (benzonatate), diphenhydramine HCl, and Mucinex DM (guaifenesin and dextromethorphan hydrobromide)
narcotic agents	Depress the cough center located in the medulla, thereby raising its threshold for incoming cough impulse. EXAMPLES: codeine and hydrocodone bitartrate

Classification of Drug	Description and Examples
expectorants	Promote and facilitate the removal of mucus from the lower respiratory tract. Refer to Figure 10.25. EXAMPLES: Robitussin (guaifenesin) and Mucinex DM (guaifenesin and dextromethorphan hydrobromide)
mucolytics	Break chemical bonds in mucus, thereby lowering its thickness. Refer to Figure 10.25. EXAMPLE: acetylcysteine
bronchodilators	Used to improve pulmonary airflow by dilating air passages. Refer to Figure 10.25. EXAMPLES: Proventil HFA (albuterol sulfate), ephedrine sulfate, aminophylline, Theo-24 (theophylline), and Spiriva (thiotropium)
inhalational glucocorticoids	Used in the treatment of bronchial asthma and in seasonal or perennial allergic conditions when other forms of treatment are not effective. Refer to Figure 10.25. EXAMPLES: Beconase AQ (beclomethasone dipropionate monohydrate), Nasacort AQ (triamcinolone acetonide), Flovent HFA (fluticasone propionate), and flunisolide
antituberculosis agents	Used in the long-term treatment of tuberculosis (9 months to 1 year). They are often used in combination of three or more drugs and the primary drug regimen for active tuberculosis combines the drugs Myambutol (ethambutol HCl), isoniazid, Rifadin, Rimactane (rifampin), pyrazenamide, or Rifater (isoniazid, pyrazinamide, rifampin)

Diagnostic *and* Laboratory Tests

Test	Description
acid-fast bacilli (AFB) (ăs´ĭd-făst´ bă-sĭl´ī)	Test performed on sputum to detect the presence of *Mycobacterium tuberculosis*, an acid-fast bacilli. Positive results indicate tuberculosis.
antistreptolysin O (ASO titer) (ăn˝ tī-strĕp-tŏ-lī´ sĭn)	Test performed on blood serum to detect the presence of streptolysin enzyme O, which is secreted by beta-hemolytic streptococcus. Positive results indicate streptococcal infection.
arterial blood gases (ABGs) (ăr-tēr´ ē-ăl)	Test measures the acidity (pH) and the levels of oxygen and carbon dioxide in the blood. This test is used to check how well the lungs are able to move oxygen into the blood and remove carbon dioxide from the blood. Important in determining respiratory acidosis and/or alkalosis and metabolic acidosis and/or alkalosis.

Test	Description
bronchoscopy (brŏng-kŏs´ kō-pē)	Visual examination of the larynx, trachea, and bronchi via a flexible bronchoscope. With the use of biopsy forceps, tissues and secretions can be removed for further analysis. See Figure 10.26.

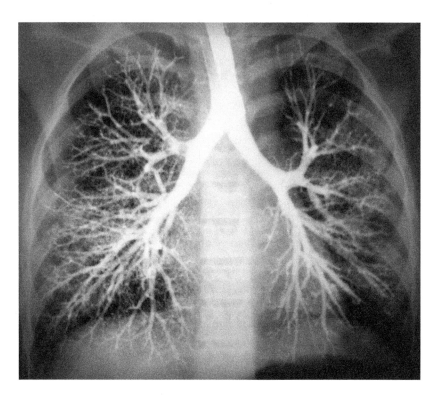

FIGURE 10.26 Image of healthy lungs obtained by bronchoscopy.
Source: Guzel Studio/Shutterstock

Test	Description
culture, sputum (spū´ tŭm)	Examination of the sputum to determine the presence of pathogenic microorganisms. Abnormal results can indicate tuberculosis, bronchitis, pneumonia, bronchiectasis, and other infectious respiratory diseases (RDs).
culture, throat	Test that identifies the presence of pathogenic microorganisms in the throat, especially beta-hemolytic streptococci.
laryngoscopy (lăr˝ ĭn-gŏs´ kō-pē)	Visual examination of the larynx via a laryngoscope.

Test	Description
pulmonary function test (pŭl′ mō-nĕ-rē)	Series of tests performed to determine the diffusion of oxygen and carbon dioxide across the cell membrane in the lungs, including tidal volume (TV), vital capacity (VC), expiratory reserve volume (ERV), inspiratory capacity (IC), residual volume (RV), forced inspiratory volume (FIV), functional residual capacity (FRC), maximal voluntary ventilation (MVV), total lung capacity (TLC), and flow volume loop (F-V loop). Abnormal results can indicate various respiratory diseases and conditions. See Figure 10.27.

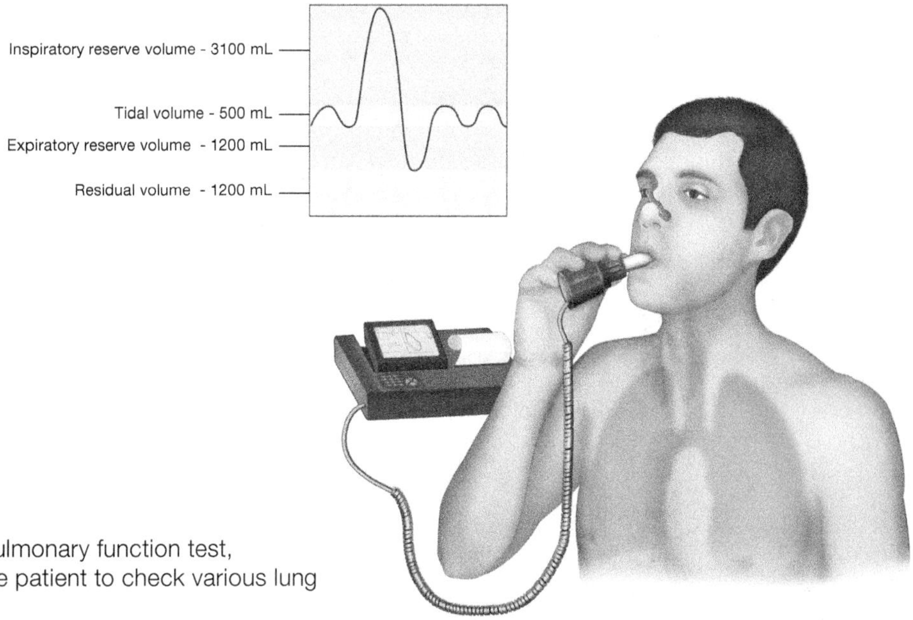

Inspiratory reserve volume - 3100 mL
Tidal volume - 500 mL
Expiratory reserve volume - 1200 mL
Residual volume - 1200 mL

FIGURE 10.27 As part of a pulmonary function test, a spirometer is being used by the patient to check various lung volume capacities.

QuantiFERON-TB Gold (QFT)	Blood test that aids in the detection of *Mycobacterium tuberculosis*, the bacteria that causes tuberculosis (TB). QFT is an interferon-gamma (IFN-γ) release assay, commonly known as an IGRA, and is a modern alternative to the tuberculin skin test (Mantoux). It is specific and sensitive, and a positive result is predictive of an infection with *Mycobacterium tuberculosis*.
rhinoscopy (rī-nŏs′ kō-pē)	Visual examination of the nasal passages.

Abbreviations *and* Acronyms

Abbreviation/ Acronym	Meaning	Abbreviation/ Acronym	Meaning
AAP	American Academy of Pediatrics	ARD	acute respiratory disease
ABGs	arterial blood gases	ARDS	acute respiratory distress syndrome
ACIP	Advisory Committee of Immunization Practices	ASO	antistreptolysin O
AFB	acid-fast bacilli	CDC	Centers for Disease Control and Prevention

Abbreviation/ Acronym	Meaning	Abbreviation/ Acronym	Meaning
CF	cystic fibrosis	NRDS	neonatal respiratory distress syndrome
CO_2	carbon dioxide	NSCLC	non-small-cell lung cancer
COPD	chronic obstructive pulmonary disease	O_2	oxygen
CXR	chest x-ray	PCV13	pneumococcal conjugate vaccine
DTaP	diphtheria, tetanus, and pertussis	PPSV23	pneumococcal polysaccharide vaccine
ERV	expiratory reserve volume	QFT	QuantiFERON-TB Gold
ET	endotracheal	R	respiration
FIV	forced inspiratory volume	RD	respiratory disease
FRC	functional residual capacity	RDS	respiratory distress syndrome
F-V loop	flow volume loop	RSV	respiratory syncytial virus
HMD	hyaline membrane disease	RV	residual volume
IC	inspiratory capacity	SARS	severe acute respiratory syndrome
IGRA	interferon-gamma (IFN-γ) release assay	SOB	shortness of breath
IRDS	infant respiratory distress syndrome	TB	tuberculosis
IRV	inspiratory reserve volume	Tdap	tetanus, diphtheria, and pertussis
IV	intravenous	TLC	total lung capacity
LTBI	latent TB infection	TV	tidal volume
MVV	maximal voluntary ventilation	VC	vital capacity

Study and Review III

Building Medical Terms

Using the following word parts, fill in the blanks to build the correct medical terms.

dys-	rhin/o	-ectasis	-pnea	-osis
pharyng	thorac/o	-staxis	-ectomy	

Definition	Medical Term
1. The collapse of an alveolus, a lobule, or a larger lung unit	atel_____
2. Literally means *difficulty in breathing*	_____pnea
3. Nosebleed	epi_____

Definition	Medical Term
4. Abnormally deep and rapid breathing	hyper_____
5. Inflammation of the pharynx	_____itis
6. Surgical excision of the left or right lung	pneumon_____
7. Surgical repair of the nose	_____plasty
8. Rapid breathing	tachy_____
9. Incision into the chest wall	_____tomy
10. Infectious disease caused by the tubercle bacillus	tubercul_____

Combining Form Challenge

Using the combining forms provided, write the medical term correctly.

anthrac/o	hem/o	olfact/o
bronch/o	laryng/o	orth/o

1. Lung condition caused by inhalation of coal dust and silica: _____osis

2. Medical instrument used to visually examine the bronchi: _____scope

3. Spitting up blood: _____ptysis

4. Medical instrument used to visually examine the larynx: _____scope

5. Process of smelling: _____ion

6. Inability to breathe unless in an upright or straight position: _____pnea

Select the Right Term

Select the correct answer, and write it on the line provided.

1. Disease of the bronchi characterized by wheezing and dyspnea is _____.

    anthracosis   asphyxia   asthma   atelectasis

2. Acute respiratory disease characterized by a barking cough is _____.

    cough   croup   cystic fibrosis   dysphonia

3. Condition of deficient amounts of oxygen in the inspired air is _____.

    eupnea   hyperpnea   hypoxemia   inhalation

4. Acute, infectious disease characterized by a cough with a "whooping" sound is _____.

laryngitis   pneumonia   pharyngitis   pertussis

5. Abnormal sound heard on auscultation of the chest; a crackling sound is _____.

rale   rhonchus   stridor   wheeze

6. One of the subgroup of viruses that causes the common cold is _____.

syncytial   rhinovirus   rhinorrhea   influenza

Drug Highlights

Match the appropriate lettered description or examples of drug(s) with the class of drug.

_____ 1. antitussives (non-narcotic)

_____ 2. antihistamines

_____ 3. mucolytics

_____ 4. antituberculosis agents

_____ 5. bronchodilators

_____ 6. decongestants

_____ 7. expectorants

_____ 8. antitussives (narcotic)

_____ 9. inhalational gluco-corticoids

_____ 10. examples of antihistamines

a. Break chemical bonds in mucus, thereby lowering its thickness

b. Used in the treatment of bronchial asthma and in seasonal or perennial allergic conditions when other forms of treatment are not effective

c. Promote and facilitate the removal of mucus from the lower respiratory tract; examples include Robitussin (guaifenesin) and Mucinex DM (guaifenesin and dextromethorphan hydrobromide)

d. Codeine depresses the cough center located in the medulla, thereby raising its threshold for incoming cough impulse

e. Often used in combination of three or more drugs; the primary drug regimen for active disease combines the drugs Myambutol (ethambutol HCl), isoniazid, Rifadin, Rimactane (rifampin), pyrazenamide, or Rifater (isoniazid, pyrazinamide, rifampin)

f. Agents that anesthetize the stretch receptors located in the respiratory passages, lungs, and pleura by dampening their activity and thereby reducing the cough reflex at its source

g. Improve pulmonary airflow by dilating air passages

h. Used to treat allergy symptoms, prevent or control motion sickness, and in combination with cold remedies to decrease mucus secretion and produce bedtime sedation

i. Agents used to provide temporary relief of nasal congestion associated with the common cold, hay fever, other upper respiratory allergies, and sinusitis; examples include Sudafed and Afrin

j. Benadryl (diphenhydramine HCl), Dimetane (brompheniramine maleate), Allegra (fexofenadine), Claritin (loratadine), Zyrtec (cetirizine)

Diagnostic and Laboratory Tests

Select the best answer to each multiple-choice question. Circle the letter of your choice.

1. Test performed on sputum to detect the presence of *Mycobacterium tuberculosis*.

   a. antistreptolysin O titer
   b. acid-fast bacilli
   c. pulmonary function test
   d. bronchoscopy

2. Visual examination of the nasal passages.

   a. bronchoscopy
   b. laryngoscopy
   c. rhinoscopy
   d. rhinoplasty

3. Test that is important in determining respiratory acidosis and/or alkalosis and metabolic acidosis and/or alkalosis.

   a. acid-fast bacilli
   b. antistreptolysin O titer
   c. arterial blood gases
   d. pulmonary function test

4. Series of tests to determine the diffusion of oxygen and carbon dioxide across the cell membrane in the lungs.

   a. acid-fast bacilli
   b. antistreptolysin O titer
   c. arterial blood gases
   d. pulmonary function test

5. Visual examination of the larynx, trachea, and bronchi via a flexible scope.

   a. bronchoscopy
   b. laryngoscopy
   c. laryngoscope
   d. rhinoscopy

Abbreviations and Acronyms

Write the correct word, phrase, or abbreviation/acronym in the space provided.

1. acid-fast bacilli _____
2. CF _____
3. TLC _____
4. chronic obstructive pulmonary disease _____
5. ET _____
6. hyaline membrane disease _____
7. respiration _____
8. SARS _____
9. shortness of breath _____
10. TB _____

Practical Application

Medical Record Analysis

This exercise contains information, abbreviations/acronyms, and medical terminology from an actual medical record or case study that has been adapted for this text. The names and any personal information have been created by the author. Read and study each form or case study and then answer the questions that follow. You may refer to Appendix III, *Abbreviations, Acronyms, and Symbols*.

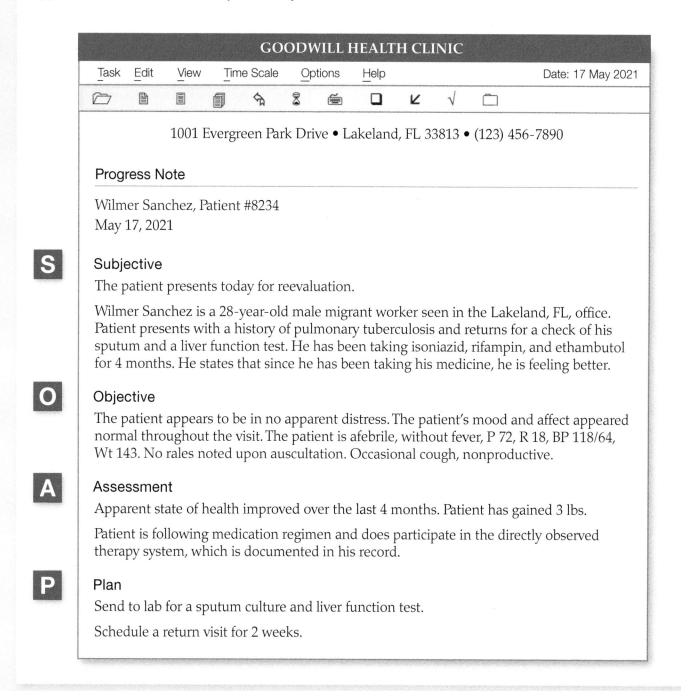

GOODWILL HEALTH CLINIC

| Task | Edit | View | Time Scale | Options | Help | | Date: 17 May 2021 |

1001 Evergreen Park Drive • Lakeland, FL 33813 • (123) 456-7890

Progress Note

Wilmer Sanchez, Patient #8234
May 17, 2021

S **Subjective**

The patient presents today for reevaluation.

Wilmer Sanchez is a 28-year-old male migrant worker seen in the Lakeland, FL, office. Patient presents with a history of pulmonary tuberculosis and returns for a check of his sputum and a liver function test. He has been taking isoniazid, rifampin, and ethambutol for 4 months. He states that since he has been taking his medicine, he is feeling better.

O **Objective**

The patient appears to be in no apparent distress. The patient's mood and affect appeared normal throughout the visit. The patient is afebrile, without fever, P 72, R 18, BP 118/64, Wt 143. No rales noted upon auscultation. Occasional cough, nonproductive.

A **Assessment**

Apparent state of health improved over the last 4 months. Patient has gained 3 lbs.

Patient is following medication regimen and does participate in the directly observed therapy system, which is documented in his record.

P **Plan**

Send to lab for a sputum culture and liver function test.

Schedule a return visit for 2 weeks.

Medical Record Exercise

Select the appropriate lettered function/description for each of the following words.

_____ **1.** afebrile

_____ **2.** rales

_____ **3.** auscultation

_____ **4.** sputum culture

_____ **5.** antituberculosis agents

a. Test to determine the presence of pathogenic microorganisms

b. Using a stethoscope to listen to sounds within the body

c. Isoniazid, rifampin, ethambutol

d. A crackling, rattling, or bubbling sound

e. Without fever

MyLab Medical Terminology™

MyLab Medical Terminology is a premium online homework management system that includes a host of features to help you study. Registered users will find:

- A multitude of quizzes and activities built within the MyLab platform
- Powerful tools that track and analyze your results—allowing you to create a personalized learning experience
- Videos and audio pronunciations to help enrich your progress
- Streaming lesson presentations (guided lectures) and self-paced learning modules
- A space where you and your instructor can check your progress and manage your assignments

11 Urinary System

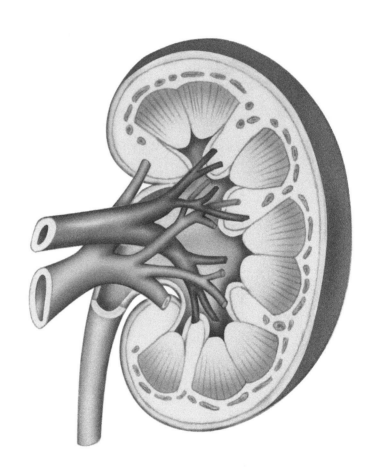

Learning Outcomes

On completion of this chapter, you will be able to:

1. Name the organs of the urinary system.
2. Identify the primary functions of the organs of the urinary system.
3. Define urinalysis and explain its role as a diagnostic tool.
4. Identify normal and abnormal constituents of urine.
5. Analyze, build, spell, and pronounce medical words.
6. Classify the drugs highlighted in this chapter.
7. Describe diagnostic and laboratory tests related to the urinary system.
8. Identify and define selected abbreviations and acronyms.

Anatomy and Physiology

The urinary system consists of two kidneys, two ureters, one bladder, and one urethra. It is also called the *excretory*, *genitourinary (GU)*, or *urogenital (UG) system* and is the organ system that produces, stores, and eliminates urine. The vital function of the urinary system is to extract certain wastes from the bloodstream, convert these materials to urine, transport the urine from the kidneys via the ureters to the bladder, and eliminate it (void) at appropriate intervals via the urethra. Through this vital function, homeostasis of body fluids is maintained. Table 11.1 provides an at-a-glance look at the urinary system. See Figure 11.1.

TABLE 11.1	Urinary System at-a-Glance
Organ/Structure	**Primary Functions/Description**
Kidneys	Produce urine, control body fluids, and help regulate the body by doing the following:
	• Remove waste and extra fluid from the body
	• Remove acid that is produced by the cells
	• Maintain healthy balance of water, salts, and minerals
	• Filter and return to the bloodstream about 200 quarts of fluid every 24 hours
	• Make erythropoietin (EPO), a hormone that stimulates the bone marrow to make red blood cells
	• Convert vitamin D into its active form (calcitriol), which is needed to maintain healthy bones
	• Make renin, an enzyme that helps regulate blood pressure
	• Make angiotensin, a protein that signals the body to retain sodium and water
Ureters	Transport urine from the kidneys to the bladder
Urinary bladder	Serves as a reservoir for urine
Urethra	Passageway of urine to the outside of the body; in the male conveys both urine and semen

Kidneys

The **kidneys** are reddish-brown, bean-shaped organs that lie against the dorsal body wall in a retroperitoneal position (behind the parietal peritoneum) in the superior lumbar region. See Figure 11.2. The kidneys extend from the thoracic vertebra (T12) to the lumbar vertebra (L3). Sitting atop each kidney is an adrenal gland, which is part of the endocrine system (discussed in Chapter 12).

Kidneys remove wastes and extra fluid from the body. As water intake decreases, the kidneys adjust accordingly and leave water in the body instead of helping to excrete it. The kidneys also remove acid that is produced by the cells of the body as they metabolize, and they remove acid that we ingest from the foods we eat. Some foods increase the acid in our body; some foods neutralize it. Kidneys help maintain a healthy balance of water, salts, and minerals—such as sodium, calcium, phosphorus, and potassium—in the blood. Without this balance, nerves, muscles, and other tissues in the body would not work properly.

The kidneys perform their life-sustaining job of filtering and returning to the bloodstream about 200 quarts of fluid every 24 hours. The kidneys produce urine; about 2 quarts of fluid are excreted from the body in the form of urine, which has been stored in

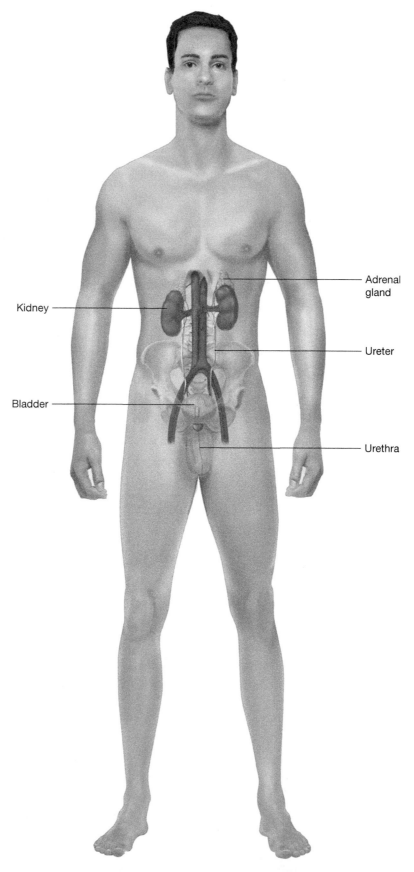

FIGURE 11.1 The urinary system: kidneys, ureters, bladder, and urethra (including the adrenal glands, which sit atop the kidneys but are part of the endocrine system).

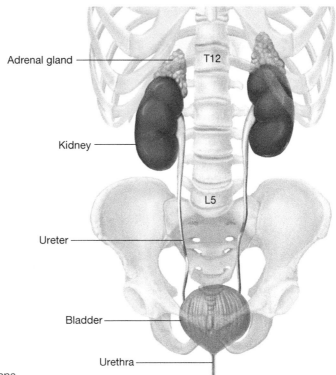

Adrenal gland

T12

Kidney

L5

Ureter

Bladder

Urethra

FIGURE 11.2 Position of the urinary organs.

the bladder for 1–8 hours. The kidneys also make erythropoietin (EPO), a hormone that stimulates the bone marrow to make red blood cells; converts vitamin D into its active form (calcitriol), which is needed to maintain healthy bones, and also helps to regulate blood pressure. The kidneys make renin, an enzyme that helps regulate blood pressure, and angiotensin, a protein that signals the body to retain sodium and water.

External Structure

Each kidney has a *concave* border and a *convex* border. The center of the concave border opens into a notch called the **hilum**. The renal artery and vein, nerves, and lymphatic vessels enter and leave through the hilum. The ureters arise from the *renal pelvis*, a saclike collecting area, located within the hilum of the kidney. The renal pelvis receives urine from the major calyces (cuplike extensions) within the kidney. Urine is collected in these calyces before it flows on into the urinary bladder. See Figure 11.3.

Internal Structure

When a cross-section is made through the kidney, two distinct areas can be seen: the **cortex**, which is the outer layer, and the **medulla** or inner portion (refer to Figure 11.3). The cortex is composed of arteries, veins, convoluted tubules, and glomerular capsules. The medulla is composed of the renal pyramids, conelike masses with papillae projecting into calices of the pelvis.

Microscopic Anatomy

Microscopic examination of the kidney reveals about 1 million **nephrons**, which are the structural and functional units of the organ (refer to Figure 11.3). Each nephron consists of two main structures, a renal corpuscle and a renal **tubule**. Each renal corpuscle consists of a **glomerulus**, which is a cluster of intertwining capillaries, and a cup-shaped hollow structure that completely surrounds the glomerulus. This portion of the renal corpuscle is called the **glomerular capsule** or *Bowman capsule*.

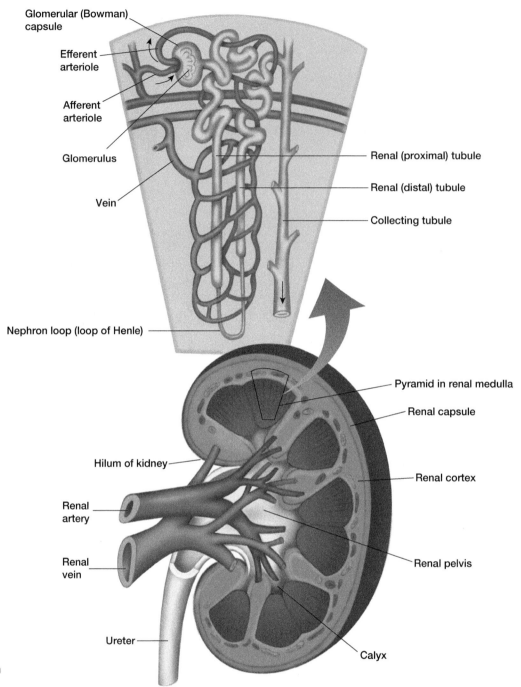

FIGURE 11.3 Kidney with an expanded view of a nephron.

The vital function of the *nephron* is to regulate, control, and then remove the waste products of metabolism from the blood plasma. These waste products are urea (chief nitrogenous constituent of urine), uric acid, and creatinine, as well as any excess sodium chloride (NaCl) and potassium ions and ketone bodies. The nephron plays a vital role in the maintenance of normal fluid balance in the body by regulated **reabsorption** of water and selected electrolytes back into the blood. Approximately 1000–1200 milliliters (mL) of blood flows through the kidney per minute. At a rate of 1000 mL of blood per minute, about 1.5 million mL flows through the kidney in each 24-hour day.

The nephrons work through a two-step process: the glomerulus filters blood, and the renal tubule (consists of three regions: proximal tubule, nephron loop [also called loop of Henle], and distal tubule) returns needed substances to blood and removes wastes. See Figure 11.4. As blood flows into each nephron, it enters a cluster of intertwining

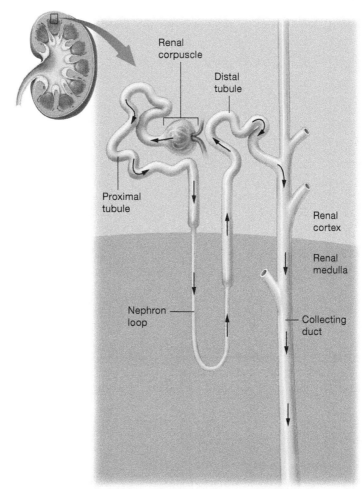

FIGURE 11.4 Nephron and collecting system. Nephrons filter the blood in the renal corpuscle and modify it as it passes through the renal tubules. The fluid then leaves the nephron and drains into the tubules of the collecting system, where it is further modified until it finally becomes urine.
Source: AMERMAN, ERIN C., HUMAN ANATOMY & PHYSIOLOGY, 2nd Ed., ©2019. Reprinted and Electronically reproduced by permission of Pearson Education, Inc., New York, NY.

capillaries, the glomerulus. The thin walls of the glomerulus allow smaller molecules, wastes, and fluid, mostly water, to pass into the tubule. Larger molecules, such as proteins and blood cells, stay in the blood vessel. A blood vessel runs alongside the renal tubule. As the filtered fluid moves along the renal tubule, the blood vessel reabsorbs almost all of the water, along with minerals and nutrients the body needs. **Glomerular filtration** is the first step in making urine. It is the process that the kidneys use to filter excess fluid and waste products out of the blood into the urine-collecting tubules of the kidney. The renal tubule helps remove excess acid from the blood. The remaining fluid and wastes in the tubule become urine.

fyi At 10 weeks' gestation, urine forms and enters the bladder of the fetus. At about the third month the fetal kidneys begin to secrete urine. The amount increases gradually as the fetus matures. The newborn's kidneys are immature and lack the ability to concentrate urine. Glomerular filtration and reabsorption are relatively low until the child is 1 or 2 years of age.

Ureters

Each kidney has a **ureter**. They are narrow, muscular tubes that drain urine from the kidneys to the bladder (refer to Figures 11.1 and 11.2). They are from 28 to 34 centimeters (cm) long and vary in diameter from 1 millimeter (mm) to 1 cm. The walls of the ureters consist of three layers: an inner coat of mucous membrane, a middle coat of smooth muscle, and an outer coat of fibrous tissue.

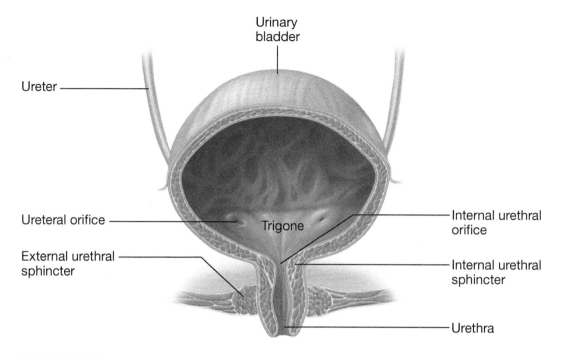

FIGURE 11.5 Structure of the female urinary bladder.
Source: MARIEB, ELAINE N.; KELLER, SUZANNE M., ESSENTIALS OF HUMAN ANATOMY & PHYSIOLOGY, 12th Ed., ©2018. Reprinted and Electronically reproduced by permission of Pearson Education, Inc., New York, NY.

Urinary Bladder

The **urinary bladder** is the muscular, membranous sac that serves as a reservoir for urine. See Figure 11.5. It is located in the anterior portion of the pelvic cavity (refer to Figures 11.1 and 11.2 for location) and consists of a lower portion, the neck, which is continuous with the urethra, and an upper portion, the apex, which is connected with the umbilicus by the median umbilical ligament. The **trigone** is a small triangular area near the base of the bladder between the openings of the two ureters and the opening of the urethra. The wall of the bladder consists of four layers: an inner layer of epithelium, a muscular coat of smooth muscle, an outer layer composed of longitudinal muscle (*detrusor urinae*), and a fibrous layer. An empty bladder feels firm as the muscular wall becomes thick.

The muscles of the bladder wall remain relaxed while the bladder fills with urine. As the bladder fills to capacity, signals sent to the brain tell a person to urinate soon. During urination, the bladder empties through the urethra, located at the bottom of the bladder.

Urethra

The **urethra** is the musculomembranous tube extending from the bladder to the outside of the body. The external urinary opening is the **urinary meatus**. The male urethra is approximately 20 cm or about 8 inches long and is divided into three sections: *prostatic, membranous,* and *penile.* It conveys both urine and semen out of the body. The female urethra is approximately 4 cm or about 1½ inches long. The urinary meatus is situated between the clitoris and the opening of the vagina. The female urethra conveys urine out of the body. See Figure 11.6.

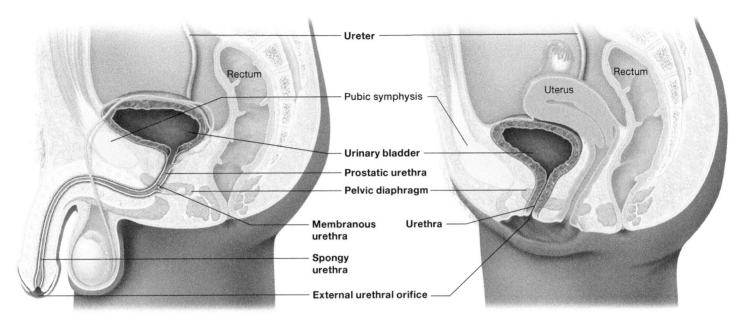

A Sagittal section through male pelvis   **B** Sagittal section through female pelvis

FIGURE 11.6 Urinary tract anatomy showing the urethra in the male and female.
Source: AMERMAN, ERIN C., HUMAN ANATOMY & PHYSIOLOGY, 2nd Ed., ©2019. Reprinted and Electronically reproduced by permission of Pearson Education, Inc., New York, NY.

 fyi **Urinary tract infections (UTIs)** are common in children. The microorganisms *Escherichia coli*, *Klebsiella*, and *Proteus* cause most urinary tract infections seen in children. The signs and symptoms of a urinary tract infection are age related. Infants can experience fever, weight loss, nausea and vomiting, increased urination (process of voiding urine), strong-smelling urine, persistent diaper rash, and failure to thrive. Older children can have frequent and/or painful urination, abdominal pain, hematuria, fever, chills, and bedwetting episodes in a trained child.

Urine

The kidneys filter unwanted substances from the blood and in this process, **urine** is produced. The three main steps of urine formation include glomerular *filtration*, *reabsorption*, and *secretion*. See Figure 11.7. These processes ensure that only waste and excess water are removed from the body. Nitrogenous wastes excreted in urine include urea, creatinine, ammonia, and uric acid. Ions such as sodium, potassium, hydrogen, and calcium are also excreted.

Urine consists of 95% water and 5% solid substances. It is secreted by the kidneys and transported by the ureters to the bladder, where it is stored before being discharged from the body via the urethra.

An average normal adult feels the need to void when the bladder contains around 300–350 mL of urine. An average of 1000–1500 mL of urine is voided daily. Normal urine is clear and yellow to amber in color and has a faintly aromatic odor, a specific gravity of 1.003–1.030, and a slightly acid pH (hydrogen ion concentration).

 fyi Changes noted in the urinary system of the older adult are loss of muscle tone in the ureters, bladder, and urethra. Bladder capacity can be reduced by half, and the older adult could have to make frequent trips to the bathroom. **Urge incontinence** (or the inability to retain urine voluntarily) is a concern for older adults. There is a leakage of urine due to bladder muscles that contract inappropriately. In men, urge incontinence can be caused by benign prostatic hyperplasia (BPH) or by prostate cancer. In most cases of urge incontinence, no specific cause can be identified. Although urge incontinence may occur in anyone at any age, it is more common in women and older adults.

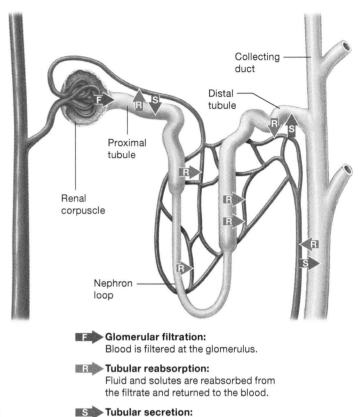

FIGURE 11.7 Sites of glomerular filtration, tubular reabsorption, and tubular secretion, the three physiological processes carried out by the kidneys to produce urine.

F **Glomerular filtration:**
Blood is filtered at the glomerulus.

R **Tubular reabsorption:**
Fluid and solutes are reabsorbed from the filtrate and returned to the blood.

S **Tubular secretion:**
Substances are secreted from the blood into the filtrate.

Urinalysis

Urinalysis (UA) is a laboratory test that evaluates the physical, chemical, and microscopic properties of urine. A freshly voided urine specimen provides for more accurate test results. A urine sample that is left standing for an extended period of time will deteriorate. If the urinalysis cannot be performed on the specimen within 1 hour of the time voided, it should be refrigerated, with the time of collection written on the label of the container. Urine should be collected in a clean, dry, disposable container. A clean-catch urine sample is preferred. The clean-catch method is used to prevent germs from the penis or vagina from getting into a urine sample. To collect the urine, the healthcare provider may give the patient a special clean-catch kit that contains a cleansing solution and sterile wipes. The patient should follow instructions exactly so that the results will be accurate.

When a bacteriological culture is to be done on urine, the specimen should be collected by **catheterization**. A urinary catheterization is the process of introducing a catheter through the urethra into the bladder for withdrawal of urine. This is a sterile procedure and performed by individuals trained and skilled in the proper technique.

Urinalysis is a valuable diagnostic tool. It can help detect substances or cellular material in the urine associated with different metabolic (glycosuria), kidney (proteinuria), and liver (biliuria) disorders. It is used to detect UTIs and other disorders of the urinary tract (nitrituria, proteinuria). See Table 11.2.

TABLE 11.2	Normal and Abnormal Constituents of Urine	
Constituent	**Normal**	**Abnormal/Significance**
Color	Yellow to amber	Red or reddish—due to presence of red blood cells
		Greenish-brown or black—due to presence of bile pigments
		Pink—due to presence of crystals
		The color of urine darkens upon standing.
Appearance	Clear	Milky—due to presence of fat globules, pus, bacteria
		Smoky—due to presence of blood cells
		Hazy—due to the formation of crystals during refrigeration
Reaction	Between 4.6 and 8.0 pH, with an average of 6.0	High acidity—due to diabetic acidosis, fever, dehydration
		Alkaline—due to UTI, renal failure
Specific gravity (sp. gr.)	Between 1.003 and 1.030	Low (1.001–1.002)—due to diabetes insipidus, kidney failure, excessive fluid intake, damage to kidney tubular cells
		High (over 1.030)—due to diabetes mellitus, hepatic disease, congestive heart failure, dehydration (due to diarrhea or vomiting)
Odor	Faintly aromatic	Fruity/sweet—due to presence of acetone, associated with diabetes mellitus
		Unpleasant—due to decomposition of drugs, foods, alcohol
		Strong/strange—due to presence of bacterial infection
Quantity	Around 1000–1500 mL per day	High—due to excessive intake of fluids, diabetes mellitus, diabetes insipidus, diuretic use
		Low—due to dehydration, acute nephritis, heart disease, diarrhea, vomiting
		None—due to uremia, end-stage renal disease (ESRD)
Protein	Negative	Positive (proteinuria)—due to renal disease, pyelonephritis, high blood pressure, kidney infection or disease, heart disease, diabetes, lupus, malaria
Glucose	Negative	Positive (glycosuria)—due to diabetes mellitus
Ketones	Negative	Positive (ketonuria)—due to uncontrolled diabetes mellitus; high-protein, low-carbohydrate diet; starvation
Bilirubin	Negative	Positive (biliuria)—due to liver disease, biliary obstruction, congestive heart failure
Blood	Negative	Positive (hematuria)—due to renal disease, trauma
Nitrites	Negative	Positive (nitrituria)—due to bacteriuria
Urobilinogen	0.1–1.0	Absent—due to biliary obstruction
		Reduced—due to antibiotic therapy
		Increased—early warning of hepatic or hemolytic disease

Study *and* Review I

Anatomy and Physiology

Write your answers to the following questions.

1. List the organs of the urinary system.

   a. _____   c. _____

   b. _____   d. _____

2. State the vital function of the urinary system. _____

   _____

3. Define *hilum*. _____

4. Define *renal pelvis*. _____

5. The medulla is the _____ portion of the kidney.

6. Define *nephron*. _____

7. Each nephron consists of a _____ and a _____.

8. The renal corpuscle consists of the _____ and the _____

   _____.

9. The three main steps of urine formation include glomerular filtration, _____, and
   secretion.

10. An average of _____ to _____ mL of urine is voided daily.

11. Describe the ureters and state their function. _____

    _____

12. Describe the urinary bladder and state its function. _____

    _____

13. The external urinary opening is the _____.

14. Define *urinalysis*. _____

    _____

15. Give the normal constituents for the physical examination of urine.

    a. Color _____   **d.** Specific gravity _____

    b. Appearance _____   **e.** Odor _____

    c. Reaction _____   **f.** Quantity _____

16. Urine that has a fruity, sweet odor can indicate _____

_____.

17. Under chemical examination, the presence of protein in urine is an important sign of _____

_____.

▶ **ANATOMY LABELING**   **Identify the structures shown below by filling in the blanks.**

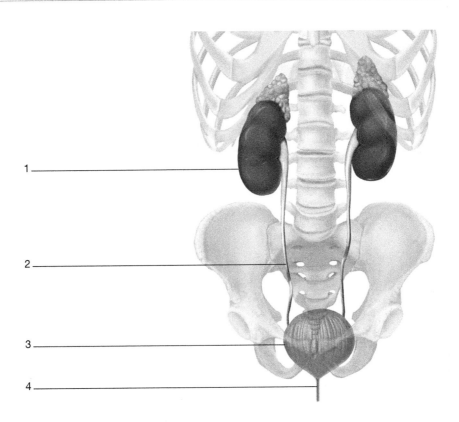

1. _____

2. _____

3. _____

4. _____

Building Your Medical Vocabulary

This section provides the foundation for learning medical terminology. Review the alphabetized list of medical terms in the following pages. Note how common prefixes and suffixes are repeatedly applied to word roots and combining forms to create different meanings. A combining form is a word root plus a vowel. The chart below lists the combining forms and word roots used in this chapter and can help to strengthen your understanding of how medical words are built and spelled.

You will find that some terms have not been divided into word parts. These are common words or specialized terms that are included to enhance your medical vocabulary.

Combining Forms

albumin/o	protein	nephr/o	kidney
bacteri/o	bacteria	noct/o	night
bil/i	bile	perine/o	perineum
calc/i	calcium	peritone/o	peritoneum
corpor/o	body	py/o	pus
cutane/o	skin	pyel/o	renal pelvis
cyst/o	bladder	ren/o	kidney
glomerul/o	glomerulus, little ball	scler/o	hardening
glycos/o	glucose, sugar	son/o	sound
hem/o	blood	ur/o	urine, urinate, urination
hemat/o	blood	ureter/o	ureter
keton/o	ketone	urethr/o	urethra
lith/o	stone	urinat/o	urine
meat/o	passage		

Word Roots

contin	to hold	strict	to draw, to bind
excretor	sifted out	uret	urine
log	study		

Medical Word	Word Parts		Definition
	Part	**Meaning**	
albuminuria (ăl-bū″ mĭ-noo′ rē-ă)	**albumin** **-uria**	protein urine	Indicates the presence of serum protein in the urine. Albumin is the major protein in blood plasma. When detected in urine (*albuminuria*), it may indicate a leak in the glomerular membrane, which allows albumin to enter the renal tubule and pass into the urine.
antidiuretic (ăn″ tĭ-dī″ ū-rĕt′ ĭk)	**anti-** **di(a)-** **uret** **-ic**	against complete, through urine pertaining to	Pertaining to a medication that decreases urine production and secretion
anuria (ăn-ū′ rē-ă)	**an-** **-uria**	without urine	Literally means *without the formation of urine*; lack of urine production
bacteriuria (băk-tēr″ ē-ū′ rē-ă)	**bacteri** **-uria**	bacteria urine	Presence of bacteria in the urine
calciuria (kăl″ sĭ-ū′ rē-ă)	**calc/i** **-uria**	calcium urine	Presence of calcium in the urine
calculus (kăl′ kū-lŭs)			Pebble; any abnormal concretion (*stone*); plural: calculi. See Figure 11.8.

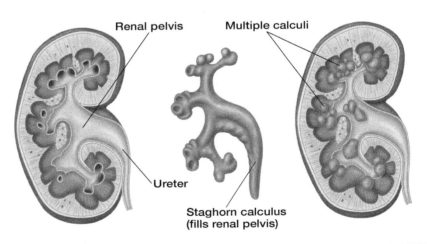

FIGURE 11.8 Urinary calculi.

Medical Word	Word Parts		Definition
	Part	Meaning	
catheter (kăth´ ĕ-tĕr)			Tube of plastic, silicone, rubber, or plastic that is inserted into a body cavity to remove fluid or to inject fluid. See Figure 11.9.

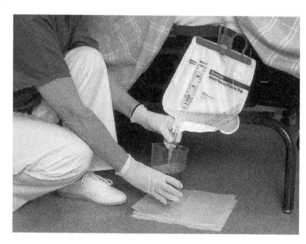

FIGURE 11.9 Closed urinary drainage system. Urine being measured after it leaves patient's body via catheter.
Source: Pearson Education, Inc.

Medical Word	Word Parts		Definition
chronic kidney disease (CKD)			Disease that results from any condition that causes gradual loss of kidney function. When the kidneys are damaged and cannot filter blood as well as healthy kidneys, waste from the blood remains in the body. CKD can lead to kidney failure. Diabetes and high blood pressure are the most common causes of CKD. See *dialysis* and *renal transplantation* for treatment options.
cystectomy (sĭs-tĕk´ tō-mē)	cyst -ectomy	bladder surgical excision	Surgical excision of the bladder or part of the bladder
cystitis (sĭs-tī´ tĭs)	cyst -itis	bladder inflammation	Inflammation of the bladder, usually occurring secondarily to ascending urinary tract infections. More than 85% of cases of cystitis are caused by *Escherichia coli*, a bacillus found in the lower gastrointestinal tract.

 fyi Cystitis is very common and occurs in more than 3 million Americans a year. It frequently affects sexually active women age 20–50 but can also occur in those who are not sexually active or in young girls and older adults. Females are more prone to cystitis because of their shorter urethra (bacteria do not have to travel as far to enter the bladder) and because of the short distance between the opening of the urethra and the anus.

Interstitial cystitis (IC) is a painful inflammation of the bladder wall. Approximately 1.3 million Americans suffer from this condition and, of those, 90% are women. Symptoms can vary from mild to severe. The cause is unknown, and IC does not respond well to antibiotic therapy.

Medical Word	Word Parts		Definition
	Part	**Meaning**	
cystocele (sĭs´ tō-sēl)	**cyst/o** **-cele**	bladder hernia	Hernia of the bladder that protrudes into the vagina
cystogram (sĭs´ tō-grăm)	**cyst/o** **-gram**	bladder a mark, record	An x-ray record of the bladder

> **! ALERT!**
>
> How many words can you build using the root **cyst** and the combining form **cyst/o**?

Medical Word	Word Parts		Definition
cystolith (sĭs´ tō-lĭth)	**cyst/o** **-lith**	bladder stone	A bladder stone; a vesical calculus
cystoscope (sĭst´ ŏ-skōp)	**cyst/o** **-scope**	bladder instrument for examining	Medical instrument used for visual examination of the bladder
dialysis (dī-ăl´ ĭ-sĭs)	**dia-** **-lysis**	complete, through destruction, separation	Medical procedure to separate waste material from the blood and to maintain fluid, electrolyte, and acid-base balance in impaired kidney function or in the absence of a kidney. The two main types of dialysis, hemodialysis (HD) (refer to Figure 11.12) and peritoneal dialysis (PD) (refer to Figure 11.16), remove wastes from the blood in different ways.
diuresis (dī˝ ū-rē´ sĭs)	**di(a)-** **ur** **-esis**	complete, through urinate condition	Pathological condition of increased or excessive flow of urine; occurs in conditions such as diabetes mellitus and diabetes insipidus. Diuretics can also produce diuresis.

fyi   *Diabetes mellitus* is a disease characterized by elevated levels of glucose in the blood and urine. In this disease there is a defect in insulin production, insulin secretion, or both.

   Diabetes insipidus is a disease in which the secretion of or response to vasopressin, a pituitary hormone, is impaired. With this disease a very large quantity of urine is produced, often with dehydration and insatiable thirst occurring.

Medical Word	Word Parts		Definition
dysuria (dĭs-ū´ rē-ă)	**dys-** **-uria**	difficult, painful urine	Difficult or painful urination
edema (ĕ-dē´ mă)			Pathological condition in which the body tissues contain an accumulation of fluid
enuresis (ĕn˝ ū-rē´ sĭs)	**en-** **ur** **-esis**	within urinate condition	Condition of involuntary emission of urine; *bedwetting*

Medical Word	Word Parts		Definition
	Part	**Meaning**	
excretory (ĕks´ krĕ-tōr˝ ē)	**excretor** **-y**	sifted out pertaining to	Pertaining to the elimination of waste products from the body
extracorporeal shock wave lithotripsy (ESWL) (ĕks˝ tră-kor-por´ ē-ăl lĭth´ ō-trip˝ sē)	**extra-** **corpor** **-eal** **lith/o** **-tripsy**	outside, beyond body pertaining to stone crushing	Process whereby a medical device is used to crush kidney stones (*renal calculi*). The patient is usually sedated and a computerized x-ray machine is used to pinpoint the location of the stone within the kidney. A series of shock waves (several hundred to two thousand) is administered to the stone, pounding it until it crumbles into small pieces. These pieces are generally flushed out with urine. See Figure 11.10.

(ESWL)
Extracorporeal Shock Wave Lithotripsy

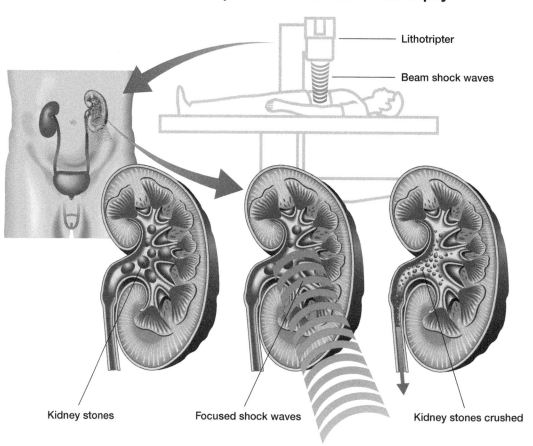

FIGURE 11.10 Illustration of extracorporeal shock wave lithotripsy.
Source: Roberto Biasini/123RF

Medical Word	Word Parts		Definition
	Part	**Meaning**	
glomerular (glō-měr′ ū-lăr)	**glomerul** **-ar**	glomerulus, little ball pertaining to	Literally means *pertaining to the glomerulus*; a network of blood vessels located within the glomerular (Bowman) capsule that permits a greater surface area for filtration

> **! ALERT!**
>
> To change *glomerulus* to its singular form, you change *us* to *i* to make *glomeruli*.

Medical Word	Word Parts		Definition
glomerulitis (glō-měr″ ū-lī′ tĭs)	**glomerul** **-itis**	glomerulus, little ball inflammation	Inflammation of the renal glomeruli
glomerulonephritis (glō-měr″ ū-lō-ně-frī′ tĭs)	**glomerul/o** **nephr** **-itis**	glomerulus, little ball kidney inflammation	Inflammation of the kidney involving primarily the glomeruli. There are three types: acute glomerulonephritis (AGN), chronic glomerulonephritis (CGN), and subacute glomerulonephritis.

fyi   **Acute nephritic syndrome (ANS)** is a group of symptoms that occur with some disorders that cause glomerulonephritis. It is often caused by an immune response triggered by an infection (causing inflammation) or other disease. The inflammation affects the function of the glomerulus, the part of the kidney that filters blood to make urine and remove waste. As a result, blood and protein appear in the urine and excess fluid builds up in the body. Swelling of the body occurs when the blood loses a protein called *albumin*, which keeps fluid in the blood vessels. When it is lost, fluid collects in the body tissues. Blood loss from the damaged kidney structures leads to blood in the urine. Acute nephritic syndrome may be related to acute kidney/renal failure and high blood pressure.

    Common symptoms of nephritic syndrome include blood in the urine (hematuria); dark, tea-colored, or cloudy urine; decreased urine output (oliguria); lack of urine output; and swelling (edema) of the face, eyes, legs, arms, hands, feet, abdomen, or other areas.

Medical Word	Word Parts		Definition
glycosuria (glī″ kō-soo′ rē-ă)	**glycos** **-uria**	glucose, sugar urine	Presence of glucose in the urine

Medical Word	Word Parts		Definition
	Part	Meaning	
hematuria (hē″ mă-toor′ ē-ă)	**hemat** **-uria**	blood urine	Presence of red blood cells (erythrocytes) in the urine. In microscopic hematuria, the urine appears normal to the naked eye, but examination with a microscope shows a high number of RBCs. Gross hematuria can be seen with the naked eye—the urine is red or the color of cola. If white blood cells are found in addition to red blood cells, then it is a sign of urinary tract infection. See Figure 11.11.

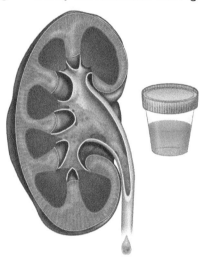

FIGURE 11.11 Hematuria. Note the color of urine in the specimen container.

Medical Word	Word Parts		Definition
hemodialysis (HD) (hē″ mō-dī-ăl′ ĭ-sĭs)	**hem/o** **dia-** **-lysis**	blood through, complete separation	Use of an artificial kidney to separate waste from the blood. The blood is circulated through tubes made of semi-permeable membranes, and these tubes are continually bathed by solutions that remove waste. See Figure 11.12.

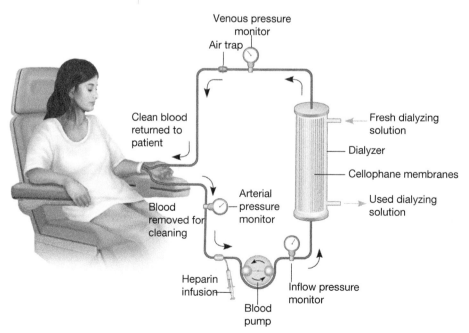

FIGURE 11.12 Schematic of hemodialysis machine.

Medical Word	Word Parts		Definition
	Part	Meaning	
hydronephrosis (hī″ drō-něf-rō′ sĭs)	hydro- nephr -osis	water kidney condition	Pathological condition in which urine collects in the renal pelvis because of an obstructed outflow, thereby causing distention and damage to the kidney; can be caused by renal calculi, tumor, or hyperplasia of the prostate gland. See Figure 11.13.

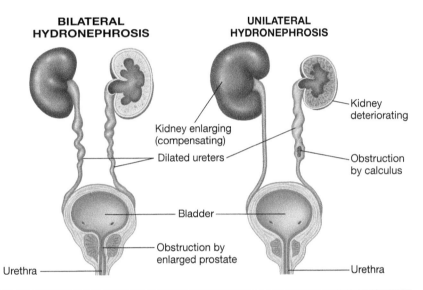

BILATERAL HYDRONEPHROSIS

UNILATERAL HYDRONEPHROSIS

Kidney enlarging (compensating)

Dilated ureters

Kidney deteriorating

Obstruction by calculus

Bladder

Obstruction by enlarged prostate

Urethra

Urethra

FIGURE 11.13 Hydronephrosis.

Medical Word	Word Parts		Definition
hypercalciuria (hī″ pěr-kăl″ sĭ-ū′ rē-ă)	hyper- calci -uria	excessive calcium urine	Excessive amount of calcium in the urine
incontinence (ĭn-kŏn′ tĭ-nens)	in- contin -ence	not to hold state	Inability to hold or control urination or defecation
interstitial cystitis (IC) (ĭn″ ter-stĭsh′ al sĭs-tī′ tĭs)			Chronically irritable and painful inflammation of the bladder wall
ketonuria (kē″ tō-nūr′ ē-ă)	keton -uria	ketone urine	Presence of ketones in the urine resulting from breakdown of fats due to faulty or inadequate carbohydrate metabolism. It occurs primarily as a complication of diabetes mellitus but can occur in dieting and starvation.
lithotripsy (lĭth′ ō-trĭp″ sē)	lith/o -tripsy	stone crushing	Crushing of a kidney stone (refer to Figures 11.10 and 11.15)
meatotomy (mē″ ă-tŏt′ ō-mē)	meat/o -tomy	passage incision	Incision of the urinary meatus to enlarge the opening
meatus (mē-ā′ tŭs)			Opening or passage; the external opening of the urethra

Medical Word	Word Parts		Definition
	Part	Meaning	
nephrectomy (nĕ-frĕk´ tō-mē)	**nephr** **-ectomy**	kidney surgical excision	Surgical excision of a kidney
nephritis (nĕ-frīt´ ĭs)	**nephr** **-itis**	kidney inflammation	Inflammation of the kidneys
nephrolithiasis (nĕf″ rō-lĭ-thī´ ă-sĭs)	**nephr/o** **lith** **-iasis**	kidney stone, calculus condition	Commonly called *kidney stones*; usually deposits of mineral salts, called *calculi*, in the kidney. These stones can pass into the ureter, irritate kidney tissue, and block urine flow. Kidney stones occur when the urine has a high level of minerals (usually calcium) that form stones. See Figure 11.14.

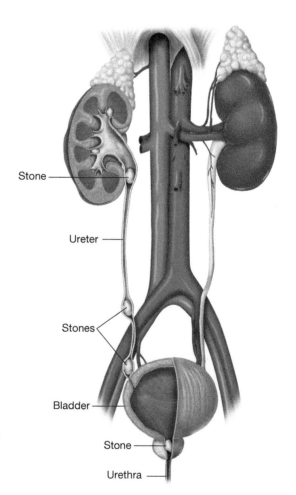

Stone

Ureter

Stones

Bladder

Stone

Urethra

FIGURE 11.14 Renal calculi (stones) can form in several areas within the urinary tract. When they form in the kidney, they usually arise within the renal pelvis, forming the condition called nephrolithiasis. Stones can also form obstructions in the ureter, bladder, or urethra.

Medical Word	Word Parts		Definition
	Part	Meaning	

fyi Kidney stones are a common and painful disorder of the urinary tract. Men tend to be affected more frequently than women. Most kidney stones pass out of the body without any intervention, but stones that cause lasting symptoms or other complications should be treated. Two treatment techniques used are **extracorporeal shock wave lithotripsy (ESWL)** (refer to Figure 11.10) or **percutaneous ultrasonic lithotripsy (PUL)** (refer to Figure 11.15).

Usually, the first symptom of a kidney stone is extreme pain, which begins suddenly when a stone moves in the urinary tract, causing irritation or blockage. A sharp, cramping pain in the back and side in the area of the kidney or in the lower abdomen is felt; nausea and vomiting may occur. If the stone is too large to pass easily, pain continues and blood may appear in the urine.

Medical Word	Part	Meaning	Definition
nephrology (ně-frŏl´ ō-jē)	**nephr/o** **-logy**	kidney study of	Literally means *study of the kidney*; study of kidney function as well as diagnosis and treatment of renal diseases
nephroma (ně-frō´ mă)	**nephr** **-oma**	kidney tumor	Kidney tumor
nephron (něf´ rŏn)			Basic structural and functional unit of the kidney
nephropathy (ně-frŏp´ ă-thē)	**nephr/o** **-pathy**	kidney disease	Pathological disease of the kidney
nephrosclerosis (něf˝ rō-sklě-rō´ sĭs)	**nephr/o** **scler** **-osis**	kidney hardening condition	Condition of hardening of the kidney

fyi **Nephrotic syndrome**, also known as **nephrosis**, is a group of symptoms that includes protein in the urine (proteinuria), low blood protein levels (hypoalbuminemia), and swelling (edema). It may affect anyone regardless of age, gender, or race. Some of the causes are nephropathy and systemic diseases such as untreated/uncontrolled hypertension, diabetes, and lupus erythematosus (an autoimmune disease in which the body's immune system mistakenly attacks healthy tissue). Nephrotic syndrome can be termed *primary*, specific to the kidneys, or can be termed *secondary*, a renal manifestation of a systemic disease. In all cases, damage to the glomeruli is an essential feature, leading to the release of too much protein into the urine. The most common symptom is swelling (edema) in the face and around the eyes; in the arms and legs, especially the feet and ankles; and in the abdominal area.

Medical Word	Part	Meaning	Definition
nocturia (nŏk-tū´ rē-ă)	**noct** **-uria**	night urine	Urination during the night

Medical Word	Word Parts		Definition
	Part	Meaning	
oliguria (ŏl-ĭg-ū′ rē-ă)	olig- -uria	scanty urine	Scanty, decreased amount of urine. The decreased production of urine may be a sign of dehydration, renal failure, hypovolemic shock, multiple organ dysfunction syndrome, or urinary obstruction/urinary retention. It can be contrasted with anuria, which represents a more complete suppression of urination.
percutaneous ultrasonic lithotripsy (PUL) (pĕr″ kū-tā′ nē-ŭs ŭl-tră-sŏn′ ĭk lĭth′ ō-trĭp″ sē)	per- cutane -ous ultra- son -ic lith/o -tripsy	through skin pertaining to beyond sound pertaining to stone crushing	Crushing of a kidney stone by using ultrasound. This is an invasive surgical procedure performed by using a nephroscope. See Figure 11.15.

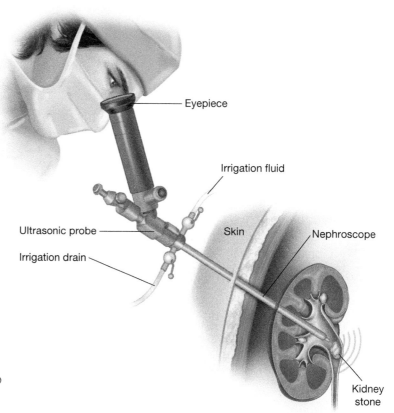

FIGURE 11.15 Percutaneous ultrasonic lithotripsy. A nephroscope is inserted into the renal pelvis, and ultrasound waves are used to fragment the stones. The fragments are then removed through the nephroscope.

Medical Word	Word Parts		Definition
	Part	Meaning	
peritoneal dialysis (PD) (pĕr″ĭ-tō-nē′ ăl dī-ăl′ ĭ-sĭs)	peritone -al dia- -lysis	peritoneum pertaining to complete, through to separate	Separation of waste from the blood by using a peritoneal catheter and dialysis. Fluid is introduced into the peritoneal cavity, and wastes from the blood pass into this fluid. The fluid and waste are then removed from the body. Types of peritoneal dialysis are IPD (intermittent) and CAPD (continuous ambulatory). See Figure 11.16.

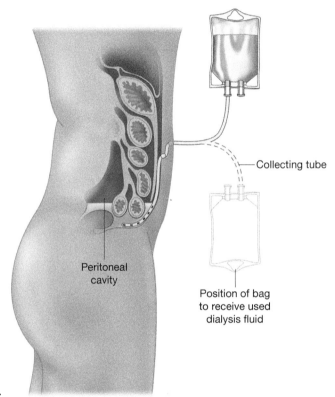

Collecting tube

Peritoneal cavity

Position of bag to receive used dialysis fluid

FIGURE 11.16 Peritoneal dialysis.

periurethral (pĕr″ĭ-ū-rē′ thrăl)	peri- urethr -al	around urethra pertaining to	Literally means *pertaining to around the urethra*; the immediate area surrounding the urethra
polyuria (pŏl″ē-ūr′ ē-ă)	poly- -uria	much urine	Literally means *much urine*; frequent urination; occurs in diabetes mellitus, chronic nephritis, and nephrosclerosis; can be induced with diuretics and following excessive intake of liquids
pyelitis (pī″ ĕ-lī′ tĭs)	pyel -itis	renal pelvis inflammation	Inflammation of the renal pelvis

Medical Word	Word Parts		Definition
	Part	Meaning	
pyelolithotomy (pī″ ĕ-lō-lĭth-ŏt′ ō-mē)	**pyel/o** **lith/o** **-tomy**	renal pelvis stone incision	Surgical incision into the renal pelvis for removal of a stone
pyelonephritis (pī″ ĕ-lō-nĕ-frīt′ ĭs)	**pyel/o** **nephr** **-itis**	renal pelvis kidney inflammation	Inflammation of the kidney and renal pelvis. It is usually caused by bacteria entering the kidneys from the bladder. *Escherichia coli* is a bacillus that is normally found in the large intestine. These infections usually spread from the lower urinary tract via the urethra, to the ureters, and then into the renal pelvis. See Figure 11.17.

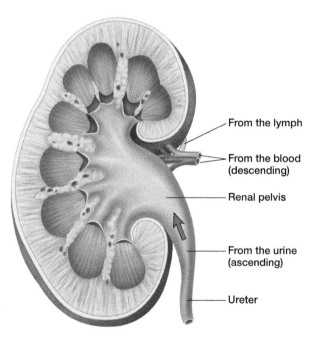

FIGURE 11.17 Routes of infection for pyelonephritis.

pyuria (pī-ūr′ ē-ă)	**py** **-uria**	pus urine	Pus or white blood cells in the urine; caused by infection (most commonly bacterial) or response to an inflammatory process in the body
renal (rē′ năl)	**ren** **-al**	kidney pertaining to	Pertaining to the kidney
renal colic (kŏl′ ĭk)			Sharp, severe pain in the lower back over the kidney, radiating forward into the groin. It usually accompanies forcible dilation of a ureter, followed by spasm as a stone is lodged or passed through it.
renal failure			Pathological failure of the kidney to function; also referred to as *kidney failure*

Medical Word	Word Parts		Definition
	Part	Meaning	
renal transplantation			The organ transplant of a healthy donor kidney into a patient with end-stage renal disease. The transplanted kidney takes over the work of the two kidneys that failed, so dialysis is no longer needed. Also called *kidney transplantation*. See Figure 11.18.

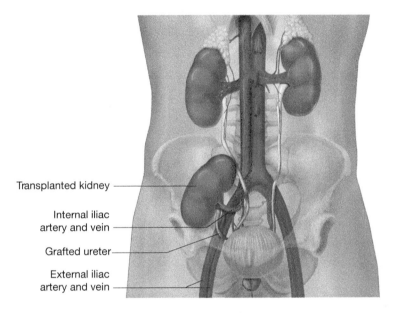

Transplanted kidney

Internal iliac artery and vein

Grafted ureter

External iliac artery and vein

FIGURE 11.18 Placement of transplanted kidney.

Medical Word	Word Parts		Definition
renin (rĕn´ ĭn)			An enzyme produced by the kidney that stimulates vasoconstriction and secretion of aldosterone. The blood renin level is elevated in some types of hypertension.
sediment (sĕd´ ĭ-mĕnt)			Substance that settles at the bottom of a liquid; a precipitate; can be produced by centrifuging urine or other body fluids
sterile (stĕr´ ĭl)			State of being free from living microorganisms; *aseptic*
uremia (ū-rē´ mē-ă)	ur -emia	urine blood condition	Excess of urea, creatinine, and other nitrogenous end products of protein and amino acid metabolism accumulated in the blood; also referred to as *azotemia*. In current usage, it refers to the syndrome associated with end-stage renal failure.
ureteroplasty (ū-rē´ tĕr-ō-plăs˝ tē)	ureter/o -plasty	ureter surgical repair	Surgical repair of a ureter

Medical Word	Word Parts		Definition
	Part	Meaning	
ureterostomy (ū-rē″tĕr-ŏs′ tō-mē)	ureter/o -stomy	ureter new opening	Surgical creation of a new opening into the ureter to provide an alternate route for drainage of urine. Example: cutaneous ureter is the surgical implantation of the ureter into the skin.
urethral stricture (ū-rē′ thrăl strĭk′ chŭr)	urethr -al strict -ure	urethra pertaining to to draw, to bind process	Narrowing or constriction of the urethra
urethroperineal (ū-rē″ thrō-pĕr″ ĭ-nē′ ăl)	urethr/o perine -al	urethra perineum pertaining to	Pertaining to the urethra and perineum

> **! ALERT!**
>
> Note the difference between the combining forms **ureter/o** and **urethr/o**. The *ureters* are tubes that lead from the kidney to the bladder and the *urethra* is a tube that leads from the bladder to the outside of the body. What a difference a few letters make!

urgency			Sudden need to void, urinate
urination (ūr″ ĭ-nā′ shŏn)	urinat -ion	urine process	The release of urine from the bladder through the urethra to the outside of the body; to void
urobilin (ū″ rō-bī′ lĭn)	ur/o bil -in	urine, urinate, urination bile substance	Brown pigment formed by the oxidation of urobilinogen; may be formed in the urine after exposure to air
urochrome (ū′ rō-krōm)			Pigment that gives urine the normal yellow color
urologist (ū-rŏl′ ō-jĭst)	ur/o log -ist	urination study one who specializes	Physician who specializes in the study of the urinary system
urology (ū-rŏl′ ō-jē)	ur/o -logy	urination study of	Study of the urinary system

Study *and* Review II

Word Parts

Prefixes Give the definitions of the following prefixes.

1. an- _____

2. anti- _____

3. dia- _____

4. dys- _____

5. en- _____

6. hydro- _____

7. extra- _____

8. in- _____

9. olig- _____

10. per- _____

11. ultra- _____

12. poly- _____

Combining Forms Give the definitions of the following combining forms.

1. albumin/o _____

2. bacter/i _____

3. calc/i _____

4. corpor/o _____

5. cyst/o _____

6. glomerul/o _____

7. glycos/o _____

8. hemat/o _____

9. keton/o _____

10. lith/o _____

11. meat/o _____

12. nephr/o _____

13. noct/o _____

14. perine/o _____

15. peritone/o _____

16. pyel/o _____

17. ren/o _____

18. son/o _____

19. ur/o _____

20. ureter/o _____

21. urethr/o _____

22. urinat/o _____

Suffixes Give the definitions of the following suffixes.

1. -a _____

2. -ar _____

3. -cele _____

4. -y _____

5. -ous _____

6. -ectomy _____

7. -emia _____

8. -gram _____

9. -ic _____

10. -in _____

11. -ion _____

12. -ist _____

13. -itis _____

14. -lith _____

15. -logy _____

16. -lysis _____

17. -tripsy _____

18. -ure _____

19. -oma _____

20. -osis _____

21. -pathy _____

22. -plasty _____

23. -scope _____

24. -esis _____

25. -stomy _____

26. -tomy _____

27. -uria _____

Identifying Medical Terms

In the spaces provided, write the medical terms for the following meanings.

1. _____ Pertaining to a medication that decreases urine production and secretion

2. _____ Surgical excision of the bladder or part of the bladder

3. _____ Inflammation of the bladder

4. _____ Difficult or painful urination

5. _____ Inflammation of the renal glomeruli

6. _____ Excessive amount of calcium in the urine

7. _____ Process of voiding urine

8. _____ Kidney stones

9. _____ Pertaining to around the urethra

10. _____ Pus in the urine

Matching

Select the appropriate lettered meaning for each of the following words.

_____ 1. ESWL

_____ 2. hemodialysis

_____ 3. lithotripsy

_____ 4. peritoneal dialysis

_____ 5. renal colic

_____ 6. urethral stricture

_____ 7. urgency

_____ 8. urination

_____ 9. urochrome

_____ 10. urology

a. Sharp, severe pain in the lower back over the kidney radiating forward into the groin caused by a stone in a ureter

b. Crushing of a kidney stone

c. Process of voiding urine

d. Medical device used to crush kidney stones

e. Use of an artificial kidney to separate waste from the blood

f. Separation of waste from the blood by using a peritoneal catheter and dialysis

g. Narrowing or constriction of the urethra

h. Pigment that gives urine its normal yellow color

i. Study of the urinary system

j. Sudden need to void, urinate

Medical Case Snapshots

This learning activity provides an opportunity to relate the medical terminology you are learning to sample patient case presentations. In the spaces provided, write in your answers.

Case 1

A 10-year-old girl is referred to an urologist. She complained that "It hurts me every time I have to go to the bathroom and I go a lot at night." The medical term _____ means painful urination and the term _____ means urination during the night. The clean-catch urine specimen appeared smoky and had an unpleasant odor. Under microscopic examination, the urine was found to contain red blood cells. This condition is called _____.

Case 2

The physician ordered a complete UA, an abbreviation for _____. The results show: *color* (reddish), which indicated the presence of _____; *reaction* 9.0 pH (alkaline urine), which is indicative of _____ _____ _____; and *nitrites positive*, indicating _____ (presence of bacteria in the urine). The diagnosis of _____ (inflammation of the bladder) was confirmed.

Case 3

A 30-year-old male is seen in the ER. He complains of sharp, severe pain in the lower back, over the kidney, radiating forward into his groin. Because of the patient's symptoms, the physician wants to evaluate him for

_____ (commonly called kidney stones). Two treatment techniques that can be

used are: ESWL, which stands for _____ _____

_____ lithotripsy, and PUL, or percutaneous _____

lithotripsy.

Drug Highlights

Classification of Drug	Description and Examples
diuretics	Decrease in reabsorption of sodium chloride by the kidneys, thereby increasing the amount of salt and water excreted in the urine. This action reduces the amount of fluid retained in the body and prevents edema. Diuretics are classified according to site and mechanism of action. The following are different types of diuretics.
thiazide	Appear to act by inhibiting sodium and chloride reabsorption in the early portion of the distal tubule. EXAMPLES: Diuril (chlorothiazide), hydrochlorothiazide, and indapamide
loop	Act by inhibiting the reabsorption of sodium and chloride in the ascending loop of Henle. EXAMPLES: bumetanide and Lasix (furosemide)
potassium sparing	Act by inhibiting the exchange of sodium for potassium in the distal tubule; inhibits potassium excretion. EXAMPLES: Aldactone (spironolactone) and Dyrenium (triamterene)
osmotic	Capable of being filtered by the glomerulus but has a limited capability of being reabsorbed into the bloodstream. EXAMPLE: Osmitrol (mannitol)
carbonic anhydrase inhibitor	Acts to increase the excretion of bicarbonate (HCO_3) ion, which carries out sodium (Na), water (H_2O), and potassium (K). EXAMPLE: Diamox (acetazolamide)

Classification of Drug	Description and Examples
urinary tract antibacterials	Sulfonamides are generally the drugs of choice for treating acute, uncomplicated urinary tract infections, especially those caused by *Escherichia coli* and *Proteus mirabilis* bacterial strains. They exert a bacteriostatic effect against a wide range of gram-positive and gram-negative microorganisms. EXAMPLES: sulfadiazine, Bactrim, and Septra, which are mixtures of trimethoprim and sulfamethoxazole
urinary tract antiseptics	May inhibit the growth of microorganisms by bactericidal, bacteriostatic, anti-infective, and/or antibacterial action. EXAMPLES: Furadantin and Macrodantin (nitrofurantoin), methenamine hippurate, and Cipro (ciprofloxacin HCl)
additional drugs	Treat disorders of the lower urinary tract by either stimulating or inhibiting smooth muscle activity, thereby improving urinary bladder functions. These functions are the storage of urine and its subsequent excretion from the body. EXAMPLES: flavoxate HCl and Urecholine (bethanechol chloride)
	Used in the treatment of interstitial cystitis. EXAMPLE: Rimso-50 (dimethyl sulfoxide)
	Reduces dysuria, nocturia, and urinary frequency. EXAMPLE: flavoxate HCl
	Treats nocturnal enuresis in children. EXAMPLE: Tofranil (imipramine HCl)
	Relaxes the muscles in the bladder, thereby decreasing the occurrence of wetting accidents. EXAMPLE: Ditropan XL (oxybutynin chloride)
	Helps control involuntary contractions of the bladder muscle. EXAMPLE: Detrol (tolterodine tartrate)

Diagnostic *and* Laboratory Tests

Test	Description
blood urea nitrogen (BUN) (ū-rē´ ă nī´ trō-jěn)	Blood test to determine the amount of urea excreted by the kidneys. Abnormal results indicate renal dysfunction.
computed tomography of kidneys, ureters, bladder (CT KUB)	CT KUB has surpassed all other imaging modalities to become the gold standard in detection of ureteric calculi (stones). In computed tomography, the x-ray beam moves in a circle around the body. This allows many different views of the same organ or structure. The x-ray information is sent to a computer that interprets the x-ray data and displays it in a two-dimensional (2D) form on a monitor.

Test	Description
creatinine clearance (krē-ăt´ ĭ-nēn)	Urine test to determine the *glomerular filtration rate (GFR)*. Abnormal results indicate renal dysfunction.

fyi Kidney function is measured by how well the kidneys clean the blood. The GFR tests how well the kidneys are working. The main factor in estimating the GFR is determining the level of creatinine in the blood. When kidneys are functioning, they remove creatinine from the blood. As kidney function slows, blood levels of creatinine rise. This test is also used to determine the patient's stage of kidney disease.

GFR Classification of Chronic Kidney Disease

Stage	Description	GFR
3	Moderately decreasing GFR	30–59 mL/min
4	Severely decreasing GFR	15–29 mL/min
5	Kidney failure	<15 mL/min

Note: Normal GFR is >60 mL/min

culture, urine	Urine test to determine the presence of microorganisms. Abnormal results indicate urinary tract infection.

fyi A few white blood cells are normally present in urine and usually give a negative chemical test result. When the number of WBCs in urine increases significantly, a clinical urine test, such as urinalysis or urine culture, will become positive. Results of this test will be considered along with a microscopic examination for WBCs in the urine.

When a test is positive and/or the WBC count in urine is high, it may indicate that there is inflammation in the urinary tract or kidneys. The most common cause for WBCs in urine (leukocyturia) is a bacterial UTI, such as a bladder or kidney infection. In addition to WBCs, bacteria and red blood cells (RBCs) may also be seen in the microscopic examination. If bacteria are present, the chemical test for nitrite may also be positive.

cystoscopy (cysto) (sĭs-tŏs´ kŭ-pē)	Visual examination of the bladder and urethra via a lighted cystoscope. Abnormal results can indicate the presence of renal calculi, a tumor, prostatic hyperplasia, and/or bleeding.
intravenous pyelography (pyelogram) (IVP) (ĭn-tră-vē´ nŭs pī˝ ĕ-lŏg´ ră-fē)	Test to visualize the kidneys, ureters, and bladder. A radiopaque substance is intravenously injected, and x-rays are taken. Abnormal results can indicate renal calculi, kidney or bladder tumors, and kidney disease.
renal biopsy	Removal of tissue from the kidney. Abnormal results can indicate kidney cancer, kidney transplant rejection, and glomerulonephritis.

Test	Description
retrograde pyelography (RP) (rĕt´rō-grād)	X-ray recording of the kidneys, ureters, and bladder following the injection of a contrast medium backward through a urinary catheter into the ureters and the calyces of the pelvis of the kidneys. Useful in locating urinary stones and obstructions. See Figure 11.19.

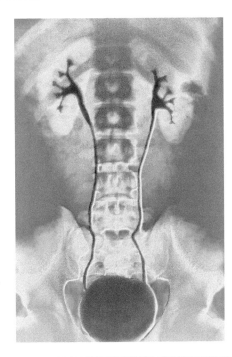

FIGURE 11.19 Retrograde pyelography. Note the contrasting of the renal calyces, ureters, and bladder following an injection of a contrast medium.
Source: CNRI/Science Source

Test	Description
serum creatinine (krē-ăt´ ĭ-nēn)	Test to determine the amount of creatinine present in the blood. Creatinine is a chemical waste product that is produced by muscle metabolism and, to a smaller extent, by eating meat. If the kidneys are not functioning properly, an increased level of creatinine may accumulate in the blood. The result of this test is useful, as it is an important marker of how well the kidneys are working. Abnormal results indicate renal dysfunction.
ultrasonography, kidneys (ŭl-tră-sŏn-ŏg´ ră-fē)	Use of high-frequency sound waves to visualize the kidneys. The sound waves (echoes) are recorded on an oscilloscope and film. Abnormal results can indicate kidney tumors, cysts, abscess, and kidney disease.

Abbreviations *and* Acronyms

Abbreviation/ Acronym	Meaning	Abbreviation/ Acronym	Meaning
AGN	acute glomerulonephritis	**CAPD**	continuous ambulatory peritoneal dialysis
ANS	acute nephritic syndrome		
BPH	benign prostatic hyperplasia	**CGN**	chronic glomerulonephritis
BUN	blood urea nitrogen	**CKD**	chronic kidney disease

Abbreviation/ Acronym	Meaning	Abbreviation/ Acronym	Meaning
CLIA	Clinical Laboratory Improvement Amendments	IVP	intravenous pyelogram
		K	potassium
cm	centimeter	Ml	milliliter
CT KUB	computed tomography of kidneys, ureters, bladder	mm	millimeter
		Na	sodium
cysto	cystoscopy	NaCl	sodium chloride
ESRD	end-stage renal disease		
ESWL	extracorporeal shock wave lithotripsy	PD	peritoneal dialysis
GFR	glomerular filtration rate	pH	hydrogen ion concentration
GU	genitourinary	PUL	percutaneous ultrasonic lithotripsy
HCO_3	bicarbonate	RP	retrograde pyelography
HD	hemodialysis	sp. gr.	specific gravity
H_2O	water	UA	urinalysis
IC	interstitial cystitis	UG	urogenital
IPD	intermittent peritoneal dialysis	UTI	urinary tract infection

Study and Review III

Building Medical Terms

Using the following word parts, fill in the blanks to build the correct medical terms.

olig-	continence	nephr/o	-ion
cyst/o	meat/o	ren	-uria

Definition	Medical Term
1. Indicates the presence of serum protein in the urine	albumin_____
2. X-ray record of the bladder	_____gram
3. Inability to hold or control urination or defecation	in_____
4. Incision of the urinary meatus to enlarge the opening	_____tomy
5. Difficult or painful urination	dys_____
6. Kidney stones	_____lithiasis

Definition	Medical Term
7. Scanty, decreased amount of urine	_____uria
8. Literally means excessive secretion and discharge of urine	poly_____
9. Pertaining to the kidney	_____al
10. To void	urinat_____

Combining Form Challenge

Using the combining forms provided, write the medical term correctly.

cyst/o   lith/o   noct/o
glycos/o   nephr/o   ureter/o

1. Hernia of the bladder that protrudes into the vagina: _____cele

2. Presence of glucose in the urine: _____uria

3. Crushing of a kidney stone: _____tripsy

4. Kidney tumor: _____oma

5. Urination during the night: _____uria

6. Disease of the ureter: _____pathy

Select the Right Term

Select the correct answer, and write it on the line provided.

1. Presence of calcium in the urine is _____.

    anuria   calciuria   calculus   calcuria

2. Pathological condition in which the body tissues contain an accumulation of fluid is _____.

    excretory   dieresis   enuresis   edema

3. Presence of red blood cells in the urine is _____.

    glycosuria   hematuria   calciuria   ketonuria

4. Condition of hardening of the kidney is _____.

    nephrology   nephrectomy   nephritis   nephrosclerosis

5. Inflammation of the kidney and renal pelvis is _____.

    pyelitis   pyelolithotomy   pyelonephritis   pyelcystitis

6. Sharp, severe pain in the lower back over the kidney is _____.

    renal failure   renal colic   rennin   stricture

Drug Highlights

Match the appropriate lettered description or examples of drug(s) with the class of drug.

_____ **1.** carbonic anhydrase inhibitor

_____ **2.** diuretics

_____ **3.** urinary tract antiseptics

_____ **4.** loop diuretics

_____ **5.** osmotic diuretic

_____ **6.** urinary tract antibacterials

_____ **7.** potassium sparing diuretics

_____ **8.** thiazide diuretics

a. Inhibit the growth of microorganisms by bactericidal, bacteriostatic, anti-infective, and/or antibacterial action

b. Osmitrol (mannitol)

c. Exert a bacteriostatic effect against gram-positive and gram-negative microorganisms

d. Inhibit the exchange of sodium for potassium in the distal tubule; inhibit potassium excretion

e. Decrease the reabsorption of sodium chloride by the kidneys, thus reducing the amount of fluid retained in the body

f. Diuril (chlorothiazide), hydrochlorothiazide, and indapamide

g. Increases the excretion of bicarbonate (HCO_3) ion, which carries out sodium (Na), water (H_2O), and potassium (K)

h. Act by inhibiting the reabsorption of sodium and chloride in the ascending loop of Henle

Diagnostic and Laboratory Tests

Select the best answer to each multiple-choice question. Circle the letter of your choice.

1. Urine test to determine the glomerular filtration rate.

    a. BUN

    b. creatinine

    c. creatinine clearance

    d. CT KUB

2. Urine test to determine the presence of microorganisms.

    a. BUN   **c.** urine culture

    b. creatinine   **d.** CT KUB

3. Test to visualize the kidneys, ureters, and bladder. A radiopaque substance is used and x-rays are taken.

    a. cystoscopy   **c.** CT KUB

    b. intravenous pyelography   **d.** renal biopsy

4. Use of high-frequency sound waves to visualize the kidneys.

    a. retrograde pyelography   **c.** ultrasonography

    b. intravenous pyelography   **d.** cystoscopy

5. In this test of the kidneys, ureters, and bladder, the x-ray beam moves in a circle around the body.

    a. cystoscopy   **c.** BUN

    b. CT KUB   **d.** retrograde pyelography

Abbreviations and Acronyms

Write the correct word, phrase, or abbreviation/acronym in the space provided.

1. acute glomerulonephritis _____

2. BUN _____

3. chronic kidney disease _____

4. cysto _____

5. GU _____

6. HD _____

7. intravenous pyelogram _____

8. PD _____

9. pH _____

10. urinalysis _____

Practical Application

Medical Record Analysis

This exercise contains information, abbreviations/acronyms, and medical terminology from an actual medical record or case study that has been adapted for this text. The names and any personal information are made up by the author. Read and study each form or case study and then answer the questions that follow. You may refer to Appendix III, *Abbreviations, Acronyms, and Symbols*.

Note: Congress passed the Clinical Laboratory Improvement Amendments (CLIA) in 1988, establishing quality standards for all laboratory testing to ensure the accuracy, reliability, and timeliness of patient test results regardless of where the test was performed.

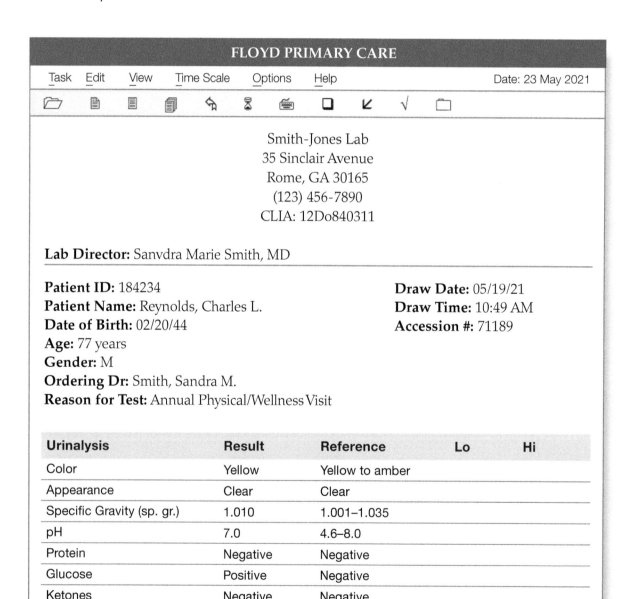

FLOYD PRIMARY CARE

| Task | Edit | View | Time Scale | Options | Help | Date: 23 May 2021 |

Smith-Jones Lab
35 Sinclair Avenue
Rome, GA 30165
(123) 456-7890
CLIA: 12Do840311

Lab Director: Sanvdra Marie Smith, MD

Patient ID: 184234
Patient Name: Reynolds, Charles L.
Date of Birth: 02/20/44
Age: 77 years
Gender: M
Ordering Dr: Smith, Sandra M.
Reason for Test: Annual Physical/Wellness Visit

Draw Date: 05/19/21
Draw Time: 10:49 AM
Accession #: 71189

Urinalysis	Result	Reference	Lo	Hi
Color	Yellow	Yellow to amber		
Appearance	Clear	Clear		
Specific Gravity (sp. gr.)	1.010	1.001–1.035		
pH	7.0	4.6–8.0		
Protein	Negative	Negative		
Glucose	Positive	Negative		
Ketones	Negative	Negative		

Urinalysis	Result	Reference	Lo	Hi
Bilirubin	Negative	Negative		
Blood	Negative	Negative		
Nitrites	Negative	Negative		
Urobilinogen	0.	0.1–1.0 mg/dL		

Action: Patient to be notified of results   **Reviewed by:** SJR   **Date:** 05/23/21

Medical Record Questions

Write the correct answer in the space provided.

1. What is the normal color of urine? _____

2. Define *specific gravity* and give the normal sp. gr. of urine. _____

3. This patient's pH was 7.0. Is this higher or lower than the average pH? _____

4. This patient's report indicated a urobilinogen of 0. Is this within normal range? _____

5. What would a positive result of glucose in the urine most likely indicate? _____

MyLab Medical Terminology™

MyLab Medical Terminology is a premium online homework management system that includes a host of features to help you study. Registered users will find:

- A multitude of quizzes and activities built within the MyLab platform
- Powerful tools that track and analyze your results—allowing you to create a personalized learning experience
- Videos and audio pronunciations to help enrich your progress
- Streaming lesson presentations (guided lectures) and self-paced learning modules
- A space where you and your instructor can check your progress and manage your assignments

12 Endocrine System

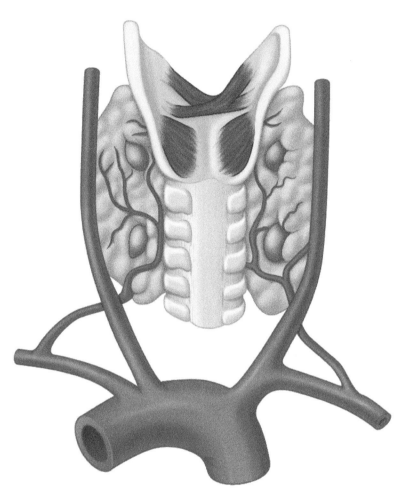

Learning Outcomes

On completion of this chapter, you will be able to:

1. Describe the major function of the endocrine system.
2. Identify the primary functions of the organs of the endocrine system.
3. Identify the various hormones secreted by the endocrine glands and their hormonal function.
4. Analyze, build, spell, and pronounce medical words.
5. Classify the drugs highlighted in this chapter.
6. Describe diagnostic and laboratory tests related to the endocrine system.
7. Identify and define selected abbreviations and acronyms.

Anatomy and Physiology

The endocrine system is made up of glands, each of which secretes a type of hormone into the bloodstream. The glands of the endocrine system and the hormones they release influence almost every cell, organ, and function of the body. Although the endocrine glands are the body's main hormone producers, some other organs such as the brain, heart, lungs, liver, skin, thymus, and the gastrointestinal mucosa, as well as the placenta during pregnancy, produce and release hormones. The primary glands of the endocrine system are the pituitary, pineal, thyroid, parathyroid, pancreas (pancreatic islets), adrenals, ovaries in the female, and testes in the male.

A major function of the endocrine system involves the production and regulation of chemical substances called *hormones*. A hormone is a chemical transmitter that is released in small amounts and transported via the bloodstream to a target organ or other cells. The word *hormone* is derived from the Greek language and means *to excite* or *to urge on*. As the body's chemical messengers, hormones transfer information and instructions from one set of cells to another. They regulate growth, development, mood, tissue function, homeostasis, metabolism, and sexual function in the male and female. Table 12.1 provides an at-a-glance look at the endocrine system. Figure 12.1 shows the primary glands of the endocrine system.

TABLE 12.1	Endocrine System at-a-Glance
Gland	**Primary Functions/Description**
Pituitary (hypophysis)	Master gland; has regulatory effects on other endocrine glands
Anterior lobe (adenohypophysis)	Influences growth and sexual development, thyroid function, adrenocortical function; regulates skin pigmentation
Posterior lobe (neurohypophysis)	Stimulates the reabsorption of water and elevates blood pressure; stimulates the uterus to contract during labor, delivery, and parturition (childbirth); stimulates the release of milk during suckling
Pineal	Helps regulate the release of gonadotropin and influences the body's internal clock
Thyroid	Plays vital role in metabolism; regulates the body's metabolic processes; influences bone and calcium metabolism; helps maintain plasma calcium homeostasis
Parathyroid	Maintains normal serum calcium level; plays a role in the metabolism of phosphorus
Pancreas (pancreatic islets)	Regulates blood glucose levels; plays a vital role in metabolism of carbohydrates, proteins, and fats
Adrenals (suprarenals)	
Adrenal cortex	Regulates carbohydrate metabolism; provides anti-inflammatory effect; helps body cope during stress; regulates electrolyte and water balance; promotes development of male characteristics
Adrenal medulla	Synthesizes, secretes, and stores catecholamines (sympathomimetic hormones: dopamine, epinephrine, norepinephrine)
Ovaries	Promote growth, development, and maintenance of female sex organs
Testes	Promote growth, development, and maintenance of male sex organs

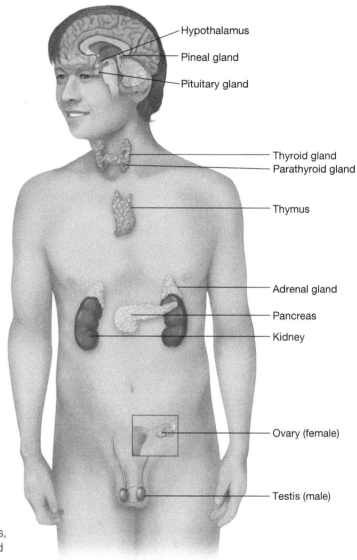

Hypothalamus

Pineal gland

Pituitary gland

Thyroid gland
Parathyroid gland

Thymus

Adrenal gland

Pancreas

Kidney

Ovary (female)

Testis (male)

FIGURE 12.1 Glands of the endocrine system (including the kidneys, which are below the adrenal glands and are part of the urinary system).

fyi Most of the structures and glands of the endocrine system develop in the fetus during the first 3 months of pregnancy. The endocrine system of the newborn is supplemented by hormones that cross the placental barrier. Both male and female newborns may have swelling of the breasts and genitalia from maternal hormones.

Hormonal Function of the Endocrine System

Hyposecretion or hypersecretion of specific hormones of the endocrine system cause or are associated with many pathological conditions. Too much or too little of any hormone can be harmful to the body. Controlling the production of or replacing specific hormones can treat many hormonal disorders and/or conditions.

The endocrine system and the nervous system work closely together to help maintain homeostasis (a state of equilibrium that is maintained within the body's internal environment). The **hypothalamus**, a collection of specialized cells that are located in the lower central part of the brain, is the primary link between the endocrine and nervous system (refer to Figure 12.1). Nerve cells in the hypothalamus control the pituitary gland by producing chemicals that either stimulate or suppress hormone secretions from the pituitary. The hypothalamus is recognized as an endocrine organ because it produces several hormones and synthesizes and secretes releasing hormones such as thyrotropin-releasing hormone (TRH) and gonadotropin-releasing hormone (GnRH) and releasing factors such as corticotropin-releasing factor (CRF), growth hormone–releasing factor (GHRF), prolactin-releasing factor (PRF), and melanocyte-stimulating hormone–releasing factor (MRF).

The hypothalamus also exerts direct nervous control over the adrenal medulla and controls the secretion of the hormones epinephrine and norepinephrine. See Table 12.2 for an overview of the endocrine glands, hormones, and hormonal functions.

TABLE 12.2 Summary of the Endocrine Glands, Hormones, and Hormonal Functions

Endocrine Glands	Hormones	Hormonal Functions
Pituitary gland		
Anterior lobe	Growth hormone (GH) (also called *somatotropin hormone [STH]*)	Promotes growth and development of bones, muscles, and other organs; enhances protein synthesis, decreases the use of glucose, and promotes fat destruction (lipolysis)
	Adrenocorticotropin hormone (ACTH)	Stimulates growth and development of the adrenal cortex
	Thyroid-stimulating hormone (TSH)	Stimulates growth and development of the thyroid gland
	Follicle-stimulating hormone (FSH)	Stimulates the growth of ovarian follicles in the female and sperm in the male
	Luteinizing hormone (LH)	Stimulates the development of the corpus luteum in the female and the production of testosterone in the male
	Prolactin hormone (PRL) (also called *lactogenic hormone [LTH]*)	Stimulates the development and growth of the mammary glands; important in the initiation and maintenance of milk production during pregnancy. Following childbirth, the act of suckling provides the stimulus for prolactin synthesis and release. When suckling ceases, prolactin secretion slows and milk production decreases and then stops.
	Melanocyte-stimulating hormone (MSH)	Regulates skin pigmentation and promotes the deposit of melanin in the skin after exposure to sunlight
Posterior lobe	Antidiuretic hormone (ADH) (also called *vasopressin [VP]*)	Stimulates the reabsorption of water by the renal tubules and has a pressor (stimulating) effect that elevates the blood pressure
	Oxytocin	Stimulates the uterus to contract during labor, delivery, and parturition; stimulates the release of milk during suckling
Pineal gland	Melatonin	Helps regulate the release of gonadotropin and influences the body's internal clock
	Serotonin	Stimulates neurotransmitter, vasoconstrictor, and smooth muscle; acts to inhibit gastric secretion
Thyroid gland	Thyroxine (T_4)	Maintains and regulates the basal metabolic rate (BMR); influences growth and development, both physical and mental, and the metabolism of fats, proteins, carbohydrates, water, vitamins, and minerals; can be synthetically produced or extracted from animal thyroid glands in crystalline form to be used in the treatment of thyroid dysfunction, especially congenital hypothyroidism (formerly called cretinism), myxedema, and Hashimoto disease

(continued)

TABLE 12.2 Summary of the Endocrine Glands, Hormones, and Hormonal Functions (*continued*)

Endocrine Glands	Hormones	Hormonal Functions
	Triiodothyronine (T$_3$)	Influences the basal metabolic rate and is more biologically active than thyroxine
	Calcitonin	Influences bone and calcium metabolism and helps maintain plasma calcium homeostasis; also known as thyrocalcitonin
Parathyroid glands	Parathyroid hormone (PTH) (also called *parathormone*)	Plays a role in maintenance of a normal serum calcium level and in the metabolism of phosphorus
Pancreas		
Pancreatic islets (islets of Langerhans)	Glucagon	Facilitates the breakdown of glycogen to glucose
	Insulin	Plays a role in maintenance of normal blood sugar. It promotes the entry of glucose into the cells, thereby lowering the blood glucose (BG) level.
	Somatostatin	Suppresses the release of glucagon and insulin
Adrenal glands		
Cortex	Cortisol	Regulates carbohydrate, protein, and fat metabolism; needed for gluconeogenesis; increases blood sugar level; provides anti-inflammatory effect; helps body cope during times of stress
	Corticosterone	Necessary for normal use of carbohydrates, the absorption of glucose, and gluconeogenesis; also influences potassium (K) and sodium (Na) metabolism
	Aldosterone	Necessary in regulating electrolyte and water balance by promoting sodium and chloride reabsorption and potassium excretion
	Testosterone	Influences development of male secondary sex characteristics
	Androsterone	Influences development of male secondary sex characteristics
Medulla	Dopamine	Dilates systemic arteries, elevates systolic blood pressure, increases cardiac output, increases urinary output
	Epinephrine (also called *adrenaline*)	Acts as vasoconstrictor, vasopressor, cardiac stimulant, antispasmodic, and sympathomimetic
	Norepinephrine (also called *noradrenaline*)	Acts as vasoconstrictor, vasopressor, and neurotransmitter
Ovaries	Estrogens (estradiol, estrone, and estriol)	Necessary for the growth, development, and maintenance of female sex organs and secondary sex characteristics; promote the development of the mammary glands; play a vital role in a woman's emotional well-being and sexual drive
	Progesterone	Prepares the uterus for pregnancy
Testes	Testosterone	Necessary for normal growth and development of the male accessory sex organs; plays a vital role in the erection process of the penis and thus is necessary for the sexual act, *copulation* (sexual intercourse)

(continued)

TABLE 12.2 Summary of the Endocrine Glands, Hormones, and Hormonal Functions *(continued)*

Endocrine Glands	Hormones	Hormonal Functions
Thymus gland	Thymosin	Promotes the maturation process of T lymphocytes
	Thymopoietin	Influences the production of lymphocyte precursors and aids in their process of becoming T lymphocytes
Gastrointestinal mucosa	Gastrin	Stimulates gastric acid secretion
	Secretin	Stimulates pancreatic juice, bile, and intestinal secretion
	Cholecystokinin	Causes contraction and emptying of the gallbladder and secretion of pancreatic enzymes, increases bile acid production in the liver, delays gastric emptying, and induces digestive enzyme production in the pancreas
	Enterogastrone	Regulates gastric secretions

Pituitary Gland (Hypophysis)

The **pituitary gland**, also called *hypophysis*, is a small gray gland located at the base of the brain (refer to Figure 12.1). It lies in a shallow depression of the sphenoid bone known as the *sella turcica*. It is attached by the infundibulum stalk to the hypothalamus. The pituitary is approximately 1 centimeter (cm) in diameter and weighs approximately 0.6 gram (g). It is divided into the anterior lobe (*adenohypophysis*) and the posterior lobe (*neurohypophysis*). The pituitary is also called the **master gland** of the body because of its regulatory effects on the other endocrine glands.

Anterior Lobe

The **anterior lobe** secretes several hormones that are necessary for the growth and development of bones, muscles, other organs, sex glands, the thyroid gland, and the adrenal cortex. The hormones secreted by the anterior lobe and their functions are described in Table 12.2 and selected hormones are shown in Figure 12.2.

Posterior Lobe

The **posterior lobe** stores and secretes two important hormones that are synthesized in the hypothalamus. Selected hormones secreted by the posterior lobe and their functions are described in Table 12.2.

Pineal Gland

The **pineal gland** is a small, pine cone–shaped gland located near the posterior end of the corpus callosum (refer to Figure 12.1). It is less than 1 cm in diameter and weighs approximately 0.1 g. The pineal gland secretes **melatonin** and **serotonin**. Melatonin is a peptide hormone that influences sleep–wake cycles and helps regulate the release of gonadotropin. It is believed to coordinate the hormones of fertility and to inhibit the reproductive system until the body matures. Serotonin is a hormone that is a neurotransmitter, vasoconstrictor, and smooth muscle stimulant and acts to inhibit gastric secretion.

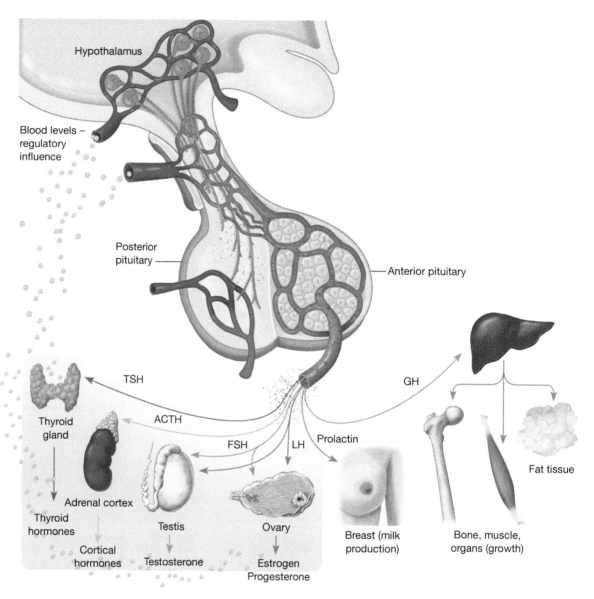

FIGURE 12.2 The pituitary gland with some examples of the many hormones it produces, showing their target cells, tissues, and/or organs.

Thyroid Gland

The **thyroid gland** is a large, bilobed gland located in the neck. It is anterior to the trachea and just below the thyroid cartilage (refer to Figure 12.1). The thyroid is approximately 5 cm long and 3 cm wide and weighs approximately 30 g. See Figure 12.3. It plays a vital role in metabolism and regulates the body's metabolic processes. The hormones secreted by the thyroid gland and their functions are described in Table 12.2.

Hyposecretion of the thyroid hormones T_3 and T_4 results in congenital **hypothyroidism** (underactive thyroid) during infancy, **myxedema** during adulthood (refer to Figure 12.17), and **Hashimoto disease**. Hypersecretion of the thyroid hormones T_3 and T_4 results in **hyperthyroidism** (overactive thyroid), which is more common in women, people with other thyroid problems, and those over 60 years of age. Graves disease, an autoimmune disorder, is the most common cause of hyperthyroidism. Other causes include thyroid nodules, thyroiditis, consuming too much iodine, and taking too much synthetic thyroid hormone.

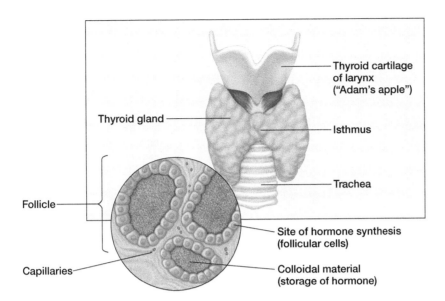

FIGURE 12.3 Thyroid gland.

Simple or **endemic goiter** is an enlargement of the thyroid gland caused by a deficiency of iodine in the diet.

Parathyroid Glands

The **parathyroid glands** are small, yellowish-brown bodies occurring as two pairs located in the neck on the posterior surface of the thyroid gland (refer to Figure 12.1). Each parathyroid gland is approximately 6 mm in diameter and weighs approximately 0.033 g. See Figure 12.4. The hormone secreted by the parathyroid is *parathyroid hormone (PTH)*, which is also called *parathormone*. This hormone and its functions are described in Table 12.2.

Hyposecretion of PTH can result in **hypoparathyroidism**, which can cause **tetany** (intermittent cramp or tonic muscular contractions). See Figure 12.5. Hypersecretion of PTH can result in **hyperparathyroidism**, which can cause **osteoporosis**, **kidney stones**, and **hypercalcemia**.

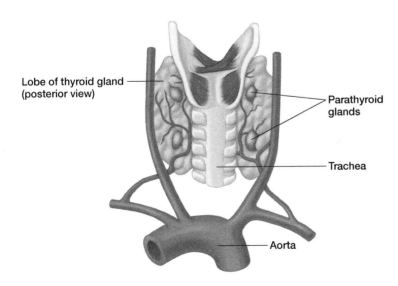

FIGURE 12.4 Parathyroid glands.

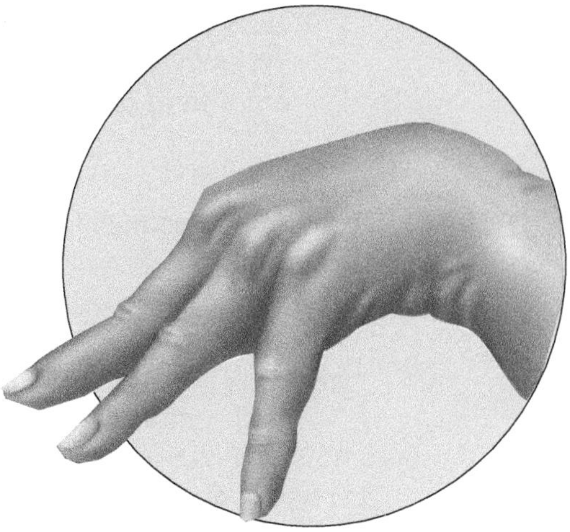

FIGURE 12.5 Tetany of the hand as a result of hypoparathyroidism.

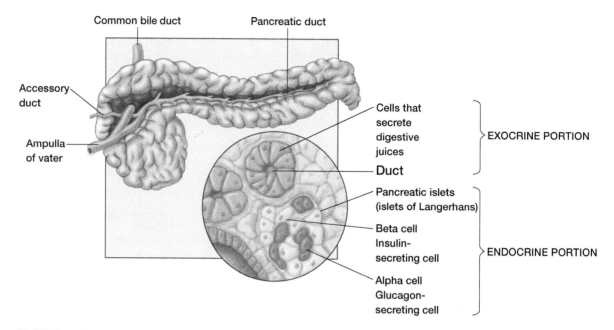

FIGURE 12.6 Pancreas—an endocrine and exocrine gland. The inset shows the pancreatic islets. The alpha cells secrete glucagon, which raises the blood glucose level. The beta cells secrete insulin, which lowers the blood glucose level.

Pancreas

Within the pancreas are small clusters of cells called **pancreatic islets** (also called *islets of Langerhans*). See Figures 12.1 and 12.6. They are composed of three major types of cells: **alpha**, **beta**, and **delta**. The alpha cells secrete the hormone glucagon, which facilitates the breakdown of glycogen to glucose, thereby elevating blood sugar.

The beta cells secrete the hormone insulin (refer to Figure 12.6), which is necessary for the maintenance of normal blood sugar (fasting: 70–99 mg/dL). Insulin is necessary to life. It acts to regulate the metabolism of glucose and the process necessary for the intermediary metabolism of carbohydrates, fats, and proteins. It promotes the entry of glucose into the cells, thereby lowering the blood glucose (BG) level. Hyposecretion or inadequate use of insulin may result in **diabetes mellitus (DM)**. Hypersecretion of insulin may result in **hyperinsulinism**. The delta cells secrete a hormone, *somatostatin*, which suppresses the release of glucagon and insulin.

Untreated diabetes mellitus or complications of diabetes can result in various multisystem effects. See Figure 12.7. Progressive complications include **hyperglycemia** (excessive amount of sugar in the blood) and **hypoglycemia** (deficient amount of sugar in the blood).

---

fyi **Type 1 diabetes mellitus** is usually diagnosed in children and young adults and was previously known as juvenile diabetes. In type 1 DM, the body does not produce insulin. Insulin is a hormone that is needed to convert sugar (glucose), starches, and other food into energy needed for daily life. The classic symptoms of DM—**polyuria** (frequent urination), **polydipsia** (excessive thirst), and **polyphagia** (extreme hunger)—appear more rapidly in children.

DM is the most common endocrine system disorder of childhood. The rate of occurrence is highest among 5- to 7-year-olds and 11- to 15-year-olds. It is noted that childhood obesity predisposes to insulin resistance and **type 2 diabetes mellitus**, a chronic metabolic disorder characterized by high blood sugar, insulin resistance, and lack of insulin. Obesity in children is a complex disorder. Its prevalence has increased so significantly in recent years that many consider it a major health concern of the developed world.

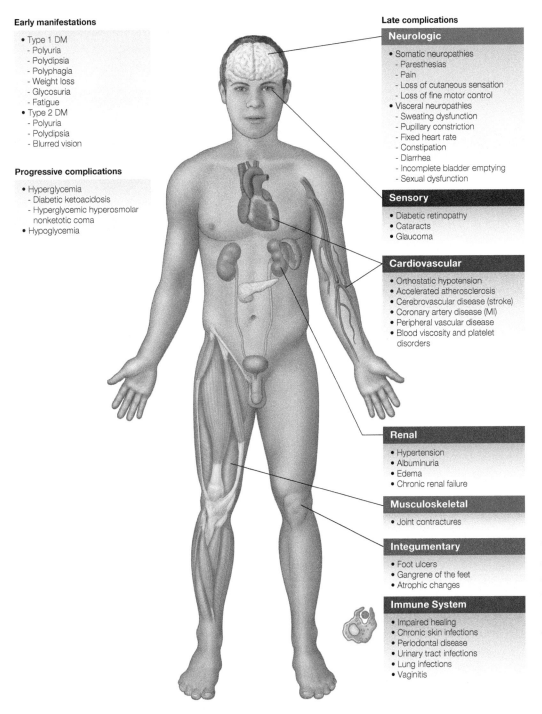

Early manifestations

- Type 1 DM
  - Polyuria
  - Polydipsia
  - Polyphagia
  - Weight loss
  - Glycosuria
  - Fatigue
- Type 2 DM
  - Polyuria
  - Polydipsia
  - Blurred vision

Progressive complications

- Hyperglycemia
  - Diabetic ketoacidosis
  - Hyperglycemic hyperosmolar nonketotic coma
- Hypoglycemia

Late complications

Neurologic

- Somatic neuropathies
  - Paresthesias
  - Pain
  - Loss of cutaneous sensation
  - Loss of fine motor control
- Visceral neuropathies
  - Sweating dysfunction
  - Pupillary constriction
  - Fixed heart rate
  - Constipation
  - Diarrhea
  - Incomplete bladder emptying
  - Sexual dysfunction

Sensory

- Diabetic retinopathy
- Cataracts
- Glaucoma

Cardiovascular

- Orthostatic hypotension
- Accelerated atherosclerosis
- Cerebrovascular disease (stroke)
- Coronary artery disease (MI)
- Peripheral vascular disease
- Blood viscosity and platelet disorders

Renal

- Hypertension
- Albuminuria
- Edema
- Chronic renal failure

Musculoskeletal

- Joint contractures

Integumentary

- Foot ulcers
- Gangrene of the feet
- Atrophic changes

Immune System

- Impaired healing
- Chronic skin infections
- Periodontal disease
- Urinary tract infections
- Lung infections
- Vaginitis

FIGURE 12.7 Multisystem effects of diabetes mellitus. Source: PEARSON EDUCATION; SERVICES, PEARSON; PEARSON EDUCATION, . ., NURSING: A CONCEPT-BASED APPROACH TO LEARNING, VOLUME I, 1st Ed., ©2019. Reprinted and Electronically reproduced by permission of Pearson Education, Inc., New York, NY.

Hyperglycemia can lead to **diabetic ketoacidosis** (accumulation of ketones and acids in the body due to faulty metabolism of carbohydrates and the improper burning of fats). A coma may develop when the blood sugar is too high or an insufficient amount of insulin has been received. Hypoglycemia occurs when too much insulin has been taken by the patient. Insulin shock is a severe form of hypoglycemia and requires an immediate dose of glucose. Convulsions, coma, and death can occur if the patient is not treated.

Adrenal Glands (Suprarenals)

The **adrenal glands** are two small, triangular-shaped glands located on top of each kidney (refer to Figure 12.1). Each gland weighs about 5 g and consists of an outer portion or *cortex* and an inner portion called the *medulla*. See Figure 12.8.

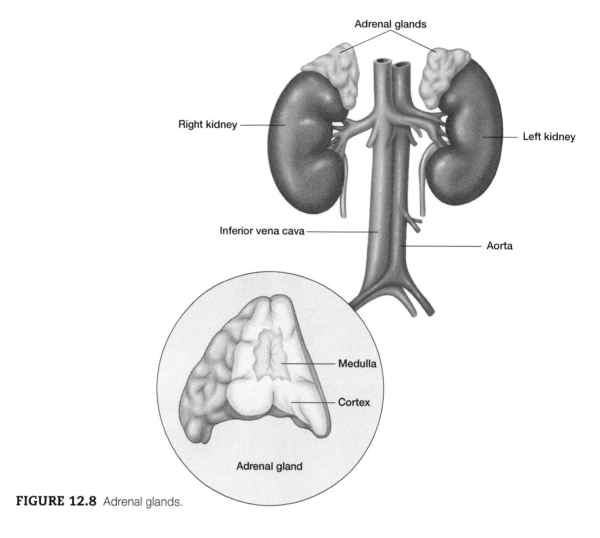

FIGURE 12.8 Adrenal glands.

Adrenal Cortex

The **adrenal cortex** is necessary to life due to its secretion of groups of hormones, the glucocorticoids, the mineralocorticoids, and the androgens. The hormones secreted by the adrenal cortex and their functions are described in Table 12.2 and a discussion of these substances and their effects on the body follows.

Glucocorticoids

The two glucocorticoid hormones are *cortisol* and *corticosterone*. Cortisol is the principal steroid hormone secreted by the cortex. Hyposecretion of cortisol can result in Addison disease; hypersecretion can result in Cushing disease.

Corticosterone is a steroid hormone secreted by the adrenal cortex. It is necessary for the normal use of carbohydrates, the absorption of glucose, and the formation of glycogen in the liver and tissues. It also influences potassium and sodium metabolism.

Mineralocorticoids

Aldosterone is the principal mineralocorticoid secreted by the adrenal cortex. It is necessary in regulating electrolyte and water balance by promoting sodium and chloride reabsorption and potassium excretion. Hyposecretion of this hormone can result in a reduced plasma volume, and hypersecretion can result in a condition known as primary aldosteronism. In primary aldosteronism, the adrenal glands produce too much aldosterone, causing the individual to lose potassium and retain sodium. The excess sodium in turn holds onto water, increasing the blood volume and blood pressure. Treatment options for people with primary aldosteronism include medications, lifestyle modifications, and surgery.

Androgens

Androgen refers to a substance or hormone that promotes the development of male characteristics. The two main androgen hormones are *testosterone* and *androsterone*. They are necessary for the development of the male secondary sex characteristics.

Adrenal Medulla

The **adrenal medulla** synthesizes, secretes, and stores catecholamines, specifically dopamine, epinephrine, and norepinephrine. The hormones secreted by the adrenal medulla and their functions are described in Table 12.2 and a discussion of these substances and their effects on the body follows.

Dopamine

Dopamine is a naturally occurring sympathetic nervous system neurotransmitter that is a precursor of norepinephrine. Dopamine can be supplied as a medication that acts on the sympathetic nervous system. It can be given to increase the amount of dopamine in the brains of patients with Parkinson disease. Dopamine has varying vasoactive effects depending on the dose at which it is administered. It can act to dilate systemic arteries, increase cardiac output, and increase urinary output.

Epinephrine

Epinephrine (*adrenaline*) acts as a vasoconstrictor, vasopressor, cardiac stimulant, antispasmodic, and sympathomimetic. Its main function is to assist in regulating the sympathetic branch of the autonomic nervous system. It can be synthetically produced and administered *parenterally* (by an injection), *topically* (on a local area of the skin), or by *inhalation* (by nose or mouth). The following are some of the known influences and functions of epinephrine:

- Elevates the systolic blood pressure
- Increases the heart rate and cardiac output
- Increases glycogenolysis (conversion of glycogen into glucose), thereby hastening the release of glucose from the liver; this action elevates the blood sugar level and provides the body a spurt of energy; referred to as the *fight-or-flight response*
- Dilates the bronchial tubes and relaxes air passageways
- Dilates the pupils to see more clearly

Norepinephrine

Norepinephrine (*noradrenaline*) acts as a vasoconstrictor, vasopressor, and neurotransmitter. It elevates systolic and diastolic blood pressure, increases the heart rate and cardiac output, and increases glycogenolysis.

Ovaries

The **ovaries** (refer to Figure 12.1) produce *estrogens* (*estradiol*, *estrone*, and *estriol*) and *progesterone*. Estrogen is the female sex hormone secreted by the graafian follicles of the ovaries. Progesterone is a steroid hormone secreted by the corpus luteum.

Testes

The **testes** (refer to Figure 12.1) produce the male sex hormone *testosterone*, which is important for sexual development, sexual behavior, and libido; supporting spermatogenesis; and erectile function.

Placenta

During pregnancy, the **placenta**, containing separate vascular systems of the mother and fetus, serves as an endocrine gland. It produces *chorionic gonadotropin hormone, estrogen,* and *progesterone*.

Gastrointestinal Mucosa

The **gastrointestinal mucosa** of the pyloric area of the stomach secretes the hormone *gastrin*, which stimulates gastric acid secretion. Gastrin also affects the gallbladder, pancreas, and small intestine secretory activities.

The gastrointestinal mucosa of the duodenum and jejunum secretes the hormone *secretin*, which stimulates pancreatic juice, bile, and intestinal secretion. The mucosa of the duodenum also secretes *cholecystokinin*, which stimulates the pancreas. *Enterogastrone*, a hormone that regulates gastric secretions, is also secreted by the duodenal mucosa.

Thymus

The **thymus** is a bilobed body located in the mediastinal cavity in front of and above the heart (refer to Figure 12.1). It is composed of lymphoid tissue and is a part of the lymphatic system. It is a ductless glandlike body and secretes the hormones *thymosin* and *thymopoietin*. See Figure 12.9. Thymosin promotes the maturation process of T lymphocytes (thymus dependent), white blood cells that play an important role in cell-mediated immunity. Thymopoietin is a hormone that influences the production of lymphocyte precursors and aids in their process of becoming T lymphocytes.

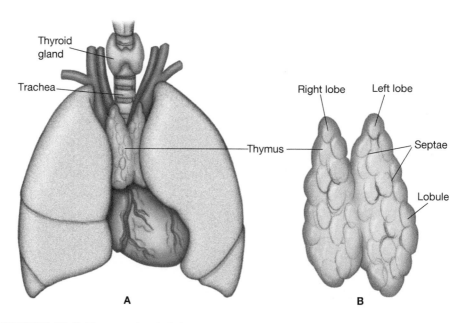

FIGURE 12.9 Thymus gland. **A** Appearance and position; **B** with anatomic structures.

Leptin and Ghrelin: Different Types of Hormones

As a growing number of people suffer from obesity, understanding the mechanisms by which various hormones and neurotransmitters have influence on energy balance has been a subject of intensive research. *Leptin* and *ghrelin* are two hormones recognized to have a major influence on energy level. These hormones are not produced by endocrine cells or glands, but are secreted by adipose tissue throughout the body. Leptin is a peptide hormone that is produced by fat cells and plays a role in body weight regulation by acting on the hypothalamus to suppress appetite and burn fat stored in adipose tissue. Ghrelin, on the other hand, is a fast-acting hormone that seems to play a role in meal initiation. In obese subjects, the circulating level of leptin is increased. It is now established that obese patients are leptin-resistant. However, the manner in which both leptin and ghrelin contribute to the development or maintenance of obesity is as yet unclear.

The American Medical Association has reclassified obesity from a condition to a disease. More than one-third of the adult population of the United States is obese. The Centers for Disease Control and Prevention (CDC) now defines normal weight, overweight, and obesity according to body mass index (BMI) rather than the traditional height/weight charts. BMI is a person's weight in kilograms (kg) divided by his or her height in meters squared. *Overweight* is defined as a BMI between 25 and 29.9 in adults. *Obesity* is defined as excessive amount of body fat with a BMI of 30 or above.

Study *and* Review I

Anatomy and Physiology

Write your answers to the following questions.

1. Name the primary glands of the endocrine system.

    a. _____   e. _____

    b. _____   f. _____

    c. _____   g. _____

    d. _____   h. _____

2. State the major function of the endocrine system. _____

_____

3. Define *hormone*._____

4. State the vital role of the hypothalamus in regulating endocrine functions. _____

_____

_____

_____

5. Why is the pituitary gland known as the master gland of the body? _____

_____

6. Name the hormones secreted by the anterior lobe (*adenohypophysis*) of the pituitary gland.

a. _____   e. _____

b. _____   f. _____

c. _____   g. _____

d. _____

7. Name the hormones secreted by the posterior lobe (*neurohypophysis*) of the pituitary gland.

a. _____   b. _____

8. The pineal gland secretes the hormones _____ and _____.

9. State the vital role of the thyroid gland. _____

10. Name the hormones stored and secreted by the thyroid gland.

a. _____   c. _____

b. _____

11. Parathyroid hormone (*parathormone*) is necessary for the maintenance of a normal level of
_____ and also plays a role in the metabolism of _____.

12. Insulin is necessary for the maintenance of a normal level of _____.

13. The adrenal cortex secretes a group of hormones known as the _____,
the _____, and the _____.

14. Name four functions of cortisol.

a. _____   c. _____

b. _____   d. _____

15. Name four functions of corticosterone.

    a. _____   **c.** _____

    b. _____   **d.** _____

16. _____ is the principal mineralocorticoid secreted by the adrenal cortex.

17. Define _androgen_. _____

18. Name the three main catecholamines synthesized, secreted, and stored by the adrenal medulla.

    a. _____   **c.** _____

    b. _____

19. Name three functions of the hormone epinephrine.

    a. _____

    b. _____

    c. _____

20. Name the two types of hormones produced by the ovaries: _____ and

    _____.

21. The testes produce the hormone _____.

22. Name the two hormones secreted by the thymus.

    a. _____   **b.** _____

23. Name the four hormones secreted by the gastrointestinal mucosa.

    a. _____   **c.** _____

    b. _____   **d.** _____

▶ **ANATOMY LABELING**   Identify the structures shown below by filling in the blanks.

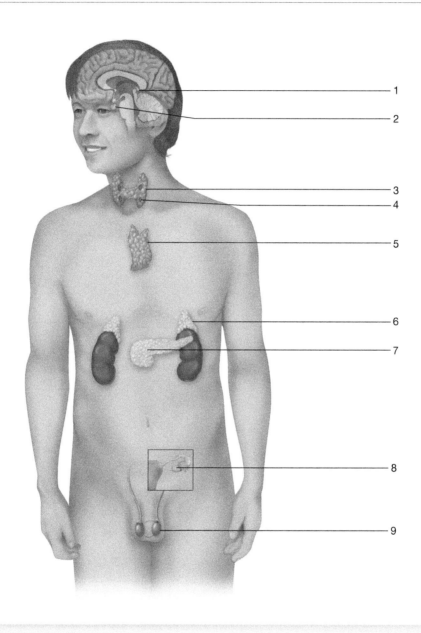

1 _____

2 _____

3 _____

4 _____

5 _____

6 _____

7 _____

8 _____

9 _____

Building Your Medical Vocabulary

This section provides the foundation for learning medical terminology. Review the alphabetized list of medical terms in the following pages. Note how common prefixes and suffixes are repeatedly applied to word roots and combining forms to create different meanings. A combining form is a word root plus a vowel. The chart below lists the combining forms and word roots used in this chapter and can help to strengthen your understanding of how medical words are built and spelled.

You will find that some terms have not been divided into word parts. These are common words or specialized terms that are included to enhance your medical vocabulary.

Combining Forms

acid/o	acid		kal/i	potassium (K)
acr/o	extremity, point		myx/o	mucus
aden/o	gland		nephr/o	kidney
adren/o	adrenal gland		neur/o	nerve
andr/o	man		ophthalm/o	eye
cortic/o	cortex		pancreat/o	pancreas
crin/o	to secrete		somat/o	body
estr/o	female		test/o	testicle
ger/o	old age		thym/o	thymus
gigant/o	giant		thyr/o(x)	thyroid, shield
gluc/o	sweet, sugar		toxic/o	poison
gonad/o	seed		trop/o	turning
hirsut/o	hairy		vas/o	vessel
hydr/o	water		viril/o	masculine
insulin/o	insulin			

Word Roots

cortis	cortex		letharg	drowsiness
dwarf	small		log	study
esthes	sensation		pine	pine cone
gester	to bear		pituitar	pituitary gland
glandul	little acorn		press	to press
insul	insulin		ster	solid

Medical Word	Word Parts		Definition
	Part	Meaning	
acidosis (ăs″ ĭ-dō′ sĭs)	acid -osis	acid condition	Condition of excessive acidity of body fluids
acromegaly (ăk″ rō-mĕg′ ă-lē)	acr/o -megaly	extremity enlargement, large	Characterized (in the adult) by marked enlargement and elongation of the bones of the face, jaw, and extremities. See Figure 12.10.

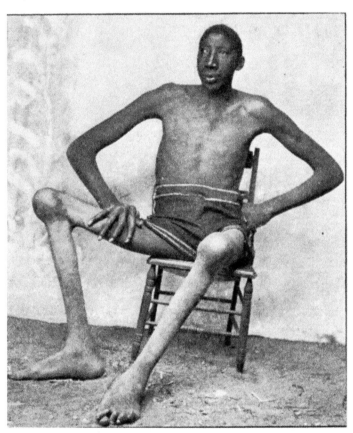

FIGURE 12.10 A man with acromegaly.
Source: Patrick Guenette/123RF

 fyi Overproduction of growth hormone, which is almost always caused by a noncancerous (benign) pituitary tumor, causes excessive growth. In adults, the condition is called *acromegaly*. In children, the condition is called *gigantism*. Children develop great stature; adults develop enlarged and elongated bones but do not grow taller. Heart failure, weakness, and vision problems are common.

Diagnosis is based on blood tests and imaging of the skull and hands; computed tomography (CT) or magnetic resonance imaging (MRI) of the head are done to look for the cause. A combination of surgery, radiation therapy, and drug therapy is used to treat the overproduction of growth hormone.

Medical Word	Word Parts		Definition
	Part	Meaning	
Addison disease (ăd´ ĭ-sŭn)			Results from a deficiency in the secretion of adrenocortical hormones; also called *adrenal insufficiency*. The most common cause of this condition is the result of the body attacking itself (autoimmune disease). For unknown reasons, the immune system views the adrenal cortex as a foreign body, something to attack and destroy. Other causes of Addison disease include infections of the adrenal glands, spread of cancer to the glands, and hemorrhage into the glands.
adenectomy (ăd´ ĕn-ĕk´ tō-mē)	aden -ectomy	gland surgical excision	Surgical excision of a gland
adenoma (ăd´ ĕ-nō´ mă)	aden -oma	gland tumor	Tumor of a gland

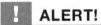 **ALERT!**

The root **aden** means *gland* and the root **adren** means *adrenal gland*. What a difference a letter makes!

Medical Word	Word Parts		Definition
adrenal (ă-drē´ năl)	adren -al	adrenal gland pertaining to	Pertaining to the adrenal glands, triangular bodies that cover the superior surface of the kidneys; also called *suprarenal glands*
adrenalectomy (ă-drē˝ nă-lĕk´ tō-mē)	adren -al -ectomy	adrenal gland pertaining to surgical excision	Surgical excision of an adrenal gland
androgen (ăn´ drō-jĕn)	andr/o -gen	man formation, produce	Hormones that produce or stimulate the development of male characteristics. The two major androgens are testosterone and androsterone.
congenital hypothyroidism (kŏn-jĕn´ ĭ-tăl hī˝ pō-thī´ royd-ĭzm)	hypo- thyr -oid -ism	deficient thyroid, shield resemble condition	A severe deficiency of thyroid hormone (iodine) in newborns, this condition causes impaired neurological function, stunted growth, and physical deformities; previously known as *cretinism*

Medical Word	Word Parts		Definition
	Part	Meaning	
cortisone (kor´ tĭ-sōn)	**cortis** **-one**	cortex hormone	Glucocorticoid (steroid) hormone secreted by the adrenal cortex; used as an anti-inflammatory agent
Cushing disease (koosh´ ĭng)			Results from hypersecretion of cortisol; symptoms include fatigue, muscular weakness, and changes in body appearance. Prolonged administration of large doses of ACTH can cause Cushing syndrome. A *buffalo hump* and a *moon face* are characteristic signs of this condition. See Figure 12.11.

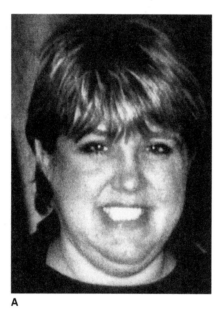 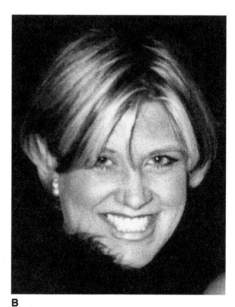

A   B

FIGURE 12.11 A woman with Cushing syndrome **A** before and **B** after treatment.
Source: Courtesy of Sharmyn McGraw

diabetes (dī˝ ă-bē´ tēz)	**dia-** **-betes**	through to go	General term used to describe diseases characterized by polyuria (excessive discharge of urine)

Medical Word	Word Parts		Definition
	Part	Meaning	
diabetes mellitus (DM) (dī″ ă-bē′ tēz mĕl′ ĭ-tŭs)	**dia-** **-betes**	through to go	Group of metabolic diseases characterized by hyperglycemia resulting from defects in insulin production, insulin secretion, or both. There are three major types of diabetes mellitus: type 1, type 2, and gestational diabetes, which occurs as a result of pregnancy. DM is the seventh highest cause of death in the United States.

fyi In the second century, Aretaeus, a Greek physician from Cappadocia who practiced in Rome, Italy, and Alexandria, Egypt, was confronted with a patient who had polyuria (excessive urination). He chose a Greek word, *diabetes* (that which passes through), to define what he considered to be the most dominant clinical sign in his patient. Later, the word *diabetes* was combined with *mellitus*, a word of Latin origin that means "honey." In 1670, in those suffering from polyuria, a distinction was made between those patients who had sweet-tasting urine (diabetes mellitus [DM]) and those patients whose urine had no taste (diabetes insipidus [DI]).

In DM the body is no longer able to control blood glucose, leading to abnormally high levels of blood sugar (hyperglycemia). Most of the food that we eat is turned into glucose, a simple sugar, for the body to use for energy. Insulin, made by the pancreas, helps glucose get into the cells of the body. When a person has DM, the body either does not make enough insulin or cannot use insulin as well as it should, causing sugar to build up in the blood. Persistently elevated blood glucose levels can cause damage to the body's tissues, including the nerves (neuropathy), blood vessels, and tissues in the eyes. **Sensory neuropathy** occurs if the body's sensory nerves become damaged. It may also be called *polyneuropathy* (**poly-** [*many*], **neuro** [*nerve*], **-pathy** [*disease*]) as it affects a number of different nerve centers. Sensory neuropathy starts from the feet or hands and can develop to affect the legs and arms. The following are symptoms of sensory neuropathy:

- Numbness
- Reduced ability to sense pain or extreme temperatures
- Tingling feeling
- Unexplained burning sensations
- Sharp stabbing pains, which may be more noticeable at night
- Dysesthesia (**dys-** [*difficult, painful*], **esthes** [*sensation*], **-ia** [*condition*])

In addition, poor circulation may occur in the legs and feet, which can weaken the healing process, contribute to infection, and lead to the formation of ulcers. The possibility of amputation of an extremity is a great concern for diabetics.

Refer to Figure 12.7 for the multisystem effects of diabetes mellitus.

Medical Word	Word Parts		Definition
	Part	Meaning	
dwarfism (dwor´ fĭzm)	dwarf -ism	small condition	Condition of being abnormally small. It is a medical disorder characterized by an adult height less than 4 feet 10 inches (147 cm) and is usually classified as to the underlying condition that is the cause for the short stature. Dwarfism is not necessarily caused by any specific disease or disorder; it can simply be a naturally occurring consequence of a person's genetic makeup. See Figure 12.12.

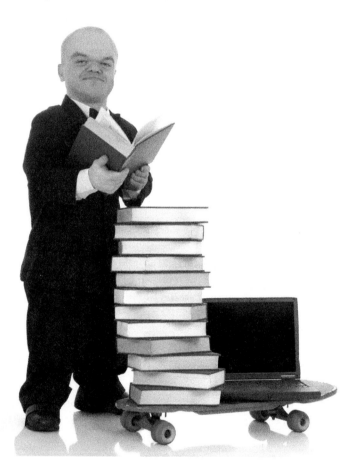

FIGURE 12.12 A man with dwarfism.
Source: sam100/Shutterstock

Medical Word	Word Parts		Definition
endocrinologist (ĕn˝ dō-krĭn-ŏl´ ō-gĭst)	endo- crin/o log -ist	within to secrete study one who specializes	Physician who specializes in the study of the endocrine system

Medical Word	Word Parts		Definition
	Part	**Meaning**	
endocrinology (ĕn″ dō-krĭn-ŏl′ ō-jē)	**endo-** **crin/o** **-logy**	within to secrete study of	Study of the endocrine system
epinephrine (ĕp″ ĭ-nĕf′ rĭn)	**epi-** **nephr** **-ine**	upon kidney substance	Hormone produced by the adrenal medulla; used as a vasoconstrictor and cardiac stimulant to relax bronchospasm and to relieve allergic symptoms; also called *adrenaline*
estrogen (ĕs′ trō-jĕn)	**estr/o** **-gen**	female formation, produce	Hormones produced by the ovaries, including estradiol, estrone, and estriol; female sex hormones important in the development of secondary sex characteristics and regulation of the menstrual cycle
euthyroid (ū-thī′ royd)	**eu-** **thyr** **-oid**	good, normal thyroid, shield resemble	Normal activity of the thyroid gland
exocrine (ĕks′ ō-krĭn)	**exo-** **-crine**	out, away from to secrete	Pertains to a type of gland that secretes into ducts (duct glands); examples include sweat glands, salivary glands, mammary glands, stomach, liver, and pancreas
exophthalmic (ĕks″ ŏf-thăl′ mĭk)	**ex-** **ophthalm** **-ic**	out, away from eye pertaining to	Pertaining to an abnormal condition characterized by a marked protrusion of the eyeballs as often seen in exophthalmic goiter or exophthalmos seen in Graves disease. People with Graves ophthalmopathy develop eye problems, including bulging, red, or swollen eyes, sensitivity to light, and blurring or double vision.
gigantism (jī′ găn-tĭzm)	**gigant** **-ism**	giant condition	Pathological condition of being abnormally large due to the overproduction of growth hormone (GH). In children, the condition is called gigantism. In adults, it is called acromegaly.
glandular (glăn′ jŭ-lăr)	**glandul** **-ar**	little acorn pertaining to	Pertaining to a gland
glucocorticoid (gloo″ kō-kort′ ĭ-koyd)	**gluc/o** **cortic** **-oid**	sweet, sugar cortex resemble	General classification of the adrenal cortical hormones: cortisol (hydrocortisone) and corticosterone

Medical Word	Word Parts		Definition
	Part	Meaning	
hirsutism (hĭr′ sŭ-tizm)	hirsut -ism	hairy condition	Abnormal condition characterized by excessive growth of hair, especially as occurring in women. See Figure 12.13.

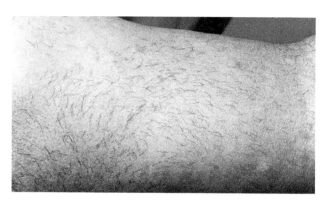

FIGURE 12.13 Hirsutism.
Source: Courtesy of Jason L. Smith, MD

Medical Word	Word Parts		Definition
hydrocortisone (hī″ drō-kŏr′ tĭ-sōn)	hydr/o cortis -one	water cortex hormone	Glucocorticoid (steroid) hormone produced by the adrenal cortex; used as an anti-inflammatory agent
hypergonadism (hī″ pĕr-gō′ năd-ĭzm)	hyper- gonad -ism	excessive seed condition	Condition of excessive secretion of the sex glands
hyperinsulinism (hī″ pĕr-in′ sŭ-lĭn-ĭzm)	hyper- insulin -ism	excessive insulin condition	Condition of excessive amounts of insulin in the blood, causing low blood sugar
hyperkalemia (hī″ pĕr-kă-lē′ mē-ă)	hyper- kal -emia	excessive potassium (K) blood condition	Condition of excessive amounts of potassium in the blood
hyperthyroidism (hī″ pĕr-thī′ royd-ĭzm)	hyper- thyr -oid -ism	excessive thyroid, shield resemble condition	Excessive secretion of thyroid hormone (TH), a condition that can affect many body systems. The most common etiologies of hyperthyroidism are Graves disease and toxic multinodular goiter. *Graves disease* is an autoimmune disease in which antibodies produced by the immune system stimulate the thyroid to produce too much thyroxine. Other forms of hyperthyroidism can be caused by **thyroiditis**, or inflammation of the thyroid gland. Certain benign or malignant tumors can also produce too much thyroid hormone. See Figure 12.14.

Medical Word	Word Parts		Definition
	Part	**Meaning**	

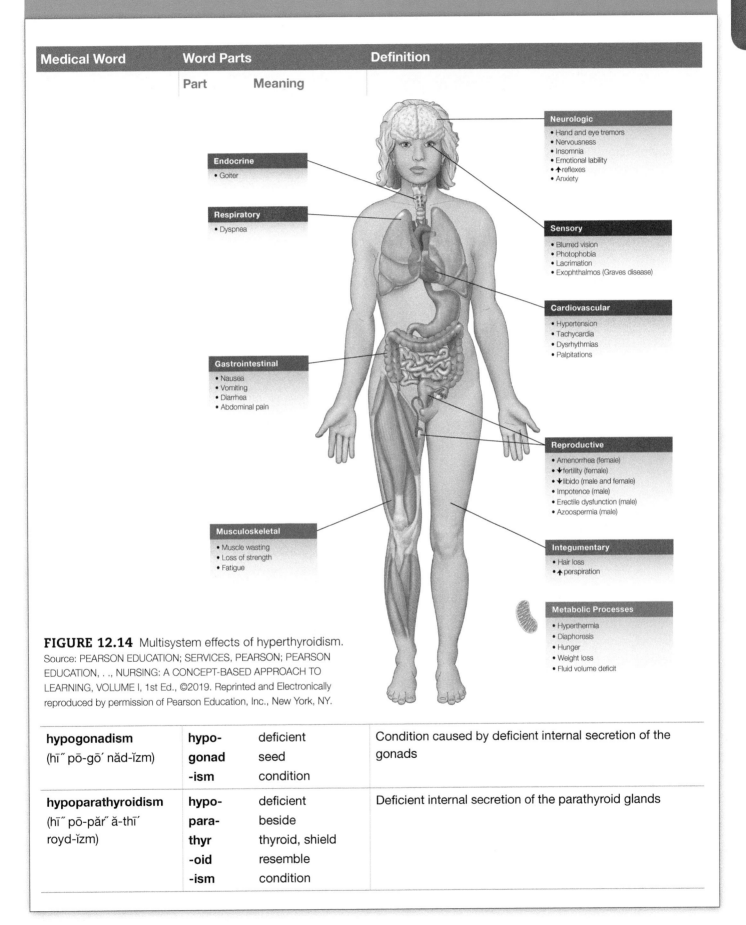

FIGURE 12.14 Multisystem effects of hyperthyroidism.
Source: PEARSON EDUCATION; SERVICES, PEARSON; PEARSON EDUCATION, . ., NURSING: A CONCEPT-BASED APPROACH TO LEARNING, VOLUME I, 1st Ed., ©2019. Reprinted and Electronically reproduced by permission of Pearson Education, Inc., New York, NY.

Medical Word	Word Parts		Definition
hypogonadism (hī″ pō-gō′ năd-ĭzm)	**hypo-**	deficient	Condition caused by deficient internal secretion of the gonads
	gonad	seed	
	-ism	condition	
hypoparathyroidism (hī″ pō-păr′ ă-thī′ royd-ĭzm)	**hypo-**	deficient	Deficient internal secretion of the parathyroid glands
	para-	beside	
	thyr	thyroid, shield	
	-oid	resemble	
	-ism	condition	

Medical Word	Word Parts		Definition
	Part	Meaning	
hypophysis (hī-pŏf´ ĭ-sĭs)	hypo- -physis	deficient, under growth	Literally means *any undergrowth*; also called the pituitary gland
hypothyroidism (hī˝ pō-thī´ royd-ĭzm)	hypo- thyr -oid -ism	deficient thyroid, shield resemble condition	Pathological condition in which the thyroid gland produces inadequate amounts of thyroid hormone. It can affect many body systems. See Figure 12.15.

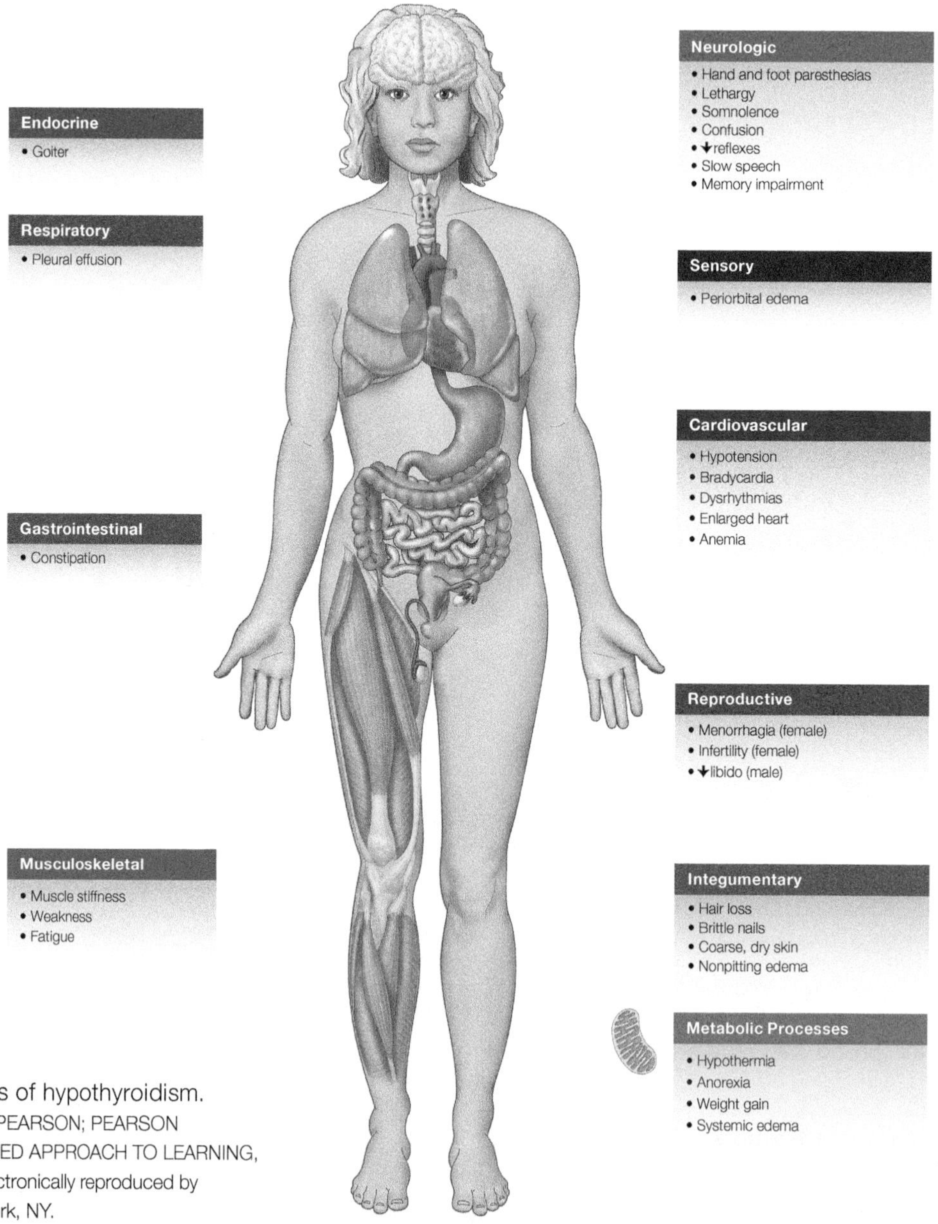

FIGURE 12.15 Multisystem effects of hypothyroidism.
Source: PEARSON EDUCATION; SERVICES, PEARSON; PEARSON EDUCATION, . ., NURSING: A CONCEPT-BASED APPROACH TO LEARNING, VOLUME I, 1st Ed., ©2019. Reprinted and Electronically reproduced by permission of Pearson Education, Inc., New York, NY.

Medical Word	Word Parts		Definition
	Part	Meaning	

 Untreated hypothyroidism can lead to a number of health problems. Constant stimulation of the thyroid to release more hormones can cause the gland to become larger, a condition known as **goiter**. Hashimoto thyroiditis, an autoimmune disease of the thyroid, is one of the most common causes of goiter. Another type of goiter is an *endemic goiter* that develops in certain geographic regions where the iodine content in food and water is deficient (Figure 12.16).

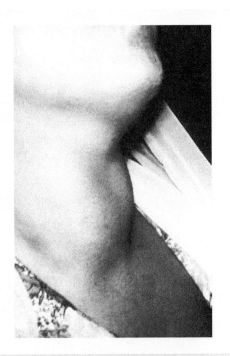

FIGURE 12.16 A man with goiter due to iodine deficiency.
Source: Centers for Disease Control and Prevention.

Medical Word	Word Parts		Definition
insulin (ĭn′ sŭ-lĭn)	**insul** **-in**	insulin substance	Hormone produced by the beta cells of the pancreatic islets in the pancreas; acts to regulate the metabolism of glucose and the process necessary for the intermediary metabolism of carbohydrates, fats, and proteins; used in the management of diabetes mellitus
insulinogenic (ĭn″ sŭ-lĭn″ ō-jĕn′ ĭk)	**insulin/o** **-genic**	insulin formation, produce	Formation or production of insulin
iodine (ī′ ŏ-dīn)			Trace mineral that aids in the development and functioning of the thyroid gland
lethargic (lĕ-thar′ jĭk)	**letharg** **-ic**	drowsiness pertaining to	Pertaining to drowsiness; sluggish

Medical Word	Word Parts		Definition
	Part	Meaning	
myxedema (mĭks″ ĕ-dē´ mă)	**myx** **-edema**	mucus swelling	Literally means *condition of mucus swelling*; it is the most severe form of hypothyroidism, characterized by marked edema of the face, a somnolent look, and hair that is stiff and without luster. Without treatment, coma and death can occur. See Figure 12.17.

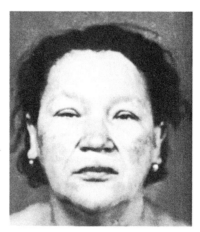 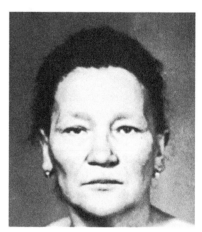

A   B

FIGURE 12.17 A A 62-year-old patient with myxedema exhibiting marked edema of the face and a somnolent look. The hair is stiff and without luster. **B** The same patient after 3 months of treatment with thyroxine.
Source: Pearson Education, Inc.

Medical Word	Word Parts		Definition
norepinephrine (nor-ĕp″ ĭ-nĕf´ rĭn)	**nor-** **epi-** **nephr** **-ine**	not upon kidney substance	Hormone produced by the adrenal medulla; used as a vasoconstrictor of peripheral blood vessels in acute hypotensive states
pancreatic (păn″ krē-ăt´ ĭk)	**pancreat** **-ic**	pancreas pertaining to	Pertaining to the pancreas
pineal (pĭn´ ē-ăl)	**pine** **-al**	pine cone pertaining to	Endocrine gland shaped like a small pine cone
pituitarism (pĭ-too´ ĭ-tă-rĭzm)	**pituitar** **-ism**	pituitary gland condition	Any condition of the pituitary gland
pituitary (pĭ-too´ ĭ-ter″ ē)	**pituitar** **-y**	pituitary gland pertaining to	Pertaining to the pituitary gland, the hypophysis

Medical Word	Word Parts		Definition
	Part	Meaning	
prediabetes (prē″ dī″ ă-bē′ tēz)	pre- dia- -betes	before through to go	Condition that occurs when a person's blood glucose levels are higher than normal but not high enough for a diagnosis of type 2 diabetes. It is estimated that at least 86 million Americans have prediabetes, in addition to the 29 million with diabetes. Without lifestyle changes, most people who have prediabetes will progress to type 2 diabetes within 10 years.

 fyi Another precursor condition to developing type 2 diabetes is called **metabolic syndrome**. The underlying causes are overweight, obesity, physical inactivity, and genetic factors. People with metabolic syndrome are at increased risk of coronary heart disease, other diseases related to plaque buildup in artery walls (e.g., stroke and peripheral vascular disease), and type 2 diabetes. Metabolic syndrome is characterized by a group of metabolic risk factors and has become increasingly common in the United States. It is closely associated with a generalized metabolic disorder called **insulin resistance syndrome**, in which the body can't use insulin efficiently.

Medical Word	Part	Meaning	Definition
progeria (prō-jē′ rē-ă)	pro- ger -ia	before old age condition	Pathological condition of premature old age occurring in childhood
progesterone (prō-jěs′ tě-rōn)	pro- gester -one	before to bear hormone	Hormone produced by the corpus luteum of the ovary, the adrenal cortex, or the placenta; released during the second half of the menstrual cycle
Simmonds disease (sĭm′ mŏnds)			Pathological condition in which complete atrophy of the pituitary gland causes loss of function of the thyroid, adrenals, and gonads; symptoms include premature aging, hair loss, and cachexia; also called *panhypopituitarism*
somatotropin (sō-măt′ ō-trō″ pĭn)	somat/o trop -in	body turning substance	Growth-stimulating hormone produced by the anterior lobe of the pituitary gland
steroids (stěr′ oydz)	ster -oid	solid resemble	Group of chemical substances that includes hormones, vitamins, sterols, cardiac glycosides, and certain drugs
testosterone (těs-tŏs′ tě-rōn)	test/o ster -one	testicle solid hormone	Hormone produced by the testes; male sex hormone important in the development of secondary sex characteristics and masculinization
thymectomy (thī-měk′ tō-mē)	thym -ectomy	thymus surgical excision	Surgical excision of the thymus gland

Medical Word	Word Parts		Definition
	Part	Meaning	
thymitis (thī-mī′ tĭs)	**thym** -**itis**	thymus inflammation	Inflammation of the thymus gland
thyroid (thī′ royd)	**thyr** -**oid**	thyroid, shield resemble	Endocrine gland located in the neck; its shape resembles a shield. See Figure 12.18.

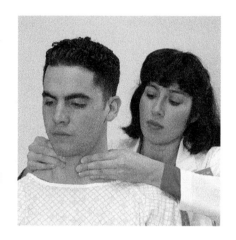

FIGURE 12.18 Palpating the thyroid gland from behind the patient is a most effective way of assessing the gland for abnormality.
Source: Pearson Education, Inc.

Medical Word	Word Parts		Definition
thyroidectomy (thī″ royd-ĕk′ tō-mē)	**thyr** -**oid** -**ectomy**	thyroid, shield resemble surgical excision	Surgical excision of the thyroid gland. See Figure 12.19.

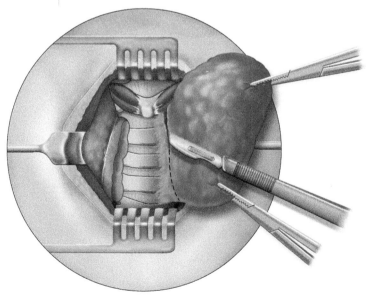

FIGURE 12.19 Thyroidectomy.

Medical Word	Word Parts		Definition
thyroiditis (thī″ royd-īt′ ĭs)	**thyr** -**oid** -**itis**	thyroid, shield resemble inflammation	Inflammation of the thyroid gland

Medical Word	Word Parts		Definition
	Part	Meaning	
thyrotoxicosis (thī″ rō-tŏk″ sĭ-kō′ sĭs)	thyr/o toxic -osis	thyroid, shield poison condition	Literally means *a poisonous condition of the thyroid gland*; pathological condition caused by an acute oversecretion of thyroid hormones
thyroxine (T₄) (thī-rŏks′ ēn)	thyro(x) -ine	thyroid, shield substance	Hormone produced by the thyroid gland; important in growth and development and regulation of the body's metabolic rate and metabolism of carbohydrates, fats, and proteins
vasopressin (VP) (văs″ ō-prĕs′ ĭn)	vas/o press -in	vessel to press substance	Hormone produced by the hypothalamus and stored in the posterior lobe of the pituitary gland; also called *antidiuretic hormone (ADH)*. Hyposecretion of this hormone can result in **diabetes insipidus (DI)**, a condition characterized by excessive thirst (*polydipsia*) and excretion of large amounts of diluted urine (*polyuria*). *Insipidus* means *tasteless*, reflecting very dilute and watery urine.
virilism (vĭr′ ĭl-ĭzm)	viril -ism	masculine condition	Pathological condition in which secondary male characteristics, such as growth of hair on face and/or body and deepening of the voice, are produced in a female, usually as the result of adrenal dysfunction or hormonal imbalance or taking medications (androgens)

Study *and* Review II

Word Parts

Prefixes   Give the definitions of the following prefixes.

1. dia- _____   6. hyper- _____

2. endo- _____   7. hypo- _____

3. eu- _____   8. para- _____

4. ex- _____   9. pro- _____

5. exo- _____   10. epi- _____

Combining Forms   Give the definitions of the following combining forms.

1. acid/o _____

2. acr/o _____

3. aden/o _____

4. adren/o _____

5. andr/o _____

6. cortic/o _____

7. crin/o _____

8. estr/o _____

9. ger/o _____

10. gigant/o _____

11. gluc/o _____

12. gonad/o _____

13. hirsut/o _____

14. insulin/o _____

15. kal/i _____

16. myx/o _____

17. pancreat/o _____

18. test/o _____

19. thym/o _____

20. thyr/o _____

21. toxic/o _____

22. viril/o _____

Suffixes   Give the definitions of the following suffixes.

1. -al _____

2. -gen _____

3. -ar _____

4. -betes _____

5. -ectomy _____

6. -edema _____

7. -emia _____

8. -genic _____

9. -ia _____

10. -ic _____

11. -ism _____

12. -ist _____

13. -itis _____

14. -logy _____

15. -one _____

16. -megaly _____

17. -oid _____

18. -oma _____

19. -osis _____

20. -pathy _____

21. -ine _____

22. -physis _____

23. -in _____

24. -y _____

Identifying Medical Terms

In the spaces provided, write the medical terms for the following meanings.

1. _____ Tumor of a gland

2. _____ Congenital deficiency in secretion of the thyroid hormones characterized by arrested physical and mental development

3. _____ General term used to describe diseases characterized by excessive discharge of urine

4. _____ Study of the endocrine system

5. _____ Normal activity of the thyroid gland

6. _____ Pertains to a type of gland that secretes into ducts (duct glands)

7. _____ Pathological condition of being abnormally large

8. _____ General classification of the adrenal cortex hormones

9. _____ Condition of excessive amounts of potassium in the blood

10. _____ Condition caused by deficient internal secretion of the gonads

Matching

Select the appropriate lettered meaning for each of the following words.

_____ 1. aldosterone

_____ 2. androgen

_____ 3. progesterone

_____ 4. cortisone

_____ 5. dopamine

_____ 6. epinephrine

_____ 7. insulin

_____ 8. iodine

_____ 9. thyroxine

_____ 10. vasopressin

a. Also called *antidiuretic hormone, ADH*

b. Hormone released during the second half of the menstrual cycle

c. Acts to regulate the metabolism of glucose

d. Hormone produced by the thyroid gland

e. Necessary in regulating electrolyte and water balance by promoting sodium and chloride reabsorption and potassium excretion

f. Hormones that produce or stimulate the development of male characteristics

g. Glucocorticoid (steroid) hormone used as an anti-inflammatory agent

h. Intermediate substance in the synthesis of norepinephrine

i. Also called *adrenaline*

j. Trace mineral that aids in the development and functioning of the thyroid gland

Medical Case Snapshots

This learning activity provides an opportunity to relate the medical terminology you are learning to sample patient case presentations. In the spaces provided, write in your answers.

Case 1

A 54-year-old female presents with fatigue, muscular weakness, and a round, red face. These are symptoms associated with _____ (disease that results from the hypersecretion of cortisol). Prolonged administration of large doses of ACTH can also cause this condition. Two characteristic signs of this condition are a _____ and a moon face.

Case 2

A 15-year-old male complains of being "thirsty, hungry, and frequent urination." The medical terms for his complaints are _____ or excessive thirst, _____ or extreme hunger, and _____ or frequent urination.

Case 3

The patient is a 48-year-old female presenting with marked protrusion of the eyeballs indicative of _____ goiter, sometimes called _____ disease. People with this condition develop eye problems including bulging, red, or _____ eyes, sensitivity to _____, and _____ or double vision.

Drug Highlights

Classification of Drug	Description and Examples
thyroid hormones	Increase metabolic rate, cardiac output, oxygen consumption, body temperature, respiratory rate, blood volume, and carbohydrate, fat, and protein metabolism; influence growth and development at cellular level. Thyroid hormones are used as supplements or replacement therapy in hypothyroidism, myxedema, and congenital hypothyroidism. EXAMPLES: Synthroid (levothyroxine sodium), Cytomel (liothyronine sodium), and Thyrolar (liotrix)
antithyroid hormones	Inhibit the synthesis of thyroid hormones by decreasing iodine use in manufacture of thyroglobin and iodothyronine; do not inactivate or inhibit thyroxine or triiodothyronine. They are used in the treatment of hyperthyroidism. EXAMPLES: Tapazole (methimazole), potassium iodide solution, and propylthiouracil

Classification of Drug	Description and Examples
insulin preparations for injection	Insulin is given by subcutaneous injection and is available in various forms such as rapid-acting, intermediate-acting, and long-acting preparations.
oral hypoglycemic agents	Stimulate insulin secretion from pancreatic cells in noninsulin-dependent diabetics with some pancreatic function. They are agents of the sulfonylurea class. EXAMPLES: Glucotrol (glipizide), DiaBeta (glyburide), and Glucophage (metformin)
hyperglycemic agents	Cause an increase in blood glucose of diabetic patients with severe hypoglycemia (insulin shock). In patients with mild hypoglycemia, the administration of an oral carbohydrate such as orange juice, candy, or a lump of sugar generally corrects the condition. If comatose, the patient is given dextrose solution IV. For management of severe hypoglycemia, the following agents may be used. EXAMPLES: Glucagon (an insulin antagonist) and Proglycem (diazoxide)

Diagnostic *and* Laboratory Tests

Test	Description
catecholamines (kăt″ĕ-kōl′ă-mēns)	Test performed on urine to determine the amount of epinephrine and norepinephrine present. These adrenal hormones increase in times of stress.
corticotropin, corticotropin-releasing factor (CRF) (kor″tĭ-kō-trō′ pin)	Test performed on blood plasma to determine the amount of corticotropin present. Increased levels can indicate stress, adrenal cortical hypofunction, and/or pituitary tumors. Decreased CRF levels can indicate adrenal neoplasms and/or Cushing syndrome.
fasting blood sugar (FBS)	Test performed on blood to determine the level of sugar in the bloodstream. It is done after fasting 8–12 hrs (NPO [nothing by mouth] after midnight) and should be performed the next morning. A FBS of 100–125 mg/dL indicates prediabetes. A FBS of 126 mg/dL may indicate diabetes mellitus. Also referred to as *fasting blood glucose (FBG)*.
glucose tolerance test (GTT) (gloo′ kōs)	Blood sugar test performed at specified intervals after the patient has been given a significant amount of glucose. Blood samples are drawn, and the glucose level of each sample is measured. It is more accurate than other blood sugar tests and is used to diagnose diabetes mellitus. A GTT of 140–199 mg/dL indicates prediabetes. A GTT at 200 mg/dL or higher indicates diabetes mellitus.
Hb A1C test	The Hb A1C test is a blood test used to diagnose diabetes, to identify people at risk of developing diabetes, and to monitor how well blood sugar levels are being controlled by the diabetic patient. For someone who doesn't have diabetes, a normal A1C level can range from 4.5 to 6%. An A1C level of 6.5% or higher on two separate tests indicates diabetes. A result between 5.7 and 6.4% is considered prediabetes, which indicates a high risk of developing diabetes. For most people who have previously diagnosed diabetes, an A1C level of 7% or less is a common treatment target.

Test	Description
17-hydroxycorticosteroids (17-OHCS) (hī-drŏk″ sē-kor tĭ-kō-stĕr′ oyds)	Test performed on urine to identify adrenocorticosteroid hormones and to determine adrenal cortical function.
17-ketosteroids (17-KS) (kē″ tō-stĕr′ oyds)	Test performed on urine to determine the amount of 17-KS present, the end product of androgens that are secreted from the adrenal glands and testes. It is used to diagnose adrenal tumors.
protein-bound iodine (PBI)	Test performed on serum to indicate the amount of iodine that is attached to serum protein. It can be used to indicate thyroid function.
radioactive iodine uptake (RAIU) (rā″ dē-ō-ăk′ tĭv ī′ ō-dīn)	Test to measure the ability of the thyroid gland to concentrate ingested iodine. Increased level can indicate hyperthyroidism, cirrhosis, and/or thyroiditis. Decreased level can indicate hypothyroidism.
thyroid scan (thī′ royd)	Test to detect tumors of the thyroid gland. The patient is given radioactive iodine 131, which localizes in the thyroid gland, which is then visualized with a scanner device. See Figures 12.20 and 12.21.

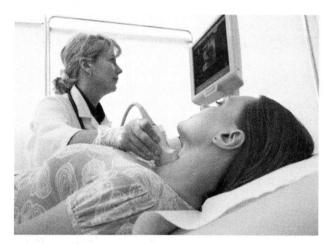

FIGURE 12.20 Doctor performing a thyroid scan on a patient.
Source: Alexander Raths/Shutterstock

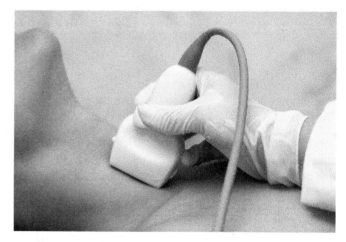

FIGURE 12.21 Scanning a man's thyroid.
Source: Bork/Shutterstock

thyroxine (T₄) (thī-rŏks′ ēn)	Test performed on blood serum to determine the amount of thyroxine present. Increased levels can indicate hyperthyroidism; decreased levels can indicate hypothyroidism.
total calcium	Test performed on blood serum to determine the amount of calcium present. Increased levels can indicate hyperparathyroidism; decreased levels can indicate hypoparathyroidism.
triiodothyronine uptake (T₃U) (trī″ ī-ō″ dō-thī′ rō-nĭn)	Test performed on blood serum to determine the amount of triiodothyronine present. Increased levels can indicate thyrotoxicosis, toxic adenoma, and/or Hashimoto thyroiditis. Decreased levels can indicate starvation, severe infection, and severe trauma.
ultrasonography (ŭl-tră-sŏn-ŏg′ ră-fē)	Use of high-frequency sound waves as a screening test or as a diagnostic tool to visualize the structure being studied; can be used to visualize the pancreas, thyroid, and any other gland

Abbreviations *and* Acronyms

Abbreviation/ Acronym	Meaning
17-KS	17-ketosteroids
17-OHCS	17-hydroxycorticosteroids
ACTH	adrenocorticotropin hormone
ADH	antidiuretic hormone
BG	blood glucose
BMI	body mass index
BMR	basal metabolic rate
cm	centimeter
CRF	corticotropin-releasing factor
DI	diabetes insipidus
DM	diabetes mellitus
FBG	fasting blood glucose
FBS	fasting blood sugar
FSH	follicle-stimulating hormone
g	gram
GH	growth hormone
GHRF	growth hormone-releasing factor
GnRF	gonadotropin-releasing factor
GTT	glucose tolerance test
IDDM	insulin-dependent diabetes mellitus
K	potassium
kg	kilogram
LH	luteinizing hormone

Abbreviation/ Acronym	Meaning
LTH	lactogenic hormone
MIF	melanocyte-stimulating hormone release-inhibiting factor
MRF	melanocyte-stimulating hormone-releasing factor
MSH	melanocyte-stimulating hormone
Na	sodium
NIDDM	non-insulin-dependent diabetes mellitus
NPO, npo	nothing by mouth (*nil per os*)
PBI	protein-bound iodine
PIF	prolactin release-inhibiting factor
PRF	prolactin-releasing factor
PRL	prolactin hormone
PTH	parathyroid hormone
RAIU	radioactive iodine uptake
STH	somatotropin hormone
T$_3$	triiodothyronine
T$_3$U	triiodothyronine uptake
T$_4$	thyroxine
TH	thyroid hormone
TRH	thyrotropin-releasing hormone
TSH	thyroid-stimulating hormone
VP	vasopressin

Study *and* Review III

Building Medical Terms

Using the following word parts, fill in the blanks to build the correct medical terms.

hypo-	dwarf	-one	-in	-al
adren	letharg	-ism	-edema	

Definition	Medical Term
1. Pertaining to the adrenal glands; also called suprarenal glands	_____al
2. Glucocorticoid hormone secreted by the adrenal cortex	cortis_____
3. Condition of being abnormally small	_____ism
4. Pathological condition of being abnormally large	gigant_____
5. Abnormal condition characterized by excessive growth of hair	hirsut_____
6. Literally means *any undergrowth*; also called the pituitary gland	_____physis
7. Hormone produced by the beta cells of the islets of Langerhans	insul_____
8. Pertaining to drowsiness, sluggish	_____ic
9. Literally means *condition of mucus swelling*	myx_____
10. Endocrine gland shaped like a small pine cone	pine_____

Combining Form Challenge

Using the combining forms provided, write the medical term correctly.

aden/o	estr/o	thym/o
andr/o	insulin/o	thyr/o

1. Any disease condition of a gland: _____osis

2. Hormone that produces the development of male characteristics: _____gen

3. Female sex hormone produced in the ovaries: _____gen

4. Formation or production of insulin: _____genic

5. Surgical excision of the thymus gland: _____ectomy

6. Endocrine gland located in the neck: _____oid

Select the Right Term

Select the correct answer, and write it on the line provided.

1. Characterized (in the adult) by marked enlargement and elongation of the bones of the face, jaw, and extremities is _____.

    Addison disease   acidosis   acromegaly   adenoma

2. General term used to describe diseases characterized by excessive discharge of urine is _____.

    diabetes   hypothyroidism   Cushing   exophthalmic

3. Hormone produced by the adrenal medulla, also called adrenaline, is _____.

    dopamine   epinephrine   estrogen   norepinephrine

4. Pathological condition in which the thyroid gland produces inadequate amounts of thyroid hormone is _____.

    hyperthyroidism   hypophysis   hypothyroidism   hypogonadism

5. Pathological condition of premature old age occurring in childhood is _____.

    myxedema   lethargic   pituitarism   progeria

6. Pathological condition in which secondary male characteristics are produced in a female is _____.

    thyrotoxicosis   progeria   hypoparathyroidism   virilism

Drug Highlights

Match the appropriate lettered description or examples of drug(s) with the class of drug.

_____ 1. hyperglycemic agents

_____ 2. thyroid hormones

_____ 3. insulin preparations for injection

_____ 4. oral hypoglycemic agents

_____ 5. antithyroid hormones

_____ 6. examples of thyroid hormones

a. Agents of the sulfonylurea class, they stimulate insulin secretion from pancreatic cells in non-insulin-dependent diabetics with some pancreatic function

b. Inhibit the synthesis of thyroid hormones by decreasing iodine use in manufacture of thyroglobin and iodothyronine; used in the treatment of hyperthyroidism

c. Synthroid (levothyroxine sodium), Cytomel (liothyronine sodium), and Thyrolar (liotrix)

d. Used as supplements or replacement therapy in hypothyroidism, myxedema, and congenital hypothyroidism

e. Available in rapid-acting, intermediate-acting, and long-acting preparations

f. Cause an increase in blood glucose of diabetic patients with severe hypoglycemia (insulin shock)

Diagnostic and Laboratory Tests

Select the best answer to each multiple-choice question. Circle the letter of your choice.

1. A test performed on urine to determine the amount of epinephrine and norepinephrine present.

    a. catecholamines

    b. corticotropin

    c. protein-bound iodine

    d. total calcium

2. Increased levels can indicate prediabetes or diabetes mellitus.

    a. protein-bound iodine

    b. total calcium

    c. fasting blood sugar

    d. thyroid scan

3. Test used to detect tumors of the thyroid gland.

    a. thyroxine

    b. total calcium

    c. thyroid scan

    d. protein-bound iodine

4. Blood sugar test performed at specific intervals after the patient has been given a certain amount of glucose.

   a. fasting blood sugar

   b. glucose tolerance test

   c. protein-bound iodine

   d. corticotropin

5. A test used in the diagnosing of adrenal tumors.

   a. 17-HCS

   b. 17-OHCS

   c. 17-KS

   d. 17-HDL

Abbreviations and Acronyms

Write the correct word, phrase, or abbreviation/acronym in the space provided.

1. basal metabolic rate _____

2. diabetes mellitus _____

3. FBS _____

4. GTT _____

5. protein-bound iodine _____

6. PTH _____

7. BMI _____

8. somatotropin hormone _____

9. TSH _____

10. VP _____

Practical Application

Case Study Analysis

This exercise contains information, abbreviations/acronyms, and medical terminology from an actual medical record or case study that has been adapted for this text. The names and any personal information have been created by the author. Read and study each form or case study and then answer the questions that follow. You may refer to Appendix III, *Abbreviations, Acronyms, and Symbols*.

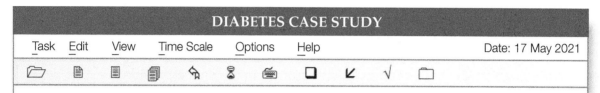

DIABETES CASE STUDY						
Task Edit View Time Scale Options Help						Date: 17 May 2021

Meet Matthew J. Marshall

Matthew is a 15 y/o white male c/o being "thirsty, hungry, and urinating a lot." He states, "I am tired and just don't have any energy. I eat like a horse, but I stay hungry. I am afraid that I have diabetes. My dad and my grandfather both take insulin."

Signs and Symptoms: Polydipsia, polyphagia, polyuria, and fatigue. Family history is notable for type 1 diabetes in father and paternal grandfather; his maternal grandmother has heart disease.

Allergies: NKDA. Typically, for a patient with this complaint and history, type 2 diabetes would be considered.

The pertinent findings on physical exam:

Vital Signs: T: 98.4°F; P: 78; R: 18; BP: 132/70

Ht: 5'5"

Wt: 160 lb

General Appearance: Overweight for age. BMI: 26.6

Heart: Regular rate and rhythm. No murmurs.

Lungs: CTA.

Abd: Noted excessive adipose tissue. Soft, nontender, no masses, no liver enlargement.

Skin: Warm and dry, no lesions, no discoloration of lower extremities.

Plan for Diagnosis and Treatment:

1. Send to lab for Hb A1C and schedule FBS.

2. Recommend that Matthew attend the next health education seminar. One or both parents are to attend the seminar with him. Explain that individuals who are overweight, have a BMI greater than or equal to 25, and who have immediate family members with diabetes are at a higher risk of developing diabetes. Note: For more information on diabetes, call (800) DIABETES.

3. Patient is to return in 1 week for test results. If indicated, proper medication regimen will be initiated for Matthew.

Case Study Questions

Write the correct answer in the space provided.

1. Why is Matthew concerned that he may have diabetes?_____

_____

2. To rule out diabetes mellitus, the physician ordered a _____ test

   and a _____.

3. What are the three classic symptoms of diabetes mellitus that Matthew stated?

   _____ _____ _____

4. What does the abbreviation *FBS* mean? _____ _____

   _____

5. A BMI over _____ may indicate a higher risk of developing diabetes.

6. The _____ test is a blood test used to diagnose diabetes.

MyLab Medical Terminology™

MyLab Medical Terminology is a premium online homework management system that includes a host of features to help you study. Registered users will find:

- A multitude of quizzes and activities built within the MyLab platform
- Powerful tools that track and analyze your results—allowing you to create a personalized learning experience
- Videos and audio pronunciations to help enrich your progress
- Streaming lesson presentations (guided lectures) and self-paced learning modules
- A space where you and your instructor can check your progress and manage your assignments

13 Nervous System

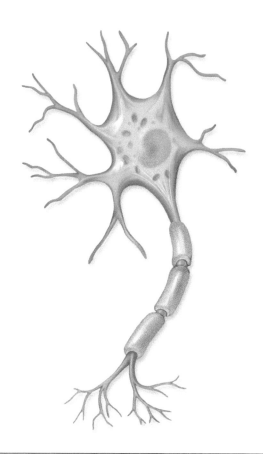

∨ Learning Outcomes

On completion of this chapter, you will be able to:

1. Identify the primary functions of the organs/structures of the nervous system.
2. Describe the principal tissues of the nervous system.
3. List the major divisions of the brain and their functions.
4. Describe the peripheral nervous system.
5. Describe the autonomic nervous system.
6. Analyze, build, spell, and pronounce medical words.
7. Classify the drugs highlighted in this chapter.
8. Describe diagnostic and laboratory tests related to the nervous system.
9. Identify and define selected abbreviations and acronyms.

Anatomy and Physiology

The nervous system is an intricate network of nerves and cells that carry messages to and from the brain and spinal cord to various parts of the body. These messages may involve communication, higher mental function and emotional expression, perception, and control or regulation of bodily functions. Along with the endocrine system, the nervous system regulates many aspects of homeostasis, such as respiratory rate, blood pressure, body temperature, and the sleep–wake cycle.

The nervous system can be described as having two interconnected divisions: the central nervous system (CNS) and the peripheral nervous system (PNS). The autonomic nervous system (ANS) is a part of the peripheral nervous system and is divided into the sympathetic division and the parasympathetic division. The CNS includes the brain and spinal cord. It is enclosed by the bones of the skull and spinal column. The PNS consists of the network of nerves and neural tissues branching throughout the body from 12 pairs of cranial nerves and 31 pairs of spinal nerves. Table 13.1 provides an at-a-glance look at the nervous system, including the CNS, the PNS, and the ANS. See Figure 13.1.

TABLE 13.1   Nervous System at-a-Glance

Organ/Structure	Primary Functions/Description
Neurons (nerve cells)	Structural and functional units of the nervous system act as specialized conductors of impulses that enable the body to interact with its internal and external environments
Neuroglia	Act as supporting tissue
Nerve fibers and tracts	Conduct impulses from one location to another
Central nervous system	Receives impulses from throughout the body, processes the information, and responds with an appropriate action
Brain	Governs sensory perception, emotions, consciousness, memory, and voluntary movements
Spinal cord	Conducts sensory impulses to the brain and motor impulses from the brain to body parts; also serves as a reflex center for impulses entering and leaving the spinal cord without involvement of the brain
Peripheral nervous system	Links the central nervous system with other parts of the body
Cranial nerves (12 pairs)	Provide sensory input and motor control or a combination of these
Spinal nerves (31 pairs)	Carry impulses to the spinal cord and to muscles, organs, and glands
Autonomic nervous system (sympathetic division and parasympathetic division)	Controls involuntary bodily functions such as sweating, secretion of glands, arterial blood pressure, smooth muscle tissue, and the heart. Also stimulates the adrenal gland to release epinephrine (adrenaline), the hormone that causes the familiar adrenaline rush or the fight-or-flight response.

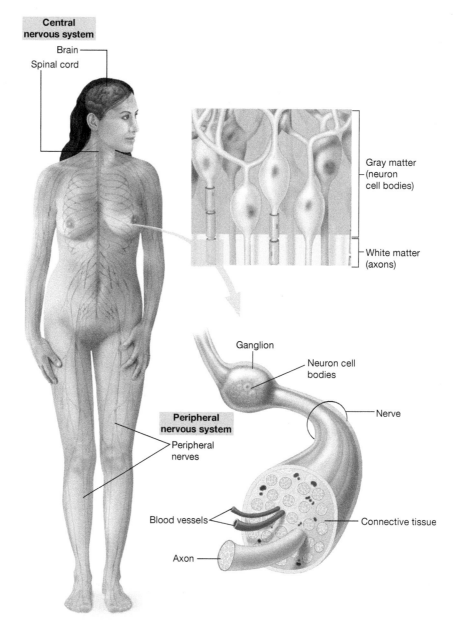

FIGURE 13.1 The nervous system is described as having two interconnected divisions: the central nervous system (CNS) consisting of the brain and spinal cord and the peripheral nervous system (PNS) consisting of peripheral nerves.

Tissues of the Nervous System

The nervous system has two principal tissue types. These tissues are made up of **neurons** or nerve cells and their supporting tissues, collectively called **neuroglia**. See Figure 13.2. Neurons are the structural and functional units of the nervous system. These cells are specialized conductors of impulses that enable the body to interact with its internal and external environments. There are several types of neurons, three of which are described in the following sections.

Motor Neurons

Motor neurons cause contractions in muscles and secretions from glands and organs. They also act to inhibit the actions of glands and organs, thereby controlling most of the body's functions. Motor neurons can be described as being *efferent processes* because they transmit impulses away from the neural cell body to the muscles or organs to be

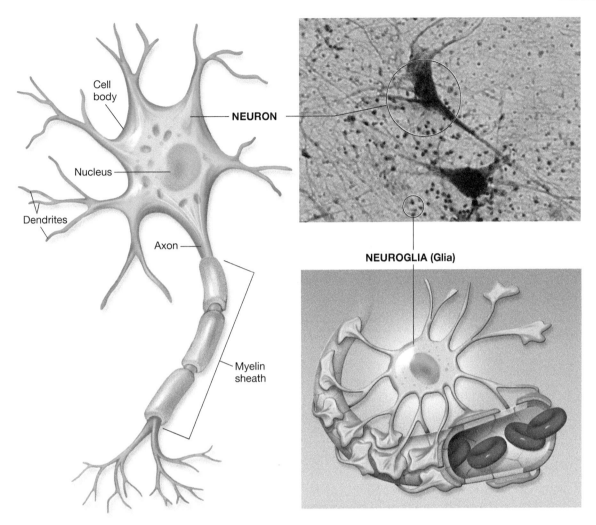

Cell
body

NEURON

Nucleus

Dendrites

Axon

NEUROGLIA (Glia)

Myelin
sheath

FIGURE 13.2 Two main types of nerve cells.

innervated. Motor neurons consist of a nucleated cell body with protoplasmic processes extending away from it in several directions.

These processes are known as **axons** and **dendrites**. An axon is a single extension of a neuron that is defined as a process that can generate and conduct action potentials. The axons of certain neurons can carry a signal both toward and away from the cell body, although most axons carry information away from the cell body. Depending on the type of neuron, the axon may range in length from short to very long. Most axons are covered with a fatty substance, the myelin sheath, which acts as an insulator and increases the transmission velocity of the nerve fiber it surrounds. Dendrites resemble the branches of a tree, are short, and transmit impulses to the cell body. Neurons may have several dendrites with only a single axon.

Sensory Neurons

Sensory neurons differ in structure from motor neurons because they do not have true dendrites. The processes transmitting sensory information to the cell bodies of these neurons are called *peripheral processes,* are sheathed, and resemble axons. They are attached to sensory receptors and transmit impulses to the CNS. After processing the information, the CNS can stimulate motor neurons in response to this sensory information. Sensory neurons are referred to as *afferent nerves* because they carry impulses from the sensory receptors to the synaptic endings in the central nervous system.

Interneurons

Interneurons are called *central* or *associative neurons* and are located entirely within the CNS. They function to mediate impulses between sensory and motor neurons.

Nerve Fibers, Nerves, and Tracts

The terms *nerve fiber, nerve,* and *tract* are used to describe neuronal processes conducting impulses from one location to another.

Nerve Fibers

A **nerve fiber** is a single elongated process, the axon of a neuron. Nerve fibers of the peripheral nervous system are wrapped by protective membranes called **sheaths**. The PNS has two types of sheaths: *myelinated* and *unmyelinated,* which are formed by accessory cells. Myelinated fibers have an inner sheath of myelin, a thick, fatty substance, and an outer sheath, or **neurilemma**, composed of *Schwann cells*. Unmyelinated fibers lack myelin and are sheathed only by the neurilemma. Nerve fibers of the central nervous system do not contain Schwann cells.

Nerves

A **nerve** is a collection of nerve fibers, outside the central nervous system. Nerves are usually described as being sensory or **afferent** (conducting to the CNS) or motor or **efferent** (conducting away from the CNS to muscles, organs, and glands).

Tracts

Groups of nerve fibers within the CNS are sometimes referred to as **tracts** when they have the same origin, function, and termination. The spinal cord contains afferent sensory tracts ascending to the brain and efferent motor tracts descending from the brain. The brain itself contains numerous tracts, the largest of which is the *corpus callosum* joining the left and right hemispheres.

Transmission of Nerve Impulses

The transmission of an impulse by a nerve fiber is based on the **all-or-none principle**. This means that no transmission occurs until the stimulus reaches a set minimum strength, which can vary for different receptors. Once the minimum stimulus or threshold is reached, a maximum impulse is produced. The impulse is then transmitted via a **synapse**, a specialized knoblike branch ending, with the help of certain chemical agents, across a space separating the axon's end knobs from the dendrites of the next neuron or from a motor end plate attached to a muscle. This space is called a **synaptic cleft**, and the chemical agents released are called **neurotransmitters**.

Central Nervous System

Consisting of the brain and spinal cord, the **central nervous system (CNS)** receives impulses from throughout the body, processes the information, and responds with an appropriate action. This activity can be at the conscious or unconscious level, depending on the source of the sensory stimulus. Both the brain and spinal cord can be divided into **gray matter** and **white matter**. The gray matter consists of unsheathed cell bodies and true dendrites. The white matter is composed of myelinated nerve fibers. In the spinal cord, the arrangement of white and gray matter results in an H-shaped core of gray cell bodies surrounded by tracts of nerve fibers interconnected to the brain. The reverse is generally true of the brain where the surface layer or cortex is gray matter and most of the internal structures are white matter.

 fyi Neural tube development occurs about the third to fourth week of embryonic life. This development becomes the central nervous system. At 6 weeks, a developing fetus's brain waves are measurable. At 28 weeks, the fetal nervous system begins some regulatory functions. By 32 weeks, the developing fetal nervous system is capable of sustaining rhythmic respirations and regulating body temperature. The growth rate of brain and nerve cells is at its most rapid pace up to about 4 years of age.

Brain

The nervous tissue of the **brain** consists of millions of nerve cells and fibers. It is the largest mass of nervous tissue in the body, weighing about 1380 g in the male and 1250 g in the female. The brain is enclosed by three membranes known collectively as the **meninges**. See Figure 13.3. From the outside in, these are the *dura mater, arachnoid,* and *pia mater*. The major structures of the brain are the *cerebrum, cerebellum, diencephalon,* and the *brainstem,* which is composed of the *midbrain, pons,* and *medulla oblongata*. See Figure 13.4 and Table 13.2.

CEREBRUM

Representing seven-eighths of the brain's total weight, the cerebrum contains nerve centers that evaluate and control all sensory and motor activity, including sensory perception, emotions, consciousness, memory, and voluntary movements.

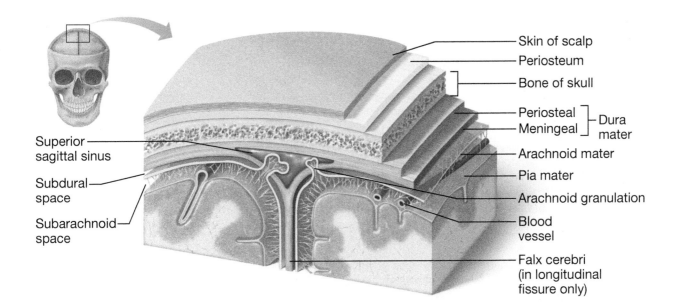

FIGURE 13.3 The meninges from the outside in: dura mater, arachnoid, and pia mater. Also showing the superior sagittal sinus, subdural space, and subarachnoid space.
Source: MARIEB, ELAINE N.; KELLER, SUZANNE M., ESSENTIALS OF HUMAN ANATOMY & PHYSIOLOGY, 12th Ed., ©2018. Reprinted and Electronically reproduced by permission of Pearson Education, Inc., New York, NY.

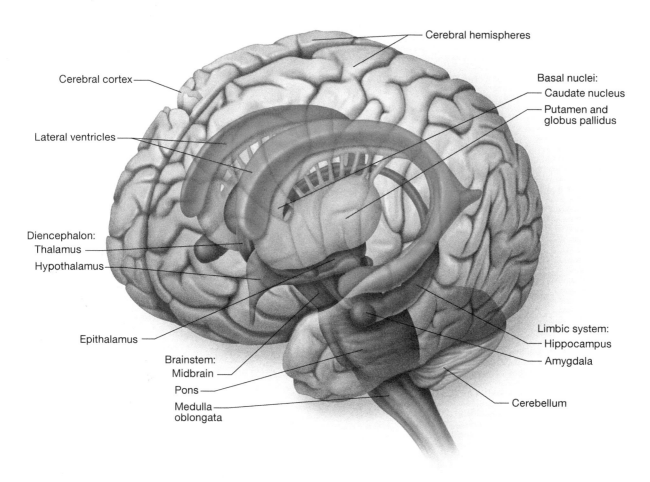

FIGURE 13.4 Major structures of the brain.

Source: AMERMAN, ERIN C., HUMAN ANATOMY & PHYSIOLOGY, 2nd Ed., ©2019. Reprinted and Electronically reproduced by permission of Pearson Education, Inc., New York, NY.

TABLE 13.2	Major Divisions of the Brain and Their Functions
Brain Area (Refer to Figure 13.4)	**Functions**
Cerebrum	Evaluates and controls all sensory and motor activity: sensory perception, emotions, consciousness, memory, and voluntary movements.
Cerebellum	Plays an important role in the integration of sensory perception and motor output. Its neural pathways link with the motor cortex, which sends information to the muscles causing them to move, and the spinocerebellar tract, which provides feedback on the position of the body in space (proprioception). The cerebellum integrates these pathways using the constant feedback on body position to fine-tune motor movements. Research shows that the cerebellum also has a broader role in a number of key cognitive functions, including attention and the processing of language, music, and other sensory temporal stimuli.
Diencephalon	
Epithalamus	Involved in the maintenance of circadian rhythm, basically a 24-hour internal clock that cycles between sleepiness and alertness at regular intervals. Functions include the secretion of melatonin by the pineal gland and regulation of motor pathways and emotions.
Thalamus	Relay center for all sensory impulses (except olfactory) being transmitted to the sensory areas of the cortex, and relays motor impulses from the cerebellum and the basal ganglia to motor areas of the cortex, thought to be involved with emotions and arousal mechanisms.

(continued)

TABLE 13.2 Major Divisions of the Brain and Their Functions (*continued*)

Brain Area (Refer to Figure 13.4)	Functions
Hypothalamus	Serves as the principal regulator of autonomic nervous activity that is associated with behavior and expression; also contains hormones that are important for the control of certain metabolic activities such as maintenance of water balance, sugar and fat metabolism, regulation of body temperature, sleep-cycle control, appetite, and sexual arousal.
Brainstem	
Midbrain	Two-way conduction pathway that acts as a relay center for visual and auditory impulses; found in the midbrain are four small masses of gray cells known collectively as the *corpora quadrigemina*. The upper two, called the *superior colliculi*, are associated with visual reflexes. The lower two, or *inferior colliculi*, are involved with the sense of hearing.
Pons	Links the cerebellum and medulla to higher cortical areas; plays a role in somatic and visceral motor control; contains important centers for regulating breathing.
Medulla oblongata	Acts as the cardiac, respiratory, and vasomotor control center; regulates and controls breathing, swallowing, coughing, sneezing, and vomiting as well as heartbeat and arterial blood pressure, thereby exerting control over the circulation of blood.

The cerebrum is divided by the longitudinal fissure into two cerebral hemispheres, the right and left, that are joined by large fiber tracts (*corpus callosum*) that allow information to pass from one hemisphere to the other. The surface or *cortex* of each hemisphere is arranged in folds creating bulges and shallow furrows. Each bulge is called a **gyrus** or **convolution**. A furrow is known as a **sulcus**. This surface is composed of gray, unmyelinated cell bodies and is known as the **cerebral cortex**. The cortex has been divided into lobes as a means of identifying certain locations. These lobes correspond to the overlying bones of the skull and are the *frontal, parietal, temporal,* and *occipital lobes*.

The hippocampus is an extension of the cerebral cortex, situated deep in the temporal lobe (refer to Figure 13.4). It is part of the limbic system, which is considered to be like a "primitive brain" that is involved with basic emotions and reactions, such as fear, anger, hunger, pleasure, sex, motivation, mood, pain, appetite, and memory. The hippocampus is currently one of the most studied areas of the brain. Studies have found that patients with conditions such as Alzheimer disease (AD), depression, and schizophrenia show signs of hippocampal atrophy (shrinkage or volume reduction). In fact, all people with AD show some amount of hippocampal atrophy, and in individuals experiencing depression, the duration of the depressed state has been correlated with the severity of hippocampal atrophy. Evidence suggests that atrophy thus produced may be permanent even though the depression has undergone remission. Hippocampal atrophy is one of the most consistent findings found in MRIs of schizophrenic patients along with functional and biochemical abnormalities.

Electrical stimulation of the various areas of the cortex during neurosurgery has identified specialized cell activity within the different lobes. The **frontal lobe** has been identified as the brain's major motor area and the site for personality and speech. The **parietal lobe** contains centers for sensory input from all parts of the body and is known as the *somesthetic area* and the site for the interpretation of language. Temperature, pressure, touch, and an awareness of muscle control are some of the sensory activities localized in this area. The **temporal lobe** contains centers for hearing, smell, and language input, and the **occipital lobe** is the primary interpretive processing area for vision. The occipital lobe is directly posterior to the temporal lobe. Refer to Table 13.2. See Figure 13.5.

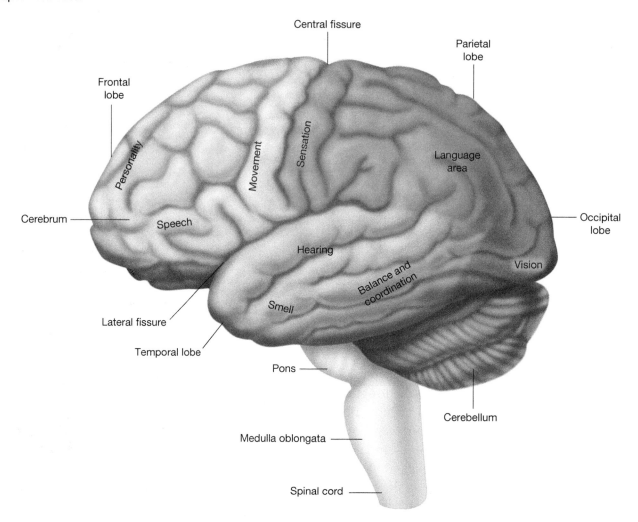

FIGURE 13.5 The brain, showing the cerebrum and its lobes with their functional centers identified.

CEREBELLUM

The cerebellum is the second largest part of the brain. It occupies a space in the back of the skull, inferior to the cerebrum and dorsal to the pons and medulla oblongata. The cerebellum is oval in shape and is divided into lobes by deep fissures. It has a cortex of gray cell bodies, and its interior contains nerve fibers and white matter connecting it to every part of the CNS. The cerebellum plays an important part in the coordination of voluntary and involuntary complex patterns of movement and adjusts muscles to maintain posture. Refer to Table 13.2.

DIENCEPHALON

The word **diencephalon** means *second portion of the brain* and refers to the epithalamus (a part of the dorsal forebrain including the pineal gland and a region in the roof of the third ventricle of the brain), thalamus, and hypothalamus. Refer to Table 13.2 and Figure 13.4.

Epithalamus. The dorsal posterior segment of the diencephalon, the **epithalamus** is involved in the maintenance of circadian rhythms and serves as a connection between the limbic system and other parts of the brain. Some functions of its components include the secretion of melatonin by the pineal gland and regulation of motor pathways and emotions.

Thalamus. The **thalamus** is the largest structure derived from the embryonic diencephalon; it is the larger of the two divisions of the diencephalon and is actually two large masses of gray cell bodies joined by a third or intermediate mass. The thalamus serves as a relay center for all sensory impulses (except olfactory) being transmitted to the sensory areas of the cortex. Besides its sensory function, the thalamus also relays motor impulses from the cerebellum and the basal ganglia to motor areas of the cortex. Some impulses related to emotional behavior are also passed from the hypothalamus, through the thalamus, to the cerebral cortex.

Hypothalamus. The **hypothalamus** lies beneath the thalamus and is a principal regulator of autonomic nervous activity that is associated with behavior and emotional expression. It also produces neurosecretions for the control of water balance, sugar and fat metabolism, regulation of body temperature, and other metabolic activities. The pituitary gland is attached to the hypothalamus by a narrow stalk, the *infundibulum*.

BRAINSTEM

The brainstem is the lower part of the brain, adjoining and structurally continuous with the spinal cord. The brainstem provides the main motor and sensory innervation to the face and neck via the cranial nerves. It consists of three structures: the mesencephalon or *midbrain*, the pons, and the medulla oblongata. The brainstem processes visual, auditory, and sensory information and plays an important role in the regulation of cardiac and respiratory function. It also regulates the CNS and is pivotal in maintaining consciousness and regulating the sleep cycle. Refer to Table 13.2.

Midbrain. The **midbrain** is located below the cerebrum and above the pons. The midbrain has four small masses of gray cells known collectively as the **corpora quadrigemina**. The upper two of these masses, called the **superior colliculi**, are associated with visual reflexes such as the tracking movements of the eyes. The lower two, or **inferior colliculi**, are involved with the sense of hearing.

Pons. The **pons** is a broad band of white matter located anterior to the cerebellum and between the midbrain and the medulla oblongata. The pons is composed of fiber tracts linking the cerebellum and medulla oblongata to higher cortical areas. It also plays a role in somatic and visceral motor control and contains important centers for regulating breathing.

Medulla Oblongata. The **medulla oblongata** connects the pons and the rest of the brain to the spinal cord. All afferent and efferent tracts from the spinal cord either pass through or terminate in the medulla oblongata. It contains nerve centers for regulation and control of breathing, swallowing, coughing, sneezing, vomiting, heartbeat, and blood pressure.

Spinal Cord

The **spinal cord** has an H-shaped gray area of cell bodies encircled by an outer region of white matter. The white matter consists of nerve tracts and fibers providing sensory input to the brain and conducting motor impulses from the brain to spinal neurons. The adult spinal cord is about 44 centimeters (cm) long and extends down the vertebral canal from the medulla oblongata to terminate near the junction of the first (L1) and second (L2) lumbar vertebrae. See Figure 13.6.

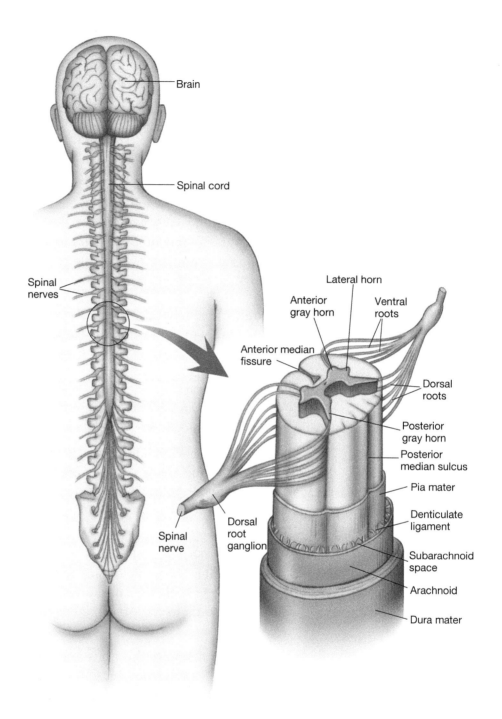

FIGURE 13.6 Brain, spinal cord, and spinal nerves with an expanded view of a spinal nerve.

Between the 12th thoracic vertebra (T12) and L1 is a region known as the **conus medullaris**, where the spinal cord becomes conically tapered. The **filum terminale** or terminal thread of fibrous tissue extends from the conus medullaris to the second sacral vertebra. The **cauda equina** (known as the horse's tail) is the terminal portion of the spinal cord that forms the nerve fibers that are the lumbar, sacral, and coccygeal spinal nerves.

The functions of the spinal cord are to conduct sensory impulses to the brain, to conduct motor impulses from the brain, and to serve as a reflex center for impulses entering and leaving the spinal cord without direct involvement of the brain.

Cerebrospinal Fluid

The brain and spinal cord are surrounded by **cerebrospinal fluid (CSF)**. This colorless fluid is produced as a filtrate of blood by the *choroid plexuses* within the *ventricles* of the brain. Cerebrospinal fluid circulates through the ventricles, the central canal, and the subarachnoid space.

The normal adult will have between 120 and 150 milliliters (mL) of cerebrospinal fluid in circulation. The fluid serves to cushion the brain and spinal cord from shocks that could cause injury. It also helps to support the brain by allowing it to float within the supporting liquid. It also contains neurotransmitters such as monoamines, acetylcholine (ACh), and neuropeptides.

Peripheral Nervous System

The network of nerves branching throughout the body from the brain and spinal cord is known as the **peripheral nervous system (PNS)**. There are 12 pairs of cranial nerves that attach to the brain and 31 pairs of spinal nerves connected to the spinal cord.

Cranial Nerves

The nerves described in the following sections attach to the brain and provide sensory input, motor control, or a combination of these functions. They are arranged symmetrically, 12 to each side of the brain, and are generally named for the area or function they serve. See Figure 13.7 and Table 13.3.

Spinal Nerves

There are 31 pairs of **spinal nerves** distributed along the length of the spinal cord and emerging from the vertebral canal on either side through the intervertebral foramina. At the point of attachment, each nerve is divided into two roots (refer to Figure 13.6). The **dorsal** or **sensory root** is composed of afferent fibers carrying impulses to the cord, and the **ventral root** contains motor fibers carrying efferent impulses to muscles and organs. Named for the region of the vertebral column from which they exit, there are eight pairs of **cervical spinal nerves**, 12 pairs of **thoracic spinal nerves**, five pairs of **lumbar spinal nerves**, five pairs of **sacral spinal nerves**, and one pair of **coccygeal spinal nerves**. See Figure 13.8.

A short distance from the cord, the fibers of the two roots unite to form a spinal nerve. Having formed a single nerve composed of afferent and efferent fibers, each spinal nerve then branches into several smaller nerves. The two primary branches from each spinal nerve are the **dorsal rami** and **ventral rami**. The dorsal rami (*branches*) carry motor and sensory fibers to the muscles and skin of the back and serve an area from the back of the head to the coccyx. The ventral rami, serving a much larger area, carry both motor and sensory fibers to the muscles and organs of the body, including the arms, legs, hands, and feet.

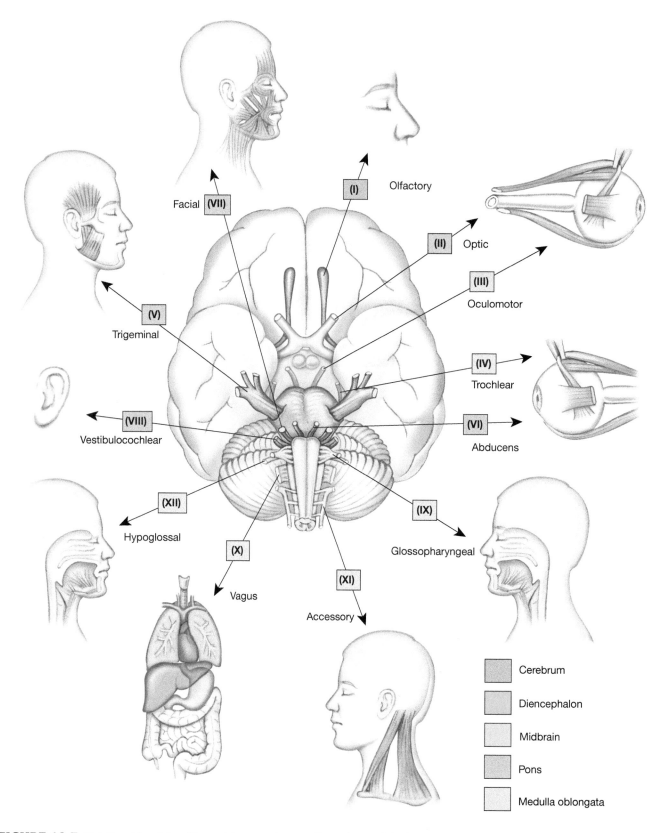

Olfactory (I)

Facial (VII)

Optic (II)

Oculomotor (III)

Trigeminal (V)

Trochlear (IV)

Vestibulocochlear (VIII)

Abducens (VI)

Hypoglossal (XII)

Vagus (X)

Glossopharyngeal (IX)

Accessory (XI)

Cerebrum

Diencephalon

Midbrain

Pons

Medulla oblongata

FIGURE 13.7 Relationship of the 12 cranial nerves to specific regions of the brain.

TABLE 13.3   Cranial Nerves and Functions

Nerve/Number	Function
Olfactory (I)	Detects and provides the sense of smell
Optic (II)	Provides vision
Oculomotor (III)	Conducts motor impulses to four of the six external muscles of the eye and to the muscle that raises the eyelid
Trochlear (IV)	Conducts motor impulses to control the superior oblique muscle of the eyeball
Trigeminal (V)	Provides sensory input from the face, nose, mouth, forehead, and top of the head; motor fibers to the muscles of the jaw (chewing)
Abducens (VI)	Conducts motor impulses to the lateral rectus muscle of the eyeball
Facial (VII)	Controls the muscles of the face and scalp; the lacrimal glands of the eye and the submandibular and sublingual salivary glands; input from the tongue for the sense of taste
Vestibulocochlear (Acoustic) (VIII)	Provides input for hearing and equilibrium
Glossopharyngeal (IX)	Provides general sense of taste; regulates swallowing; controls secretion of saliva
Vagus (X)	Controls muscles of the pharynx, larynx, thoracic, and abdominal organs; responsible for swallowing, voice production, slowing of heartbeat, acceleration of peristalsis
Accessory (XI)	Controls the trapezius and sternocleidomastoid muscles, permitting movement of the head and shoulders
Hypoglossal (XII)	Controls the tongue; tongue movements

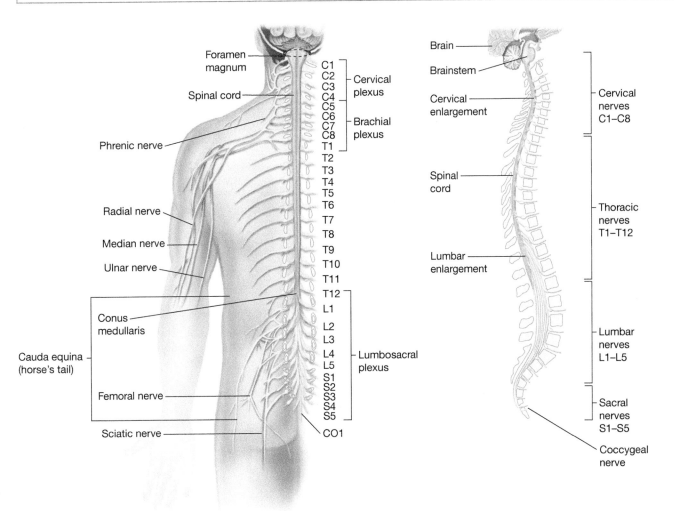

FIGURE 13.8 The 31 pairs of spinal nerves.

Autonomic Nervous System

Actually a part of the peripheral nervous system, the **autonomic nervous system (ANS)** controls involuntary bodily functions such as sweating, secretions of glands, arterial blood pressure, smooth muscle tissue, and the heart. The autonomic nervous system is primarily composed of efferent fibers from certain cranial and spinal nerves and can be functionally divided into two divisions, the **sympathetic** and **parasympathetic**. These two divisions counteract each other's activity to keep the body in a state of homeostasis. See Figure 13.9.

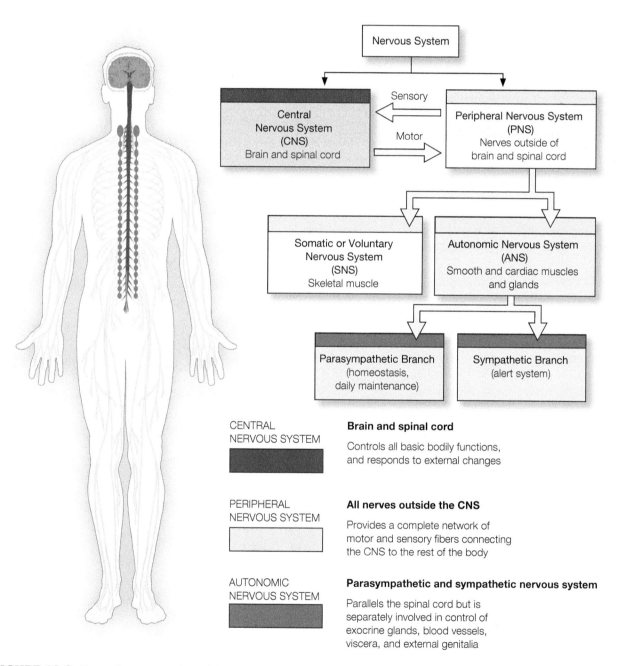

FIGURE 13.9 General representation of the nervous system.

Sympathetic Division

Branches from the ventral roots of the 12 thoracic and the first three lumbar spinal nerves form the first part of the **sympathetic division**. The cell bodies of these nerve fibers are located in the *gray matter* of the spinal cord. Just outside the spinal cord, axons of these nerve cells leave the spinal nerves and enter almost immediately into masses of nerve cell bodies, the **sympathetic ganglia**, which form a chain that runs next to the vertebral column. This chain of about 23 ganglia runs from the base of the head to the coccyx and is known as the **sympathetic trunk**. Within the ganglia of the sympathetic trunk, fibers from the spinal nerves synapse with ganglionic nerve cell bodies. These ganglionic neurons produce long axons that reach to the parts of the body to be innervated. This arrangement, characteristic of autonomic nerves, creates a two-neuron chain as opposed to single-neuron control of regular motor nerves.

Because of the arrangement in which *sympathetic fibers* from spinal nerves synapse with many cell bodies in the sympathetic ganglia, they tend to produce widespread innervation when activated. This condition has been described as preparing the individual for fight or flight. During the *fight-or-flight response*, a person experiences increased alertness, increased metabolic rate, decreased digestive and urinary function, an increase in respiration, blood pressure, and heart rate, and a corresponding warming of the body that can activate the sweat glands. The sympathetic system stimulates the adrenal glands to release epinephrine (adrenaline), the hormone that causes the familiar adrenaline rush.

Parasympathetic Division

Very long fibers branching from cranial nerves III, VII, IX, and X, along with long fibers of sacral nerves II, III, and IV, form the first stage of the **parasympathetic division**. Cell bodies for these long fibers are located in the brain and spinal cord. These long fibers extend to ganglia located near the organs to be innervated.

The parasympathetic division works to conserve energy and innervate the digestive system. When activated, it stimulates the salivary and digestive glands, decreases the metabolic rate, slows the heart rate, reduces blood pressure, and promotes the passage of material through the intestines along with absorption of nutrients by the blood.

Study *and* Review I

Anatomy and Physiology

Write your answers to the following questions.

1. Name the two interconnected divisions of the nervous system.

    a. _____   b. _____

2. _____ are the structural and functional units of the nervous system.

3. Describe an axon. _____

4. Describe a dendrite. _____

5. State an action of sensory neurons. _____

6. Define the following terms:

    a. Nerve fiber _____

    b. Nerve _____

    c. Tracts _____

7. The central nervous system consists of the _____ and the

    _____.

8. Name the three meninges enclosing the brain.

    a. _____   **c.** _____

    b. _____

9. Name four major structures of the brain.

    a. _____   **c.** _____

    b. _____   **d.** _____

10. The _____ has been identified as the brain's major motor area.

11. The parietal lobe is also known as the _____.

12. The temporal lobe contains centers for _____ and

    _____ input.

13. The occipital lobe is the primary area for _____.

14. State the functions of the thalamus.

    a. _____   **b.** _____

15. State three functions of the hypothalamus.

    a. _____   **c.** _____

    b. _____

16. The cerebellum plays an important role in the integration of _____ and

    _____.

17. State five functions of the medulla oblongata.

    a. _____   **d.** _____

    b. _____   **e.** _____

    c. _____

18. State the three functions of the spinal cord.

    a. _____   **c.** _____

    b. _____

19. The normal adult has between _____ and _____ mL of cerebrospinal fluid in circulation.

20. State four functions of the autonomic nervous system.

    a. _____   **c.** _____

    b. _____   **d.** _____

21. Name the two divisions of the autonomic nervous system.

    a. _____   **b.** _____

▶ **ANATOMY LABELING**   Identify the structures shown below by filling in the blanks.

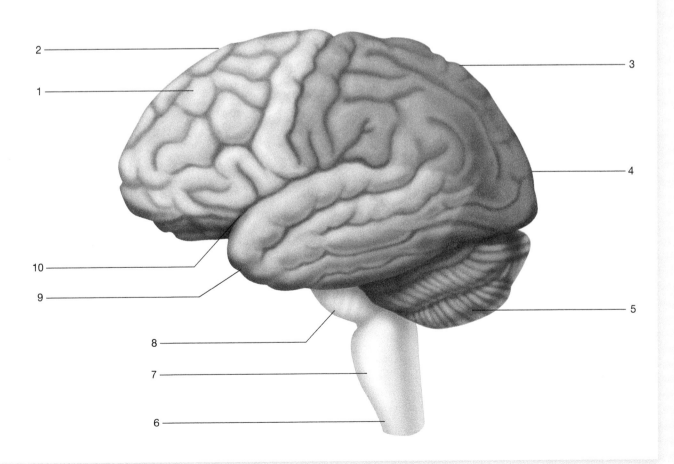

Building Your Medical Vocabulary

This section provides the foundation for learning medical terminology. Review the alphabetized list of medical terms in the following pages. Note how common prefixes and suffixes are repeatedly applied to word roots and combining forms to create different meanings. A combining form is a word root plus a vowel. The chart below lists the combining forms and word roots used in this chapter and can help to strengthen your understanding of how medical words are built and spelled.

You will find that some terms have not been divided into word parts. These are common words or specialized terms that are included to enhance your medical vocabulary.

Combining Forms

cephal/o	head	**lob/o**	lobe
cerebell/o	little brain	**mening/i**	membrane, meninges
cerebr/o	cerebrum	**mening/o**	membrane, meninges
cran/i	skull	**ment/o**	mind
crani/o	skull	**my/o**	muscle
cyt/o	cell	**myel/o**	spinal cord
dendr/o	tree	**narc/o**	numbness, sleep, stupor
disk/o	disk	**neur/o**	nerve
dur/o	dura, hard	**pallid/o**	globus pallidus
electr/o	electricity	**papill/o**	papilla
encephal/o	brain	**poli/o**	gray
esthesi/o	feeling	**scler/o**	hardening
fibr/o	fiber	**somn/o**	sleep
gli/o	glue	**spin/o**	thorn, spine
hypn/o	sleep	**spondyl/o**	vertebra
lamin/o	thin plate	**vag/o**	vagus, wandering
later/o	side	**ventricul/o**	ventricle

Word Roots

ambul	to walk	**log**	study
concuss	shaken violently	**mnes**	memory
ganglion	knot	**sympath**	sympathy

Medical Word	Word Parts		Definition
	Part	Meaning	
acetylcholine (ACh) (ăs″ ĕ-tĭl-kō′ lēn)			Cholinergic neurotransmitter; plays an important role in the transmission of nerve impulses at synapses and myoneural junctions
akathisia (ăk″ ă-thĭ′ zhē-ă)			Inability to remain still; motor restlessness and anxiety
akinesia (ă″ kĭ-nē′ zhē-ă)	a- -kinesia	lack of motion, movement	Loss or lack of voluntary motion
Alzheimer disease (AD) (ahlts′ hī-mer)			A progressive degeneration of brain tissue that usually begins after age 60. It is the most common cause of dementia among older adults. Symptoms of AD can be described as the 4 A's: anger, aggression, anxiety, and apathy. It is a disease that causes a slow decline in memory, thinking, and reasoning skills.
amnesia (ăm-nē′ zhă)	a- mnes -ia	lack of memory condition	Condition in which there is a loss or lack of memory
amyotrophic lateral sclerosis (ALS) (ā-mī″ ō-trō′ fĭk lăt′ ĕr-ăl sklĕ-rō′ sĭs)	a- my/o -troph(y) -ic later -al scler -osis	lack of muscle nourishment pertaining to side pertaining to hardening condition	Muscular weakness, atrophy, with spasticity caused by degeneration of motor neurons of the spinal cord; also called *Lou Gehrig disease*
analgesia (ăn″ ăl-jē′ zē-ă)	an- -algesia	lack of condition of pain	Condition in which there is a lack of the sensation of pain
anesthesia (ăn″ ĕs-thē′ zhă)	an- -esthesia	lack of feeling	Literally means *loss or lack of the sense of feeling*; a pharmacologically induced reversible state of amnesia, analgesia, loss of responsiveness, loss of skeletal muscle reflexes, and decreased stress response
anesthesiologist (ăn″ ĕs-thē″ zē-ŏl′ ō-jĭst)	an- esthesi/o log -ist	lack of feeling study one who specializes	Physician who specializes in the science of anesthesia
aphagia (ă-fā′ jē-ă)	a- -phagia	lack of to eat, swallow	Loss or lack of the ability to eat or swallow

Medical Word	Word Parts		Definition
	Part	Meaning	
aphasia (ă-fā′ zē-ă)	a- -phasia	lack of to speak, speech	Literally means *a lack of the ability to speak*. It is a language disorder in which there is an impairment of producing or comprehending spoken or written language due to brain damage. It can be caused by a stroke, traumatic brain injury, or other brain injury, or it may develop slowly, as in the case of a brain tumor or progressive neurological disease, such as in Alzheimer or Parkinson diseases.
apraxia (ā-prăk′ sē-ă)	a- -praxia	lack of action	Loss or lack of the ability to use objects properly and to recognize common ones; inability to perform motor tasks or activities of daily living (ADL), such as dressing and bathing
asthenia (ăs-thē′ nē-ă)	a- -sthenia	lack of strength	Loss or lack of strength
astrocytoma (ăs″ trō-sī-tō′ mă)	astro- cyt -oma	star-shaped cell tumor	A primary tumor of the brain composed of astrocytes (star-shaped neuroglial cells) characterized by slow growth, cyst formation, metastasis, and malignant glioblastoma within the tumor mass. Surgical intervention is possible in the early developmental stage of the tumor; also called *astrocytic glioma.*
ataxia (ă-tăk′ sē-ă)	a- -taxia	lack of order, coordination	Literally means *loss or lack of order*; neurological sign and symptom consisting of lack of coordination of muscle movements. It implies dysfunction of parts of the nervous system that coordinate movement, such as the cerebellum.
bradykinesia (brăd″ ĭ-kĭ-nē′ sē-ă)	brady- -kinesia	slow motion, movement	Abnormal slowness of motion
cephalalgia (sĕf″ ă-lăl′ jē-ă)	cephal -algia	head pain	Head pain; *headache*
cerebellar (sĕr″ ĕ-bĕl′ ăr)	cerebell -ar	little brain pertaining to	Pertaining to the cerebellum
cerebral palsy (CP) (sĕr′ ă-brĭl pawl′ zē)			Disorder of movement and posture caused by damage to the motor control centers of the developing brain and can occur during gestation, during childbirth, or after birth up to about age 3. Most common permanent disorder of childhood involving four motor dysfunctions: spastic, dyskinetic, ataxic, and mixed. See Figure 13.10.

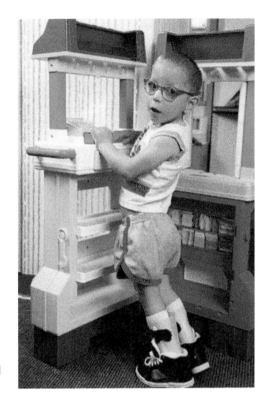

FIGURE 13.10 Child with cerebral palsy has abnormal muscle tone and lack of physical coordination.

GOOD TO KNOW ▶

Bell palsy is another form of palsy. It is a temporary facial paralysis resulting from damage or trauma to the facial nerve. The facial nerve is also called the 7th cranial nerve and travels through a narrow, bony canal (called the *Fallopian canal*) in the skull, beneath the ear, to the muscles on each side of the face.

Symptoms of Bell palsy can vary and range in severity from mild weakness to total paralysis. They include twitching, weakness, or paralysis on one or rarely both sides of the face, drooping of the eyelid and corner of the mouth, drooling, dryness of the eye or mouth, impairment of taste, and excessive tearing in one eye. Most often these symptoms, which usually begin suddenly and reach their peak within 48 hours, lead to significant facial distortion. See Figure 13.11.

Although the exact cause of Bell palsy is unknown, it is believed that a viral infection such as viral meningitis or herpes simplex may cause this disorder.

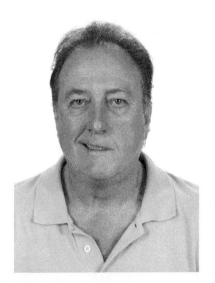

FIGURE 13.11 A man with Bell palsy.
Source: Steven Frame/123RF

Medical Word	Word Parts		Definition
	Part	**Meaning**	
cerebrospinal (sĕr″ĕ-brō-spī′năl)	**cerebr/o** **spin** **-al**	cerebrum spine pertaining to	Pertaining to the cerebrum and the spinal cord
chorea (kō-rē′ă)			Abnormal involuntary movement disorder, one of a group of neurological disorders called *dyskinesias*; characterized by episodes of rapid, jerky involuntary muscular twitching of the limbs or facial muscles
coma (kō′mă)			Unconscious state or stupor from which the patient cannot be aroused; may occur as a complication of an underlying illness or as a result of injuries to the brain. Coma rarely lasts more than 2–4 weeks, although it can last for years. The outcome for coma depends on the cause, severity, and site of the damage.
concussion (brain) (kŏn-kŭsh′ŭn)	**concuss** **-ion**	shaken violently process	Head injury with a transient loss of brain function; may also be called *mild brain injury*, *mild traumatic brain injury (MTBI)*, *mild head injury (MHI)*, and *minor head trauma (MHT)*

fyi **Chronic traumatic encephalopathy (CTE)** is a type of traumatic brain injury that can occur in individuals who participate in contact sports and receive repeated blows to the head. CTE injuries are associated with memory disturbances, behavioral and personality changes, Parkinsonism, and speech and gait abnormalities. CTE involves progressive damage to nerve cells, which results in visible changes to the brain.

Over recent years there has been increasing attention focused on the neurological sequelae of sports-related traumatic brain injury, particularly concussion. *Concussion* is a frequent occurrence in contact sports: 1.6 to 3.8 million sports-related concussions occur annually in the United States. Repetitive closed head injury occurs in a wide variety of contact sports, including football, boxing, wrestling, rugby, hockey, lacrosse, soccer, and skiing. Furthermore, in collision sports such as football and boxing, players may experience thousands of subconcussive hits over the course of a single season. *Subconcussive* (below the threshold of concussion) impacts are repetitive, but less forceful impacts to the head. Also at risk are military personnel (and civilians) who experience explosive blasts that may cause subconcussive impacts to the head.

Medical Word	Word Parts		Definition
craniectomy (krā″nē-ĕk′tō-mē)	**cran/i** **-ectomy**	skull surgical excision	Surgical excision of a portion of the skull (*cranium*), which encases the brain

Medical Word	Word Parts		Definition
	Part	Meaning	
craniotomy (krā″ nē-ŏt′ ō-mē)	crani/o -tomy	skull incision	Literally means *surgical incision into the skull*. It is a surgical operation in which a bone flap is removed from the skull to access the brain. Used to repair defects associated with traumatic head injuries or to repair a cerebral aneurysm. See Figure 13.12.

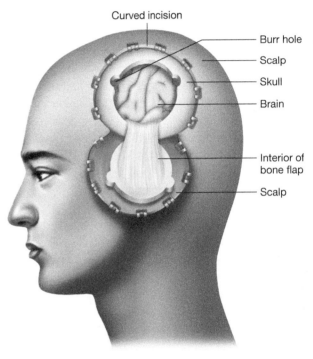

FIGURE 13.12 In a craniotomy, a portion of the skull and overlying scalp is pulled back to allow access to the brain.

| deep brain stimulation (DBS) | | | A surgical procedure used to treat a variety of disabling neurological symptoms—most commonly the symptoms of Parkinson disease (PD), such as tremor, rigidity, stiffness, slowed movement, and walking problems; it is also used to treat essential tremor, a common neurological movement disorder. Currently, DBS is used only for patients whose symptoms cannot be adequately controlled with medications. |

Medical Word	Word Parts		Definition
	Part	**Meaning**	
dementia (di-men´ chă)	**de-** **ment** **-ia**	down mind condition	Group of symptoms marked by memory loss and loss of other cognitive functions such as perception, thinking, reasoning, and remembering

fyi

There are several types of dementia other than Alzheimer disease (AD). A recently recognized brain disorder that mimics the clinical features of AD is being called *limbic-predominant age-related TDP-43 encephalopathy (LATE)*. Its name refers to the area in the brain most likely to be affected (the limbic region), as well as the protein at the center of it (TDP-43). TDP-43 (transactive response DNA binding protein 43 kDa) is a protein that normally helps to regulate gene expression in the brain and other tissues. Recent research shows that a buildup of abnormally folded TDP-43 protein is not uncommon in older adults. Roughly 25% of individuals over 85 years of age have enough misfolded TDP-43 protein to affect their memory and/or thinking abilities. LATE, which affects the brain differently and develops more slowly than AD, may be more common than AD among people in their 80s.

Abnormalities in the TDP protein have also been linked to other types of dementia, including *frontotemporal lobar degeneration (FTLD)* and *frontotemporal dementia (FTD)*, which are characterized by the shrinking or atrophying of the brain's frontal and temporal lobes caused by the damage and death of the neurons (nerve cells) in the lobes. Thinking and behaviors normally controlled by these parts of the brain are affected; symptoms including unusual behaviors, emotional problems, trouble communicating, inability to work, and difficulty with walking. Scientists think that FTLD is the most common cause of dementia in people younger than age 60. Approximately 60% of people with FTLD are 45–64 years old. The disorders are progressive, meaning symptoms get worse over time. No cure or treatments that slow or stop the progression of frontotemporal disorders are available today.

TDP-43 pathology is also commonly associated with *hippocampal sclerosis*, the severe shrinkage of the hippocampal region of the brain—the part of the brain that deals with learning and memory. Hippocampal sclerosis and its clinical symptoms of cognitive impairment can be very similar to the effects of AD.

Another type of dementia is called *Lewy body dementia (LBD)*, a disease associated with abnormal deposits of a protein, *alpha-synuclein*, in the brain. These deposits, called *Lewy bodies*, affect chemicals in the brain whose changes, in turn, can lead to problems with thinking, movement, behavior, and mood. LBD, the second most common type of dementia after AD, is a progressive disease that lasts an average of 5–8 years from the time of diagnosis to death, although the time span can range from 2–20 years. How quickly symptoms develop and worsen varies greatly from person to person.

diskectomy (dĭs-kĕk´ tō-mē)	**disk** **-ectomy**	a disk surgical excision	Surgical excision of an intervertebral disk
dyslexia (dĭs-lĕk´ sē-ă)	**dys-** **-lexia**	difficult diction, word, phrase	Difficulty reading and writing words even though vision and intelligence are unimpaired

Medical Word	Word Parts		Definition
	Part	Meaning	
dysphasia (dĭs-fā′ zē-ă)	dys- -phasia	difficult speak, speech	Impairment of speech that may be caused by a brain lesion
electromyography (ē-lĕk″ trō-mī-ŏg′ ră-fē)	electr/o my/o -graphy	electricity muscle recording	Process of recording the contraction of a skeletal muscle as a result of electrical stimulation; used in diagnosing disorders of nerves supplying muscles
encephalitis (ĕn-sĕf″ ă-lī′ tĭs)	encephal -itis	brain inflammation	Inflammation of the brain. There are numerous types of encephalitis, many of which are caused by viral infection. Symptoms include sudden fever, headache, vomiting, photophobia (abnormal sensitivity to light), stiff neck and back, confusion, drowsiness, clumsiness, unsteady gait, and irritability.
encephalopathy (ĕn-sĕf″ ă-lŏp′ ă-thē)	encephal/o -pathy	brain disease	Any pathological dysfunction of the brain. HIV encephalopathy is called *AIDS dementia complex*.
endorphins (ĕn-dor′ fĭns)			Chemical substances produced in the brain that act as natural analgesics (opiates) and provide feelings of pleasure
epidural (ĕp″ ĭ-dū′ răl)	epi- dur -al	upon dura, hard pertaining to	Literally means *pertaining to situated on the dura mater*; often used to refer to a form of regional anesthesia involving injection of medication via a catheter into the epidural space. This causes both a loss of sensation (anesthesia) and a loss of pain (analgesia), by blocking the transmission of signals through nerves in or near the spinal cord.

! ALERT!

The prefix **epi-** means *upon*. How many words in this chapter begin with **epi-**?

Medical Word	Word Parts		Definition
epiduroscopy (ep″ ĭ-dū-rŏs′ kō-pē)	epi- dur/o -scopy	upon dura, hard visual examination, to view, examine	Minimally invasive form of surgery that introduces medication via an endoscope into the epidural space; used for back pain relief when all other conservative treatments have failed

Medical Word	Word Parts		Definition
	Part	Meaning	
epilepsy (ĕp´ ĭ-lĕp˝ sē)	epi- -lepsy	upon seizure	A neurological disorder involving repeated seizures of any type. Seizures are episodes of disturbed brain function that cause changes in attention and/or behavior. The types of seizures experienced by those with epilepsy are classified into four main categories: **Partial seizures** (focal seizures)—electrical disturbances are localized to areas of the brain near the source or focal point of the seizure. **Generalized seizures** (bilateral, symmetrical)—widespread electrical discharge that involves both the right and left hemispheres of the brain. **Unilateral seizures**—electrical discharge is predominantly confined to one of the two hemispheres of the brain. **Unclassified seizures**—cannot be placed into one of the other three categories because of incomplete data.

fyi

The majority of epilepsy cases are idiopathic (cause not identified) and symptoms begin during childhood or early adolescence. A child who has a seizure while standing should be gently assisted to the floor and placed in a side-lying position. See Figure 13.13. In adults, epilepsy can occur after severe neurological trauma.

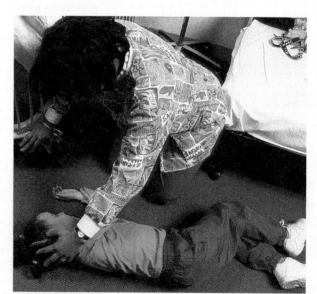

FIGURE 13.13 A child having a seizure is gently assisted to the floor and placed in a side-lying position.
Source: Pearson Education, Inc.

ganglionectomy (gang˝ lē-ō-nĕk´ tō-mē)	ganglion -ectomy	knot surgical excision	Surgical excision of a ganglion (a mass of nerve tissue outside the brain and spinal cord)

Medical Word	Word Parts		Definition
	Part	Meaning	
glioma (glī-ō′ mă)	gli -oma	glue tumor	Tumor composed of neuroglial tissue
Guillain-Barré syndrome (gē-yăn′ bă-rā′)			Pathological condition in which the myelin sheaths covering peripheral nerves are destroyed, resulting in decreased nerve impulses, loss of reflex response, and sudden muscle weakness. Generally an acute viral infection occurs 1–3 weeks before the onset of the syndrome; also called *infectious polyneuritis*, *acute febrile polyneuritis*, or *acute idiopathic polyneuritis*.
hemiparesis (hĕm″ ē-păr′ ĕ-sĭs)	hemi- -paresis	half weakness	Weakness on one side of the body that can be caused by a stroke, cerebral palsy, brain tumor, multiple sclerosis, and other brain and nervous system diseases
hemiplegia (hĕm″ ē-plē′ jē-ă)	hemi- -plegia	half stroke, paralysis	Paralysis of one-half of the body when it is divided along the median sagittal plane; total paralysis of the arm, leg, and trunk on the same side of the body. Stroke is the most common cause of this condition. See Figure 13.14B.

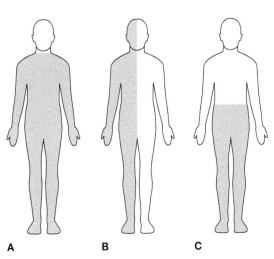

FIGURE 13.14 Types of paralysis: **A** Quadriplegia is complete or partial paralysis of the upper extremities and complete paralysis of the lower part of the body. **B** Hemiplegia is paralysis of one half of the body when it is divided along the median sagittal plane. **C** Paraplegia is a paralysis of the lower part of the body.

A   B   C

Medical Word	Word Parts		Definition
	Part	Meaning	
herniated disk syndrome (HDS) (hĕr´ nē-āt˝ ĕd)			Condition in which part or all of the soft, gelatinous central portion of an intervertebral disk (the nucleus pulposus) is forced through a weakened part of the disk. Compression on the nerves can cause *sciatica* or severe lumbar back pain that radiates down one or both legs; also called *herniated intervertebral disk*, *ruptured disk*, *herniated nucleus pulposus (HNP)*, or *slipped disk*. See Figure 13.15.

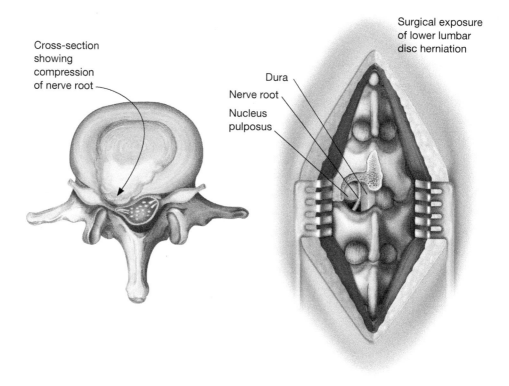

Cross-section showing compression of nerve root

Surgical exposure of lower lumbar disc herniation

Dura

Nerve root

Nucleus pulposus

FIGURE 13.15 Herniated intervertebral disk showing the herniated nucleus pulposus (on the left) applying pressure against the nerve root and surgical intervention (on the right).

Medical Word	Word Parts		Definition
	Part	Meaning	
herpes zoster (hĕr´ pēz zŏs´ tĕr)			Viral disease characterized by painful vesicular eruptions along a segment of the spinal or cranial nerves; also called *shingles*. See Figure 13.16.

FIGURE 13.16 Herpes zoster.
Source: Courtesy of Jason L. Smith, MD

GOOD TO KNOW ▶

Shingles is caused by the varicella-zoster virus, the same virus that causes chickenpox. In people who have had chickenpox, the virus is never fully cleared from the body. Instead, the virus remains dormant in the nerve tissues. When the immune system is weakened, the virus reactivates and spreads along the nerve fibers to the particular area of skin supplied by the involved nerve.

Shingles is a painful rash that usually develops on one side of the body, often the face or torso. The rash consists of blisters that typically scab over in 7–10 days and clears up within 2–4 weeks. Some people describe the pain as an intense burning sensation. For some people, the pain can last for months or even years after the rash goes away. This long-lasting pain is called *postherpetic neuralgia (PHN)* and is the most common complication of shingles. The risk of getting shingles and PHN increases as one gets older. The Centers for Disease Control and Prevention (CDC) recommends that healthy adults 50 years and older get two doses of Shingrix (recombinant zoster vaccine), 2–6 months apart. Shingrix provides strong protection against shingles and PHN and is the preferred vaccine over Zostavax, a shingles vaccine in use since 2006. Zostavax may still be used to prevent shingles in healthy adults 60 years or older.

Medical Word	Word Parts		Definition
	Part	**Meaning**	
hydrocephalus (hī″ drō-sĕf′ ă-lŭs)	**hydro-**	water	Condition in which there is an increased amount of cerebrospinal fluid within the ventricles of the brain, causing the head to be enlarged. Treatment involves the surgical placement of an artificial shunt, which drains the fluid into the abdominal cavity. See Figure 13.17.
	cephal	head	
	-us	pertaining to	

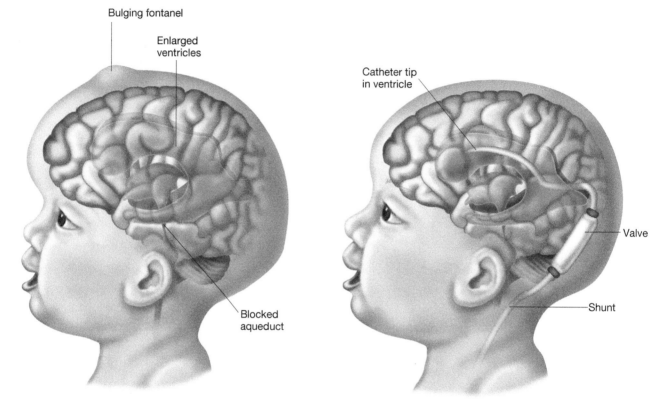

FIGURE 13.17 Hydrocephalus. The figure on the right shows a shunt inserted to send the excess cerebrospinal fluid to the abdominal cavity.

hyperesthesia (hī″ pĕr-ĕs-thē′ zhē-ă)	**hyper-**	excessive	Increased feelings of sensory stimuli, such as pain, touch, or sound
	-esthesia	feeling	
hyperkinesis (hī″ pĕr-kĭn-ē′ sĭs)	**hyper-**	excessive	Increased muscular movement and motion; inability to be still; also known as *hyperactivity*
	-kinesis	motion	
hypnosis (hĭp-nō′ sĭs)	**hypn**	sleep	Artificially induced trancelike state resembling somnambulism (sleepwalking)
	-osis	condition	
intracranial (ĭn″ tră-krā′ nē-ăl)	**intra-**	within	Pertaining to within the skull
	crani	skull	
	-al	pertaining to	
laminectomy (lăm″ ĭ-nĕk′ tō-mē)	**lamin**	thin plate	Surgical excision of a vertebral posterior arch
	-ectomy	surgical excision	
lobotomy (lō-bŏt′ ō-mē)	**lob/o**	lobe	Surgical incision into the prefrontal or frontal lobe of the brain
	-tomy	incision	

Medical Word	Word Parts		Definition
	Part	Meaning	
meningioma (měn-ĭn″ jē-ō′ mă)	mening/i	membrane, meninges	Tumor of the meninges that originates in the arachnoidal tissue
	-oma	tumor	
meningitis (měn″ ĭn-jī′ tĭs)	mening	membrane, meninges	Inflammation of the meninges of the spinal cord or brain. With early diagnosis and prompt treatment, most patients recover from meningitis. Individuals with bacterial meningitis are usually hospitalized for treatment.
	-itis	inflammation	

GOOD TO KNOW ▶

Any type of illness caused by *Neisseria meningitidis* bacteria is termed meningococcal disease. With proper immunization, meningitis may be prevented. There are two types of meningococcal vaccines available in the United States:

1. Meningococcal conjugate vaccines (Menactra and Menveo)

   The CDC recommends routine meningococcal conjugate vaccination as follows:

   • All 11- to 12-year-olds should be vaccinated. A booster dose is recommended at age 16 years.

   • Also, children and adults at increased risk for meningococcal disease should be vaccinated.

2. Serogroup B meningococcal vaccines (Bexsero and Trumenba)

   The CDC recommends routine serogroup B meningococcal vaccination for:

   • Teens and young adults (16- to 23-year-olds) should be vaccinated.

| meningocele (měn-ĭn′ gō-sēl) | mening/o | membrane, meninges | Congenital hernia (saclike protrusion) in which the meninges protrude through a defect in the skull or spinal column. See Figure 13.18. |
| | -cele | hernia | |

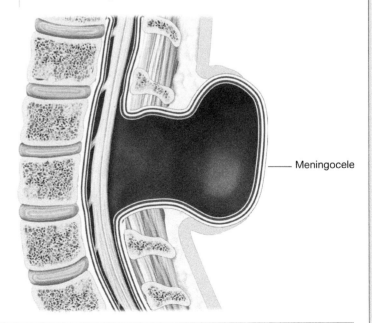

Meningocele

FIGURE 13.18 Meningocele, a congenital abnormality of the spine.

Medical Word	Word Parts		Definition
	Part	Meaning	
meningomyelocele (mĕ-nĭng″ gō-mī″ ĕ-lō-sēl)	mening/o	membrane, meninges	Congenital herniation of the spinal cord and meninges through a defect in the vertebral column
	myel/o	spinal cord	
	-cele	hernia	
microcephaly (mī″ krō-sĕf′ ă-lē)	micro-	small	Abnormally small head; congenital anomaly characterized by an abnormal smallness of the head in relation to the rest of the body. See Figure 13.19.
	cephal	head	
	-y	pertaining to	

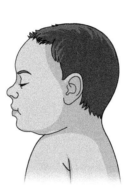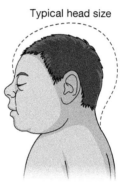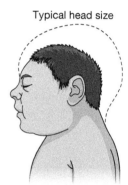

Typical head size   Typical head size

Baby with typical head size   **Baby with microcephaly**   **Baby with severe microcephaly**

FIGURE 13.19 One of the most devastating outcomes of Zika infection during pregnancy is microcephaly. This illustration compares a baby with a typical head size to a baby with microcephaly and a severe form of microcephaly.
Source: Centers for Disease Control and Prevention (CDC)

 fyi The Zika virus is transmitted to humans primarily through the bite of an infected *Aedes* species mosquito (refer to Figure 3.10). Zika infection during pregnancy can cause fetuses to have a birth defect of the brain called *microcephaly*. Other problems have been detected among fetuses and newborns infected with Zika virus, such as defects of the eye, hearing deficits, and impaired growth.

Medical Word	Word Parts		Definition
	Part	Meaning	
multiple sclerosis (MS) (mŭl´ tĭ-pl sklĕ-rō´ sĭs)	scler -osis	hardening condition	Chronic disease of the central nervous system marked by damage to the myelin sheath. Plaques occur in the brain and spinal cord, causing tremor, weakness, incoordination, paresthesia, and disturbances in vision and speech. The multiple effects of MS are shown in Figure 13.20.

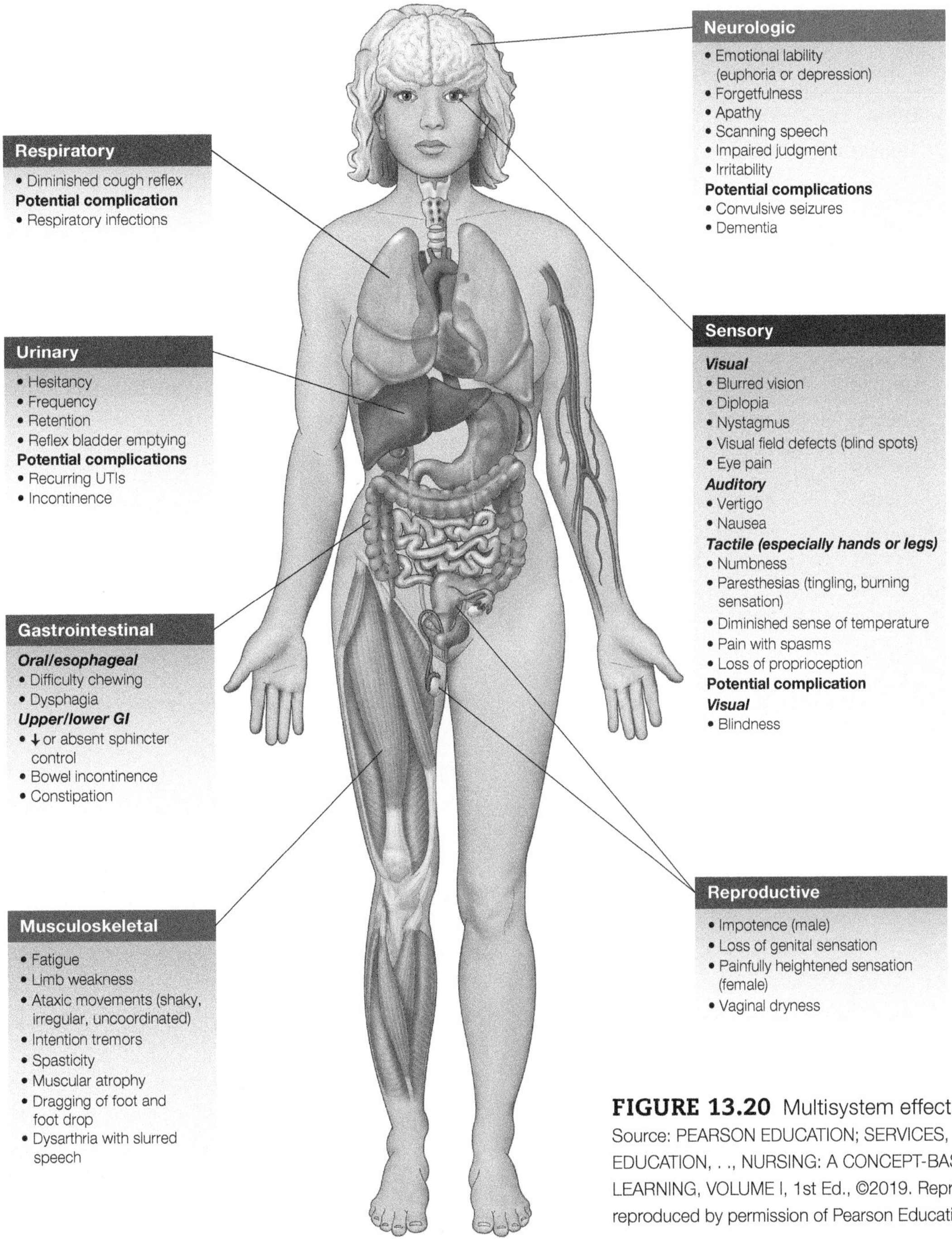

Respiratory
- Diminished cough reflex
Potential complication
- Respiratory infections

Urinary
- Hesitancy
- Frequency
- Retention
- Reflex bladder emptying
Potential complications
- Recurring UTIs
- Incontinence

Gastrointestinal
Oral/esophageal
- Difficulty chewing
- Dysphagia
Upper/lower GI
- ↓ or absent sphincter control
- Bowel incontinence
- Constipation

Musculoskeletal
- Fatigue
- Limb weakness
- Ataxic movements (shaky, irregular, uncoordinated)
- Intention tremors
- Spasticity
- Muscular atrophy
- Dragging of foot and foot drop
- Dysarthria with slurred speech

Neurologic
- Emotional lability (euphoria or depression)
- Forgetfulness
- Apathy
- Scanning speech
- Impaired judgment
- Irritability
Potential complications
- Convulsive seizures
- Dementia

Sensory
Visual
- Blurred vision
- Diplopia
- Nystagmus
- Visual field defects (blind spots)
- Eye pain
Auditory
- Vertigo
- Nausea
Tactile (especially hands or legs)
- Numbness
- Paresthesias (tingling, burning sensation)
- Diminished sense of temperature
- Pain with spasms
- Loss of proprioception
Potential complication
Visual
- Blindness

Reproductive
- Impotence (male)
- Loss of genital sensation
- Painfully heightened sensation (female)
- Vaginal dryness

FIGURE 13.20 Multisystem effects of multiple sclerosis.
Source: PEARSON EDUCATION; SERVICES, PEARSON; PEARSON EDUCATION, . ., NURSING: A CONCEPT-BASED APPROACH TO LEARNING, VOLUME I, 1st Ed., ©2019. Reprinted and Electronically reproduced by permission of Pearson Education, Inc., New York, NY.

Medical Word	Word Parts		Definition
	Part	**Meaning**	
myelitis (mī″ ĕ-lī′ tĭs)	**myel** **-itis**	spinal cord inflammation	Inflammation of the spinal cord
narcolepsy (năr′ kō-lĕp″ sē)	**narc/o** **-lepsy**	numbness, sleep, stupor seizure	Chronic condition with recurrent attacks of uncontrollable drowsiness and sleep
neuralgia (noo-ral′ jă)	**neur** **-algia**	nerve pain	Pain in a nerve or nerves
neurasthenia (noor″ ăs-thē′ nē-ă)	**neur** **-asthenia**	nerve weakness	Pathological condition characterized by weakness, exhaustion, and prostration that often accompanies severe depression
neurectomy (noo-rĕk′ tō-mē)	**neur** **-ectomy**	nerve surgical excision	Surgical excision of a nerve
neuritis (noo-rī′ tĭs)	**neur** **-itis**	nerve inflammation	Inflammation of a nerve
neuroblast (noor′ ŏ-blast″)	**neur/o** **-blast**	nerve germ cell	Germ (embryonic) cell from which nervous tissue is formed
neuroblastoma (noor″ ō-blăs-tō′ mă)	**neur/o** **-blast** **-oma**	nerve germ cell tumor	Malignant tumor composed of cells resembling neuroblasts; occurs mostly in infants and children
neurofibroma (noor″ ō-fī-brō′ mă)	**neur/o** **fibr** **-oma**	nerve fiber tumor	Fibrous connective tissue tumor of a nerve. See Figure 13.21.

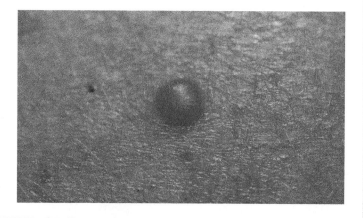

FIGURE 13.21 Neurofibroma.
Source: Courtesy of Jason L. Smith, MD

Medical Word	Word Parts		Definition
	Part	**Meaning**	
neuroglia (noo-rŏg´ lē-ă)	**neur/o** **-glia**	nerve glue	Supporting or connective tissue cells of the central nervous system (*astrocytes*, *oligodendroglia*, *microglia*, and *ependymal cells*)
neurologist (nū-rŏl´ ō-jĭst)	**neur/o** **log** **-ist**	nerve study one who specializes	Physician who specializes in the study of the nervous system
neurology (Neuro) (nū-rŏl´ ŏ-jē)	**neur/o** **-logy**	nerve study of	Study of the nervous system
neuroma (noor-ō´ mă)	**neur** **-oma**	nerve tumor	Tumor of nerve cells and nerve fibers
neuropathy (noo-rŏp´ ă-thē)	**neur/o** **-pathy**	nerve disease	Any pathological nervous tissue disease
neurotransmitter (noor˝ ō-trans-mit´ ĕr)			Chemical substances, such as dopamine and acetylcholine, that carry electrical impulses across a synapse between two neurons
oligodendroglioma (ŏl˝ ĭ-gō-dĕn˝ drō-glī-ō´ mă)	**oligo-** **dendr/o** **gli** **-oma**	little tree glue tumor	Malignant tumor composed of oligodendroglia (a type of cell that makes up one component of the tissue of the CNS)
pain			A symptom of a physical or emotional condition. Pain has been described as unpleasant bodily sensations or a complex of sensations resulting from injury or disease that cause physical discomfort or emotional distress.
pallidotomy (păl˝ ĭ-dŏt´ ō-mē)	**pallid/o** **-tomy**	globus pallidus incision	Surgical destruction of the globus pallidus of the brain done to treat involuntary movements or muscular rigidity in Parkinson disease
papilledema (păp˝ ĭl-ĕ-dē´ mă)	**papill** **-edema**	papilla swelling	Swelling of the optic disk, usually caused by increased intracranial pressure (ICP); also called *choked disk*
paraplegia (păr˝ ă-plē´ jē-ă)	**para-** **-plegia**	beside stroke, paralysis	Paralysis of the lower part of the body and of both legs. Refer to Figure 13.14C.
paresis (păr´ ĕ-sĭs)			Slight, partial, or incomplete paralysis

Medical Word	Word Parts		Definition
	Part	Meaning	
paresthesia (păr″ ĕs-thē′ zhē-ă)	**par-** **-esthesia**	beside feeling	Abnormal sensation, feeling of numbness, prickling, or tingling
Parkinson disease (păr′ kĭn-sŭn)			A progressive neurological disorder caused by degeneration of nerve cells in the part of the brain that controls movement. This degeneration creates a shortage of the brain signaling chemical (neurotransmitter) known as *dopamine*, causing the movement impairments that characterize the disease. Often the first symptom of Parkinson disease is tremor (trembling or shaking) of a limb, especially when the body is at rest. The tremor often begins on one side of the body, frequently in one hand. Other common symptoms include slow movement (*bradykinesia*), an inability to move (*akinesia*), rigid limbs, a shuffling gait, and a stooped posture. Also called *paralysis agitans* or *shaking palsy*.
poliomyelitis (pō″ lē-ō-mī″ ĕl-īt′ ĭs)	**poli/o** **myel** **-itis**	gray spinal cord inflammation	Inflammation of the gray matter of the spinal cord
polyneuritis (pŏl″ ē nū-rī′ tĭs)	**poly-** **neur** **-itis**	many nerve inflammation	Literally means *inflammation involving many nerves*
quadriplegia (kwŏd″ rĭ plē′ jē-ă)	**quadri-** **-plegia**	four stroke, paralysis	Paralysis of all four extremities and usually the trunk due to injury to the spinal cord in the cervical spine; also called *tetraplegia*. Refer to Figure 13.14A.
Reye syndrome (rī sĭn′drōm)			Acute disease that causes edema of the brain and increased intracranial pressure, hypoglycemia, and fatty infiltration of the liver and other vital organs; occurs in children and has a relation to aspirin administration; can be viral in origin
sciatica (sī-ăt′ ĭ-kă)			Severe pain along the course of the sciatic nerve
sleep			State of rest for the body and mind; has two distinct types: rapid eye movement (REM), sometimes called *dream sleep*, and non-rapid eye movement (NREM)

Medical Word	Word Parts		Definition
	Part	Meaning	

 fyi Sleep problems, including snoring, sleep apnea, insomnia, sleep deprivation, and restless legs syndrome, are common. One factor that plays an essential role in sleep is an individual's *circadian* (means *around day* or *24-hour cycle*) *rhythm* or "body clock." Circadian rhythms are physical, mental, and behavioral changes that follow a roughly 24-hour cycle, responding primarily to light and darkness in an organism's environment. They are important in determining human sleep patterns and sleep–wake cycles, hormone release, body temperature, and other important bodily functions. Abnormal circadian rhythms have been associated with sleep disorders, such as insomnia, as well as obesity, diabetes, depression, bipolar disorder, and seasonal affective disorder.

Some Common Circadian Rhythm Disorders

Jet lag or rapid time zone change syndrome: Consists of symptoms that include excessive sleepiness and a lack of daytime alertness in people who travel across time zones.

Shift-work sleep disorder: Affects people who frequently rotate shifts or work at night.

Delayed sleep-phase syndrome (DSPS): Disorder of sleep timing. People with DSPS tend to fall asleep very late at night and have difficulty waking up in the morning.

Advanced sleep-phase disorder (ASPD): Disorder in which a person goes to sleep earlier and wakes earlier than desired.

Non-24-hour sleep–wake disorder: Frequently affects those who are totally blind since the circadian clock is set by the light and dark cycle over a 24-hour period. The disorder results in drastically reduced sleep time and sleep quality at night and problems with sleepiness during the day.

Medical Word	Word Parts		Definition
	Part	Meaning	
somnambulism (sŏm-năm′ bū-lĭzm)	**somn** **ambul** **-ism**	sleep to walk condition	Condition of sleepwalking
spondylosyndesis (spŏn″ dĭ-lō-sĭn-dĕ′ sĭs)	**spondyl/o** **syn-** **-desis**	vertebra together binding	Surgical procedure to bind vertebrae after removal of a herniated disk; also called *spinal fusion*
stroke			Death of focal brain tissue that occurs when the brain does not get sufficient blood and oxygen; also called *cerebrovascular accident (CVA)* or *brain attack*. If the flow of blood in an artery supplying the brain is interrupted for longer than a few seconds, brain cells can die, causing permanent damage. The interruption can be caused either by bleeding (hemorrhagic stroke) or blood clots in the brain. See Figures 13.22 and 13.23. A *transient ischemic attack (TIA)* is a temporary interference in the blood supply to the brain. It sometimes is referred to as a *ministroke*, and symptoms can last for a few minutes or several hours.

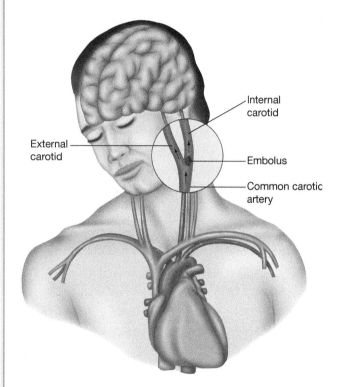

FIGURE 13.22 Embolus traveling to the brain.

External carotid

Internal carotid

Embolus

Common carotic artery

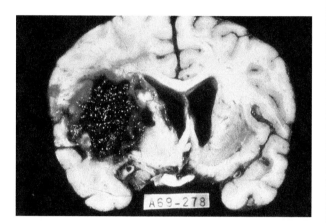

A69-278

FIGURE 13.23 Cross-section of brain showing cerebrovascular accident.

fyi

The risk of stroke doubles with each decade after age 55. Stroke occurs in men more often than in women. A very common cause of stroke is atherosclerosis. Fatty deposits and blood platelets collect on the wall of the arteries, forming plaques. Over time, the plaques slowly begin to block the flow of blood. The plaque itself can block the artery enough to cause a stroke.

In some cases, the plaque causes the blood to flow abnormally, which leads to a blood clot. A clot can stay at the site of narrowing and prevent blood flow to all of the smaller arteries it supplies. This type of clot, which does not travel, is called a **thrombus**. In other cases, the clot can travel and wedge into a smaller vessel. A clot that travels is called an **embolism** (refer to Figure 13.22). Strokes caused by embolisms are commonly associated with cardiovascular pathology, especially heart disorders.

The following sudden symptoms are the warning signs of stroke:

- Numbness or weakness of face, arm, or leg, especially on one side of the body.
- Confusion; trouble speaking or understanding.
- Trouble seeing in one or both eyes.
- Trouble walking, dizziness, loss of balance or coordination.
- Severe headache with no known cause.

The FAST test helps spot symptoms of stroke. FAST stands for:

- **F**ace: Ask for a smile. Does one side droop?
- **A**rms: When raised, does one side drift down?
- **S**peech: Can the person repeat a simple sentence? Does he or she have trouble speaking or slur words?
- **T**ime: Time is critical. Call 911 immediately if any symptoms are present.

Medical Word	Word Parts		Definition
	Part	**Meaning**	
subdural (sŭb-dū´ răl)	**sub-** **dur** **-al**	below dura, hard pertaining to	Pertaining to below the dura mater
sundowning (sŭn´ down-ĭng)			Increased agitation or restlessness that occurs in the late afternoon or early evening in patients with cognitive impairment; most common with Alzheimer-type dementia and Parkinson disease
sympathectomy (sĭm˝ pă-thĕk´ tō-mē)	**sympath** **-ectomy**	sympathy surgical excision	Surgical excision of a portion of the sympathetic nervous system, such as a nerve or ganglion
transcutaneous electrical nerve stimulation (TENS) (trăns-kū-tā´ nē-ŭs)			Use of mild electrical stimulation to interfere with the transmission of painful stimuli; has proved useful in relieving pain in some patients
vagotomy (vā-gŏt´ ō-mē)	**vag/o** **-tomy**	vagus, wandering incision	Surgical incision of the vagus nerve
ventriculogram (vĕn-trĭk´ ū-lō-grăm)	**ventricul/o** **-gram**	ventricle record	X-ray of the cerebral ventricles

Study *and* Review II

Word Parts

Prefixes   Give the definitions of the following prefixes.

1. a-́ _____

2. an- _____

3. astro- _____

4. brady- _____

5. de- _____

6. dys- _____

7. epi- _____

8. hemi- _____

9. hydro- _____

10. hyper- _____

11. intra- _____

12. micro- _____

13. oligo- _____

14. par- _____

15. para- _____

16. poly- _____

17. quadri- _____

18. sub- _____

Combining Forms   Give the definitions of the following combining forms.

1. cephal/o _____

2. cerebell/o _____

3. cerebr/o _____

4. crani/o _____

5. dendr/o _____

6. disk/o _____

7. dur/o _____

8. electr/o _____

9. encephal/o _____

10. esthesi/o _____

11. hypn/o _____

12. lamin/o _____

13. mening/o _____

14. myel/o _____

15. narc/o _____

16. neur/o _____

17. pallid/o _____

18. poli/o _____

19. somn/o _____

20. spin/o _____

21. spondyl/o _____

22. vag/o _____

23. ventricul/o _____

Suffixes   Give the definitions of the following suffixes.

1. -al _____

2. -algesia _____

3. -algia _____

4. -ar _____

5. -asthenia _____

6. -blast _____

7. -cele _____

8. -desis _____

9. -ectomy _____

10. -edema _____

11. -esthesia _____

12. -glia _____

13. -gram _____

14. -graphy _____

15. -ia _____

16. -ic _____

17. -ion   _____

18. -ism   _____

19. -ist   _____

20. -itis   _____

21. -kinesia   _____

22. -kinesis   _____

23. -lepsy   _____

24. -lexia   _____

25. -logy   _____

26. -troph(y)   _____

27. -scopy   _____

28. -oma   _____

29. -osis   _____

30. -paresis   _____

31. -pathy   _____

32. -phagia   _____

33. -phasia   _____

34. -praxia   _____

35. -sthenia   _____

36. -taxia   _____

37. -tomy   _____

38. -us   _____

39. -y   _____

Identifying Medical Terms

In the spaces provided, write the medical terms for the following meanings.

1. _____ Condition in which there is a loss or lack of memory

2. _____ Condition in which there is a lack of the sensation of pain

3. _____ Loss or lack of the ability to eat or swallow

4. _____ Neurological sign and symptom consisting of lack of coordination of muscle movements

5. _____ Head pain; headache

6. _____ Pertaining to the cerebellum

7. _____ Surgical excision of a portion of the skull

8. _____ Condition in which an individual has difficulty reading and writing words even though vision and intelligence are unimpaired

9. _____ Inflammation of the brain

10. _____ Literally means pertaining to situated on the dura mater

Matching

Select the appropriate lettered meaning for each of the following words.

_____ 1. acetylcholine

_____ 2. Alzheimer disease

_____ 3. stroke

_____ 4. endorphins

_____ 5. epilepsy

_____ 6. Bell palsy

_____ 7. diskectomy

_____ 8. epiduroscopy

_____ 9. dementia

_____ 10. sciatica

a. Group of symptoms marked by memory loss and other cognitive functions

b. Chemical substances produced in the brain that act as natural analgesics (*opiates*) and provide feelings of pleasure

c. Cerebrovascular accident

d. The most common cause of dementia among older adults

e. A neurological disorder involving repeated seizures of any type

f. Used for back pain relief when all other conservative treatments have failed

g. Cholinergic neurotransmitter

h. Temporary facial paralysis resulting from damage or trauma to the facial nerve

i. Severe pain along the course of the sciatic nerve

j. Surgical excision of an intervertebral disk

Medical Case Snapshots

This learning activity provides an opportunity to relate the medical terminology you are learning to sample patient case presentations. In the spaces provided, write in your answers.

Case 1

An 8-year-old girl was accompanied by her mother to the doctor's office. The mother states that, about 2 years ago, her daughter was diagnosed with _____, which is a neurological disorder involving repeated seizures. The majority of diagnosed cases of this disorder are _____ as their causes cannot be identified.

Case 2

The 74-year-old male was seen by his physician. He was in acute pain and complaining of severe itching around his waistline. Examination of his torso revealed evidence of a viral disease characterized by painful vesicular eruptions. This disease, known as _____ _____, is caused by the varicella-zoster virus, the same virus that causes _____. The common name for this condition is _____.

Case 3

A 70-year-old male diagnosed with Parkinson disease was seen by a neurologist. The patient had moderate to severe tremor (worse in the left hand than the right), difficulty in movement with _____ or abnormal slowness of motion, with freezing in place or _____. The physician discussed with the patient and his wife the possibility of a surgical procedure known as a _____, wherein there is destruction of the globus pallidus of the brain.

Drug Highlights

Classification of Drug	Description and Examples
analgesics	Inhibit ascending pain pathways in the central nervous system. They increase pain threshold and alter pain perception.
narcotic	EXAMPLES: codeine sulfate, Dilaudid (hydromorphone HCl), Demerol (meperidine HCl), morphine sulfate, Norco (hydrocodone), Vicodin (hydrocodone), and Lorcet (hydrocodone)
non-narcotic	EXAMPLES: butorphanol tartrate and nalbuphine HCl
analgesics–antipyretics	Act to relieve pain (analgesic effect) and reduce fever (antipyretic effect).
	EXAMPLES: Tylenol (acetaminophen), aspirin, Advil/Motrin (ibuprofen), and Naprosyn/Aleve (naproxen)
sedatives and hypnotics	Depress the central nervous system by interfering with the transmission of nerve impulses. Depending on the dosage, barbiturates, benzodiazepines, and certain other drugs can produce either a sedative or a hypnotic effect. When used as a sedative, the dosage is designed to produce a calming effect without causing sleep. Used as a hypnotic, the dosage is sufficient to cause sleep.
barbiturate	EXAMPLE: Seconal sodium (secobarbital)
nonbarbiturate	EXAMPLES: lorazepam HCl, Restoril (temazepam), and Halcion (triazolam)
antiparkinsonism drugs	Used for palliative relief from such major symptoms as bradykinesia, rigidity, tremor, and disorder of equilibrium and posture. Therapy involves an attempt to replenish dopamine levels and/or inhibit the effects of the neurotransmitter acetylcholine.
	EXAMPLES: Sinemet 25–100 (25 mg of carbidopa and 100 mg of levodopa), levodopa, trihexyphenidyl HCl, Cogentin (benztropine mesylate), Requip (ropinirole), Tasmar (tolcapone), and Stalevo (carbidopa, levodopa, and entacapone)

Classification of Drug	Description and Examples
anticonvulsants	Inhibit the spread of seizure activity in the motor cortex.
	EXAMPLES: Dilantin (phenytoin), Depakene (valproic acid), Tegretol (carbamazepine), Klonopin (clonazepam), and Mysoline (primidone)
	Selected anticonvulsants are used to help control the type of pain caused by damaged nerves and can help quiet the burning, stabbing, or shooting pain often caused by neuropathy. These drugs can be prescribed for diabetic neuropathy, shingles, trigeminal neuralgia, and/or damaged nerves due to chemotherapy, herniated disk, or fibromyalgia.
	EXAMPLES: Carbatrol, Tegretol (carbamazepine), and Neurontin (gabapentin)
cholinesterase inhibitors	Increase the brain's levels of acetylcholine, which helps to restore communication between brain cells. These medications can be used to improve global functioning (including activities of daily living [ADL]), behavior, and cognition) in some patients with Alzheimer disease.
	EXAMPLES: Aricept (donepezil hydrochloride) and Exelon (rivastigmine tartrate)

 fyi

To date, no treatment can stop Alzheimer disease (AD). However, for some people in the early and middle stages of the disease, the drugs donepezil (Aricept), rivastigmine (Exelon), galantamine (Razadyne), or memantine (Namenda) can help prevent some symptoms from becoming worse for a limited time. Also, some medicines can help control behavioral symptoms of AD such as sleeplessness, agitation, wandering, anxiety, and depression.

During the 2018 Alzheimer's Association International Conference in Chicago, the results of a promising clinical trial were presented. A new drug, an antibody called BAN2401, achieved a first in a large clinical trial by simultaneously reducing the characteristic Alzheimer plaques—beta amyloid clusters—in the brains of patients, and slowing the formulation of new ones. It lessened existing clusters by 70% on average. In sum, the drug could be the first to successfully attack both the brain changes and the symptoms of the memory-crippling disease.

anesthetics	Interfere with the conduction of nerve impulses and are used to produce loss of sensation, loss of pain, muscle relaxation, and/or complete loss of consciousness; block nerve transmission in the area to which they are applied.
local	Block nerve transmission in the area to which they are applied.
	EXAMPLES: Xylocaine (lidocaine HCl) and Marcaine (bupivacaine HCl)
general	Affect the central nervous system and produce either partial or complete loss of consciousness. They also produce analgesia, skeletal muscle relaxation, and reduction of reflex activity.
	EXAMPLES: Suprane (desflurane), isoflurane, Sojourn, and Ultane (Sevoflurane)

fyi

Every day, more than 130 people in the United States die after overdosing on opioids. The misuse of and addiction to opioids—including prescription pain relievers, heroin, and synthetic opioids such as fentanyl—is a serious national crisis that affects public health as well as social and economic welfare and has led to what is now termed *the opioid epidemic*. The CDC estimates that the total economic burden of prescription opioid misuse alone in the United States is $78.5 billion a year, including the costs of healthcare, lost productivity, addiction treatment, and criminal justice involvement. See Figure 13.24.

THE OPIOID EPIDEMIC BY THE NUMBERS
2016 and 2017 Data

 130+
People died every day from opioid-related drug overdoses[3] (estimated)

 11.4 m
People misused prescription opioids[1]

 42,249
People died from overdosing on opioids[2]

 2 million
People misused prescription opioids for the first time[1]

 2.1 million
People had an opioid use disorder[1]

 17,087
Deaths attributed to overdosing on commonly prescribed opioids[2]

 886,000
People used heroin[1]

 19,413
Deaths attributed to overdosing on synthetic opioids other than methadone[2]

 81,000
People used heroin for the first time[1]

 15,469
Deaths attributed to overdosing on heroin[2]

SOURCES
1. 2017 National Survey on Drug Use and Health, Mortality in the United States, 2016
2. NCHS Data Brief No. 293, December 2017
3. NCHS, National Vital Statistics System. Estimates for 2017 and 2018 are based on provisional data.

FIGURE 13.24 Opioid epidemic data for 2016 and 2017.
Source: U.S. Department of Health and Human Services

 fyi

According to the National Institute of Drug Abuse, Naloxone is a medication designed to rapidly reverse opioid overdose. It is an *opioid antagonist*, meaning that it binds to opioid receptors and can reverse and block the effects of other opioids. It can very quickly restore normal respiration to a person whose breathing has slowed or stopped as a result of overdosing with heroin or prescription opioid pain medications. Naloxone is available as an injectable, an autoinjectable, and a prepackaged nasal spray.

Diagnostic *and* Laboratory Tests

Test	Description
cerebral angiography (sĕr´ ĕ-brăl ăn-jē-ŏg´ ră-fē)	Process of making an x-ray record of the cerebral arterial system. A radiopaque substance is injected into an artery of the arm or neck, and x-ray films of the head are taken to visualize cerebral aneurysms, tumors, or ruptured blood vessels.
cerebrospinal fluid (CSF) analysis (sĕr˝ ĕ-brŏ-spī´ năl)	Examination of spinal fluid for color, pressure, pH, and the levels of protein, glucose, and leukocytes. Abnormal results can indicate hemorrhage, tumor, and various disease processes.
computed tomography (CT) (kŏm-pū´ tĕd tō-mŏg˝ ră-fē)	Diagnostic procedure used to study the structure of the brain. Computerized three-dimensional x-ray images allow the radiologist to differentiate among intracranial tumors, cysts, edema, and hemorrhage.
echoencephalography (ĕk˝ ō-ĕn-sĕf-ă-lŏg´ ră-fē)	Process of using ultrasound to determine the presence of a centrally located mass in the brain.
electroencephalography (EEG) (ē-lĕk˝ trō-ĕn-sĕf˝ ă-lŏg´ ră-fē)	Process of measuring the electrical activity of the brain via an electroencephalograph. Abnormal results can indicate epilepsy, brain tumor, infection, abscess, hemorrhage, and/or coma; brain "death" can also be determined by an EEG.
lumbar puncture (LP) (lŭm´ băr)	Insertion of a needle into the lumbar subarachnoid space for removal of spinal fluid. The fluid is examined for color, pressure, level of protein, chloride, glucose, and leukocytes. See Figure 13.25.

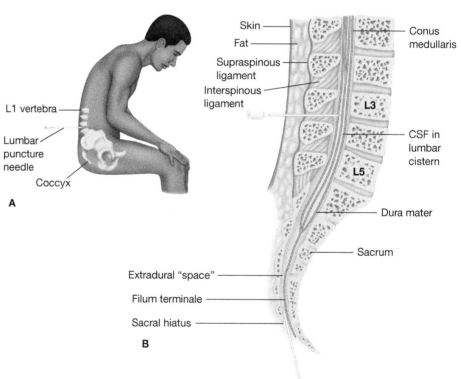

FIGURE 13.25 A Lumbar puncture, also known as *spinal tap*; **B** section of the vertebral column showing the spinal cord and membranes with a lumbar puncture needle at L3–L4 and in the sacral hiatus.

myelogram (mī´ ĕ-lō-grăm)	X-ray of the spinal canal after the injection of a radiopaque dye. Useful in diagnosing spinal lesions, cysts, herniated disks, tumors, and nerve root damage.

Test	Description
neurological examination (noo-rŏ-loj′ ĭ-kăl)	Assessment of a patient's vision; hearing; sense of taste, smell, touch, and pain; position; temperature; gait; and muscle strength, coordination, and reflex action to determine neurological status.
positron emission tomography (PET) (pŏz′ ĭ-trŏn ē-mĭsh′ ŭn tō-mŏg′ră-fē)	Computer-based nuclear imaging procedure that can produce three-dimensional pictures of actual organ functioning. Useful in locating brain lesion, identifying blood flow and oxygen metabolism in stroke patients, showing metabolic changes in Alzheimer disease, and studying biochemical changes associated with mental illness.
ultrasonography, brain (ŭl-tră-sŏn-ŏg′ ră-fē)	Use of high-frequency sound waves to produce an image on a computer screen. Used as a screening test or diagnostic tool.

Abbreviations *and* Acronyms

Abbreviation/Acronym	Meaning	Abbreviation/Acronym	Meaning
ACh	acetylcholine	ICP	intracranial pressure
AD	Alzheimer disease	LATE	limbic-predominant age-related TDP-43 encephalopathy
ADL	activities of daily living		
ALS	amyotrophic lateral sclerosis	LBD	Lewy body dementia
ANS	autonomic nervous system	LP	lumbar puncture
ASPD	advanced sleep phase disorder	MHI	mild head injury
CDC	Centers for Disease Control and Prevention	MHT	minor head trauma
		mL	milliliter
cm	centimeter	MRI	magnetic resonance imaging
CNS	central nervous system	MS	multiple sclerosis
CP	cerebral palsy	MTBI	mild traumatic brain injury
CSF	cerebrospinal fluid	Neuro	neurology
CT	computed tomography	NREM	non-rapid eye movement (sleep)
CTE	chronic traumatic encephalopathy	PD	Parkinson disease
CVA	cerebrovascular accident	PET	positron emission tomography
DBS	deep brain stimulation	PHN	postherpetic neuralgia
DSPS	delayed sleep phase syndrome	PNS	peripheral nervous system
EEG	electroencephalogram	REM	rapid eye movement (sleep)
FTD	frontotemporal dementia	TDP-43	transactive response DNA binding protein 43 kDa
FTLD	frontotemporal lobar degeneration		
GCS	Glasgow Coma Scale	TENS	transcutaneous electrical nerve stimulation
HDS	herniated disk syndrome		
HNP	herniated nucleus pulposus	TIA	transient ischemic attack

Study *and* Review III

Building Medical Terms

Using the following word parts, fill in the blanks to build the correct medical terms.

an-	concuss	papill	-itis	-esthesia
quadri-	neur	-kinesia	-ectomy	-tomy

Definition   **Medical Term**

1. Condition in which there is a lack of the sensation of pain   _____algesia

2. Abnormal slowness of movement   brady_____

3. Head injury with a transient loss of brain function   _____ion

4. Inflammation of the brain   encephal_____

5. Surgical excision of a vertebral posterior arch   lamin_____

6. Pain in a nerve or nerves   _____algia

7. Swelling of the optic disk, usually caused by ICP   _____edema

8. Abnormal sensation, feeling of numbness, or prickling   par_____

9. Paralysis of all four extremities and usually the trunk   _____plegia

10. Surgical incision of the vagus nerve   vago_____

Combining Form Challenge

Using the combining forms provided, write the medical term correctly.

cephal/o	encephal/o	mening/o
cran/i	hypn/o	neur/o

1. Head pain; headache: _____algia

2. Surgical excision of a portion of the skull: _____ectomy

3. Any pathological dysfunction of the brain: _____pathy

4. Artificially induced trancelike state resembling sleepwalking: _____osis

5. Inflammation of the meninges of the spinal cord or brain: _____itis

6. Supporting or connective tissue cells of the central nervous system: _____glia

Select the Right Term

Select the correct answer, and write it on the line provided.

1. Inability to remain still; motor restlessness and anxiety is _____.

    akathisia   akinesia   aphagia   apraxia

2. Literally means *loss or lack of the sense of feeling* is _____.

    analgesia   anesthesia   aphasia   asthenia

3. Unconscious state or stupor from which the patient cannot be aroused is _____.

    chorea   concussion   coma   epilepsy

4. Group of symptoms marked by memory loss and other cognitive functions is _____.

    dyslexia   dysphasia   hypnosis   dementia

5. Increased muscular movement and motion is _____.

    hyperesthesia   narcolepsy   hyperkinesis   paresis

6. Death of focal brain tissue that occurs when the brain does not get sufficient blood and oxygen is _____.

    sundowning   stroke   coma   concussion

Drug Highlights

Match the appropriate lettered description or examples of drug(s) with the class of drug.

_____ 1. sedatives and hypnotics

_____ 2. analgesics

_____ 3. antiparkinsonism drugs

_____ 4. cholinesterase inhibitors

_____ 5. local anesthetics

_____ 6. anticonvulsants

_____ 7. example of a narcotic analgesic

_____ 8. analgesics–antipyretics

_____ 9. general anesthetics

_____ 10. drugs used to treat Alzheimer disease

a. Provide palliative relief from such major symptoms as bradykinesia, rigidity, tremor, and disorder of equilibrium and posture

b. Block nerve transmission of pain in the area to which they are applied

c. Inhibit the spread of seizure activity in the motor cortex

d. Depress the central nervous system by interfering with the transmission of nerve impulses, producing either a sedative or a hypnotic effect depending on the dosage

e. Act to relieve pain (analgesic effect) and reduce fever (antipyretic effect)

f. Aricept (donepezil hydrochloride) and Exelon (rivastigmine tartrate)

g. Inhibit ascending pain pathways in the central nervous system, increasing pain threshold and altering pain perception

h. Improve global functioning (including activities of daily living, behavior, and cognition) in some patients with Alzheimer disease

i. Vicodin (hydrocodone)

j. Affect the central nervous system and produce either partial or complete loss of consciousness

Diagnostic and Laboratory Tests

Select the best answer to each multiple-choice question. Circle the letter of your choice.

1. Diagnostic procedure used to study the structure of the brain.

a. computed tomography

b. echoencephalography

c. electroencephalography

d. myelogram

2. Process of using ultrasound to determine the presence of a centrally located mass in the brain.

a. computed tomography

b. echoencephalography

c. electroencephalography

d. myelogram

3. X-ray of the spinal canal after the injection of a radiopaque dye.

a. cerebral angiography

b. computed tomography

c. myelogram

d. ultrasonography

4. Computer-based nuclear imaging procedure that can produce three-dimensional pictures of actual organ functioning.

a. electroencephalography

b. myelogram

c. ultrasonography

d. positron emission tomography

5. Use of high-frequency sound waves to produce an image on a computer screen.

a. electroencephalography

b. myelogram

c. ultrasonography

d. positron emission tomography

Abbreviations and Acronyms

Write the correct word, phrase, or abbreviation/acronym in the space provided.

1. Alzheimer disease _____

2. amyotrophic lateral sclerosis _____

3. CNS _____

4. CP _____

5. computed tomography _____

6. herniated disk syndrome _____

7. ICP _____

8. LP _____

9. MS _____

10. positron emission tomography _____

Practical Application

Medical Record Analysis

This exercise contains information, abbreviations/acronyms, and medical terminology from an actual medical record or case study that has been adapted for this text. The names and any personal information have been created by the author. Read and study each form or case study and then answer the questions that follow. You may refer to Appendix III, *Abbreviations, Acronyms, and Symbols*.

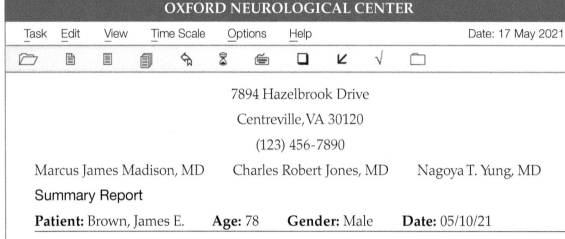

OXFORD NEUROLOGICAL CENTER

| Task | Edit | View | Time Scale | Options | Help | Date: 17 May 2021 |

7894 Hazelbrook Drive

Centreville, VA 30120

(123) 456-7890

Marcus James Madison, MD   Charles Robert Jones, MD   Nagoya T. Yung, MD

Summary Report

Patient: Brown, James E.   **Age:** 78   **Gender:** Male   **Date:** 05/10/21

James E. Brown, age 78, has advanced Parkinson disease, present for 7 years. It is affecting his activities of daily living (ADL). He has difficulty bathing and dressing and has frequent falls. He has marked hesitancy on changing directions and unsteadiness with fatigue. He can brush his teeth and wash his face.

On neurological examination he did have mild to moderate impairment in cognition and short-term memory, although he is oriented to time, place, and person. He has a mild tremor, worse in the left arm than the right. He has rigidity in the upper extremities. He has marked difficulty in movement, with long delays in initiating movement and frequent freezing in place. He has postural instability. He has mild difficulty with articulation of speech, dysarthria. His gait is characterized by shuffling strides. He can arise from a chair with difficulty only after multiple attempts. Deep tendon reflexes are symmetrical, and toes are downgoing. Cranial nerves are unremarkable.

He has been on Sinemet 25–100 mg tid for the last 6 years. I have asked him to increase his Sinemet dose to qid. Mr. Brown is to return to our office in 3 months.

Marcus James Madison, MD

Medical Record Questions

Write the correct answer in the space provided.

1. On neurological examination Mr. Brown did have mild to moderate impairment in _____ and short-term memory.

2. Mr. Brown has a mild _____, worse in the left arm than the right.

3. What does *dysarthria* mean? _____

4. Sinemet 25–100 mg is classified as a/an _____ drug.

5. Why is this drug prescribed for Mr. Brown? _____

_____

MyLab Medical Terminology™

MyLab Medical Terminology is a premium online homework management system that includes a host of features to help you study. Registered users will find:

- A multitude of quizzes and activities built within the MyLab platform
- Powerful tools that track and analyze your results—allowing you to create a personalized learning experience
- Videos and audio pronunciations to help enrich your progress
- Streaming lesson presentations (guided lectures) and self-paced learning modules
- A space where you and your instructor can check your progress and manage your assignments

14 Special Senses: The Ear

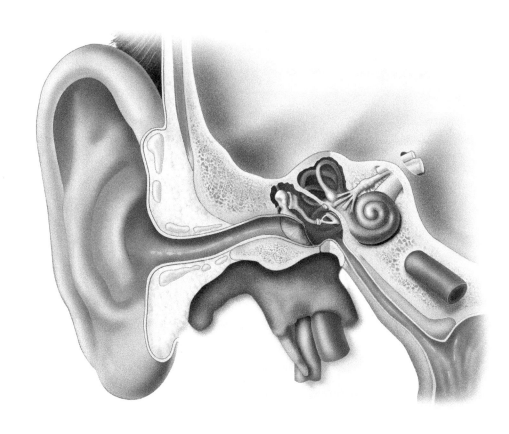

∨ Learning Outcomes

On completion of this chapter, you will be able to:

1. Describe the three distinct divisions of the ear.
2. Identify the primary functions of the ear.
3. Analyze, build, spell, and pronounce medical words.
4. Classify the drugs highlighted in this chapter.
5. Describe diagnostic and laboratory tests related to the ear.
6. Identify and define selected abbreviations and acronyms.

Anatomy and Physiology

The **ear** is generally described as having three distinct divisions: the external ear, the middle ear, and the inner ear, each with separate functions. The ear contains structures for both the sense of hearing and the sense of balance. The eighth cranial nerve, also called the acoustic or auditory nerve, carries nerve impulses for both hearing and balance from the ear to the brain. Table 14.1 provides an at-a-glance look at the ear. The ear and its anatomic structures are shown in Figure 14.1.

TABLE 14.1　Special Senses: The Ear at-a-Glance

Organ/Structure	Primary Functions/Description
External ear	
Auricle (pinna)	Collects and directs sound waves into the auditory canal and then into the tympanic membrane
External acoustic meatus (auditory canal)	Numerous glands line the canal and secrete cerumen (earwax) to lubricate and protect the ear
Tympanic membrane (eardrum)	Separates the external ear from the middle ear and is not actually part of the external ear
Middle ear	
Contains the ossicles: malleus, incus, and stapes	Transmits sound vibrations from the tympanic membrane to the cochlea
The eustachian tube is a narrow tube between the middle ear and the throat	Helps to equalize external/internal air pressure on the tympanic membrane
Inner ear	
Cochlea	Located on the basilar membrane is the *organ of Corti* containing hair cell sensory receptors for the sense of hearing
Vestibule	Contains the utricle and saccule, membranous pouches containing perilymph. The utricle communicates with the semicircular canals and contains hair cell sensory receptors connected to fibers from the eighth cranial nerve. These hair cells react to the force of gravity and movement of *otoliths* and are a part of the sense of equilibrium (state of balance).
Semicircular canals	Contain nerve endings in the form of hair cells that note changes in the position of the head and report such movement to the brain through fibers leading to the eighth cranial nerve

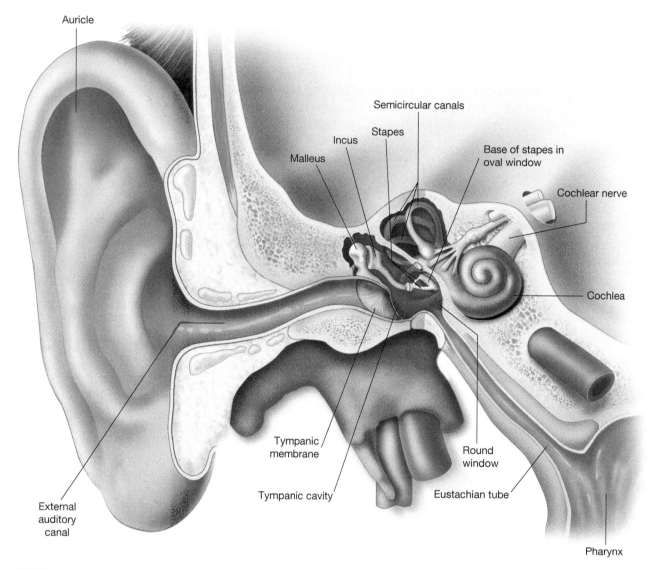

FIGURE 14.1 The ear and its anatomic structures.

External Ear

The **external ear** is the appendage on the side of the head consisting of the **auricle** or **pinna** and the *external acoustic meatus*. The auricle is the visible part of the ear that has a curved fold forming most of the rim of the external ear. This fold makes it more difficult for insects to reach the eardrum, thereby protecting the tympanic membrane. At the same time, **cerumen** (earwax) in the auditory canal also helps to keep unwanted materials like dirt and dust out of the ear. The auricle is the first part of the ear that reacts with sound. It acts like a funnel that assists in directing the sound further into the ear. It also helps to regulate the air pressure within the ear by keeping the air pressure at a moderate level, so more sound passes into the auditory canal.

Middle Ear

The **middle ear**, separated from the external ear by the eardrum, is an air-filled cavity (**tympanic cavity**) carved out of the temporal bone. The **attic** (epitympanic recess) of the middle ear is the portion lying above the tympanic cavity proper. It contains the head of

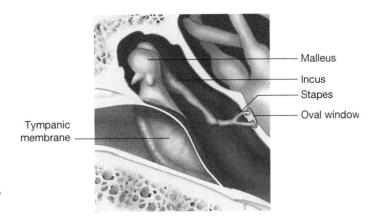

FIGURE 14.2 The ossicles of the middle ear along with the oval window and tympanic membrane.

the malleus and the short limb of the incus. The tympanic cavity contains three special-ized small bones or **ossicles** instrumental to the hearing process. These ossicles are the **malleus (hammer), incus (anvil),** and **stapes (stirrup).** See Figure 14.2. These bones mechan-ically transmit sound vibrations from the tympanic membrane, to which the malleus is attached, through the incus to the stapes, which attaches to a thin membrane covering a small opening, the oval window (refer to Figure 14.1), that marks the beginning of the inner ear. During transmission, tympanic vibrations can be amplified as much as 22 times their original force.

The tympanic cavity connects to the throat/nasopharynx via the **eustachian tube,** which is a narrow tube between the middle ear and the throat. This ear–throat connec-tion makes the ear susceptible to infection. The spread of infection from the throat along this membrane to the middle ear is called **otitis media (OM).** The continued spread of infection to one of the mastoid bones is called **mastoiditis.** The eustachian tube functions to equalize air pressure on both sides of the eardrum. Normally the walls of the tube are collapsed. Swallowing and chewing actions open the tube to allow air in or out, as needed for equalization. Equalizing air pressure ensures that the eardrum vibrates max-imally when struck by sound waves.

 At 36 weeks, the **earlobes** of the fetus are soft, and around 40 weeks they become firm. In newborns, the wall of the ear canal is pliable because of underdeveloped cartilage and bone. The eustachian tube in infants is shorter and straighter than in older children and adults. Because of this, an infant or young child is more pre-disposed to developing an ear infection. When this occurs, the child's ears should be examined very carefully.

Inner Ear

The **inner ear** consists of a membranous labyrinth or mazelike network of canals located within a bony labyrinth. These structures are called **labyrinths** because of their compli-cated shapes. The bony labyrinth, located in the temporal bone, consists of the *cochlea, vestibule,* and three *semicircular canals.* Within the bony labyrinth, but separated from it by a pale fluid called **perilymph,** is the membranous labyrinth, filled with a fluid called **endolymph.** This membranous labyrinth contains the actual hearing cells, the hair cells of the organ of Corti.

Cochlea

The **cochlea** is a spiral-shaped bony structure containing the cochlear duct; it is so named because it resembles a snail shell (refer to Figure 14.1). The spiral cavity of the bony cochlea is partitioned into three tubelike channels that run the entire length of the spiral. Two membranes form these tubelike areas. The *basilar membrane* forms the lower channel or *scala tympani,* and the *vestibular membrane (Reissner membrane)* forms the upper channel, which is called the *scala vestibuli.* Between the two scala is a space, the *cochlear duct,* formed by the vestibular membrane on top and the basilar membrane as a floor. Located on the basilar membrane is the **organ of Corti** containing hair cell sensory receptors for the sense of hearing. The fluid perilymph fills the scala vestibuli and scala tympani. A different fluid, endolymph, fills the cochlear duct.

fyi

A cochlear implant is a small, complex electronic device that can help to provide a sense of sound to a person who is profoundly deaf or severely hard of hearing. The implant consists of an external portion that sits behind the ear and a second portion that is surgically placed under the skin. See Figure 14.3. An implant does not restore normal hearing. Instead, it can give a deaf person a useful representation of sounds in the environment and help him or her to understand speech. An implant has the following parts:

- A microphone, which picks up sound from the environment.
- A speech processor, which selects and arranges sounds picked up by the microphone.
- A transmitter and receiver/stimulator, which receive signals from the speech processor and convert them into electric impulses.
- An electrode array, which is a group of electrodes that collects the impulses from the stimulator and sends them to different regions of the auditory nerve.

Children and adults can be fitted for cochlear implants. Adults who have lost all or most of their hearing later in life often can benefit from cochlear implants. Cochlear implants, coupled with intensive postimplantation therapy, can help young children, often between 2 and 6 years old, to acquire speech, language, and social skills. See Figure 14.4.

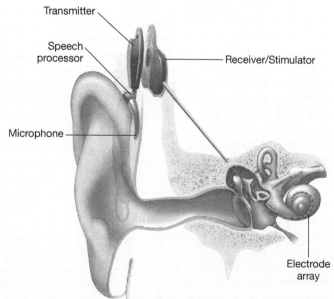

Ear with Cochlear Implant

Transmitter

Speech processor

Microphone

Receiver/Stimulator

Electrode array

FIGURE 14.3 Ear with cochlear implant.
Source: NIH Medical Arts

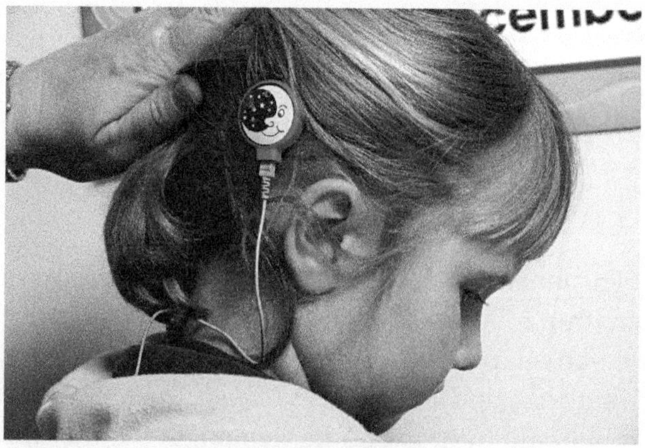

FIGURE 14.4 A young child with a cochlear implant.
Source: Pearson Education, Inc.

THE PROCESS OF HEARING

In the process of hearing, sound waves are collected by the auricle (pinna) and directed through the external auditory canal to the tympanic membrane (eardrum), causing it to vibrate. These vibrations move the three small bones of the middle ear (malleus, incus, and stapes). The movement of the stapes at the oval window sets up pressure waves in the auditory fluids (perilymph and endolymph). The waves distort the basilar membrane and cause the vibration of the hair cells of the organ of Corti. These vibrations are picked up by auditory nerve fibers that transmit an electric nerve signal to the cerebral cortex of the brain, where it is interpreted as sound. The path of sound vibrations is shown in Figure 14.5.

Vestibule

The **vestibule** is a bony structure located between the cochlea and the three semicircular canals. The bony vestibule contains the **utricle** and **saccule**, membranous pouches containing perilymph. The utricle communicates with the semicircular canals and contains hair cell sensory receptors connected to fibers from the eighth cranial nerve. These hair cells bend to the forces of gravity and movement of **otoliths** and are a part of the sense of *equilibrium*. Receptors in the utricle and saccule respond to gravity and linear acceleration. Because of their orientation in the head, the utricle is sensitive to a change in horizontal movement, and the saccule gives information about vertical acceleration (such as when in an elevator).

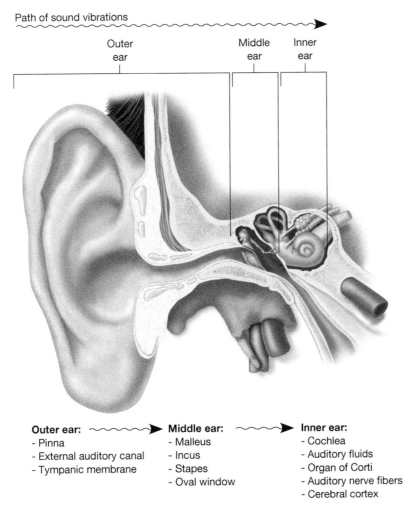

FIGURE 14.5 Path of sound vibrations.

The utricle and saccule together make the *otolith organs*. Both of these organs contain a sensory epithelium, the **macula**, which consists of hair cells and associated supporting cells. Overlying the hair cells and their hair bundles is a gelatinous layer, and above this is a fibrous structure, the **otolithic membrane**, in which are embedded crystals of calcium carbonate called **otoconia**. The crystals give the otolith organs their name: *otolith* is Greek for "ear stones."

Semicircular Canals

Located at right angles to each other are the superior, posterior, and inferior **semicircular canals**. Within the bony canals are the membranous semicircular ducts containing endolymph. At the base of each canal is an enlargement called an **ampulla** containing nerve endings in the form of hair cells. Changes in the position of the head cause the fluid in the canals to flow against these sensory receptors, which, in turn, report such movement to the brain through fibers leading to the eighth cranial nerve. Dizziness and motion sickness are associated with the continued movement of the fluid in the semicircular canals due to gravitational influences and the resulting sensory sensation in these areas.

fyi

With aging, changes occur in the external, middle, and inner ear. The skin of the auricle can become dry and wrinkled. Production of cerumen declines and it is drier. There is also dryness of the external canal, which causes itching. Hairs in the external canal become coarser and longer, especially in males. The eardrum thickens, and the bony joints in the middle ear degenerate.

Changes in the inner ear affect sensitivity to sound, understanding of speech, and balance. Degenerative changes include atrophy of the cochlea, the cochlear nerve cells, and the organ of Corti. These changes lead to the hearing loss, **presbycusis**, which is common in the older adult. Noisy surroundings make it difficult for older adults to discriminate between sounds, thereby impairing communication and socialization. The hearing distance (HD) of older adults can also be impaired.

Study *and* Review I

Anatomy and Physiology

Write your answers to the following questions.

1. The ears contain structures for both the sense of _____ and the sense of _____.

2. Name the three divisions of the ear.

a. _____ c. _____

b. _____

3. The external ear consists of the _____ and the _____.

4. Which structure of the external ear collects sound waves? _____

5. State the two functions of cerumen.

a. _____   b. _____

6. Name the three ossicles of the middle ear.

a. _____   c. _____

b. _____

7. State the function of the ossicles. _____

8. State two functions of the middle ear.

a. _____   b. _____

9. The bony labyrinth of the inner ear consists of the _____, _____, and the _____.

10. Name the three divisions of the membranous labyrinth.

a. _____   c. _____

b. _____

11. Located on the basilar membrane is the _____, containing hair cell sensory receptors for the sense of hearing.

12. The _____ is a bony structure located between the cochlea and the three semicircular canals.

13. The auditory nerve is also known as the _____.

14. Dizziness and _____ are associated with the continued movement of the fluid in the semicircular canals due to gravitational influences.

15. Name the two types of fluid found in the ear.

a. _____   b. _____

▶ **ANATOMY LABELING**   Identify the structures shown below by filling in the blanks.

Building Your Medical Vocabulary

This section provides the foundation for learning medical terminology. Review the alphabetized list of medical terms in the following pages. Note how common prefixes and suffixes are repeatedly applied to word roots and combining forms to create different meanings. A combining form is a word root plus a vowel. The chart below lists the combining forms and word roots used in this chapter and can help to strengthen your understanding of how medical words are built and spelled.

You will find that some terms have not been divided into word parts. These are common words or specialized terms that are included to enhance your medical vocabulary.

Combining Forms

audi/o	to hear	**neur/o**	nerve
aur/i	ear	**ot/o**	ear
chol/e	gall or bile	**pharyng/o**	pharynx
cochle/o	land snail	**presby/o**	old
electr/o	electricity	**py/o**	pus
labyrinth/o	maze, inner ear	**rhin/o**	nose
laryng/o	larynx, voice box	**scler/o**	hardening
mast/o	mastoid process	**staped/o**	stapes, stirrup
myring/o	eardrum, tympanic membrane	**steat/o**	fat
myc/o	fungus	**tympan/o**	eardrum, tympanic membrane

Word Roots

acoust	hearing	**log**	study
auditor	hearing	**med**	middle
fenestrat	window		

Medical Word	Word Parts		Definition
	Part	**Meaning**	
acoustic (ă-koos′tĭk)	**acoust** **-ic**	hearing pertaining to	Pertaining to the sense of hearing
audiogram (ŏ′ dē-ō-grăm″)	**audi/o** **-gram**	to hear mark, record	Record of hearing as a graph showing the results of a pure tone hearing test (audiometry); see the Diagnostic and Laboratory Tests section for more information

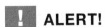 **ALERT!**

How many words can you build using the combining form **audi/o**?

Medical Word	Word Parts		Definition
	Part	**Meaning**	
audiologist (ŏ″ dē-ŏl′ ō-jĭst)	**audi/o** **log** **-ist**	to hear study one who specializes	One who specializes in diagnosing disorders of hearing
audiology (ŏ″ dē-ŏl′ ō-jē)	**audi/o** **-logy**	to hear study of	Study of hearing disorders
audiometer (ŏ″ dē-ŏm′ ĕ-tĕr)	**audi/o** **-meter**	to hear instrument to measure	Medical instrument used to measure hearing
auditory (ŏ′ dĭ-tō″ rē)	**auditor** **-y**	hearing pertaining to	Pertaining to the sense of hearing
aural (or′ ăl)	**aur** **-al**	ear pertaining to	Pertaining to the ear
auricle (or′ ĭ-kl)	**aur/i** **-cle**	ear small	External portion of the ear; also known as the *pinna*
binaural (bī-nawr′ ăl)	**bin-** **aur** **-al**	twice ear pertaining to	Pertaining to both ears
cholesteatoma (kō″ lē-stē″ ă-tō′ mă)	**chol/e** **steat** **-oma**	gall or bile fat tumor	Tumor-like mass filled with epithelial cells and cholesterol
deafness			Complete or partial loss of the ability to hear. *Hearing impairment* is often used to describe a minimal loss of hearing as compared to the use of the word *deafness* when there is complete or extensive loss of hearing. See Figure 14.6.

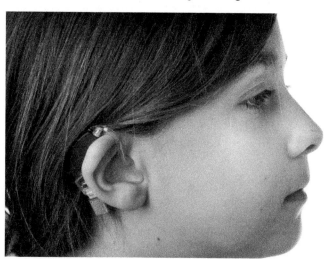

FIGURE 14.6 A child with a hearing impairment wears a hearing aid in her right ear.
Source: BCFC/Shutterstock

Medical Word	Word Parts		Definition
	Part	Meaning	

Sustained noise over 85 decibels (db, dB) can cause permanent **hearing loss**. Risk doubles with each 5-decibel increase. About two in every 10 teens have lost some of their hearing ability from exposure to noise and are not aware of it, according to a study conducted at the University of Florida. See Figure 14.7. High-pitched sounds are the first to be affected by noise exposure. As hearing loss progresses, a person can start to have difficulty hearing, particularly when there is noise in the background. Excessive noise can permanently damage the hair cell sensory receptors of the organ of Corti. These receptors are instrumental in transmitting sound to the brain.

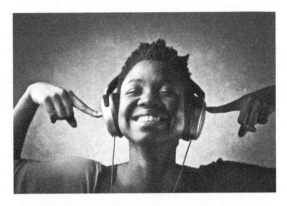

FIGURE 14.7 Listening to loud music with headphones or at rock concerts is a frequent cause of hearing loss among teenagers and young adults.
Source: ollyy/Shutterstock

Medical Word	Word Parts		Definition
	Part	Meaning	
electrocochleography (ē-lĕk″ trō-kŏk″ lē-ŏg′ ră-fē)	**electr/o** **cochle/o** **-graphy**	electricity land snail recording	Recording of the electrical activity produced when the cochlea is stimulated
endaural (end-awr′ ăl)	**end-** **aur** **-al**	within ear pertaining to	Pertaining to within the ear
endolymph (ĕn′ dō-lĭmf)	**endo-** **-lymph**	within clear fluid, serum	Clear fluid contained within the labyrinth of the ear
equilibrium (ē″ kwĭ-lĭb′ rē-ŭm)			State of balance
fenestration (fĕn″ ĕs-trā′ shŭn)	**fenestrat** **-ion**	window process	Surgical operation in which a new opening is made in the labyrinth of the inner ear to restore hearing
labyrinth (lăb′ ĭ-rĭnth)	**labyrinth**	maze, inner ear	The inner ear; made up of the *vestibule*, *cochlea*, and *semicircular canals*
labyrinthectomy (lăb″ ĭ-rĭn-thĕk′ tō-mē)	**labyrinth** **-ectomy**	maze, inner ear surgical excision	Surgical excision of the labyrinth
labyrinthitis (lăb″ ĭ-rĭn-thī′ tĭs)	**labyrinth** **-itis**	maze, inner ear inflammation	Inflammation of the labyrinth
labyrinthotomy (lăb″ ĭ-rĭn-thŏt′ ō-mē)	**labyrinth/o** **-tomy**	maze, inner ear incision	Incision of the labyrinth

Medical Word	Word Parts		Definition
	Part	**Meaning**	
malleus (măl´ ē-ŭs)			Largest of the three ossicles; also called the *hammer*
mastoiditis (măs˝ toyd-īt´ ĭs)	**mast** **-oid** **-itis**	mastoid process resemble inflammation	Inflammation of one of the mastoid bones; characterized by fever, headache, and malaise
Ménière disease (men-yār´)			An abnormality of the inner ear causing a host of symptoms, including vertigo (sensation of spinning), tinnitus (a ringing or roaring sound in the ears), fluctuating hearing loss, and the sensation of pressure or pain in the affected ear. Symptoms are associated with a change in fluid volume within the labyrinth and can occur suddenly and arise daily or as infrequently as once a year.
monaural (mŏn-awr´ ăl)	**mon(o)-** **aur** **-al**	one ear pertaining to	Pertaining to one ear
myringectomy (mĭr-ĭn-jĕk´ tō-mē)	**myring** **-ectomy**	eardrum, tympanic membrane surgical excision	Surgical excision of the tympanic membrane
myringoplasty (mĭr-ĭn´ gō-plăst˝ ē)	**myring/o** **-plasty**	eardrum, tympanic membrane surgical repair	Surgical repair of the tympanic membrane
myringoscope (mĭr-ĭn´ gō-skōp)	**myring/o** **-scope**	eardrum, tympanic membrane instrument for examining	Medical instrument used to examine the eardrum
myringotome (mĭ-rĭn´ gō-tōm)	**myring/o** **-tome**	eardrum, tympanic membrane instrument to cut	Surgical instrument used for cutting the eardrum
myringotomy (mĭr-ĭn-gŏt´ ō-mē)	**myring/o** **-tomy**	eardrum, tympanic membrane incision	Surgical incision of the tympanic membrane to remove unwanted fluids from the ear

Medical Word	Word Parts		Definition
	Part	Meaning	
otalgia (ō″ tăl′ jē-ă)	ot -algia	ear pain	Pain in the ear, earache
otic (ō′ tĭk)	ot -ic	ear pertaining to	Pertaining to the ear
otitis (ō-tī′ tĭs)	ot -itis	ear inflammation	Inflammation of the ear
otitis media (ō-tī′ tĭs mē′ dē-ă)	ot -itis med -ia	ear inflammation middle condition	Inflammation of the middle ear. Most middle ear infections are a result of an upper respiratory infection (URI) that has spread through the eustachian tube. See Figure 14.8.

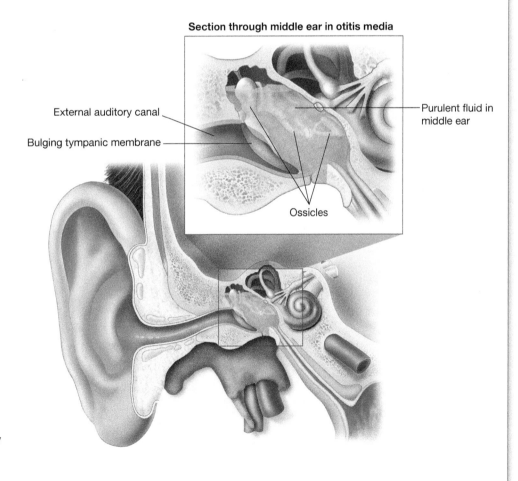

Section through middle ear in otitis media

External auditory canal

Bulging tympanic membrane

Purulent fluid in middle ear

Ossicles

FIGURE 14.8 Otitis media. In acute otitis media, the tympanic membrane is usually bulging and purulent fluid is present in the middle ear.

fyi Otitis media is often difficult to detect in children because most children affected by this disorder do not yet have sufficient speech and language skills to tell others what is bothering them. Common signs of otitis media include:

- Unusual irritability; fussiness; crying
- Difficulty sleeping; night awakening
- Tugging or pulling at one or both ears (Figure 14.9)
- Fever
- Fluid draining from the ear
- Loss of balance
- Unresponsiveness to quiet sounds or other signs of hearing difficulty such as sitting too close to the television or being inattentive

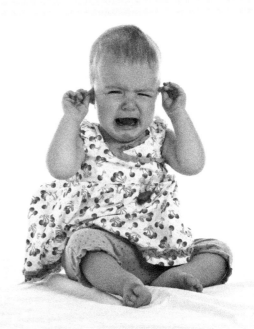

FIGURE 14.9 This young child is crying and pulling on her ears, two important signs of otitis media.
Source: John Wollwerth/Shutterstock

Terminology for Otitis Media	
antrum	Cavity or chamber in a bone
attic	Portion of the middle ear lying above the tympanic cavity proper
atticoantral	Pertaining to the attic and mastoid antrum of the ear
mastoid antrum	Cavity in the mastoid portion of the temporal bone; tympanic antrum
suppurative	Process of pus formation
tubotympanic	Pertaining to the tympanum (middle ear) and the eustachian tube

Medical Word	Word Parts		Definition
	Part	Meaning	
otolaryngologist (ō″ tō-lar″ ĭn-gŏl′ ō-jĭst)	ot/o laryng/o log -ist	ear larynx, voice box study one who specializes	Physician who specializes in the study of the ear and larynx (*voice box*)
otolaryngology (ō″ tō-lar″ ĭn-gŏl′ ō-jē)	ot/o laryng/o -logy	ear larynx, voice box study of	Study of the ear and larynx (*voice box*)
otolith (ō′ tō-lĭth)	ot/o -lith	ear stone	Ear stones
otomycosis (ō″ tō-mī-kō′ sĭs)	ot/o myc -osis	ear fungus condition	Fungal infection of the ear
otoneurology (ō″ tō-nū-rŏl′ ō-jē)	ot/o neur/o -logy	ear nerve study of	Specialized diagnosis and treatment of the ear and its neurological association
otopharyngeal (ō″ tō-fă-rĭn′ jē-āl)	ot/o pharyng -eal	ear pharynx pertaining to	Pertaining to the ear and pharynx
otoplasty (ō′ tō-plăs″ tē)	ot/o -plasty	ear surgical repair	Surgical repair of the ear
otopyorrhea (ō″ tō-pī″ ō-rē′ă)	ot/o py/o -rrhea	ear pus flow	Pus in the ear
otorhinolaryngology (ENT) (ō″ tō-rī″ nō-lăr″ ĭn-gŏl′ ō-jē)	ot/o rhin/o laryng/o -logy	ear nose larynx study of	Study of the ear, nose, and larynx (*voice box*). The medical specialty is often referred to as *ENT* (*ear, nose, throat*); in this case, *throat* is used in a broad sense instead of *larynx*.
otosclerosis (ō″ tō-sklĕ-rō′ sĭs)	ot/o scler -osis	ear hardening condition	Hardening (stiffening) condition of the ear structures characterized by progressive deafness

Medical Word	Word Parts		Definition
	Part	Meaning	
otoscope (ō′ tō-skōp)	ot/o -scope	ear instrument for examining	Medical instrument used to examine the ear. See Figure 14.10. An inspection of the walls of the auditory canal should find no sign of irritation, discharge, or a foreign object. The walls are normally pink and some cerumen is present. The tympanic membrane is usually pearly gray and translucent. It reflects light and the ossicles are visible.

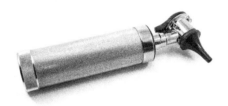

FIGURE 14.10 Otoscope.
Source: Keith Bell/Shutterstock

Medical Word	Word Parts		Definition
perilymph (pĕr′ ĭ-lĭmf)	peri- -lymph	around clear fluid, serum	Serum fluid of the inner ear
presbycusis (prĕz″ bĭ-kū′ sĭs)	presby -cusis	old hearing	Impairment of hearing that occurs with aging
stapedectomy (stā″ pĕ-dĕk′ tō-mē)	staped -ectomy	stapes, stirrup surgical excision	Surgical excision of the stapes in the middle ear to improve hearing, especially in cases of otosclerosis. The stapes is replaced by a prosthesis.
tinnitus (tĭn-ī′ tŭs)			The sensation of ringing or roaring sounds in one or both ears is a symptom associated with damage to the auditory cells in the inner ear. It can also be a symptom of other health problems.
tuning fork			Instrument used medically in a hearing test, which, when struck at the forked end, vibrates, producing a musical tone, and thus can be heard and felt. A metal instrument with a handle and two prongs or tines, tuning forks can be made of steel, aluminum, or magnesium alloy. See Figure 14.11.

FIGURE 14.11 Tuning fork. The vibrations and tone produced when the fork is struck can be used to assess a person's ability to hear various sound frequencies.
Source: Shutswis/123RF

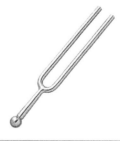

Medical Word	Word Parts		Definition
	Part	**Meaning**	
tympanectomy (tĭm″ păn-ĕk′ tō-mē)	**tympan**	eardrum, tympanic membrane	Surgical excision of the tympanic membrane (eardrum)
	-ectomy	surgical excision	
tympanic (tĭm-păn′ ĭk)	**tympan**	eardrum, tympanic membrane	Pertaining to the eardrum (tympanic membrane)
	-ic	pertaining to	
tympanitis (tĭm-păn-ī′ tĭs)	**tympan**	eardrum, tympanic membrane	Inflammation of the eardrum (tympanic membrane)
	-itis	inflammation	
tympanoplasty (tĭm″ păn-ō-plăs′ tē)	**tympan/o**	eardrum, tympanic membrane	Surgical repair of the tympanic membrane (eardrum)
	-plasty	surgical repair	
vertigo (ver′ tĭ-gō)			Sensation of instability and loss of equilibrium; patients feel like they are spinning in space or objects around them are spinning. Caused by a disturbance in the semicircular canal of the inner ear or the vestibular nuclei of the brainstem.

Study *and* Review II

Word Parts

Prefixes   Give the definitions of the following prefixes.

1. end- _____

2. endo- _____

3. peri- _____

4. bin- _____

5. mon(o)- _____

Combining Forms   Give the definitions of the following combining forms.

1. audi/o _____
2. aur/i _____
3. chol/e _____
4. cochle/o _____
5. electr/o _____
6. labyrinth/o _____
7. laryng/o _____
8. mast/o _____
9. myring/o _____

10. neur/o _____
11. ot/o _____
12. pharyng/o _____
13. presby/o _____
14. py/o _____
15. scler/o _____
16. staped/o _____
17. steat/o _____
18. tympan/o _____

Suffixes   Give the definitions of the following suffixes.

1. -al _____
2. -algia _____
3. -cusis _____
4. -ectomy _____
5. -gram _____
6. -graphy _____
7. -ic _____
8. -ist _____
9. -itis _____
10. -lith _____
11. -logy _____
12. -lymph _____
13. -meter _____

14. -oid _____
15. -oma _____
16. -osis _____
17. -plasty _____
18. -rrhea _____
19. -scope _____
20. -tome _____
21. -tomy _____
22. -y _____
23. -cle _____
24. -ion _____
25. -ia _____

Identifying Medical Terms

In the spaces provided, write the medical terms for the following meanings.

1. _____ One who specializes in diagnosing disorders of hearing

2. _____ Measurement of the hearing sense

3. _____ Pertaining to the sense of hearing

4. _____ Pertaining to within the ear

5. _____ Inflammation of the labyrinth

6. _____ Surgical repair of the tympanic membrane

7. _____ Surgical instrument used for cutting the eardrum

8. _____ Pain in the ear, earache

9. _____ Study of the ear and larynx

10. _____ Pertaining to the ear and pharynx

Matching   Select the appropriate lettered meaning for each of the following words.

_____   1. auricle   a. State of balance

_____   2. binaural   b. Inner ear

_____   3. acoustic   c. Surgical repair of the ear

_____   4. equilibrium   d. Surgical repair of the tympanic membrane

_____   5. fenestration   e. Pertaining to both ears

_____   6. labyrinth   f. Sensation of instability, loss of equilibrium

_____   7. myringotomy   g. Surgical operation in which a new opening is made in the labyrinth

_____   8. otoplasty   h. External portion of the ear

_____   9. tympanoplasty   i. Pertaining to the sense of hearing

_____   10. vertigo   j. Surgical incision of the tympanic membrane

Medical Case Snapshots

This learning activity provides an opportunity to relate the medical terminology you are learning to sample patient case presentations. In the spaces provided, write in your answers.

Case 1

The mother of a 2-year-old baby states that Takeshia has been unusually fussy for 2 days and that last night "she woke me up screaming and she felt so hot." Upon examination of the left ear the physician noted a bulging of the tympanic membrane and the presence of purulent fluid in the middle ear. In the space provided, write the medical term for this condition _____ _____.

Case 2

A 15-year-old male is seen by an otolaryngologist. He complains of ringing in the ears and is diagnosed with _____. When questioned, he admits to listening to loud music with headphones and that he likes going to rock concerts. Excessive noise can do permanent damage to the sensory receptors of the _____ _____ _____.

Case 3

The 15-year-old male was referred to a(n) _____, who specializes in diagnosing disorders of hearing. Using a(n) _____ (which is a medical instrument used to measure hearing), both ears were tested, one at a time. The patient was diagnosed with a partial loss of the ability to hear in the left ear. Loss of hearing is known as _____.

Drug Highlights

Classification of Drug	Description and Examples
analgesics	Used to relieve pain without causing loss of consciousness. EXAMPLES: Tylenol (acetaminophen), Advil/Motrin (ibuprofen), and aspirin
antipyretics	Agents that reduce fever. EXAMPLES: Tylenol (acetaminophen), aspirin Note: In children, aspirin should not be used as an analgesic or antipyretic because of the risk of Reye syndrome.
antibiotics	Used to treat infectious diseases; can be natural or synthetic substances that inhibit the growth of or destroy microorganisms, especially bacteria

Classification of Drug	Description and Examples
penicillins	Act by interfering with bacterial cell wall synthesis among newly formed bacterial cells. Penicillins are contraindicated in patients who are known to be allergic or hypersensitive to any of its varieties or to any of the cephalosporins. EXAMPLES: penicillin G, ampicillin, penicillin V, piperacillin, and amoxicillin
cephalosporins	Chemically and pharmacologically related to the penicillins, they act by inhibiting bacterial cell wall synthesis, thereby promoting the death of the developing microorganisms. Hypersensitivity to cephalosporins and/or penicillins can result in an allergic reaction. EXAMPLES: cefazolin sodium, cefaclor, Keflex (cephalexin), and Suprax (cefixime)
tetracyclines	Primarily bacteriostatic and active against a wide range of gram-negative and gram-positive microorganisms, they inhibit protein synthesis in the bacterial cell Note: Contraindicated in children 8 years of age and younger; they cause permanent discoloration of tooth enamel. EXAMPLES: tetracycline hydrochloride, demeclocycline HCl, and Doryx/Vibramycin (doxycycline)
erythromycins	Work by inhibiting protein synthesis in susceptible bacteria. These drugs can be used for patients who are allergic to penicillin. EXAMPLES: Ery-TabB, E.E.S., EryPed, and Erythrocin
drugs used to treat vertigo	Vertigo is a sensation of movement, when the person is not moving, that can be caused by a lesion or other process affecting the brain, the eighth cranial nerve, or the labyrinthine system of the ear. Drugs used for vertigo include anticholinergics, antihistamines, and antidopamines. EXAMPLES: dimenhydrinate, Benadryl (diphenhydramine HCl), meclizine HCl, and Transderm Scop (scopolamine)

Diagnostic *and* Laboratory Tests

Test	Description
auditory-evoked response (aw′dĭ-tō-rē-ĕ-vōkd′)	Response to auditory stimuli (sound) that can be measured independently of the patient's subjective response. Use of an electroencephalograph can determine the intensity of sound and presence of response. This test is useful to test the hearing of children who are too young for standard tests, autistic, hyperkinetic, and/or developmentally disabled.
electronystagmography (ENG) (ĕ-lĕk″trō-nĭs-tăg-mŏg′ră-fē)	Recording eye movement in response to specific stimuli, such as sound; used to determine the presence and location of a lesion in the vestibule of the ear, to help diagnose unilateral hearing loss of unknown origin, and to help identify the cause of vertigo, tinnitus, and dizziness

Test	Description
pure tone audiometry	Method of testing pure tones by providing calibrated tones to a person via earphones, allowing that person to increase the sound level until it can just be heard. See Figure 14.12. Various strategies are used, but pure tone audiometry with tones starting at about 125 Hz (cycles/second) and increasing by octaves, half-octaves, or third-octaves to about 8000 Hz is typical. Hearing tests of right and left ears are generally done independently. The results of such tests are summarized in audiograms. Audiograms compare hearing to the normal threshold of hearing, which varies with frequency, as illustrated by the hearing curves. The audiogram is normalized to the hearing curve so that a straight horizontal line at 0 represents normal hearing.

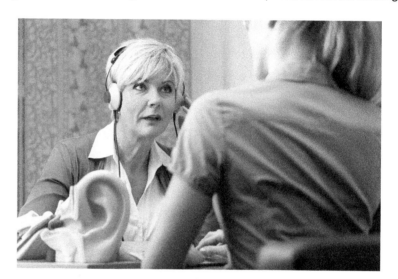

FIGURE 14.12 Woman undergoing pure tone audiometry testing.
Source: Kzenon/Shutterstock

Test	Description
otoscopy (ō-tŏs´ kō-pē)	Visual examination of the external auditory canal and the tympanic membrane via an otoscope. Pneumatic otoscopy uses a special attachment on the otoscope. This allows the examiner to direct a light stream of air toward the eardrum. The directed air current should then cause the tympanic membrane to vibrate. With dysfunction there is little or no vibration noted. See Figure 14.13.

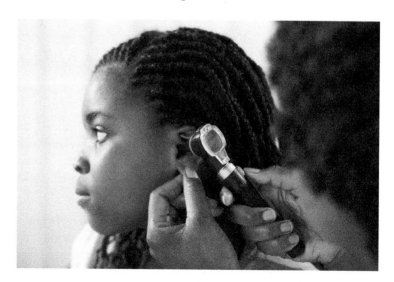

FIGURE 14.13 Otoscopy. Doctor using an otoscope to check a young girl's ear.
Source: Andrey_Popov/Shutterstock

Test	Description

 When examining the tympanic membrane with an otoscope, the position, mobility, color, and degree of translucency are evaluated and described. The normal tympanic membrane is in the neutral position (neither retracted nor bulging), pearly gray, translucent, and responds briskly to positive and negative pressure, indicating an air-filled space. An abnormal tympanic membrane can be retracted or bulging and immobile or poorly mobile in pneumatic **otoscopy**. The position of the tympanic membrane is a key for differentiating acute otitis media (AOM) and otitis media with effusion. In acute otitis media, the tympanic membrane is usually bulging and purulent fluid is present in the middle ear (refer to Figure 14.8).

tuning fork test	Method of testing hearing by the use of a tuning fork (refer to Figure 14.11). Two types of hearing loss (conductive and perceptive) can be distinguished through the use of this test. Tuning forks are used in several types of tests: the Rinne, Weber, Bing, and Schwabach tests. See Figure 14.14.

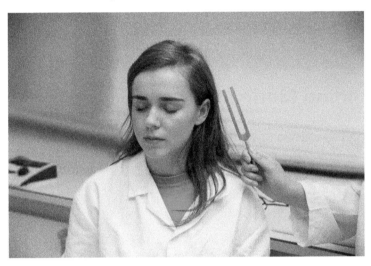

FIGURE 14.14 University student undergoing tuning fork test in audiology laboratory.
Source: Wavebreakmedia/Shutterstock

Rinne test (rĭn´ nē)	The Rinne test utilizes a tuning fork to compare bone conduction (BC) hearing with air conduction (AC). After being struck, the vibrating tuning fork is held on the mastoid process until sound is no longer heard. The fork is then immediately placed just outside the ear. Normally, the sound is audible at the ear.
tympanometry (tĭm˝ pă-nŏm´ ĕ-trē)	Measurement of the movement of the tympanic membrane and pressure in the middle ear. It is used for detecting middle ear disorders.

Abbreviations *and* Acronyms

Abbreviation/Acronym	Meaning	Abbreviation/Acronym	Meaning
AC	air conduction	HD	hearing distance
AOM	acute otitis media	Hz	cycles/second
BC	bone conduction	OM	otitis media
db, dB	decibel	TM	tympanic membrane
ENG	electronystagmography	URI	upper respiratory infection
ENT	ear, nose, throat (otorhinolaryngology)		

Study *and* Review III

Building Medical Terms

Using the following word parts, fill in the blanks to build the correct medical terms.

aur	ot/o	tympan/o	-lymph
myring/o	staped	-ic	-itis

Definition	Medical Term
1. Pertaining to the sense of hearing	acoust_____
2. Pertaining to the ear	_____al
3. Clear fluid contained within the labyrinth of the ear	endo_____
4. Surgical instrument used for cutting the eardrum	_____tome
5. Inflammation of the ear	ot_____
6. Surgical repair of the ear	_____plasty
7. Serum fluid of the inner ear	peri_____
8. Surgical excision of the stapes in the middle ear	_____ectomy
9. Pertaining to the eardrum (tympanic membrane)	tympan_____
10. Surgical repair of the tympanic membrane (eardrum)	_____plasty

Combining Form Challenge

Using the combining forms provided, write the medical term correctly.

audi/o   labyrinth/o   ot/o
aur/i   myring/o   presby/o

1. Medical instrument used to measure hearing: _____meter

2. External portion of the ear; known as the pinna: _____cle

3. Surgical excision of the labyrinth: _____ectomy

4. Surgical repair of the tympanic membrane: _____plasty

5. Pain in the ear; earache: _____algia

6. Impairment of hearing that occurs with aging: _____cusis

Select the Right Term

Select the correct answer, and write it on the line provided.

1. Record of hearing by audiometry is _____.

    acoustic   audiology   audiogram   aural

2. A state of balance is _____.

    cochlea   equilibrium   tinnitus   eustachian

3. Surgical operation in which a new opening is made in the labyrinth of the inner ear to restore hearing is _____.

    labyrinthotomy   myringectomy   fenestration   stapedectomy

4. Largest of the three ossicles, also called the hammer, is _____.

    incus   stapes   labyrinth   malleus

5. The sensation of ringing or roaring sounds in one or both ears is _____.

    tinnitus   tympanitis   presbycusis   vertigo

6. Pertaining to one ear is _____.

    endaural   aural   monaural   binaural

Drug Highlights

Match the appropriate lettered description or examples of drug(s) with the class of drug.

_____ 1. analgesics

_____ 2. penicillins

_____ 3. anticholinergics, antihistamines, antidopamines

_____ 4. erythromycins

_____ 5. tetracyclines

_____ 6. antipyretics

_____ 7. cephalosporins

_____ 8. antibiotics

a. Agents that reduce fever

b. Work by inhibiting protein synthesis in susceptible bacteria

c. Used to treat infectious diseases

d. Act by interfering with bacterial cell wall synthesis among newly formed bacterial cells

e. Related to the penicillins, they promote the death of developing microorganisms

f. Used to treat vertigo

g. Cause permanent discoloration of tooth enamel in children 8 years of age and younger

h. Used to relieve pain without causing loss of consciousness

Diagnostic and Laboratory Tests

Select the best answer to each multiple-choice question. Circle the letter of your choice.

1. The response to auditory stimuli that can be measured independent of the patient's subjective response.

   a. auditory-evoked response
   b. electronystagmography
   c. tuning fork test
   d. otoscopy

2. Recording of eye movement in response to specific stimuli.

   a. auditory-evoked response
   b. electronystagmography
   c. tympanometry
   d. otoscopy

3. Visual examination of the external auditory canal and the tympanic membrane.

   a. tuning fork test
   b. tympanometry
   c. electronystagmography
   d. otoscopy

4. Measurement of the movement of the tympanic membrane.

    a. tuning fork tests

    b. tympanometry

    c. otoscopy

    d. electronystagmography

5. This test utilizes a tuning fork to compare bone conduction (BC) hearing with air conduction (AC).

    a. Rinne test

    b. tympanometry

    c. otoscopy

    d. electronystagmography

Abbreviations and Acronyms

Write the correct word, phrase, or abbreviation/acronym in the space provided.

1. air conduction _____

2. bone conduction _____

3. db, Db _____

4. electronystagmography _____

5. ENT _____

6. hearing distance _____

7. otitis media _____

Practical Application

Medical Record Analysis

This exercise contains information, abbreviations/acronyms, and medical terminology from an actual medical record or case study that has been adapted for this text. The names and any personal information have been created by the author. Read and study each form or case study and then answer the questions that follow. You may refer to Appendix III, *Abbreviations, Acronyms, and Symbols*.

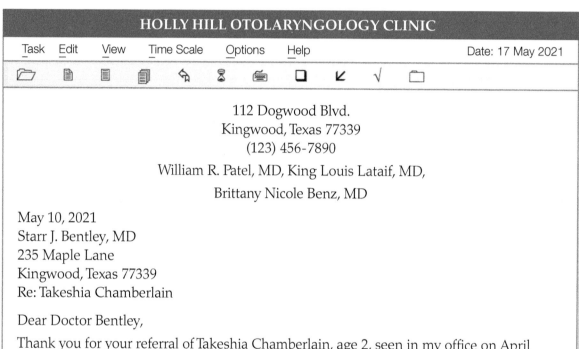

HOLLY HILL OTOLARYNGOLOGY CLINIC

| Task | Edit | View | Time Scale | Options | Help | | Date: 17 May 2021 |

112 Dogwood Blvd.
Kingwood, Texas 77339
(123) 456-7890

William R. Patel, MD, King Louis Lataif, MD,

Brittany Nicole Benz, MD

May 10, 2021
Starr J. Bentley, MD
235 Maple Lane
Kingwood, Texas 77339
Re: Takeshia Chamberlain

Dear Doctor Bentley,

Thank you for your referral of Takeshia Chamberlain, age 2, seen in my office on April 25, 2021. When seen, Takeshia had a fever of 102.2°F, with noted dark circles under both eyes and appeared to be in moderate pain. Child was pulling on her left ear and upon examination left TM red, dull, and bulging diffuse light reflex with loss of landmark. Pneumatic otoscopy revealed immobile left TM. Right TM pearly gray, landmarks intact. Nasal mucosa dark red and swollen, with moderate amount of discharge. Oral mucosa erythematous with yellow-white exudates, no lesions. Uvula rises in midline with phonation. Gag reflex present. No lymphadenopathy. Neck supple. Lungs CTA and heart normal rate and rhythm. No murmurs. Skin: no rashes or lesions, warm to the touch.

A diagnosis of acute otitis media (AOM) left ear was confirmed.

I ordered acetaminophen (Tylenol) liquid, 1.6 mL (1 teaspoon) PO every 4 hours prn for pain and fever. Amoxicillin (Amoxil) suspension 40 mg per kg per day, in three divided doses, every 8 hours for 10 days for infection. Instructed the mother on the adverse reactions to penicillin and explained that she should not give the antibiotic with soft drinks or fruit juices because the acid in these products could destroy the effectiveness of the drug. Stressed the importance of the baby taking the antibiotic as ordered for the entire 10 days and around the clock, every 8 hours. Instructed the mother to bring the baby back to the clinic if symptoms do not improve in 48–72 hours. Scheduled a follow-up visit for 3 weeks.

Best regards,

William R. Patel, MD

Medical Record Questions

Write the correct answer in the space provided.

1. In Takeshia the signs and symptoms of acute otitis media included a fever of _____ and the child was _____ on her left ear.

2. The diagnosis was determined by a visual examination of the ear called pneumatic _____, a physical examination of the child, and the signs and symptoms presented.

3. Acetaminophen (Tylenol) is classified as a(n) _____ and is given to relieve _____ and reduce _____.

4. Amoxicillin (Amoxil) is a(n) _____ and is given for _____.

5. The _____ in soft drinks and fruit juices can destroy the effectiveness of the _____ drug.

MyLab Medical Terminology™

MyLab Medical Terminology is a premium online homework management system that includes a host of features to help you study. Registered users will find:

- A multitude of quizzes and activities built within the MyLab platform
- Powerful tools that track and analyze your results—allowing you to create a personalized learning experience
- Videos and audio pronunciations to help enrich your progress
- Streaming lesson presentations (guided lectures) and self-paced learning modules
- A space where you and your instructor can check your progress and manage your assignments

15 Special Senses: The Eye

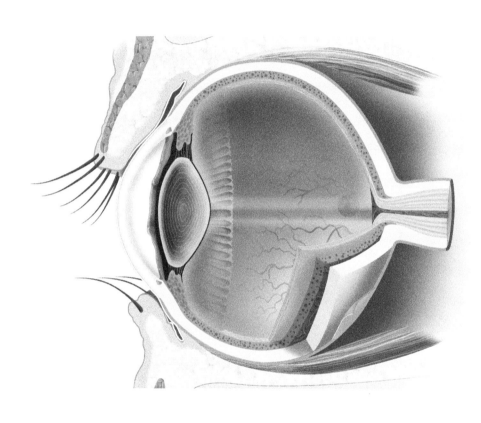

 Learning Outcomes

On completion of this chapter, you will be able to:

1. State the description and primary functions of the eye and its anatomical structures.
2. Analyze, build, spell, and pronounce medical words.
3. Classify the drugs highlighted in this chapter.
4. Describe diagnostic and laboratory tests related to the eye.
5. Identify and define selected abbreviations and acronyms.

Anatomy and Physiology

The **eye** is composed of special anatomical structures that work together to facilitate sight. Light passes through the cornea, pupil, lens, and the vitreous body to stimulate sensory receptors (*rods* and *cones*) in the **retina** or innermost layer of the eye. **Vision** is made possible through the coordinated actions of nerves that control the movement of the eyeball, the amount of light admitted by the pupil, the focusing of that light on the retina by the lens, and the transmission of the resulting sensory impulses to the brain by the optic nerve. The brain permits the perception of vision. Table 15.1 provides an at-a-glance look at the eye. Figure 15.1 shows the internal structures of the eye.

TABLE 15.1	Special Senses: The Eye at-a-Glance
Organ/Structure	**Primary Functions/Description**
Orbit	Contains the eyeball; cavity is lined with fatty tissue that cushions the eyeball and has several openings through which blood vessels and nerves pass
Muscles of the eye	Six short muscles provide support and rotary movement of the eyeball
Eyelids	Protect the eyeballs from intense light, foreign particles, and impact; permits the eye to remain moist
Conjunctiva	Acts as a protective covering for the exposed surface of the eyeball and helps keep the eyelid and eyeball moist
Lacrimal apparatus	Produces, stores, and removes tears that cleanse and lubricate the eye
Eyeball	Organ of vision
Sclera	Outer layer of the eyeball composed of fibrous connective tissue; at the front of the eye, it is visible as the white of the eye and ends at the cornea
Cornea	Transparent anterior portion of the eyeball, which bends light rays and helps to focus them on the surface of the retina
Choroid	Pigmented vascular membrane that prevents internal reflection of light
Ciliary body	Smooth muscle that forms a part of the ciliary body that governs the convexity of the lens; secretes nutrient fluids that nourish the cornea, the lens, and surrounding tissues
Iris	Colored membrane attached to the ciliary body (can appear as blue, brown, green, hazel, or gray) with a circular opening in its center, the pupil, and two muscles that contract; regulates the amount of light admitted by the pupil
Retina	Innermost layer with photoreceptive cells; translates light waves focused on its surface into nerve impulses
Lens	Sharpens the focus of light on the retina (accommodation [Acc])

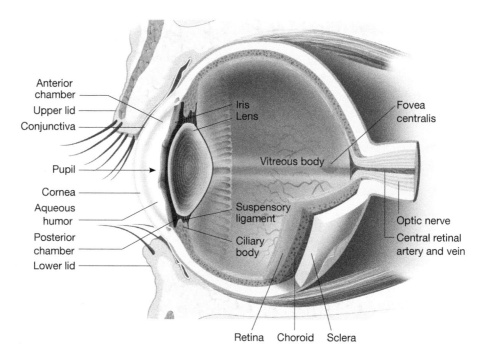

FIGURE 15.1 Structures of the eye.

External Structures of the Eye

The orbit, the muscles of the eye, the eyelids, the conjunctiva, and the lacrimal apparatus make up the external structures of the eye.

Orbit

The **orbit** is a cone-shaped cavity in the front of the skull that contains the *eyeball*. Formed by the combination of several bones, this cavity is lined with fatty tissue that cushions the eyeball and has several **foramina** (openings) through which blood vessels and nerves pass. The **optic foramen** is the short canal through the lesser wing of the sphenoid bone at the apex of the orbit that gives passage to the optic nerve and the ophthalmic artery.

Muscles of the Eye

Six eye muscles control movement of the eye, allowing it to follow a moving object and move precisely. Of the six, four are rectus muscles and two are oblique muscles. *Rectus muscles* allow a person to see up, down, right, and left. *Oblique muscles* allow the eyes to turn to see upper left and upper right, lower left and lower right. See Figure 15.2. The eye muscles also help maintain the shape of the eyeball.

Eyelids

Each eye has a pair of **eyelids** that are continuous with the skin, cover the eyeball, and protect it from intense light, foreign particles, and impact. Through their blinking motion, eyelids keep the eyeball's surface lubricated and free from dust and debris. Known as the *superior* and *inferior palpebrae*, those movable "curtains" join to form a **canthus** or angle at either corner of the eye. The slit between the eyelids is called the **palpebral fissure** through which light reaches the inner eye.

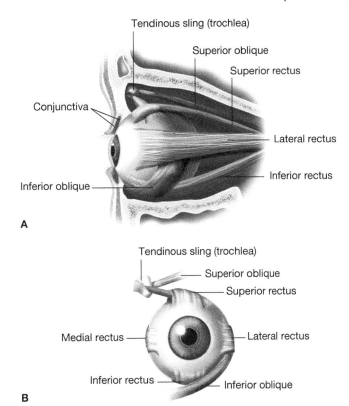

FIGURE 15.2 Eye muscles. **A** Lateral view, left eye. **B** Anterior view, left eye.

The edges of the eyelids contain eyelashes that help protect the eyeball by preventing foreign matter, such as insects, smoke, dust, or dirt particles, from coming into contact with the eyeball. Along the inner margin of the thin skin of the lid, *meibomian glands* secrete sebum, an oily substance that coats the surface of the eyes and keeps the water component of tears from evaporating (drying out). Together, the water and the oil layer make up the tear film.

A condition in which the glands are not secreting enough oil or the oil they secrete is of poor quality is called *meibomian gland dysfunction (MGD)*. MGD can cause or exacerbate dry eye symptoms and eyelid inflammation. The oil glands become blocked with thickened secretions and chronically clogged glands eventually become unable to secrete any oil, which results in permanent changes in the tear film and dry eyes. Symptoms include dryness, burning, itching, stickiness, watering, light sensitivity, red eyes, intermittent blurry vision, and chalazions (styes). Treatment usually includes warm compresses to the involved area.

Conjunctiva

Lining the underside of each eyelid and reflected onto the anterior portion of the eyeball is a mucous membrane known as the **conjunctiva**. This membrane acts as a protective covering for the exposed surface of the eyeball.

Lacrimal Apparatus

Included in the **lacrimal apparatus** are those structures that produce, store, and remove the tears that cleanse and lubricate the eye. These structures are the lacrimal gland, located in the outer corner of each eyelid, lacrimal canaliculi (ducts), the lacrimal sac, and the nasolacrimal duct, which empties into the nasal cavity. See Figure 15.3.

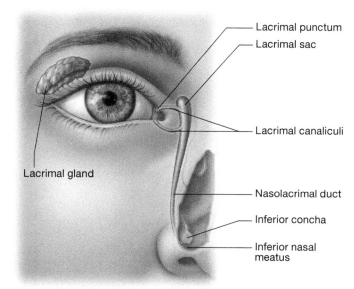

FIGURE 15.3 Lacrimal glands and lacrimal canaliculi (ducts).
Source: AMERMAN, ERIN C., HUMAN ANATOMY & PHYSIOLOGY, 2nd Ed., ©2019. Reprinted and Electronically reproduced by permission of Pearson Education, Inc., New York, NY.

Anterior view

LACRIMAL GLAND

Located above the outer corner of the eye, the lacrimal gland secretes tears through approximately 12 ducts onto the surface of the conjunctiva of the upper lid. This fluid washes across the anterior surface of the eye and is collected by the *lacrimal canaliculi* (ducts).

LACRIMAL CANALICULI

The lacrimal canaliculi are the two ducts at the inner corner of the eye that collect tears and drain into the lacrimal sac.

LACRIMAL SAC

The enlargement of the upper portion of the lacrimal duct is known as the lacrimal sac. Tears secreted by the lacrimal glands are pulled into this sac and subsequently forced into the nasolacrimal duct by the blinking action of the eyelids. The sac is dilated and pulls in fluid as the muscles associated with blinking close the lids. The sac constricts, forcing the fluid down the nasolacrimal duct as the lids are opened.

NASOLACRIMAL DUCT

The passageway draining lacrimal fluid into the nose is known as the nasolacrimal duct. The lacrimal sac is the enlarged upper portion of this duct.

The eyes begin to develop as an outgrowth of the forebrain in the 4-week-old embryo. At 24 weeks, the eyes are structurally complete. At 28 weeks, eyebrows and eyelashes are present, and the eyelids open. The newborn can see, and **visual acuity (VA)** is estimated to be around 20/400. Most newborns appear to have crossed eyes because their eye muscles are not fully developed. At first, the eyes appear to be blue or gray. Permanent coloring becomes fixed between 6 and 12 months of age. Tears do not appear until approximately 1–3 months because the lacrimal gland ducts are immature. Depth perception begins to develop around 9 months of age. Visual acuity testing is recommended for all children starting at 3 years of age. Children are farsighted until about 5 years of age.

Internal Structures of the Eye

The eyeball, its various structures, and the nerve fibers connecting it to the brain make up the internal eye (refer to Figure 15.1).

Eyeball

The **eyeball** is the organ of vision. It is globe shaped and has three layers. The eyeball contains two cavities: the **anterior cavity** and the **posterior cavity**. The anterior cavity is filled with a watery fluid known as the **aqueous humor**. Behind the lens of the eye is a much larger posterior cavity filled with a jelly-like material, the **vitreous**, which maintains the eyeball's spherical shape. The three layers forming the outer, middle, and inner surfaces of the eyeball as well as the lens and its functions are discussed in the following sections.

OUTER LAYER

The eyeball's outer layer is composed of the sclera or white of the eye and the cornea or transparent anterior portion of the eye's fibrous outer surface. The curved surface of the cornea is important because it bends light rays and helps to focus them on the surface of the retina.

MIDDLE LAYER

Known as the uvea, the middle layer of the eyeball, lying just below the sclera, consists of the iris, the ciliary body, and the choroid.

The **iris** is a colored membrane attached to the ciliary body and suspended between the lens and the cornea in the aqueous humor. It has a circular opening in its center—the **pupil**—and two muscles that contract or dilate to regulate the amount of light admitted by the pupil.

The **ciliary body** is a circular structure that is an extension of the iris. The ciliary body secretes nutrient fluids (the *aqueous humor*) that nourish the cornea, the lens, and the surrounding tissues. It also contains the ciliary muscle, which changes the shape of the lens when the eyes focus on a near object. This process is called accommodation (see further discussion in the Lens section that follows).

The **choroid** is a pigmented vascular layer of the eyeball that prevents internal reflection of light. It is located between the retina and the sclera.

INNER LAYER

The innermost layer of the eye, or retina, is richly supplied with blood vessels and contains photoreceptive cells that translate light waves focused on its surface into nerve impulses. See Figure 15.4.

The photoreceptor cells of the retina are the **rods** and **cones**. Rods are sensitive to dim light and are used for night vision. Cones are sensitive to bright light and color vision. Most of the approximately 6 million cone cells are grouped into a small area called the **macula lutea**. In the center of the macula lutea is a small depression, the **fovea centralis**, which is the central focusing point within the eye; it contains only cone cells. The eye contains approximately 120 million rods that are sensitive to dim light. They contain **rhodopsin**, a pigment necessary for night vision.

The point at which nerve fibers from the retina converge to form the optic nerve is known as the **optic disk**. At the optic disk, fibers of the optic nerve extend to the thalamus and on to the visual cortical areas of the brain. The absence of rods and cones

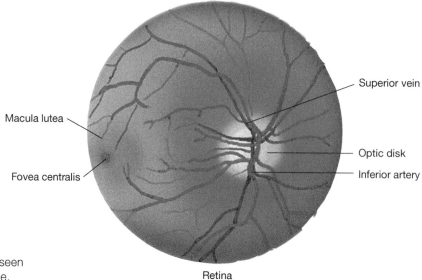

FIGURE 15.4 Retina as seen through an ophthalmoscope.

in the area of the optic disk creates a *blind spot* on the surface of the retina, located about 3 millimeters to the nasal side of the macula. It is the only part of the retina that is insensitive to light.

LENS

A colorless crystalline body biconvex in shape and enclosed in a transparent capsule, the lens is suspended by ligaments just behind the iris. Contraction and relaxation of the ciliary muscle control the tension of the suspensory ligaments to change the shape of the lens. The function of the lens is to sharpen the focus of light on the retina. This process, called *accommodation (Acc)*, is reflexive in nature and combines changes in the size of the pupil, the curvature of the lens, and the convergence of the optic axes to keep the image in the same place on both retinae. Accommodation occurs for both near and distant vision.

How Sight Occurs

Refraction is the bending of light as it passes through one object to another. Vision occurs when light rays are bent (refracted) as they pass through the cornea and the lens. The light is then focused on the retina. The retina converts the light rays into messages that are sent through the optic nerve to the brain. The brain interprets these messages into the images we see. See Figures 15.5 and 15.6.

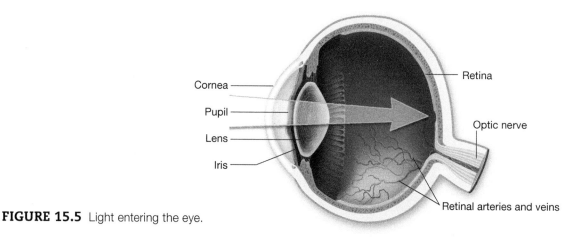

FIGURE 15.5 Light entering the eye.

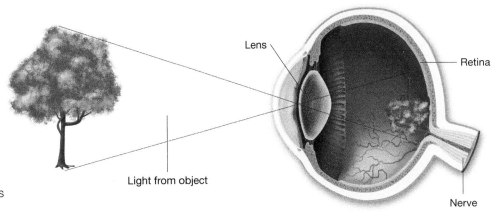

FIGURE 15.6 In normal vision, the lens focuses the inverted visual image on the retina. The brain rights the image.

The most common vision problems are refractive errors, more commonly known as *nearsightedness, farsightedness, astigmatism,* and *presbyopia.* Refractive errors occur when the shape of the eye prevents light from focusing directly on the retina. The length of the eyeball (either longer or shorter), changes in the shape of the cornea, or aging of the lens can cause refractive errors.

Study *and* Review I

Anatomy and Physiology

Write your answers to the following questions.

1. The external structures of the eye are the _____, _____, _____, _____, and _____.

2. The orbit is lined with _____, which cushions the eyeball.

3. The optic foramen is an opening for the _____ and _____.

4. State the functions of the muscles of the eye.

   a. _____

   b. _____

5. Each eye has a pair of eyelids that function to protect the eyeball from _____, _____, and _____.

6. Describe the conjunctiva and state its function. _____

7. Define *lacrimal apparatus.* _____

8. The internal structures of the eye are the _____, _____, and
_____.

9. The eyeball is the organ of _____.

10. The point at which nerve fibers from the retina converge to form the optic nerve is known as the
_____.

11. Define *accommodation*. _____

12. Match the following terms and definitions by placing the correct letter on the line provided.

_____	**1.** aqueous humor	**a.**	White of the eye
_____	**2.** vitreous humor	**b.**	Colored membrane attached to the ciliary body
_____	**3.** iris	**c.**	Watery fluid
_____	**4.** sclera	**d.**	Opening in the center of the iris
_____	**5.** uvea	**e.**	Jelly-like material
_____	**6.** pupil	**f.**	Middle layer of the eyeball
_____	**7.** retina	**g.**	Transparent anterior portion of the eyeball
_____	**8.** rods and cones	**h.**	Innermost layer of the eyeball
_____	**9.** lens	**i.**	Photoreceptor cells
_____	**10.** cornea	**j.**	Colorless crystalline body

▶ **ANATOMY LABELING**   Identify the structures shown below by filling in the blanks.

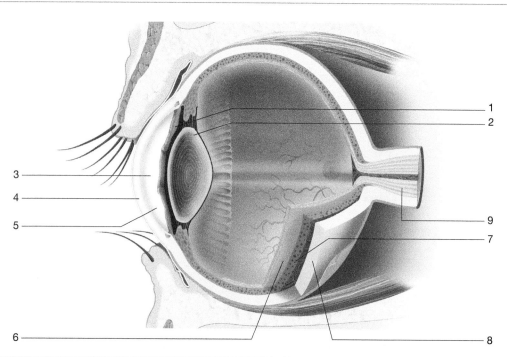

Building Your Medical Vocabulary

This section provides the foundation for learning medical terminology. Review the alphabetized list of medical terms in the following pages. Note how common prefixes and suffixes are repeatedly applied to word roots and combining forms to create different meanings. A combining form is a word root plus a vowel. The chart below lists the combining forms and word roots used in this chapter and can help to strengthen your understanding of how medical words are built and spelled.

You will find that some terms have not been divided into word parts. These are common words or specialized terms that are included to enhance your medical vocabulary.

Combining Forms

ambly/o	dull	mi/o	less, small
anis/o	unequal	ocul/o	eye
blephar/o	eyelid	ophthalm/o	eye
choroid/o	choroid	opt/o	eye
conjunctiv/o	to join together, conjunctiva	orth/o	straight
cor/o	pupil	phac/o	lens
corne/o	cornea	phak/o	lens
cry/o	cold	phot/o	light
cycl/o	ciliary body	presby/o	old
dacry/o	tear, lacrimal duct, tear duct	pupill/o	pupil
dipl/o	double	retin/o	retina
electr/o	electricity	scler/o	sclera, hardening
fibr/o	fiber	stigmat/o	point
foc/o	focus	surg/o	surgery
goni/o	angle	ton/o	tone, tension
irid/o	iris	trich/o	hair
kerat/o	cornea	trop/o	turn
lacrim/o	tear, lacrimal duct, tear duct	uve/o	uvea
lent/o	lens	xen/o	foreign material
metr/o	measure	xer/o	dry

Word Roots

coagulat	to clot	mydriat	dilate, widen
emulsificat	disintegrate	nyctal	night
enucleat	to remove the kernel of	strabism	squinting
log	study		

Medical Word	Word Parts		Definition
	Part	Meaning	
accommodation (Acc) (ă -kŏm″ ō-dā′ shŭn)			Process by which the eyes make adjustments to see objects at various distances
amblyopia (ăm″ blē-ō′ pē-ă)	**ambly** **-opia**	dull vision	Dullness of vision; reduced or dimness of vision; also called *lazy eye*

 fyi The use of dichoptic therapy (simultaneous training of both eyes), which presents different images to each eye separately, using popular children's movies, has produced improved visual acuity in young children. Dichoptic techniques combined with perceptual-learning tasks or certain video games have been shown to improve visual acuity significantly in people with amblyopia.

Medical Word	Word Parts		Definition
anisocoria (ăn-ī″ sō-kōr′ ē-ă)	**anis/o** **cor** **-ia**	unequal pupil condition	Condition in which the pupils are unequal in size
aphakia (ă-fā′ kē-ă)	**a-** **phak** **-ia**	lack of, without lens condition	Condition in which the crystalline lens is absent
astigmatism (ă-stĭg′ mă-tĭzm)	**a-** **stigmat** **-ism**	lack of, without point condition	Defect in the refractive powers of the eye in which a ray of light is not focused on the retina but is spread over an area. It is due to a misshapen curvature of the cornea and lens.
bifocal (bī-fō′ kăl)	**bi-** **foc** **-al**	two focus pertaining to	Pertaining to having two foci, as in bifocal glasses; one focus for near vision and another for far vision
blepharitis (blĕf″ ăr-ī′ tĭs)	**blephar** **-itis**	eyelid inflammation	Inflammation of the hair follicles and glands along the edges of the eyelids
blepharoplasty (blĕf′ ă-rō-plăs″ tē)	**blephar/o** **-plasty**	eyelid surgical repair	Surgical repair of the eyelid or eyelids. One of the most commonly performed facial cosmetic procedures for conditions such as tired-looking eyes, excess skin, droopy eyelids, or circles around the eyes. It can also be combined with other facial and skin rejuvenation procedures such as brow or mid-face lift and laser or chemical skin resurfacing.

Medical Word	Word Parts		Definition
	Part	Meaning	
blepharoptosis (blĕf″ ă-rŏp-tō´ sĭs)	blephar/o -ptosis	eyelid prolapse, drooping	Drooping of the upper eyelid(s)
cataract (kat´ ă-rakt´)			Opacity of the crystalline lens or its capsule; most often occurs in older adults. See Figure 15.7. The most common symptoms of a cataract are cloudy or blurry vision; problems with light, including headlights that seem too bright at night, glare from lamps or very bright sunlight, and seeing a halo around lights; colors that seem faded; poor night vision; double or multiple vision; and frequent need for changes in eyeglass or contact lens prescription. Surgery is the only effective treatment for a cataract. See *phacoemulsification*.

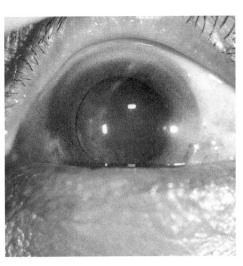

FIGURE 15.7 Cataract of the right eye.
Source: ARZTSAMUI/Shutterstock

chalazion (kă-lā´ zē-ŏn)			Small, hard, painless cyst of a sebaceous gland of the eyelids
choroiditis (kōr″ oy-dīt´ ĭs)	choroid -itis	choroid inflammation	Inflammation of the vascular coat of the eye

Medical Word	Word Parts		Definition
	Part	Meaning	
conjunctivitis (kŏn-junk″ tĭ-vī′ tĭs)	conjunctiv -itis	to join together, conjunctiva inflammation	Inflammation of the conjunctiva that can be caused by allergens, irritating substances (shampoo, dirt, smoke, pool chlorine), bacteria, viruses, or sexually transmitted infections (STIs). The type called *pinkeye* is usually infectious and contagious. See Figure 15.8.

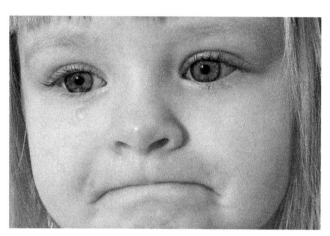

FIGURE 15.8 Child with conjunctivitis (pinkeye).
Source: Steve Snowden/Shutterstock

 fyi Symptoms of conjunctivitis include:

- Redness in the white of the eye or inner eyelid
- Increased amount of tears
- Thick yellow discharge that crusts over the eyelashes, especially after sleep (with conjunctivitis caused by bacteria)
- Other discharge from the eye (green or white)
- Itchy eyes (especially with conjunctivitis caused by allergies)
- Burning eyes (especially with conjunctivitis caused by chemicals and irritants)
- Blurred vision
- Increased sensitivity to light

Treatment is based on the cause. For example, antibiotic eyedrops or ointments are used for conjunctivitis caused by a bacterial infection. If topical antibiotics do not solve the problem, then oral antibiotics are used. Eyedrops containing antihistamines, nonsteroidal anti-inflammatory agents, or corticosteroids are used if allergies are the cause. Or, if foreign matter has caused the inflammation, it is removed.

| corneal
(kŏr′ nē-ăl) | corne
-al | cornea
pertaining to | Pertaining to the cornea |

Medical Word	Word Parts		Definition
	Part	Meaning	
corneal transplant (kŏr´ nē-ăl)			Surgical process of transferring the cornea from a donor to a patient

 fyi A corneal transplant is often referred to as *keratoplasty* or a *corneal graft*. The procedure can be used to improve sight, relieve pain, and treat severe infection or damage. One of the most common reasons for a corneal transplant is a condition called *keratoconus*, which causes the cornea to change shape. The type of corneal transplant will depend on which part of the cornea is damaged or how much of the cornea needs replacing. The options include:
- Penetrating keratoplasty (PK)—a full-thickness transplant
- Deep anterior lamellar keratoplasty (DALK)—replacing or reshaping the outer and middle (front) layers of the cornea
- Endothelial keratoplasty (EK)—replacing the deeper (back) layers of the cornea

Medical Word	Word Parts		Definition
cryosurgery (krī˝ ō-sĕr´ jĕr-ē)	cry/o surg -ery	cold surgery pertaining to	Pertaining to a type of surgery that uses extreme cold to destroy tissue or to produce well-demarcated areas of cell injury; can be used in the removal of cataracts and in the repair of retinal detachment
cycloplegia (sī˝ klō-plē´ jē-ă)	cycl/o -plegia	ciliary body stroke, paralysis	Paralysis of the ciliary muscle
dacryoma (dăk˝ rē-ō´ mă)	dacry -oma	tear, lacrimal duct, tear duct tumor	Tumor-like swelling caused by obstruction of the tear duct(s)
diplopia (dĭp-lō´ pē-ă)	dipl -opia	double sight, vision	Double vision
electroretinogram (ē-lĕk˝ trō-rĕt´ ĭ-nō-grăm)	electr/o retin/o -gram	electricity retina mark, record	Record of the electrical response of the retina to light stimulation
emmetropia (EM) (ĕm˝ ĕ-trō´ pē-ă)	em- metr -opia	in measure sight, vision	Normal or perfect vision (refer to Figure 15.6)
entropion (ĕn-trō´ pē-ŏn)	en- trop -ion	in turn process	Turning inward of the margin of the lower eyelid
enucleation (ē-nū˝ klē-ā´ shŭn)	enucleat -ion	to remove the kernel of process	Process of removing an entire part or mass without rupture, as the eyeball from its orbit

Medical Word	Word Parts		Definition
	Part	Meaning	
esotropia (ET) (ĕs″ ō-trō′ pē-ă)	**eso-** **trop** **-ia**	inward turn condition	Condition in which the eye or eyes turn inward; *crossed eyes*
exotropia (XT) (ĕks″ ō-trō′ pē-ă)	**ex(o)-** **trop** **-ia**	out turn condition	Turning outward of one or both eyes
glaucoma (glaw-kō′ mă)			A group of eye diseases that produce increased intraocular pressure (IOP) caused by a backup of fluid in the eye. When the eye pressure is increased, the optic nerve becomes damaged and the retinal ganglion cells undergo a slow process of cell death termed *apoptosis*, resulting in permanent vision loss. See Figure 15.9.

Slowly rising intraocular pressure

Rapidly rising intraocular pressure

Lens

Cornea

Anterior chamber

Iris

Trabecular meshwork

Canal of Schlemm

Congestion in trabecular meshwork reduces flow through Canal of Schlemm

Flow of aqueous humor

Normal anterior chamber

Posterior chamber

Trabecular meshwork

Canal of Schlemm

Trabecular meshwork and Canal of Schlemm blocked, preventing outflow of aqueous humor

Closed anterior angle

A

B

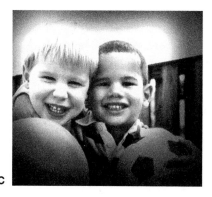

C

FIGURE 15.9 In glaucoma, the accumulation of aqueous humor in the anterior chamber of the eye causes pressure to build, resulting in eventual loss of vision. **A** and **B** show two forms of glaucoma; **C** shows the narrowing of the optic field that is a typical symptom of untreated glaucoma.

Source: Pearson Education, Inc.

Medical Word	Word Parts		Definition
	Part	Meaning	

 fyi Glaucoma, one of the leading causes of blindness, affects people of all ages and all races. Regular eye exams are very important and should include measurements of the eye's intraocular pressure. If glaucoma is recognized early, vision loss can be slowed or prevented, but once lost, it cannot be recovered. Even with treatment, about 15% of people with glaucoma will become blind in at least one eye within 20 years. The two major categories of glaucoma are open-angle (also known as primary or chronic) and primary angle-closure (acute or chronic). The following are the signs and symptoms of both types of glaucoma:

Open-Angle Glaucoma

- Patchy blind spots in peripheral or central vision, frequently in both eyes
- Tunnel vision in the advanced stages

Acute Angle-Closure Glaucoma

- Severe headaches
- Eye pain
- Nausea and vomiting
- Blurred vision
- Halos around lights
- Eye redness

Medical Word	Word Parts		Definition
gonioscope (gō′ nē-ō-skōp)	**goni/o** **-scope**	angle instrument for examining	Instrument used to examine the angle of the anterior chamber of the eye
hemianopia (hĕm″ ē-ă-nō′ pē-ă)	**hemi-** **an-** **-opia**	half lack of sight, vision	Inability (blindness) to see half of the field of vision

Medical Word	Word Parts		Definition
	Part	**Meaning**	
hyperopia (Hy) (hī″ pĕr-ō′ pē-ă)	**hyper-** **-opia**	beyond sight, vision	Vision defect in which parallel rays come to a focus beyond the retina; *farsightedness*. See Figure 15.10.

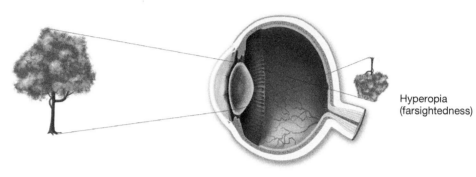

Hyperopia
(farsightedness)

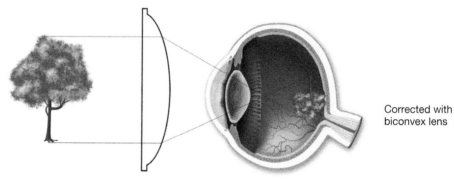

Corrected with
biconvex lens

FIGURE 15.10 Hyperopia is the inability to shorten the focal distance adequately for nearby objects, making the image on the retina blurry. This condition can be corrected by placing a biconvex lens in front of the eyes.

intraocular (ĭn″ tră-ŏk′ ū-lăr)	**intra-** **ocul** **-ar**	within eye pertaining to	Pertaining to within the eye
iridectomy (ĭr″ ĭ-dĕk′ tō-mē)	**irid** **-ectomy**	iris surgical excision	Surgical excision of a portion of the iris
iridocyclitis (ĭr″ ĭd-ō-sī-klī′ tĭs)	**irid/o** **cycl** **-itis**	iris ciliary body inflammation	Inflammation of the iris and ciliary body
keratitis (kĕr″ ă-tī′ tĭs)	**kerat** **-itis**	cornea inflammation	Inflammation of the cornea

Medical Word	Word Parts		Definition
	Part	**Meaning**	
keratoconjunctivitis (kĕr″ ă-tō-kŏn-jŭnk″ tĭ-vī″ tĭs)	**kerat/o** **conjunctiv** -itis	cornea to join together, conjunctiva inflammation	Inflammation of the cornea and the conjunctiva
keratoplasty (kĕr′ ă-tō-plăs″ tē)	**kerat/o** **-plasty**	cornea surgical repair	Surgical repair of the cornea
lacrimal (lăk′ rĭm-ăl)	**lacrim** **-al**	tear, lacrimal duct, tear duct pertaining to	Pertaining to the tears
laser (lā′ zĕr)			Acronym for *light amplification by stimulated emission of radiation*

fyi

Laser surgery can be used to treat glaucoma, including the following types:

1. *Laser peripheral iridotomy (LPI)* in which a small hole is made in the iris to allow it to fall back from the fluid channel and help the fluid drain.

2. *Argon laser trabeculoplasty (ALT)* in which a laser beam opens the fluid channels of the eye, helping the drainage system to work better.

3. *Selective laser trabeculoplasty (SLT)*, a type of laser surgery that uses a combination of frequencies, allowing the laser to work at very low levels. It treats specific cells selectively and leaves untreated portions of the trabecular meshwork (the meshlike drainage canals surrounding the iris) intact.

4. When medication and/or laser surgery does not lower the intraocular pressure of the eye, the doctor could recommend a procedure called *filtering microsurgery*. This procedure makes a tiny drainage hole in the sclera (*sclerostomy*). The new drainage hole allows fluid to flow out of the eye and thereby helps lower eye pressure. This prevents or reduces damage to the optic nerve.

Medical Word	Word Parts		Definition
	Part	Meaning	
macular degeneration (măk´ ū-lăr dē´ jĕn-ĕr˝ ā-shŭn)			Macular degeneration, or age-related macular degeneration (AMD), is a leading cause of vision loss in Americans age 55 and older. It causes severe loss of central vision, but peripheral vision is retained. AMD blurs the sharp central vision one needs for straight-ahead activities such as reading, sewing, and driving. AMD causes no pain. See Figure 15.11

Macular Degeneration

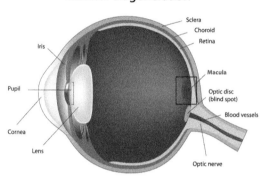

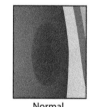 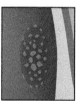

Normal   "Wet" Macular Degeneration   "Dry" Macular Degeneration

FIGURE 15.11 Macular degeneration.
Source: Alila Medical Media/Shutterstock

fyi The two basic types of macular degeneration are *dry* and *wet*. The dry form is marked by atrophy (a wasting away) and degeneration of retinal cells with the formation of small yellow deposits (drusen). There is no treatment for the dry form. The wet form results from the growth of new (neovascular) and oozing (exudative) blood vessels under the retina and macula. Wet AMD can be treated with laser surgery, photodynamic therapy, and injections into the eye. Regular comprehensive eye exams can detect macular degeneration before the disease causes vision loss. Treatment can slow vision loss, but it does not restore vision.

Medical Word	Word Parts		Definition
miotic (mī-ŏt´ ĭk)	**mi/o** **-tic**	less, small pertaining to	Pertaining to an agent that causes the pupil to contract
mydriatic (mĭd˝ rē-ăt´ ĭk)	**mydriat** **-ic**	dilate, widen pertaining to	Pertaining to an agent that causes the pupil to dilate

Medical Word	Word Parts		Definition
	Part	Meaning	
myopia (My) (mī-ō´ pē-ă)			Vision defect in which parallel rays come to a focus in front of the retina; *nearsightedness*. See Figure 15.12.

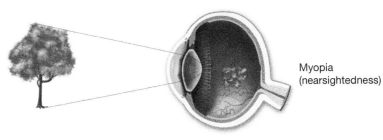

Myopia (nearsightedness)

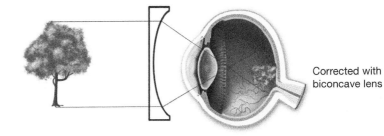

Corrected with biconcave lens

FIGURE 15.12 Myopia is the inability to lengthen the focal distance adequately for distant objects, making the image on the retina blurry. This condition can be corrected by placing a biconcave lens in front of the eyes.

fyi LASIK is a surgical procedure intended to reduce a person's dependency on glasses or contact lenses. LASIK is the acronym for *laser-assisted in situ keratomileusis* (corneal reshaping).

The procedure is used for myopia/nearsightedness and permanently changes the shape of the cornea, using an excimer laser. A mechanical microkeratome (a blade device) or a laser keratome (a laser device) is used to cut a flap in the cornea. A hinge is left at one end of this flap. The flap is folded back revealing the stroma, the middle section of the cornea. Pulses from a computer-controlled laser vaporize a portion of the stroma and the flap is replaced.

Medical Word	Part	Meaning	Definition
nyctalopia (nĭk˝ tă-lō´ pē-ă)	**nyctal** **-opia**	night sight, vision	Condition in which the individual has difficulty seeing at night; *night blindness*
nystagmus (nĭs-tăg´ mŭs)			Involuntary, constant, rhythmic movement of the eyeball
ocular (ŏk´ ū-lăr)	**ocul** **-ar**	eye pertaining to	Pertaining to the eye
ocular fundus (ŏk´ ū-lăr fŭn´ dŭs)			Posterior inner part of the eye as seen with an ophthalmoscope
ophthalmologist (ŏf˝ thăl-mŏl´ ō-jĭst)	**ophthalm/o** **log** **-ist**	eye study one who specializes	Physician who specializes in the study of the eye

Medical Word	Word Parts		Definition
	Part	Meaning	
ophthalmology (ŏf″ thăl-mŏl′ ō-jē)	**ophthalm/o** **-logy**	eye study of	Study of the eye
ophthalmoscope (ŏf″ thăl′ mō-skōp)	**ophthalm/o** **-scope**	eye instrument for examining	Medical instrument used to examine the interior of the eye (refer to Figure 15.22)
optic (op′ tĭk)	**opt** **-ic**	eye pertaining to	Pertaining to the eye

> **! ALERT!**
>
> How many words can you build using the root **opt** and the combining form **opt/o**?

Medical Word	Word Parts		Definition
optician (ŏp-tĭsh′ ăn)	**opt** **-ician**	eye specialist	One who specializes in making optical products and accessories, such as eyeglasses. This person is not a physician.
optometrist (OD) (ŏp-tŏm′ ĕ-trĭst)	**opt/o** **metr** **-ist**	eye measure one who specializes	One who specializes in examining the eyes for refractive errors and providing appropriate corrective lenses. This person is not a medical doctor (MD) but is trained and licensed as a doctor of optometry (OD). See Figure 15.13.

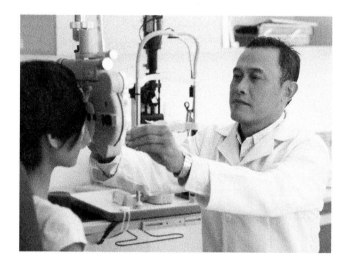

FIGURE 15.13 Optometrist examining a patient's eyes.
Source: Dinis Tolipov/123RF

Medical Word	Word Parts		Definition
orthoptics (or-thŏp′ tĭks)	**orth** **opt** **-ic(s)**	straight eye pertaining to	Study and treatment of defective binocular vision resulting from defects in ocular musculature; also a technique of eye exercises for correcting defective binocular vision
phacoemulsification (fāk″ ō-ē-mŭl′ sĭ-fĭ-kā″ shŭn)	**phac/o** **emulsificat** **-ion**	lens disintegrate process	Process of using ultrasound to disintegrate a cataract by inserting a needle through a small incision and aspirating the disintegrated cataract. See Figure 15.14.

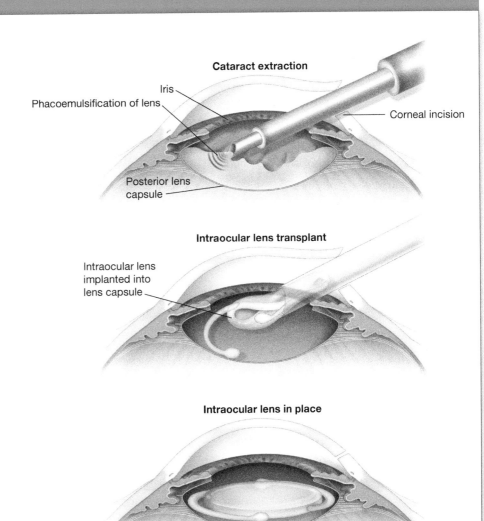

Cataract extraction

Iris

Phacoemulsification of lens

Corneal incision

Posterior lens capsule

Intraocular lens transplant

Intraocular lens implanted into lens capsule

Intraocular lens in place

FIGURE 15.14 Phacoemulsification is used to remove the cataract, then an artificial lens is implanted.

 fyi

Smaller incisions in cataract surgery have become the standard, with phacoemulsification now being the method of choice for most surgeons. Along with these advances have come improved intraocular lens materials and designs, especially for use with smaller incisions.

An *intraocular lens (IOL)* is a tiny, artificial lens for the eye. It replaces the eye's natural lens that is removed during cataract surgery. The most common type of lens used with cataract surgery is called a *monofocal IOL*. It has one focusing distance and is set to focus for up close, medium range, or distance vision.

Some IOLs, called *multifocal* and *accommodative lenses*, have different focusing powers within the same lens. These IOLs reduce dependence on glasses by giving clear vision for more than one set distance. Multifocal IOLs provide both distance and near focus at the same time. The lens has different zones set at different powers. It is designed so the brain learns to select the right focus automatically. Accommodative IOLs move or change shape inside the eye, allowing focusing at different distances. Toric© IOLs are designed for people with astigmatism, which is caused by an uneven curve in the cornea or lens.

Medical Word	Word Parts		Definition
	Part	Meaning	
phacolysis (fă-kŏl´ĭ-sĭs)	**phac/o** **-lysis**	lens destruction, to separate	Surgical destruction and removal of the crystalline lens in the treatment of a cataract
photocoagulation (fō″ tō-kō-ăg″ ū-lā´ shŭn)	**phot/o** **coagulat** **-ion**	light to clot process	Process of altering proteins in tissue by the use of light energy such as the laser beam; used to treat retinal detachment, retinal bleeding, intraocular tumors, and/or macular degeneration (wet)
photophobia (fō″ tō-fō´ bē-ă)	**phot/o** **-phobia**	light fear	Unusual intolerance to light

fyi *Computer vision syndrome (CVS)* is a condition that occurs when eye or vision problems relate to the heavy use of digital devices. Ocular symptoms associated with the syndrome include eye strain, decreased vision, burning, stinging, and photophobia. One may help avoid this syndrome by following the 20-20-20 rule. At least every 20 minutes, take a 20-second break and view something 20 feet away. It is also recommended that one should take a 15-minute break for every 2 hours spent on computers or other digital devices.

presbyopia (prĕz″ bē-ō´ pē-ă)	**presby** **-opia**	old sight, vision	Vision defect in which parallel rays come to a focus beyond the retina; occurs normally with aging; also called *hyperopia* (farsightedness). Refer to Figure 15.10.
pupillary (pū´ pĭ-lĕr-ē)	**pupill** **-ary**	pupil pertaining to	Pertaining to the pupil
radial keratotomy (rā´ dē-ăl kĕr-ă-tŏt´ ō-mē)	**kerat/o** **-tomy**	cornea incision	Surgical procedure that can be performed to correct nearsightedness (*myopia*). Delicate spokelike incisions are made in the cornea to flatten it, thereby shortening the eyeball so that light reaches the retina. Vision is not improved for all patients, and complications could lead to blindness.

Medical Word	Word Parts		Definition
	Part	Meaning	
retinal detachment (rĕt´ ĭ-năl dē-tăch´ mĕnt)			Separation of the retina from the choroid layer of the eye that can be caused by trauma or can occur spontaneously. See Figure 15.15.

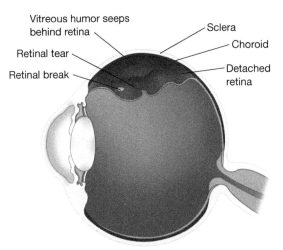

FIGURE 15.15 Retinal detachment.

> **fyi**
>
> When the retina detaches, it is lifted or pulled from its normal position. In some cases there may be small areas of the retina that are torn. These areas, called *retinal tears* or *retinal breaks*, can lead to retinal detachment. If not promptly treated, retinal detachment can cause permanent vision loss. There are three types of retinal detachment:
>
> - ***Rhegmatogenous.*** A tear or break in the retina that allows fluid to get under the retina causes it to separate from the retinal pigment epithelium (RPE), the pigmented cell layer that nourishes the retina. These types of retinal detachments are the most common.
> - ***Tractional.*** Scar tissue on the retina's surface contracts and causes the retina to separate from the RPE. This type of detachment is less common.
> - ***Exudative.*** Caused by retinal diseases, including inflammatory disorders, or injury/trauma to the eye, fluid leaks into the area underneath the retina, but there are no tears or breaks in the retina.

Medical Word	Word Parts		Definition
retinitis (rĕt´ ĭ-nī´ tĭs)	retin -itis	retina inflammation	Inflammation of the retina
retinitis pigmentosa (rĕt´ ĭ-nī´ tĭs pĭg´ mĕn-tō´ să)			Chronic progressive disease marked by bilateral primary degeneration of the retina beginning in childhood and leading to blindness by middle age. Night blindness and a reduced field of vision are early clinical signs of this disease.
retinoblastoma (rĕt´ ĭ-nō-blăs-tō´ mă)	retin/o -blast -oma	retina germ cell tumor	Malignant tumor arising from the germ cell of the retina

Medical Word	Word Parts		Definition
	Part	Meaning	
retinopathy (rĕt″ ĭn-ŏp′ ă-thē)	retin/o -pathy	retina disease	Any disease of the retina. In the United States, *diabetic retinopathy* is the leading cause of new blindness in people age 20–74. See Figures 15.16 and 15.17.

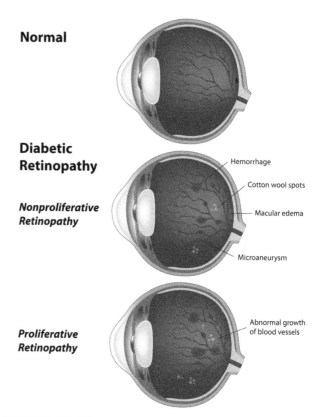

Normal

Diabetic Retinopathy

Nonproliferative Retinopathy

Hemorrhage

Cotton wool spots

Macular edema

Microaneurysm

Proliferative Retinopathy

Abnormal growth of blood vessels

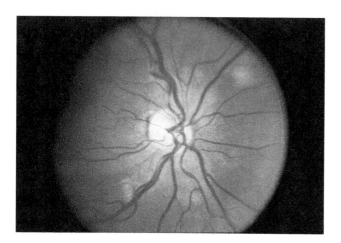

FIGURE 15.16 Appearance of the ocular fundus in diabetic retinopathy.
Source: Courtesy of the National Eye Institute, National Institutes of Health

FIGURE 15.17 Diabetic retinopathy, an eye disease due to diabetes.
Source: Alila Medical Media/Shutterstock

Medical Word	Word Parts		Definition
retrolental fibroplasia (RLF) (rĕt″ rō-lĕn′ tăl fī″ brō-plā′ sē-ă)	retro- lent -al fibr/o -plasia	behind lens pertaining to fiber formation	Disease of the retinal vessels present in premature newborns; can be caused by excessive use of oxygen in the incubator; can cause retinal detachment and blindness
scleritis (sklĕ-rī′ tĭs)	scler -itis	hardening, sclera inflammation	Inflammation of the sclera (white of the eye)

Medical Word	Word Parts		Definition
	Part	**Meaning**	
strabismus (stră-bĭz´ mŭs)	**strabism** **-us**	squinting structure	Disorder of the eye in which the optic axes cannot be directed to the same object. See Figure 15.18.

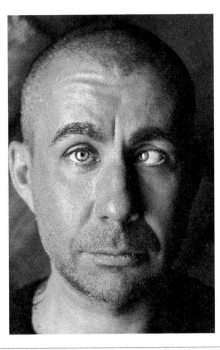

FIGURE 15.18 Man with strabismus.
Source: Andrey Kiselev/123RF

| **sty(e)** (stī) | | | Inflammation of one or more of the sebaceous glands of the eyelid; also called a *hordeolum.* See Figure 15.19. |

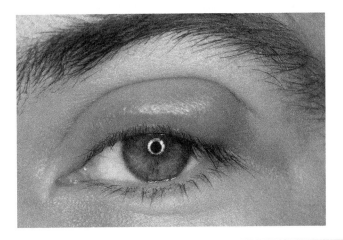

FIGURE 15.19 Person with a sty(e) on the eyelid.
Source: Pavel L Photo and Video/ Shutterstock

| **tonography** (tō-nŏg´ ră-fē) | **ton/o** **-graphy** | tone recording | Recording of intraocular pressure used in detecting glaucoma |

Medical Word	Word Parts		Definition
	Part	**Meaning**	
tonometer (tōn-ŏm´ ĕ-tĕr)	**ton/o** **-meter**	tone instrument to measure	Medical instrument used to measure intraocular pressure. See Figure 15.20.

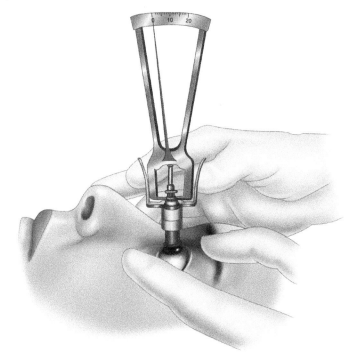

FIGURE 15.20 Schiötz tonometer for measuring intraocular pressure.

Medical Word	Word Parts		Definition
trichiasis (trĭk-ī´ ă-sĭs)	**trich** **-iasis**	hair condition	Condition of in-growing eyelashes that rub against the cornea, causing a constant irritation to the eyeball
trifocal (trī-fō´ kăl)	**tri-** **foc** **-al**	three focus pertaining to	Pertaining to having three foci
uveal (ū´ vē-ăl)	**uve** **-al**	uvea pertaining to	Pertaining to the second or vascular coat of the eye
uveitis (ū-vē-ī´ tĭs)	**uve** **-itis**	uvea inflammation	Inflammation of the uvea (consists of the iris, ciliary body, and choroid and forms the pigmented layer)
xenophthalmia (zĕn˝ ŏf-thăl´ mē-ă)	**xen** **ophthalm** **-ia**	foreign material eye condition	Inflamed eye condition caused by foreign material
xerophthalmia (zēr-ŏf-thăl´ mē-ă)	**xer** **ophthalm** **-ia**	dry eye condition	Eye condition in which the conjunctiva is dry

Study *and* Review II

Word Parts

Prefixes   Give the definitions of the following prefixes.

1. a- _____

2. bi- _____

3. en- _____

4. em- _____

5. eso- _____

6. hyper- _____

7. intra- _____

8. tri- _____

9. ex(o)- _____

10. hemi- _____

11. an- _____

12. retro- _____

Combining Forms   Give the definitions of the following combining forms.

1. ambly/o _____

2. anis/o _____

3. blephar/o _____

4. choroid/o _____

5. conjunctiv/o _____

6. cor/o _____

7. corne/o _____

8. cry/o _____

9. cycl/o _____

10. dacry/o _____

11. dipl/o _____

12. irid/o _____

13. kerat/o _____

14. lacrim/o _____

15. lent/o _____

16. mi/o _____

17. ophthalm/o _____

18. opt/o _____

19. orth/o _____

20. phac/o _____

21. phot/o _____

22. retin/o _____

23. xen/o _____

24. xer/o _____

Suffixes   Give the definitions of the following suffixes.

1. -al _____

2. -ar _____

3. -ary _____

4. -blast _____

5. -iasis _____

6. -ectomy _____

7. -gram _____

8. -graphy _____

9. -ia _____

10. -ic _____

11. -ician _____

12. -ion _____

13. -ism _____

14. -ist _____

15. -itis _____

16. -logy _____

17. -lysis _____

18. -plasia _____

19. -meter _____

20. -oma _____

21. -opia _____

22. -osis _____

23. -pathy _____

24. -phobia _____

25. -plasty _____

26. -plegia _____

27. -ptosis _____

28. -scope _____

29. -tic _____

30. -tomy _____

31. -us _____

Identifying Medical Terms

In the spaces provided, write the medical terms for the following meanings.

1. _____ Dullness of vision

2. _____ Pertaining to having two foci

3. _____ Drooping of the upper eyelid(s)

4. _____ Pertaining to the cornea

5. _____ Tumor-like swelling caused by obstruction of the tear duct(s)

6. _____ Double vision

7. _____ Normal or perfect vision

8. _____ Pertaining to within the eye

9. _____ Inflammation of the cornea

10. _____ Surgical repair of the cornea

Matching

Select the appropriate lettered meaning for each of the following words.

_____ 1. anisocoria

_____ 2. entropion

_____ 3. cataract

_____ 4. hemianopia

_____ 5. phacoemulsification

_____ 6. photocoagulation

_____ 7. radial keratotomy

_____ 8. retrolental fibroplasia

_____ 9. strabismus

_____ 10. sty(e)

a. Disorder of the eye in which the optic axes cannot be directed to the same object

b. Disease of the retinal vessels present in premature infants

c. Process of using ultrasound to disintegrate a cataract

d. Use of a laser to treat retinal detachment and/or retinal bleeding

e. Condition in which the pupils are unequal

f. Turning inward of the margin of the lower eyelid

g. Surgical procedure performed to correct myopia

h. Inability to see half of the field of vision

i. Hordeolum

j. Opacity of the crystalline lens or its capsule

Medical Case Snapshots

This learning activity provides an opportunity to relate the medical terminology you are learning to sample patient case presentations. In the spaces provided, write in your answers.

Case 1

A 63-year-old male presents with "trouble driving at night." He states that "bright lights hurt my eyes" and "I see halos around them." When opacity of the crystalline lens occurs in an older adult, it is said to be a _____. With this condition colors seem faded and the only effective treatment is known as _____, a process of using ultrasound to disintegrate the lens.

Case 2

A 17-year-old male was seen by an ophthalmologist. He complains that his eyes are really bothering him. He has been swimming every day for the past 2 weeks training for a swim meet. He is diagnosed with _____, or inflammation of the conjunctiva. With this condition some of the symptoms are _____ in the white of the eye, an increased amount of tears, a thick _____ discharge, and _____ vision.

Case 3

A 64-year-old female is seen by her physician. Her medical history includes diagnoses of hypertension and type 2 diabetes mellitus. The results of a comprehensive eye exam revealed an increased intraocular pressure, which is known as _____. With this condition there are no outward symptoms and if left untreated, permanent _____ _____ may occur.

Drug Highlights

Classification of Drug	Description and Examples
drugs used to treat glaucoma	Work by increasing the outflow of aqueous humor, by decreasing its production, or by producing both of these actions.
prostaglandin analogues	Increase the drainage of intraocular fluid, thereby decreasing intraocular pressure.
	EXAMPLES: Travatan Z (travoprost ophthalmic solution 0.004%), Lumigan (bimatoprost ophthalmic solution 0.03%), and Xalatan (latanoprost)
alpha adrenergic antagonist	Decreases production of intraocular fluid and increases drainage.
	EXAMPLE: Alphagan P (brimonidine tartrate ophthalmic solution 0.1%)
beta blockers	Decrease production of intraocular fluid.
	EXAMPLES: Akbeta (levobunolol HCl ophthalmic solution), Betoptic S (betaxolol HCl 0.25%), OptiPranolol (metipranolol), Timoptic-XE, and Betimol (timolol hemihydrate)
carbonic anhydrase inhibitors	Decrease production of intraocular fluid.
	EXAMPLES: Azopt (brinzolamide ophthalmic suspension 1%), Diamox Sequels, acetazolomide, and Trusopt (dorzolamide)
cholinergic (miotic)	Increases drainage of intraocular fluid.
	EXAMPLE: pilocarpine HCl (ophthalmic solution)
cholinesterase	Increases drainage of intraocular fluid.
	EXAMPLE: Phospholine Iodide (echothiophate)
combination of beta blocker and carbonic anhydrase inhibitor	Decreases production of intraocular fluid.
	EXAMPLE: Cosopt (dorzolomide HCl timolol maleate) (ophthalmic solution)
mydriatics	Agents used to dilate the pupil (mydriasis); can be anticholinergics or sympathomimetics.
anticholinergics	Dilate the pupil and interfere with the ability of the eye to focus properly (cycloplegia). They are used primarily as an aid in refraction, during internal examination of the eye, in intraocular surgery, and in the treatment of anterior uveitis and secondary glaucomas.
	EXAMPLES: atropine sulfate and Mydriacyl (tropicamide)

Classification of Drug	Description and Examples
sympathomimetics	Produce mydriasis without cycloplegia. Pupil dilation is obtained as the drug causes contraction of the dilator muscle of the iris. They also affect intraocular pressure by decreasing production of aqueous humor while increasing its outflow from the eye. EXAMPLES: epinephrine HCl and phenylephrine HCl
antibiotics	Used to treat infectious diseases, especially those caused by bacteria. Those used for the eye can be in the form of an ointment, cream, or solution. EXAMPLES: chloramphenicol, polymyxin B sulfate, Vigamox (moxifloxacin), and Zymar (gatifloxacin)
antifungal agent	Natacyn (natamycin) is used to treat fungal infections of the eye, such as blepharitis, conjunctivitis, and keratitis.
antiviral agents	Dendrid (idoxuridine) and Herplex (idoxuridine) are potent antiviral agents used to treat keratitis caused by the herpes simplex virus. Viroptic (trifluridine) is also used to treat viral infections of the eye and is effective in the treatment of herpes simplex infections.

Diagnostic *and* Laboratory Tests

Test	Description
color vision tests	Use of polychromatic (multicolored) charts or an *anomaloscope* (a device for detecting color blindness) to assess an individual's ability to recognize differences in color. A person who is color blind will not see the number 27 in the circle in Figure 15.21.

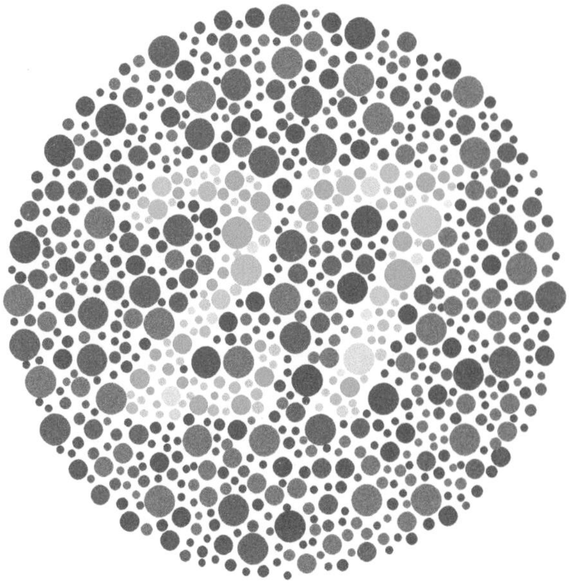

FIGURE 15.21 Color vision chart. Color blind individuals cannot see the number 27 in the circle.

Test	Description
exophthalmometry (ĕk″ sŏf-thăl-mŏm′ ĕ-trē)	Process of measuring the forward protrusion of the eye via an exophthalmometer; used to evaluate an increase or decrease in *exophthalmos* (abnormal protrusion of the eyeball) usually associated with hyperthyroidism
gonioscopy (gō″ nē-ŏs′ kō-pē)	Examination of the anterior chamber of the eye via a gonioscope; used for determining ocular motility and rotation
keratometry (kĕr″ ă-tŏm′ ĕ-trē)	Process of measuring the cornea via a keratometer
ocular ultrasonography (ŏk′ ū-lăr ŭl-tră-sŏn-ŏg′ ră-fē)	Use of high-frequency sound waves (via a small probe placed on the eye) to measure for intraocular lenses (IOL) and to detect orbital and periorbital lesions; also used to measure the length of the eye and the curvature of the cornea in preparation for surgery
ophthalmoscopy (ŏf-thăl-mŏs′ kō-pē)	Examination of the interior of the eyes via an ophthalmoscope; used to view the retina and identify changes in the blood vessels and to diagnose systemic diseases. See Figure 15.22.

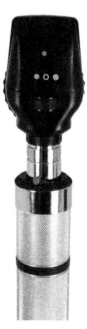

FIGURE 15.22 Ophthalmoscope.
Source: bjsites/Shutterstock

Test	Description
tonometry (tōn-ŏm′ ĕ-trē)	Measurement of the intraocular pressure (IOP) of the eye; used to screen for and detect glaucoma. By directing a quick puff of air onto the eye, or gently applying a pressure-sensitive tip near or against the eye, elevated eye pressure can be detected. Numbing drops are usually applied to the eye for this test. Refer to Figure 15.20.

Test	Description
visual acuity (VA) (vĭzh´ ū-ăl ă-kū´ ĭ-tē)	Acuteness or sharpness of vision. A Snellen eye chart can be used to test it; the patient reads letters of various sizes from a distance of 20 feet. Normal vision is 20/20. See Figure 15.23.

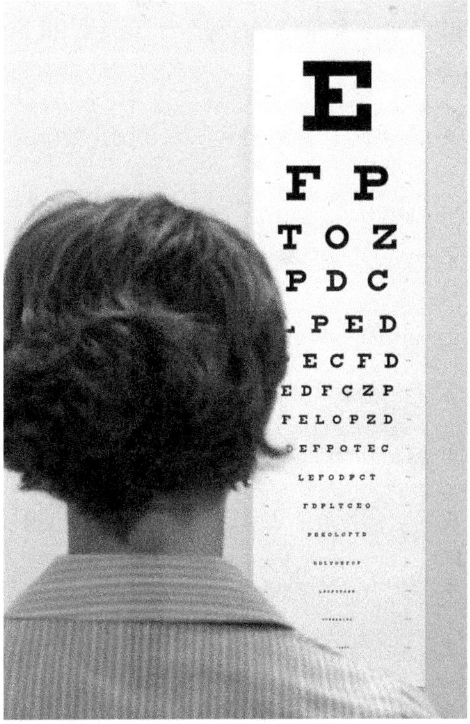

FIGURE 15.23 Woman undergoing a visual acuity test.
Source: Rtimages/Shutterstock

Abbreviations *and* Acronyms

Abbreviation/ Acronym	Meaning	Abbreviation/ Acronym	Meaning
Acc	accommodation	LPI	laser peripheral iridotomy
ALT	argon laser trabeculoplasty	MD	medical doctor
AMD	age-related macular degeneration	MGD	meibomian gland dysfunction
CVS	computer vision syndrome	My	myopia
DALK	deep anterior lamellar keratoplasty	OD	doctor of optometry, optometrist
EK	endothelial keratoplasty	PK	penetrating keratoplasty
EM	emmetropia	RLF	retrolental fibroplasia
ET	esotropia	RPE	retinal pigment epithelium
Hy	hyperopia	SLT	selective laser trabeculoplasty
IOL	intraocular lens	STIs	sexually transmitted infections
IOP	intraocular pressure	VA	visual acuity
LASIK	laser-assisted in situ keratomileusis	XT	exotropia

Study *and* Review III

Building Medical Terms

Using the following word parts, fill in the blanks to build the correct medical terms.

dipl-   nyctal   retin/o   -ectomy   -phobia
lacrim   ophthalm/o uve   -tic   -iasis

Definition	Medical Term
1. Double vision	_____opia
2. Surgical excision of a portion of the iris	irid_____
3. Pertains to tears	_____al
4. Pertaining to an agent that causes the pupil to contract	mio_____
5. Condition in which the individual has difficulty seeing at night	_____opia
6. Study of the eye	_____logy
7. Unusual intolerance to light	photo_____
8. Any disease of the retina	_____pathy
9. Condition of in-growing eyelashes that rub against the cornea	trich_____
10. Pertaining to the second or vascular coat of the eye	_____al

Combining Form Challenge

Using the combining forms provided, write the medical term correctly.

ambly/o   cycl/o   goni/o
blephar/o   dacry/o   kerat/o

1. Dullness of vision: _____opia

2. Drooping of the upper eyelid(s): _____ptosis

3. Paralysis of the ciliary muscle: _____plegia

4. Tumor-like swelling caused by obstruction of the tear duct(s): _____oma

5. Instrument used to examine the angle of the anterior chamber of the eye: _____scope

6. Inflammation of the cornea: _____itis

Select the Right Term

Select the correct answer, and write it on the line provided.

1. Process by which the eyes make adjustments to see objects at various distances is _____.

    amblyopia   accommodation   anisocoria   astigmatism

2. Opacity of the crystalline lens or its capsule is _____.

    cataract   chalazion   choroiditis   conjunctivitis

3. Turning inward of the margin of the lower eyelid is _____.

    enucleation   esotropia   entropion   exotropia

4. Disease caused by increased intraocular pressure is _____.

    nystagmus   hemianopia   gonioscope   glaucoma

5. Vision defect in which parallel rays come to a focus beyond the retina is _____.

    hyperopia   presbyopia   myopia   esotropia

6. Inflammation of one or more of the sebaceous glands of the eyelid is _____.

    scleritis   strabismus   sty(e)   xerophthalmia

Drug Highlights

Match the appropriate lettered description or examples of drug(s) with the class of drug.

_____ 1. prostaglandin analogue

_____ 2. alpha adrenergic antagonist

_____ 3. example of beta blocker that decreases production of intraocular fluid

_____ 4. example of cholinergic (miotic) that increases drainage of intraocular fluid

_____ 5. cholinesterase

_____ 6. example of an anticholinergic

_____ 7. sympathomimetic

_____ 8. mydriatics

_____ 9. example of an antifungal agent for the eye

_____ 10. example of an antiviral agent for the eye

a. Causes contraction of the dilator muscle of the iris resulting in dilation of the pupil

b. Pilocarpine HCl (ophthalmic solution)

c. Decreases production of intraocular fluid and increases drainage.

d. Agents used to dilate the pupil (mydriasis); can be anticholinergics or sympathomimetics

e. Increases the drainage of intraocular fluid, thereby decreasing intraocular pressure

f. Dendrid (idoxuridine)

g. Akbeta (levobunolol HCl ophthalmic solution)

h. Drug used to treat glaucoma

i. Natacyn (natamycin)

j. Atropine sulfate

Diagnostic and Laboratory Tests

Select the best answer to each multiple-choice question. Circle the letter of your choice.

1. Process of measuring the forward protrusion of the eye.

   a. gonioscopy

   b. keratometry

   c. exophthalmometry

   d. tonometry

2. Process of measuring the cornea.

   a. gonioscopy

   b. keratometry

   c. exophthalmometry

   d. tonometry

3. Used to identify changes in the blood vessels in the eye and to diagnose systemic diseases.

   a. exophthalmometry

   b. gonioscopy

   c. ophthalmoscopy

   d. tonometry

4. Process of measuring the intraocular pressure of the eye.

   a. exophthalmometry

   b. gonioscopy

   c. ophthalmoscopy

   d. tonometry

5. Process used to measure the acuteness or sharpness of vision.

   a. color vision tests

   b. ultrasonography

   c. tonometry

   d. visual acuity

Abbreviations and Acronyms

Write the correct word, phrase, or abbreviation/acronym in the space provided.

1. accommodation _____

2. EM _____

3. Hy _____

4. intraocular lens _____

5. esotropia _____

6. My _____

7. VA _____

8. IOP _____

9. retrolental fibroplasia _____

10. XT _____

Practical Application

Medical Record Analysis

This exercise contains information, abbreviations/acronyms, and medical terminology from an actual medical record or case study that has been adapted for this text. The names and any personal information have been created by the author. Read and study each form or case study and then answer the questions that follow. You may refer to Appendix III, *Abbreviations, Acronyms, and Symbols*.

INSTRUCTIONS FOR OUTPATIENT CATARACT SURGERY

Task	Edit	View	Time Scale	Options	Help	Date: 17 July 2021

Before Surgery

1. Your surgery has been scheduled for August 2, 2021, as an outpatient at: Dewdrop Surgery Center.

2. Report to the center the day of surgery at 7:10 A.M.

3. The afternoon before surgery and the morning of surgery, use the antibiotics Vigamox and Zymar drops in the right eye to help prevent a bacterial infection. Afternoon and evening before surgery, 1 drop at 3:00, 5:00, 7:00, and 9:00 P.M.

4. Do not eat or drink anything the morning of surgery, except a sip of water to take your medications.

5. Do not wear makeup, fingernail polish, or jewelry to the center.

6. If you are normally taking any medications in the morning, especially heart or blood pressure medications, be sure to take them before you come to the center for surgery. However, if you take insulin or diabetes medication, do not take it until you get home from surgery.

7. Go by the outpatient surgery department at Dewdrop Surgery Center to pre-admit any time before the day of surgery.

After Surgery

1. You may go home shortly after surgery. Be sure to bring someone to drive you home. You may resume normal activities but do not engage in vigorous exercise on the day of surgery. Be careful not to have a fall.

2. The shield may be removed 6 hours after surgery. **DO NOT PUT ANY PRESSURE ON YOUR EYE AND DO NOT RUB YOUR EYE**. Put the Vigamox/Zymar drops in 3 times before you go to bed.

3. Return to Dr. Cedric Emmanuel's office on August 3, 2021, at 10:25 A.M. and further instructions will be given. Bring all your eyedrops to the office with you.

4. Continue any medications that you are taking unless otherwise instructed. Resume your usual diet.

5. If you have mild pain, take Tylenol regular-strength (325 mg) acetaminophen: two tablets every 4–6 hours as needed, not to exceed 12 tablets in 24 hours. If the pain is severe, call Dr. Cedric Emmanuel: Office & beeper (123) 456-7890.

Medical Record Questions

Write the correct answer in the space provided.

1. What type of medication is Vigamox and why is it ordered for this patient? _____

_____

2. What type of medication is Zymar and why is it ordered for this patient? _____

_____

3. Should the patient take his or her heart and blood pressure medicine the morning of surgery? _____

4. When should the patient go by the Dewdrop Surgery Center to pre-admit? _____

5. If the patient has mild pain, what should he or she take? _____

MyLab Medical Terminology™

MyLab Medical Terminology is a premium online homework management system that includes a host of features to help you study. Registered users will find:

- A multitude of quizzes and activities built within the MyLab platform
- Powerful tools that track and analyze your results—allowing you to create a personalized learning experience
- Videos and audio pronunciations to help enrich your progress
- Streaming lesson presentations (guided lectures) and self-paced learning modules
- A space where you and your instructor can check your progress and manage your assignments

16 Female Reproductive System with an Overview of Obstetrics

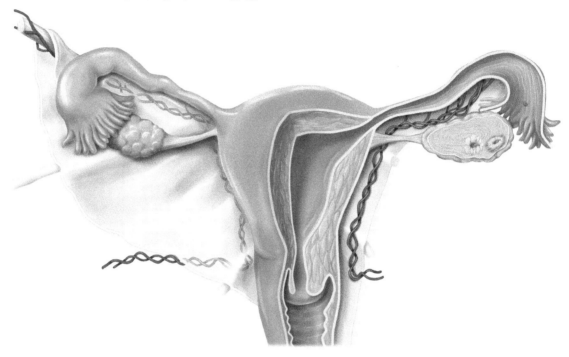

⌄ Learning Outcomes

On completion of this chapter, you will be able to:

1. State the description and primary functions of the organs/structures of the female reproductive system.
2. Describe three abnormal positions of the uterus.
3. Describe the menstrual cycle.
4. Define obstetrics and summarize the process of fertilization.
5. State the definition of pregnancy and describe its four stages.
6. Describe the three stages of labor.
7. Analyze, build, spell, and pronounce medical words.
8. Classify the drugs highlighted in this chapter.
9. Describe diagnostic and laboratory tests related to this chapter.
10. Identify and define selected abbreviations and acronyms.

Anatomy and Physiology

The female reproductive system consists of a left and a right ovary, which are the female's primary sex organs, and the following accessory sex organs: two fallopian tubes, the uterus, the vagina, the vulva, and two breasts. The female reproductive system has several functions. The ovaries produce the female egg cells, called *ova* or *oocytes*. The ova are then transported to the fallopian tube where fertilization of an ovum (singular of ova) by a spermatozoon (sperm) may occur. The fertilized egg then moves to the uterus, where the uterine lining has thickened in response to the normal hormones of the reproductive cycle. Once in the uterus the fertilized egg can implant into the thickened uterine lining and continue to develop. If fertilization does not take place, the uterine lining is shed as menstrual flow. In addition, the female reproductive system produces female sex hormones that maintain the reproductive cycle. To summarize, the functions of the female reproductive system are to:

- Produce female egg cells (ova)
- Transport ova to fallopian tube (where fertilization may occur)
- Implant fertilized egg into thickened uterine lining (site of nourishment and development of the fetus)
- Produce female sex hormones

Table 16.1 provides an at-a-glance look at the female reproductive system. See Figures 16.1 and 16.2.

TABLE 16.1	Female Reproductive System at-a-Glance
Organ/Structure	**Primary Functions/Description**
Uterus	Provides a place for the nourishment and development of the fetus during pregnancy; contracts rhythmically and powerfully to help push out the fetus during the process of birthing
Fallopian tubes	Serve as ducts to convey the ovum from the ovary to the uterus and to convey spermatozoa toward the ovary; the site of conception
Ovaries	Produce ova (oocytes) and hormones
Vagina	Female organ of copulation (sexual intercourse), serves as a passageway for the discharge of the monthly flow (menstruation) and a passageway for the birth of a fetus
Vulva	External female genitalia
Mons pubis	Provides pad of fatty tissue
Labia majora	Provides two folds of adipose tissue
Labia minora	Lying within the labia majora, encloses the vestibule
Vestibule	Serves as the entrance to the urethra, the vagina, and two excretory ducts of Bartholin glands located on either side of the vaginal opening at the base of the *labia majora*. These glands secrete mucus for lubrication.
Clitoris	Erectile tissue that is homologous to the penis of the male; produces pleasurable sensations during sexual intercourse
Breasts	Following childbirth, mammary glands produce milk

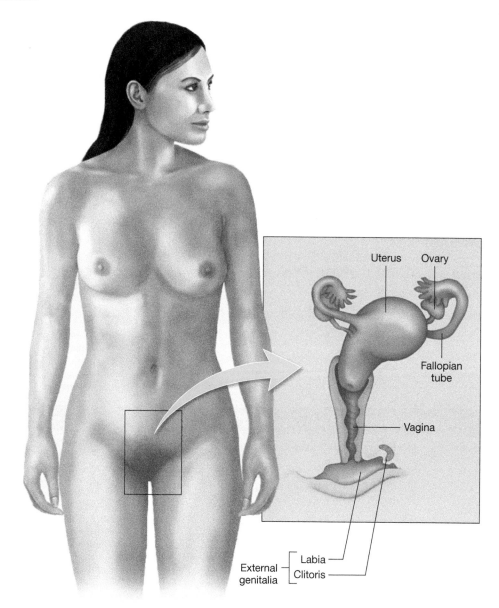

FIGURE 16.1 Female reproductive system.

Uterus

The **uterus** is a muscular, hollow, pear-shaped organ that is about 8 centimeters (cm) long, 5 cm wide, and 2.5 cm thick. The normal position of the uterus, known as **anteflexion**, is with the cervix pointing toward the lower end of the sacrum and the fundus toward the suprapubic region. See Figure 16.3. An average uterus weighs between 30 and 40 grams (g), which is 1 and 1.4 ounces (oz).

The uterus can be divided into two anatomical regions: the body and the cervix. The *uterine body* or *corpus* is the larger (upper) portion. The *fundus* is the rounded portion of the uterine body above the openings of the fallopian tubes. The uterine body ends at a constricted central area known as the *isthmus*. The cervix is the lowermost cylindrical portion of the uterus that extends from the isthmus to the vagina.

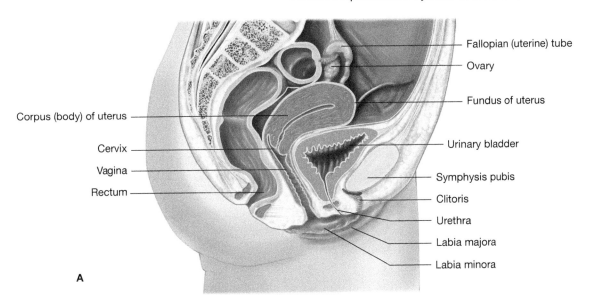

Fallopian (uterine) tube
Ovary
Fundus of uterus
Corpus (body) of uterus
Urinary bladder
Cervix
Vagina
Symphysis pubis
Rectum
Clitoris
Urethra
Labia majora
Labia minora

A

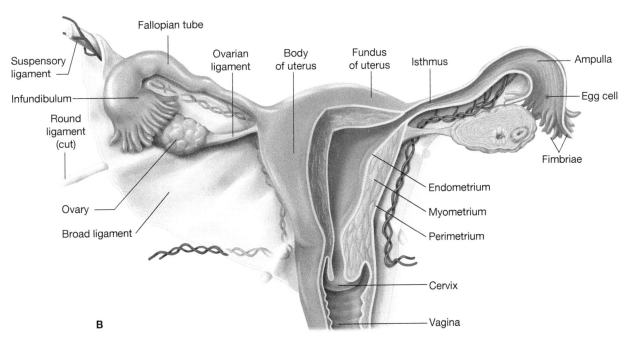

Suspensory ligament
Fallopian tube
Ovarian ligament
Body of uterus
Fundus of uterus
Isthmus
Ampulla
Infundibulum
Egg cell
Round ligament (cut)
Fimbriae
Ovary
Endometrium
Broad ligament
Myometrium
Perimetrium
Cervix
Vagina

B

FIGURE 16.2 Female organs of reproduction and associated structures. **A** Sagittal section. **B** Posterior view. The posterior organ walls have been removed on the right side to reveal the shape of the lumen of the Fallopian tube, uterus, and vagina.

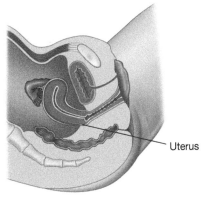

Uterus

FIGURE 16.3 Normal position of the uterus, called *anteflexion*.

Anteflexion

The uterus is suspended in the anterior part of the pelvic cavity, halfway between the sacrum and the symphysis pubis, above the bladder, and in front of the rectum. A number of ligaments support the uterus and hold it in position: two broad ligaments, two round ligaments, two uterosacral ligaments, and the ligaments that are attached to the bladder.

Uterine Wall

The wall of the uterus consists of three layers: the **perimetrium** or outer layer, the **myometrium** or muscular middle layer, and the **endometrium**, which is the mucous membrane lining the inner surface of the uterus. Refer to Figure 16.2B. The endometrium is composed of columnar epithelium and connective tissue and is supplied with blood by both straight and spiral arteries. It undergoes marked changes in response to hormonal stimulation during the menstrual cycle.

Abnormal Positions of the Uterus

The uterus can become malpositioned because of weakness of any of its supporting ligaments. Trauma, disease processes of the uterus, or multiple pregnancies can contribute to the weakening of the supporting ligaments. The following terms describe some of the abnormal positions (see Figure 16.4) of the uterus:

Retroversion. Turned backward with the cervix pointing forward toward the symphysis pubis.

Retroflexion. Bent backward at an angle with the cervix usually unchanged from its normal position.

Anteversion. Fundus turned forward toward the pubis with the cervix tilted up toward the sacrum.

Fallopian Tubes

Also called the **uterine tubes** or **oviducts**, the **fallopian tubes** extend laterally from either side of the uterus and end near each ovary. An average, normal fallopian tube is about 11.5 cm long and 0.6 cm wide. Its wall is composed of three layers: the **serosa** or outermost layer, composed of connective tissue; the **muscular layer**, containing inner circular

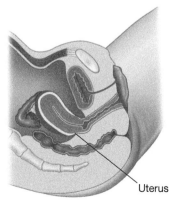
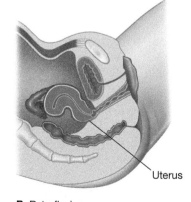
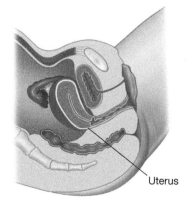

A Retroversion **B** Retroflexion **C** Anteversion

FIGURE 16.4 Displacement of the uterus within the uterine cavity. **A** Retroversion is a backward tilting. **B** Retroflexion is a backward bending. **C** Anteversion is a forward tilting.

and outer longitudinal layers of smooth muscle; and the **mucosa** or inner layer, consisting of simple columnar epithelium.

Anatomical Features of the Fallopian Tubes

The **isthmus** is the constricted portion of the fallopian tube nearest the uterus. From the isthmus, the tube continues laterally and widens to form a section called the **ampulla**. Beyond the ampulla, the tube continues to expand and ends as a funnel-shaped opening. This end of the tube is called the **infundibulum**, and its opening is the **ostium**. Surrounding each ostium are **fimbriae** or *finger-like structures* (refer to Figure 16.2) that work to propel the discharged ovum into the tube, where ciliary action aids in moving it toward the uterus. Should the ovum become impregnated by a spermatozoon while in the tube, the process of *fertilization* occurs.

Fertilization

Fertilization is the process in which a sperm penetrates an ovum and unites with it. See Figure 16.5. At this time, the 23 chromosomes from the male combine with the 23 chromosomes from the female to make a new life. Fertilization generally occurs within 24 hours following ovulation and usually takes place in the fallopian tube. A single sperm penetrates the ovum, and the resulting cell is called a **zygote**.

By this event, called **conception**, the gender and other biological traits of the new individual are determined. The fertilized ovum or zygote is genetically complete and immediately begins to divide, forming a solid mass of cells called a **morula**. See Figure 16.6. The cells of the morula continue to divide, and by the time the developing **embryo** (the term for the stage of development between weeks 2 and 8) reaches the uterus, it is a

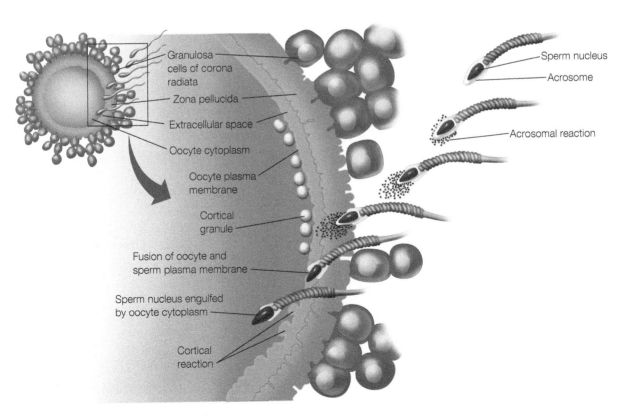

FIGURE 16.5 Sperm penetration of an ovum. The sequential steps of oocyte penetration by a sperm are depicted moving from top to bottom.

hollow ball of cells known as a **blastocyst**, which consists of an outer layer of cells and an inner cell mass. As the blastocyst develops, it forms a structure with two cavities, the **yolk sac** and **amniotic cavity**. In humans, the yolk sac is the site of formation of the first red blood cells and the cells that will become ovum and sperm.

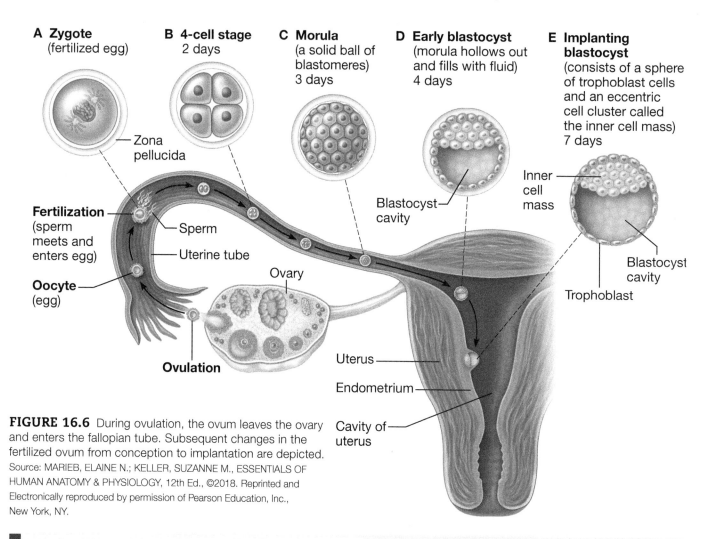

FIGURE 16.6 During ovulation, the ovum leaves the ovary and enters the fallopian tube. Subsequent changes in the fertilized ovum from conception to implantation are depicted.
Source: MARIEB, ELAINE N.; KELLER, SUZANNE M., ESSENTIALS OF HUMAN ANATOMY & PHYSIOLOGY, 12th Ed., ©2018. Reprinted and Electronically reproduced by permission of Pearson Education, Inc., New York, NY.

 fyi The sex of a child is determined at the time of fertilization. When a spermatozoon carrying the X sex chromosome fertilizes the X-bearing ovum, the result is a female child (X + X = female). When the X-bearing ovum is fertilized by the Y-bearing spermatozoon, a male child is produced (X + Y = male). Sex differentiation occurs early in the embryo. At 16 weeks, the external genitals of the fetus are recognizably male or female. This difference can be seen during ultrasonography. See Figure 16.7.

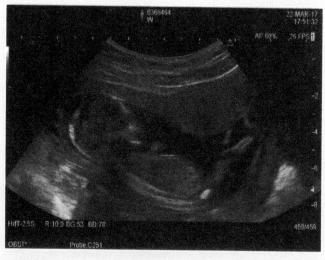

FIGURE 16.7 Ultrasonogram showing a male fetus.
Source: dreamsseeker2/Shutterstock

Ovaries

Located on either side of the uterus, the **ovaries** are almond-shaped organs attached to the uterus by the ovarian ligament. They lie close to the fimbriae of the fallopian tubes. The anterior border of each ovary is connected to the posterior layer of the broad ligament by the **mesovarium** (portion of the peritoneal fold). Each ovary is attached to the side of the pelvis by the **suspensory ligaments**. An average, normal ovary is about 4 cm long, 2 cm wide, and 1.5 cm thick. See Figure 16.8.

Microscopic Anatomy

Each ovary consists of two distinct areas: the **cortex** or outer layer and the **medulla** or inner portion. The cortex contains small secretory sacs or follicles in three stages of development. These stages are known as **primary**, **growing**, and **graafian** or *mature stage*. The ovarian medulla contains connective tissue, nerves, blood and lymphatic vessels, and some smooth muscle tissue.

Major Functions of the Ovaries

The anterior lobe of the pituitary gland, which produces the *gonadotropic hormones* FSH and LH, primarily controls the functional activity of the ovaries. These abbreviations are for *follicle-stimulating hormone*, which is instrumental in the development of the ovarian follicles, and *luteinizing hormone*, which stimulates the development of the **corpus luteum**, a small yellow mass of cells that develops within a ruptured ovarian follicle.

Two major functions have been identified for the ovaries: the production of ova (female reproductive cells) and the production of hormones.

PRODUCTION OF OVA (OOCYTES)

Each month a *graafian follicle* ruptures on the ovarian cortex, and an ovum (singular of ova) discharges into the pelvic cavity, where it enters the fallopian tube. This process is known as ovulation. In an average, normal woman more than 400 ova may be produced during her reproductive years (refer to Figure 16.8).

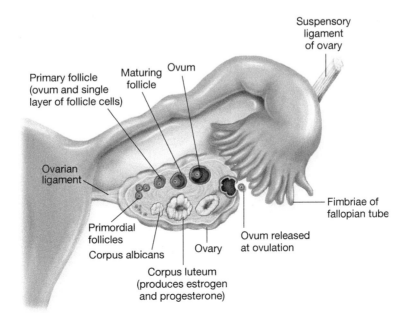

FIGURE 16.8 Ovary.

PRODUCTION OF HORMONES

The ovaries are also endocrine glands, producing estrogen, the female sex hormone secreted by the ovarian follicles, and progesterone, a steroid hormone secreted by the corpus luteum that is important in the maintenance of pregnancy. These hormones are essential in promoting growth and development and maintaining the female secondary sex organs and characteristics. These hormones also prepare the uterus for pregnancy, promote development of the mammary glands, and play a vital role in a woman's emotional well-being and sexual drive.

Vagina

The **vagina** is a musculomembranous tube extending from the vestibule to the uterus (refer to Figure 16.2). It is 8–10 cm in length and situated between the bladder and the rectum. It is lined by mucous membrane made up of *squamous epithelium*. A fold of mucous membrane, the **hymen**, partially or completely covers the external opening of the vagina, although it is sometimes absent.

Vulva

The **vulva** consists of the following five organs that comprise the external female genitalia (see Figure 16.9):

Mons pubis. A pad of fatty tissue of triangular shape and, after puberty, covered with pubic hair. It may be referred to as the *mons veneris* or *mound of Venus* and is the rounded area over the *symphysis pubis*.

Labia majora. The two folds of adipose tissue, which are large liplike structures, lying on either side of the vaginal opening.

Labia minora. Two thin folds of skin that lie within the labia majora and enclose the vestibule.

Vestibule. The cleft between the labia minora. It is approximately 4–5 cm long and 2 cm wide. Four major structures open into it: the urethra, the vagina, and two excretory ducts of the Bartholin glands.

Clitoris. A small organ consisting of sensitive erectile tissue that is homologous to the penis of the male. It is located between the anterior labial commissure and partially hidden by the anterior portion of the labia minora.

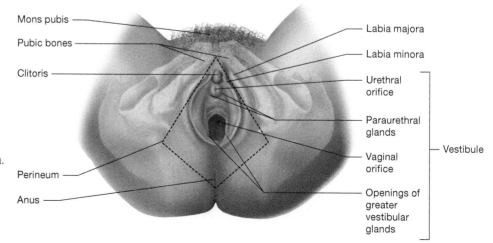

FIGURE 16.9 The female genitalia.
Source: AMERMAN, ERIN C., HUMAN ANATOMY & PHYSIOLOGY, 2nd Ed., ©2019. Reprinted and Electronically reproduced by permission of Pearson Education, Inc., New York, NY.

The **perineum** is the region bounded by the inferior edges of the pelvis. In the female, it is located between the vulva and the anus. It is a muscular sheet that forms the pelvic floor, and during childbirth it can be torn and cause injury to the anal sphincter. To avoid such an injury, an *episiotomy*, a surgical procedure to prevent tearing of the perineum and facilitate delivery of the baby, may be performed.

Breasts

The **breasts** or *mammary glands* are compound alveolar structures consisting of 15–20 glandular tissue lobes separated by septa of connective tissue. Most women have two breasts that lie anterior to the pectoral muscles and curve outward from the lateral margins of the sternum to the anterior border of the axilla. See Figure 16.10A. The size of the breast can vary greatly according to age, heredity, and adipose (fatty) tissue present.

The **areola** is the pigmented area found in the skin over each breast, and the *nipple* is the elevated area in the center of the areola. The color of the areola can range from pink to red to dark brown or nearly black, but generally tends to be paler among people with lighter skin tones and darker among people with darker skin tones. The areola is supplied with a row of small sebaceous glands that secrete an oily substance to keep it resilient. The *lactiferous glands* consist of 20–24 glands in the areola of the nipple, which convey milk to a suckling baby during **lactation** (the process of milk secretion). See Figure 16.10B.

The hormone **prolactin** is produced by the anterior lobe of the pituitary. Its primary function is to enhance breast development and initiate lactation (breastfeeding).

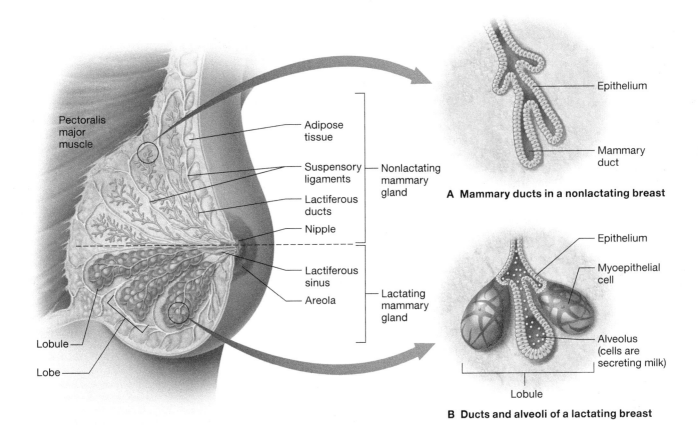

FIGURE 16.10 Internal anatomy of the female breast.

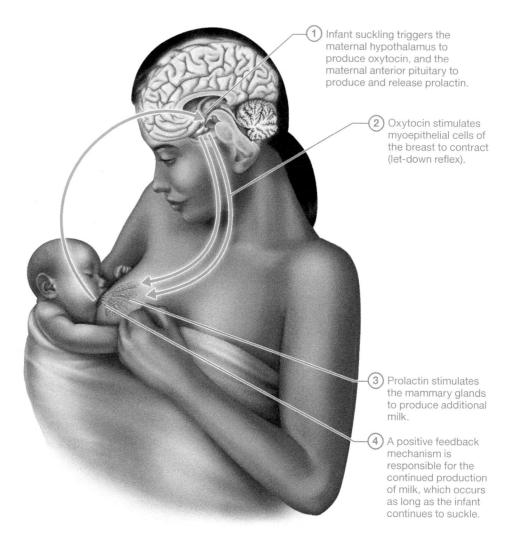

(1) Infant suckling triggers the maternal hypothalamus to produce oxytocin, and the maternal anterior pituitary to produce and release prolactin.

(2) Oxytocin stimulates myoepithelial cells of the breast to contract (let-down reflex).

(3) Prolactin stimulates the mammary glands to produce additional milk.

(4) A positive feedback mechanism is responsible for the continued production of milk, which occurs as long as the infant continues to suckle.

FIGURE 16.11 Hormonal regulation of lactation.
Source: AMERMAN, ERIN C., HUMAN ANATOMY & PHYSIOLOGY, 2nd Ed., ©2019. Reprinted and Electronically reproduced by permission of Pearson Education, Inc., New York, NY.

See Figure 16.11. Prolactin levels are normally elevated in pregnant and nursing women. Other hormones playing a role in milk production are insulin and glucocorticoids. **Colostrum**, a thin yellowish secretion, is the *first milk* and contains mainly serum and white blood cells.

Breastfeeding

Breastfeeding is the act of providing milk to a baby from the mother's breasts. Mature mother's milk and its precursor, *colostrum*, are considered to be the most balanced foods available for newborns and infants. Breast milk is easily digested, nonallergenic, and transmits maternal antibodies that protect against various infections and illnesses. In addition, the baby's suckling causes the release of **oxytocin** in the mother, which stimulates uterine contractions and promotes the return of the uterus to its normal nonpregnant size and state (refer to Figure 16.11).

fyi The American Academy of Pediatrics currently recommends that pediatricians and parents be aware that exclusive breastfeeding is sufficient to support optimal growth and development for approximately the first 6 months of life and provides continuing protection against diarrhea and respiratory tract infection. Breastfeeding should be continued for at least the first year of life.

Menstrual Cycle

The menstrual cycle is a periodic recurrent series of changes occurring in the uterus, ovaries, vagina, and breasts. It is regulated by the complex interaction of hormones: luteinizing hormone (LH) and follicle-stimulating hormone (FSH), which are produced by the pituitary gland, and the female sex hormones estrogen and progesterone, which are produced by the ovaries. The onset of the **menstrual cycle**, *menarche*, occurs at the age of **puberty** and ceases at **menopause**. The menstrual cycle occurs during a woman's reproductive years, except during **pregnancy**. The first day of bleeding is counted as the beginning of each menstrual cycle (day 1). The cycle ends just before the next menstrual period. The menstrual cycle occurs approximately every 21–35 days in an adult (the average cycle is 28 days) and has three phases: the follicular phase, ovulation, and the luteal phase. See Figure 16.12.

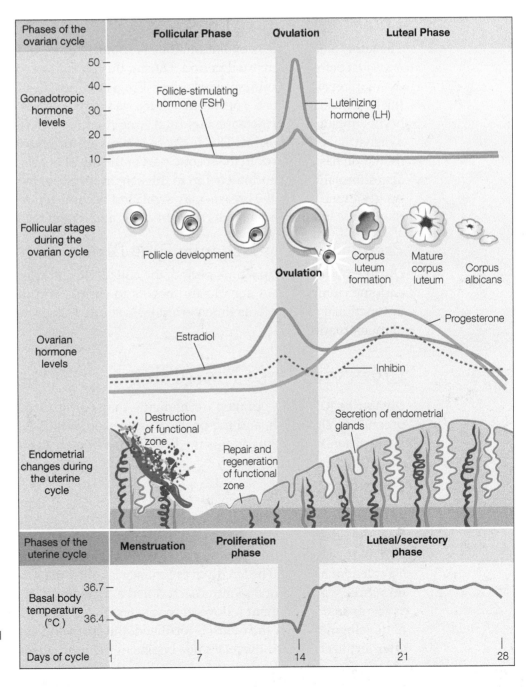

FIGURE 16.12 Hormonal regulation of the female reproductive cycle.

Follicular Phase

Menstruation, which marks the first day of the follicular phase, is characterized by the discharge of a bloody fluid from the uterus accompanied by a shedding of the endometrium. This phase averages 4–5 days and is considered to be the first to the fifth days of the cycle.

Ovulatory Phase

The **ovulatory phase** is characterized by the stimulation of estrogen, the thickening and vascularization of the endometrium, along with the maturing of the ovarian follicle. This phase begins about the fifth day and ends at the time of rupture of the graafian follicle (release of the egg), usually 36 hours after the surge in luteinizing hormone begins. About 12–24 hours after the egg is released, this surge can be detected by measuring the luteinizing hormone level in the urine. If the egg is not fertilized within 12–48 hours of being released, it disintegrates. The ovulatory phase occurs about 14 days before the onset of menstruation.

Luteal or Secretory Phase

The **luteal phase** follows ovulation. It lasts about 14 days, unless fertilization occurs, and ends just before a menstrual period. During this phase, the corpus luteum in the ovary is developing and secreting progesterone. Progesterone causes the mucus in the cervix to thicken, making the entry of sperm or bacteria into the uterus less likely. It also causes the body temperature to increase slightly during the luteal phase and remain elevated until a menstrual period begins. This increase in temperature can be used to estimate whether ovulation has occurred. In the second part of the luteal phase, the estrogen level increases, also stimulating the endometrium to thicken. In response to the increase in estrogen and progesterone levels, the breasts may swell and become tender. If the egg is not fertilized, the corpus luteum degenerates after 14 days, and a new menstrual cycle begins.

Premenstrual or Ischemic Time Period

During the **premenstrual** time period, the coiled uterine arteries become constricted, the endometrium becomes anemic and begins to shrink, and the corpus luteum decreases in functional activity. This time period lasts about 2 days and ends with the occurrence of menstruation.

Overview of Obstetrics

Obstetrics (OB) is the branch of medicine that pertains to the care of women during pregnancy, childbirth, and the postpartum period, which is also called the **puerperium**. A physician specializing in this medical field is known as an **obstetrician**.

Pregnancy

Pregnancy can be defined as a temporary condition that occurs within a woman's body from the time of conception through the embryonic and fetal periods to birth. The normal term of pregnancy is approximately 40 weeks (280 days); this equals 10 lunar months or 9⅓ calendar months. The length of pregnancy is called the **gestation period** and is divided into three segments of 3 months each called a **trimester**.

Human development follows three stages: the *preembryonic stage* is the first 14 days of development after the ovum is fertilized; the *embryonic stage* begins in the third week after fertilization; and the *fetal stage* begins in the ninth week. See Figure 16.13.

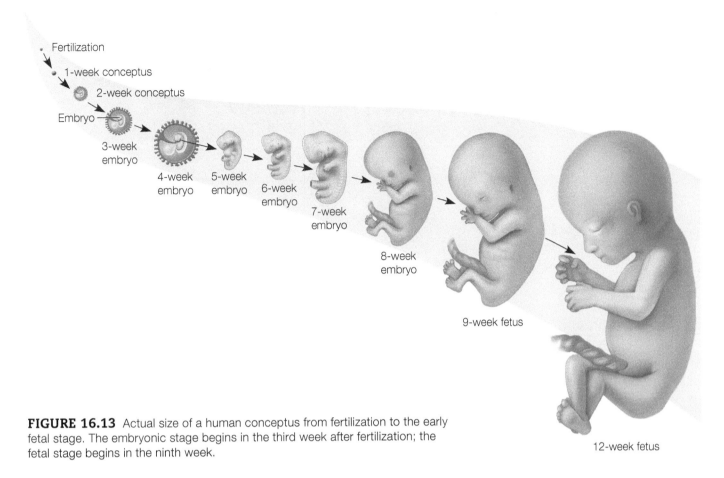

FIGURE 16.13 Actual size of a human conceptus from fertilization to the early fetal stage. The embryonic stage begins in the third week after fertilization; the fetal stage begins in the ninth week.

During the fifth week of development, the embryo has a marked C-shaped body and a rudimentary tail. At 7 weeks, the head of the embryo is rounded and nearly erect. The eyes have shifted forward and are closer together, and the eyelids begin to form. At 9 weeks, every organ system and external structure is present, and the developing embryo is now called a **fetus**.

At 14 weeks, the skin of the fetus is so transparent that blood vessels are visible beneath it. More muscle tissue and body skeleton have developed and hold the fetus more erect. At 20 weeks, the fetus weighs approximately 312 g and measures crown to rump about 16 cm. The skin is less transparent due to subcutaneous deposits of brown fat. Fingernails and toenails have developed and "woolly" hair may cover the head. See Figure 16.14.

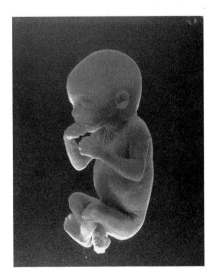

FIGURE 16.14 Fetus at 20 weeks. The fetus weighs approximately 312 g and measures about 16 cm. Subcutaneous deposits of brown fat make the skin less transparent.
Source: James Stevenson/Science Source

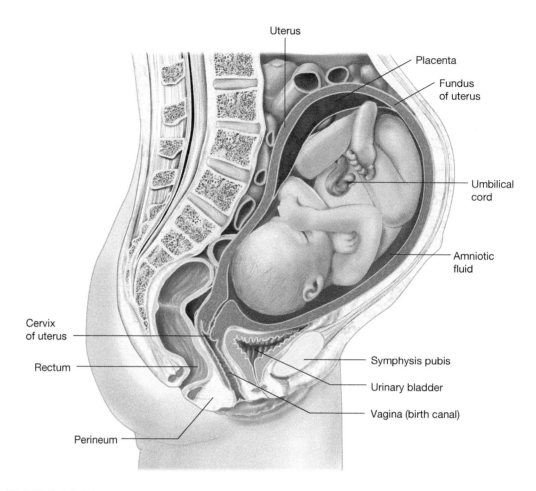

FIGURE 16.15 Position of fetus in full-term pregnancy.

Pregnancy is divided into four stages:

1. **Prenatal.** Time period between conception and onset of labor; refers to both the care of the woman during pregnancy and the growth and development of the fetus. Figure 16.15 shows the position of the fetus in a full-term pregnancy.

2. **Labor.** Time period during which forceful contractions move the fetus down the birth canal and expel it from the uterus during childbirth.

3. **Parturition.** Time period of actively giving birth; also known as **childbirth** or **delivery**.

4. **Postpartum period** or **puerperium.** Six-week time period following childbirth and expulsion of the placenta. The female reproductive organs usually return to an essentially prepregnant condition in which *involution of the uterus* (return of the uterus to normal size after childbirth) occurs.

Labor and Delivery

Labor is the process by which forceful contractions move the fetus down the birth canal and expel it from the uterus during childbirth. The signs and symptoms that labor is about to start can occur from hours to weeks before the actual onset of labor. Signs of impending labor include:

- ***Braxton Hicks contractions.*** Irregular contractions that begin in the second trimester and intensify as full term approaches.

- *Increased vaginal discharge.* Normally clear and nonirritating discharge caused by fetal pressure.
- *Lightening.* The descent of the baby into the pelvis. The expectant mother will notice that she can breathe easier and often states, "The baby has dropped." This may occur 2–3 weeks before the first stage of labor begins.
- *Bloody show.* Thick mucus mixed with pink or dark-brown blood. As the cervix softens, effaces, and dilates, the mucous plug that has sealed the uterus during pregnancy is dislodged from the cervix and small capillaries are torn, producing the bloody show.
- *Rupture of the membranes.* Occurs when the amniotic sac (bag of waters) ruptures.

  Note: When the membranes do not rupture on their own, they will be ruptured by the attending physician or midwife. This is known as **AROM: a**rtificial **r**upture **o**f **m**embranes.
- *Energy spurt or nesting.* Occurs in many women shortly before the onset of labor. They may suddenly have the energy to clean their houses and do things that they have not had the energy to do previously.
- *Weight loss.* Loss of 1–3 pounds shortly before labor can occur as hormone changes cause excretion of extra body water.

Stages of Labor

True labor is characterized by rhythmic contractions that develop a regular pattern and are more frequent, more intense, and last longer. A general feeling of discomfort is felt in the lower back and lower abdomen. A bloody show is often present, and progressive effacement and dilation of the cervix occur. Labor is divided into three stages: dilation, expulsion, and placental. See Figure 16.16.

- **First stage: Dilation.** Begins with the onset of true labor and lasts until the cervix is fully dilated to 10 cm.
- **Second stage: Expulsion.** Continues after the cervix is dilated to 10 cm until the delivery of the baby. During this stage, an **episiotomy**, a surgical procedure performed to prevent tearing of the perineum and to facilitate delivery of the fetus, may be performed.
- **Third stage: Placental.** Delivery of the placenta.

The **placenta** is a highly vascular organ that anchors the developing fetus to the uterus and provides the means by which the fetus receives its nourishment and oxygen. It also functions as an excretory, respiratory, and endocrine organ, which produces human chorionic gonadotropin (hCG). The placenta consists of a fetal portion and a maternal portion. The fetal portion has a shiny, slightly grayish appearance and is formed by a coming-together of chorionic villi in which the umbilical vein and arteries intertwine to form the **umbilical cord**. The maternal portion develops from the decidua basalis of the uterus. It has a red, beefy-looking appearance. The mature placenta is 15–18 cm (6–7 in.) in diameter and weighs approximately 450 g (about 1 lb). When expelled following parturition, it is known as the **afterbirth**.

 fyi The newborn baby usually has a cone-shaped or molded head due to its journey down the birth canal. It is covered with **vernix caseosa**, a protective cheesy substance that covers the fetus during intrauterine life. The baby will present with **lanugo**, fine downy hair that covers the body, especially the shoulders, back, forehead, and temple. The external **genitalia**, the male or female reproductive organs, are usually enlarged.

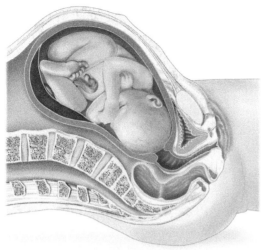

A DILATION STAGE:
Uterine contractions dilate cervix

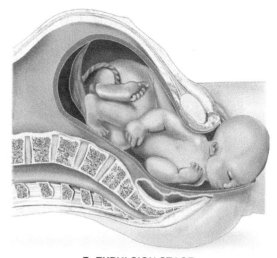

B EXPULSION STAGE:
Birth of baby or expulsion

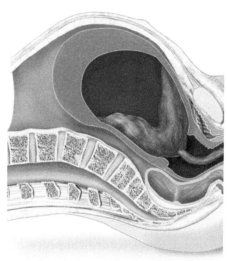

C PLACENTAL STAGE:
Delivery of placenta

FIGURE 16.16 Three stages of labor and delivery. **A** Dilation stage. **B** Expulsion stage. **C** Placental stage.

The time it takes to deliver the placenta is anywhere from 5 to 30 minutes. The placenta is expelled in one of two ways: the **Schultze mechanism**, with the fetal surface presenting, or the **Duncan mechanism** presenting the maternal surface. The placenta is examined to be certain that all of it has been expelled. Any small portion of the placenta that remains in the uterus could interfere with uterine contractions after the birth of the baby and contribute to infection. To control bleeding from the vessels that supplied the placenta during pregnancy, the uterus must contract and remain contracted after placental expulsion.

NEWBORN ASSESSMENT

The first assessment of the newborn involves using the Apgar score. It is performed immediately following the birth of the baby. This method was developed by Virginia Apgar (U.S. anesthesiologist, 1909–1974) as the first objective evaluation of newborns in 1952 and since then, the Apgar score has become the standard tool for assessing newborns.

The five assessments of the Apgar score are a mnemonic based on Virginia's last name. Ratings are based on Appearance (color), Pulse (heartbeat), Grimace (reflex), Activity (muscle tone), and Respiration (breathing). The score is taken at 1 and 5 minutes after birth, the high score being 10 and the low score being 1. See Table 16.2.

TABLE 16.2 The Apgar Score			
Sign	**0**	**1**	**2**
Heart rate	Absent	Less than 100/min	More than 100/min
Respiratory effort	Absent	Slow, irregular	Regular or crying
Reflex irritability	No response	Grimace, frown	Cry, cough
Muscle tone	Limp	Some motion, some flexion of extremities, some resistance to extension of extremities	Active, spontaneous flexion, good tone
Color	Cyanotic or pale	Body pink, extremities cyanotic	Completely pink or good color; no cyanosis

Study *and* Review I

Anatomy and Physiology

Write your answers to the following questions.

1. List the primary and accessory sex organs of the female reproductive system.

   a. _____ d. _____

   b. _____ e. _____

   c. _____ f. _____

2. The normal position of the uterus is known as _____.

3. Define *fundus*. _____

4. Name the three layers of the uterine wall.

   a. _____ c. _____

   b. _____

5. State two primary functions associated with the uterus.

   a. _____

   b. _____

6. Define the following terms.

    a. Retroflexion _____

    _____

    b. Anteversion _____

    _____

    c. Retroversion _____

    _____

7. The fallopian tubes are also called the _____ or

_____.

8. Should the ovum become impregnated by a spermatozoon while in the fallopian tube, the process of

_____ occurs.

9. State two major functions of the ovary.

    a. _____   **b.** _____

10. State three functions of the vagina.

    a. _____   **c.** _____

    b. _____

11. The breasts or _____ are compound alveolar structures.

12. The _____ is the pigmented area found in the skin over each breast, and the

_____ is the elevated area in its center.

13. Define colostrum. _____

_____

14. Name the three phases of the menstrual cycle.

    a. _____   **c.** _____

    b. _____

Overview of Obstetrics

Write your answers to the following questions.

1. _____ is the branch of medicine that pertains to the care of women during pregnancy, childbirth, and the postpartum period.

2. _____ is the process in which a sperm penetrates an ovum.

3. The fertilized ovum is also known as a _____.

4. As the blastocyst develops, it forms a structure with two cavities, the _____ and _____.

5. Pregnancy is divided into four stages. Describe each of these stages.

   a. Prenatal stage _____

   b. Labor _____

   c. Parturition _____

   d. Postpartum period _____

6. Labor is divided into three stages. Describe each of these stages.

   a. First stage _____

   b. Second stage _____

   c. Third stage _____

▶ **ANATOMY LABELING**   Identify the structures shown below by filling in the blanks.

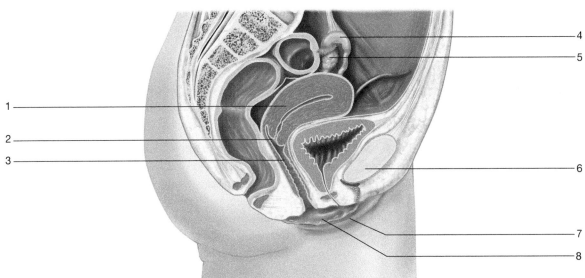

Building Your Medical Vocabulary

This section provides the foundation for learning medical terminology. Review the alphabetized list of medical terms in the following pages. Note how common prefixes and suffixes are repeatedly applied to word roots and combining forms to create different meanings. A combining form is a word root plus a vowel. The chart below lists the combining forms and word roots used in this chapter and can help to strengthen your understanding of how medical words are built and spelled.

You will find that some terms have not been divided into word parts. These are common words or specialized terms that are included to enhance your medical vocabulary.

Combining Forms

abort/o	to miscarry	**metr/o**	womb, uterus
cervic/o	cervix, neck	**metri/o**	womb, uterus
coit/o	a coming-together	**my/o**	muscle
colp/o	vagina	**o/o**	ovum, egg
culd/o	cul-de-sac	**oophor/o**	ovary
cyst/o	bladder	**pareun/o**	lying beside, sexual intercourse
fibr/o	fibrous tissue	**rect/o**	rectum
gynec/o	female	**salping/o**	fallopian tube
hyster/o	womb, uterus	**uter/o**	uterus
mamm/o	breast	**vagin/o**	vagina
mast/o	breast	**vers/o**	turning
men/o	month, menses, menstruation		

Word Roots

bartholin	Bartholin glands	**log**	study
cept	receive	**lump**	lump
genital	belonging to birth	**ovulat**	little egg
hymen	hymen	**pause**	cessation
lamp(s)	to shine		

Medical Word	Word Parts		Definition
	Part	**Meaning**	
abortion (AB) (ă-bōr´ shŭn)	**abort** **-ion**	to miscarry process	Process of miscarrying (either spontaneous or induced); termination of a pregnancy. Treatment during or after a miscarriage includes measures to prevent hemorrhage and infection. With any type of miscarriage, the patient should see her healthcare provider as soon as possible. If the abortion is incomplete and not all tissue has been expelled, a dilation and curettage (D&C), which is an expansion of the cervical canal and scraping of the uterine wall, is usually performed.

fyi

The risk for spontaneous abortion is higher in women over age 35, in women with systemic diseases such as diabetes mellitus or thyroid conditions, and in women with a history of three or more prior spontaneous abortions. The types of spontaneous abortions or miscarriages include the following:

Threatened. Uterine bleeding or spotting is accompanied by cramping or low-back pain. The cervix is not dilated. See Figure 16.17A.

Imminent or inevitable. Uterine bleeding or spotting is accompanied by cramping or low-back pain. The cervix is dilated. Miscarriage is inevitable when there is dilation or effacement of the cervix or rupture of the membranes. See Figure 16.17B.

Incomplete. Some products of conception have been expelled, but some remain in the uterus. Bleeding and cramps may persist when the miscarriage is not complete. See Figure 16.17C.

Complete. All of the products of conception are expelled. A completed miscarriage can be confirmed by an ultrasound.

Missed. A pregnancy demise in which nothing is expelled. It is not known why this occurs. Signs of this would be a loss of pregnancy symptoms and the absence of fetal heart tones.

Recurrent miscarriage (RM). Defined as three or more consecutive first-trimester miscarriages. Also referred to as *habitual abortion*.

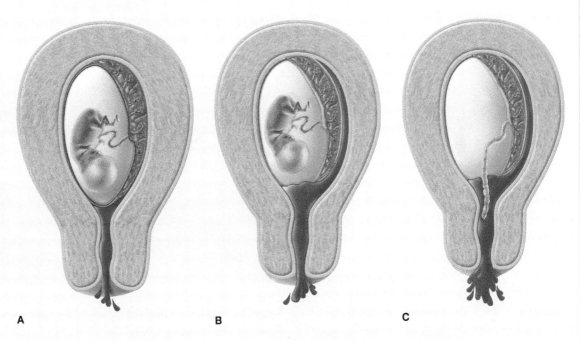

A   B   C

FIGURE 16.17 Types of spontaneous abortion. **A** Threatened: The cervix is not dilated, and the placenta is still attached to the uterine wall, but some bleeding occurs. **B** Imminent: The placenta has separated from the uterine wall, the cervix has dilated, and the amount of bleeding has increased. **C** Incomplete: The embryo or fetus has passed out of the uterus; however, the placenta remains.

Medical Word	Word Parts		Definition
	Part	Meaning	
adnexa (ăd-něk´ să)			Accessory parts of a structure; *adnexa uteri* refers to the ovaries and fallopian tubes
amenorrhea (ă-měn˝ ō-rē´ ă)	a- men/o -rrhea	lack of month, menses, menstruation flow	Lack of the monthly flow (menses or menstruation)
bartholinitis (băr˝ tō-lĭn-ī´ tĭs)	bartholin -itis	Bartholin glands inflammation	Inflammation of Bartholin glands. To check for swelling, redness, or tenderness, a Bartholin gland is palpated at the posterior labia majora.
cervicitis (sěr-vĭ-sī´ tĭs)	cervic -itis	cervix inflammation	Inflammation of the uterine cervix
cesarean section (CS, C-section)			Delivery of the fetus by means of an incision through the abdominal cavity and then into the uterus. See Figure 16.18. Elective C-section is indicated for known cephalopelvic (head to pelvis) disproportion, malpresentations, and active herpes infection. Fetal distress is the most common cause for an emergency C-section.

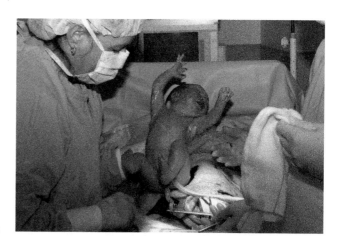

FIGURE 16.18 Cesarean birth.
Source: Francois Etienne du Plessis/Shutterstock

Medical Word	Word Parts		Definition
colposcope (kŏl´ pō-skōp)	colp/o -scope	vagina instrument for examining	Medical instrument used to examine the vagina and cervix by means of a magnifying lens

Medical Word	Word Parts		Definition
	Part	Meaning	
contraception (kŏn″ tră-sĕp′ shŭn)	contra- cept -ion	against receive process	Process of preventing conception
culdocentesis (kŭl″ dō-sĕn-tē′ sĭs)	culd/o -centesis	cul-de-sac surgical puncture	Surgical puncture of the cul-de-sac for removal of fluid
cystocele (sĭs′ tō-sēl)	cyst/o -cele	bladder hernia	Hernia of the bladder that protrudes into the vagina
Doppler ultrasound (dŏp′ lĕr ŭl′ tră-sownd)			Procedure using an audio transformation of high-frequency sounds to monitor the fetal heartbeat (FHB). See Figure 16.19.

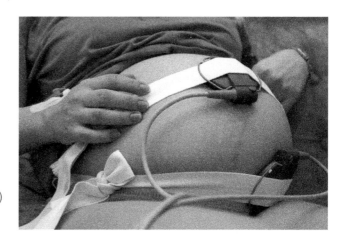

FIGURE 16.19 The fetal heartbeat (FHB) can be monitored with a Doppler device.
Source: ArtAs/iStock/Getty Images

dysmenorrhea (dĭs″ mĕn-ō-rē′ ă)	dys- men/o -rrhea	difficult, painful month, menses, menstruation flow	Difficult or painful monthly flow (menses or menstruation)
dyspareunia (dĭs″ pă-roo′ nē-ă)	dys- pareun -ia	difficult, painful lying beside, sexual intercourse condition	Difficult or painful sexual intercourse (copulation)
eclampsia (ĕ-klămp′ sē-ă)	ec- lamp(s) -ia	out to shine condition	Complication of severe preeclampsia that involves seizures; also known as *toxemia* or *pregnancy-induced hypertension (PIH)*

Medical Word	Word Parts		Definition
	Part	Meaning	
ectopic pregnancy (ĕk-tŏp´ ĭk prĕg´ năn-sē)			A pregnancy that occurs when the fertilized egg is implanted in one of various sites, the most common being a fallopian tube; also referred to as a *tubal pregnancy*. See Figure 16.20. This type of pregnancy is life-threatening to the mother and almost always fatal to her fetus.

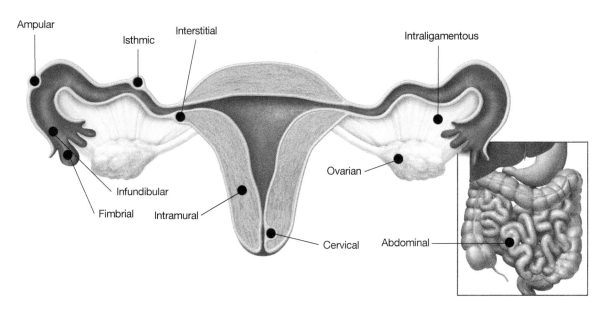

FIGURE 16.20 Various implantation sites in ectopic pregnancy. The most common site is within the fallopian tube, hence the term *tubal pregnancy*.

Medical Word	Word Parts		Definition
endometriosis (ĕn´´ dō-mē´´ trē-ō´ sĭs)	endo- metri -osis	within uterus condition	Pathological condition in which endometrial tissue has been displaced to various sites in the abdominal or pelvic cavity. This tissue responds to cyclic hormonal signals. Because it is outside the uterus and cannot be cast off each month, the tissue causes bleeding, with the formation of scars and adhesions. This is generally what causes daily or monthly cyclic pain.
fibroma (fī-brō´ mă)	fibr -oma	fibrous tissue tumor	Fibrous tissue tumor; also called *fibroid tumor*, the most common benign tumor found in women. See *uterine fibroid*.
genitalia (jĕn-ĭ-tāl´ ē-ă)	genital -ia	belonging to birth condition	Male or female reproductive organs. Refer to Figure 16.9 for female genitalia and Figure 17.2 for male genitalia.

Medical Word	Word Parts		Definition
	Part	Meaning	
gravida (grăv´ ĭ-dă)			Refers to any pregnancy, regardless of duration, including the present one; when used in the recording of an obstetrical history, indicates the number of pregnancies, for example, **nulligravida** refers to a woman who has never been pregnant and is written as gravida 0, **primigravida** refers to a woman who is pregnant for the first time and is written as gravida 1, **multigravida** refers to a woman who has been pregnant more than once and is written as gravida 2 (3, 4, 5, etc.).
group B streptococcus (GBS) (strĕp˝ tō-kŏk´ ŭs)			Type of bacterium commonly found in the vagina and intestinal tract; found in 10–25% of all pregnant women; it can cause life-threatening infections in the newborn
gynecologist (gī˝ nĕ-kŏl´ ō-jĭst)	**gynec/o** **log** **-ist**	female study one who specializes	Physician who specializes in the study of the female, especially the diseases of the female reproductive organs and the breasts
gynecology (GYN) (gī˝ nĕ-kŏl´ ō-jē)	**gynec/o** **-logy**	female study of	Study of the female, especially the diseases of the female reproductive organs and the breasts
hymenectomy (hī˝ mĕn-ĕk´ tō-mē)	**hymen** **-ectomy**	hymen surgical excision	Surgical excision of the membranous fold of tissue (the hymen) that partially or completely covers the vaginal opening. This procedure may be used to allow for the flow of the menses, allow for tampon use, and/or to allow for sexual intercourse.
hysterectomy (hĭs˝ tĕr-ĕk´ tō-mē)	**hyster** **-ectomy**	womb, uterus surgical excision	Surgical excision of the uterus

 fyi When the entire uterus, including the cervix, fallopian tubes, and ovaries, is removed during a hysterectomy, it is referred to as *total abdominal hysterectomy (TAH)* (removal of the uterus and cervix) *with bilateral salpingo-oophorectomy (BSO)* (removal of the fallopian tubes and ovaries). If a woman has not yet reached menopause, a hysterectomy stops menstruation (monthly periods) and ends her ability to become pregnant. This is referred to as *surgical menopause.*

Medical Word	Word Parts		Definition
hysteroscope (hĭs´ tĕr-ō-skōp)	**hyster/o** **-scope**	womb, uterus instrument for examining	Instrument used in the biopsy of uterine tissue before 12 weeks of gestation. This tissue is then analyzed for chromosome arrangement, DNA sequence, and genetic defects.

Medical Word	Word Parts		Definition
	Part	**Meaning**	
hysterotomy (hĭs″ tĕr-ŏt´ ō-mē)	**hyster/o** **-tomy**	womb, uterus incision	Incision into the uterus, commonly combined with a laparotomy (surgical incision into the abdomen) during a cesarean section
intrauterine (ĭn´ tră-ū´ tĕr-ĭn)	**intra-** **uter** **-ine**	within uterus pertaining to	Pertaining to within the uterus
laser ablation (lā´ zĕr ăb-lā´ shŭn)			Procedure that uses a laser to destroy the uterine lining; may also be called *endometrial ablation*. A biopsy is performed before the procedure to make sure no cancer is present. This procedure can be used to reduce excessive menstrual bleeding. It causes sterility.
linea nigra (lĭn´ ē-ă nī´ gră)			Dark line on the abdomen that runs from above the umbilicus to the pubis during pregnancy. See Figure 16.21. The term comes from Latin and literally means *black line*. It can be light and barely visible in some women or it can be much darker than the surrounding skin and stand out more clearly in other women.

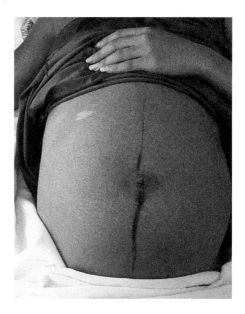

FIGURE 16.21 Linea nigra.
Source: Pearson Education, Inc.

lochia (lō´ kē-ă)			Vaginal discharge occurring after childbirth. At first it is blood-tinged (*lochia rubra*); then, after 3 or 4 days, it becomes pink and brown-tinged (*lochia serosa*); after that, it becomes yellow and then turns to white (*lochia alba*). Lochia typically last 2–4 weeks.

Medical Word	Word Parts		Definition
	Part	Meaning	
lumpectomy (lŭm-pĕkʹ tō-mē)	lump -ectomy	lump surgical excision	Surgical removal of a tumor from the breast. This procedure removes only the tumor and some surrounding tissue but no lymph nodes. See Figure 16.22.

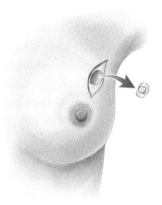

Lumpectomy

FIGURE 16.22 A lumpectomy removes only the tumor and a small margin of surrounding tissue.

Medical Word	Word Parts		Definition
mammoplasty (mămʹ ō-plăsʺ tē)	mamm/o -plasty	breast surgical repair	Surgical repair of the breast
mastectomy (măs-tĕkʹ tō-mē)	mast -ectomy	breast surgical excision	Surgical excision of the breast can involve a modified radical or a radical mastectomy. With a modified radical approach, all of the breast tissue and the underarm lymph nodes are removed but the muscles remain intact. See Figure 16.23. In a radical mastectomy (not shown), the chest muscles are removed.

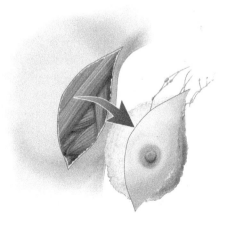

Modified radical mastectomy

FIGURE 16.23 A modified radical mastectomy removes all breast tissue and the underarm lymph nodes but leaves the underlying muscles.

Medical Word	Word Parts		Definition
	Part	Meaning	
mastitis (măs-tī′ tis)	mast	breast	Inflammation of the breast that occurs most commonly in women who are breastfeeding. See Figure 16.24. It is caused by bacteria that enter through a crack or abrasion of the nipple. Generalized symptoms include fever, chills, and headache. Localized symptoms include breast pain, redness, tenderness, and swelling.
	-itis	inflammation	

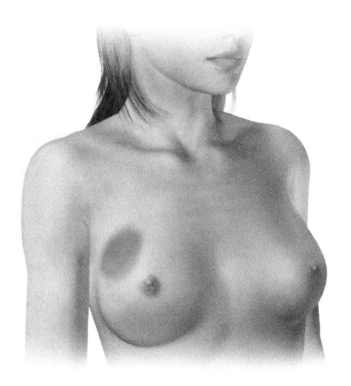

FIGURE 16.24 Mastitis. Inflammation and swelling are present in the upper outer quadrant of the breast.

menarche (mĕn-ar′ kē)	men	month, menses, menstruation	Beginning of the first monthly flow (menses, menstruation)
	-arche	beginning	

 ALERT!

How many words can you build using the root **men** and the combining form **men/o**?

Medical Word	Word Parts		Definition
	Part	Meaning	
menopause (měn´ ō-pawz)	men/o	month, menses, menstruation	Cessation of the monthly flow; also called *climacteric*
	pause	cessation	

fyi At about 50 years of age, men and women begin experiencing bodily changes that are directly related to hormonal production. In women, the ovaries cease to produce estrogen and progesterone. With decreased production of these female hormones, women enter the phase of life known as *menopause*.

The symptoms of menopause vary from being hardly noticeable to being severe and can include hot flashes, vaginal dryness, insomnia, joint pain, headache, mood changes, irritability, and depression. Breast tissue can lose its firmness, and pubic and axillary hair becomes sparse. Without estrogen, the uterus becomes smaller, the vagina shortens, and vaginal tissues become drier. There can be loss of bone mass, leading to **osteoporosis**, a condition characterized by a decrease in the density of bones causing them to become weak and fragile.

Medical Word	Word Parts		Definition
menorrhagia (měn″ ō-rā´ jē-ă)	men/o	month, menses, menstruation	Excessive uterine bleeding at the time of a menstrual period, either in number of days or amount of blood or both. Can be caused by such conditions as uterine fibroid tumors, pelvic inflammatory disease, or an endocrine imbalance.
	-rrhagia	to burst forth	
menorrhea (měn″ ō-rē´ ă)	men/o	month, menses, menstruation	Normal monthly flow (menses, menstruation)
	-rrhea	flow	
mittelschmerz (mĭt´ ěl-shmārts)			Abdominal pain that occurs midway between the menstrual periods at ovulation
myometritis (mī″ ō-mē-trī´ tĭs)	my/o	muscle	Inflammation of the muscular wall of the uterus
	metr	womb, uterus	
	-itis	inflammation	
oligomenorrhea (ŏl″ ĭ-gō-měn″ ō-rē´ ă)	oligo-	scanty	Scanty monthly flow (menses, menstruation)
	men/o	month, menses, menstruation	
	-rrhea	flow	
oogenesis (ō″ ō-jěn´ ě-sĭs)	o/o	ovum, egg	Formation of the ovum
	-genesis	formation, produce	
oophorectomy (ō″ ŏf-ō-rěk´ tō-mē)	oophor	ovary	Surgical excision of an ovary
	-ectomy	surgical excision	

Medical Word	Word Parts		Definition
	Part	Meaning	
ovulation (ŏv″ ū-lā′ shŭn)	ovulat -ion	little egg process	Process in which an ovum is discharged from the cortex of the ovary; periodic ripening and rupture of a mature graafian follicle and the discharge of an ovum from the cortex of the ovary. See Figure 16.25. Occurs approximately 14 days before the onset of the next menstrual period.

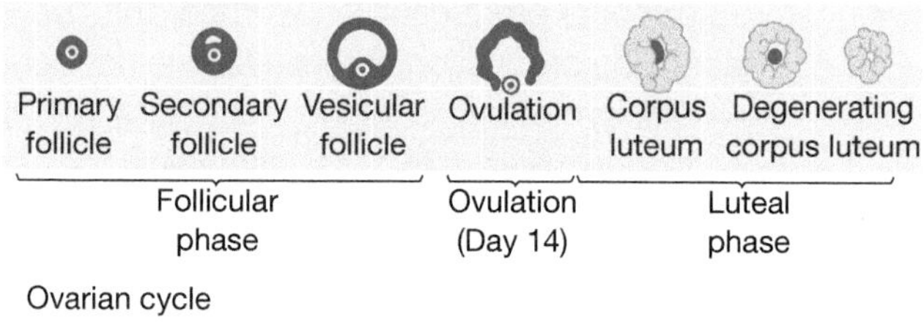

FIGURE 16.25 Changes in the ovarian follicle during the 28-day ovarian cycle.

Primary follicle | Secondary follicle | Vesicular follicle | Ovulation | Corpus luteum | Degenerating corpus luteum

Follicular phase | Ovulation (Day 14) | Luteal phase

Ovarian cycle

para			Means to bear or bring forth; refers to a woman who has given birth after a minimum of 20 weeks' gestation, regardless of whether the baby is born alive or dead

fyi When recording an obstetrical history, *para* is used to indicate the number of births. For example, **multipara** refers to a woman who has given birth to two or more children and is written as para 2 (3, 4, 5, etc.); **nullipara** refers to a woman who has not given birth after more than 20 weeks of gestation and is written as para 0; and **primipara** refers to a woman who has had one birth at more than 20 weeks' gestation, regardless of whether the infant was born alive or dead, and is written as para 1.

pelvic inflammatory disease (PID) (pĕl′ vĭk ĭn-flăm′ ă-tŏr″ ē)			Infection of the upper genital area; can affect the uterus, ovaries, and fallopian tubes

fyi *Pelvic inflammatory disease (PID)* is the most common and serious complication of sexually transmitted infections (STIs) among women. This infection of the upper genital area occurs when disease-causing organisms migrate upward from the vagina and cervix into the upper genital area. If untreated, it can cause scarring, which can lead to infertility, tubal pregnancy, chronic pelvic pain, and other serious consequences. Infertility occurs in approximately 20% of women who have had PID.

perimenopause (pĕr-ē-mĕn′ ō-pawz)	peri- men/o pause	around month, menses, menstruation cessation	Period of gradual changes that lead into menopause, affecting a woman's hormones, body, and feelings. It can be a stop–start process that can take months or years. Hormone levels fluctuate, thereby causing changes in the menstrual cycle, which becomes irregular.

Medical Word	Word Parts		Definition
	Part	Meaning	
placenta previa (plă-sĕn′ tă prē′ vē-ă)			In this condition, the placenta is improperly implanted in the lower uterine segment. The fetus receives less oxygen and the expectant mother has an increased risk of hemorrhage and infection. Placenta previa is classified as one of four degrees (Figure 16.26): **Grade 1.** The placenta is implanted in the lower uterine segment but does not reach the internal cervical os, although it is in close proximity to it (Figure 16.26A). **Grade 2.** Placental tissue reaches the margin of the internal cervical os, but does not cover it. **Grade 3.** The placenta partially covers the internal cervical os (Figure 16.26B). **Grade 4.** The placenta completely covers the internal cervical os (Figure 16.26C).

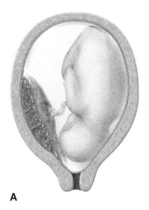
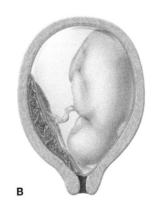
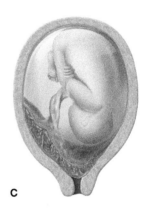

A B C

FIGURE 16.26 Placenta previa. **A** Grade 1, low-lying placental implantation. **B** Grade 3, partial placenta previa. **C** Grade 4, complete placenta previa.

fyi The most common symptom of placenta previa is painless uterine bleeding during the second half of pregnancy. Bleeding can be scanty or profuse (hemorrhage). When this occurs, the expectant mother is advised to go to the hospital.

To determine a diagnosis, a transabdominal ultrasound examination is performed to pinpoint the placenta's location. A vaginal examination is usually avoided because it could trigger heavy bleeding. A woman who has been diagnosed with placenta previa may need to stay in the hospital until delivery. If the bleeding stops, and it often does, her physician continues to monitor the expectant mother and her baby.

Medical Word	Word Parts		Definition
	Part	**Meaning**	
postcoital (pōst-kō´ ĭt-ăl)	**post-**	after	Pertaining to after sexual intercourse
	coit	a coming- together	
	-al	pertaining to	
preeclampsia (prē˝ ĕ-klămp´ sē-ă)	**pre-**	before	Serious complication of pregnancy characterized by increasing hypertension, proteinuria (abnormal concentrations of urinary protein), and edema; also known as *pregnancy-induced hypertension (PIH)*
	ec-	out	
	lamp(s)	to shine	
	-ia	condition	
premenstrual syndrome (PMS) (prē-mĕn´ stroo-ăl)			Condition that affects certain women and can cause distressful symptoms that begin 2 weeks before the onset of menstruation. The cause is unknown but may be due to the amount of prostaglandin produced, a deficient or excessive amount of estrogen or progesterone, or an interrelationship between these factors. The multisystem effects of premenstrual syndrome are presented in Figure 16.27.

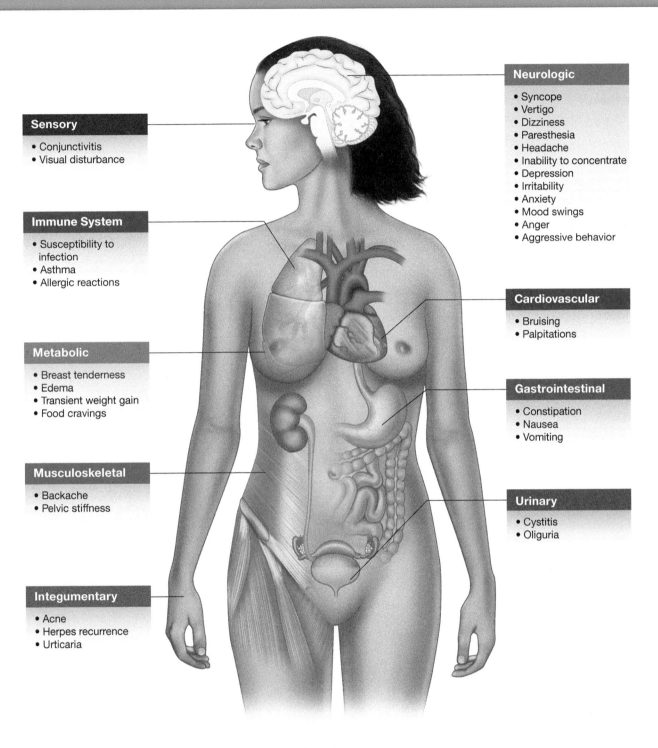

Sensory
- Conjunctivitis
- Visual disturbance

Immune System
- Susceptibility to infection
- Asthma
- Allergic reactions

Metabolic
- Breast tenderness
- Edema
- Transient weight gain
- Food cravings

Musculoskeletal
- Backache
- Pelvic stiffness

Integumentary
- Acne
- Herpes recurrence
- Urticaria

Neurologic
- Syncope
- Vertigo
- Dizziness
- Paresthesia
- Headache
- Inability to concentrate
- Depression
- Irritability
- Anxiety
- Mood swings
- Anger
- Aggressive behavior

Cardiovascular
- Bruising
- Palpitations

Gastrointestinal
- Constipation
- Nausea
- Vomiting

Urinary
- Cystitis
- Oliguria

FIGURE 16.27 Multisystem effects of premenstrual syndrome.

Medical Word	Word Parts		Definition
	Part	Meaning	
rectovaginal (rĕk″ tō-văj′ ĭ-năl)	rect/o vagin -al	rectum vagina pertaining to	Pertaining to the rectum and vagina
retroversion (rĕt″ rō-vĕr′ shŭn)	retro- vers -ion	backward turning process	Process of being turned backward, such as the displacement of the uterus with the cervix pointed forward. Refer to Figure 16.4A.
salpingectomy (săl″ pĭn-jĕk′ tō-mē)	salping -ectomy	fallopian tube surgical excision	Surgical excision of a fallopian tube
salpingitis (săl″ pĭn-jī′ tĭs)	salping -itis	fallopian tube inflammation	Inflammation of a fallopian tube
salpingo- oophorectomy (săl′ pĭng″ gō-ō″ ŏf-ō-rĕk′ tō-mē)	salping/o oophor -ectomy	fallopian tube ovary surgical excision	Surgical excision of an ovary and a fallopian tube
toxic shock syndrome (TSS)			A serious bacterial infection caused by *staphylococcus aureus* bacteria. Symptoms of TSS start suddenly with vomiting, high fever (temperature at least 102°F [38.8°C]), a rapid drop in blood pressure (with lightheadedness or fainting), watery diarrhea, headache, sore throat, and muscle aches.

Medical Word	Word Parts		Definition
	Part	**Meaning**	
uterine fibroid (ū´ tĕr-ĭn fī-broyd)	**uter** **-ine** **fibr** **-oid**	uterus pertaining to fibrous tissue resemble	Benign fibrous tumor of the uterus made up of muscle cells and other tissues that grow within the wall of the uterus; the most common benign tumors in women of childbearing age; also called *uterine leiomyoma*. See Figure 16.28. Fibroids are classified into three groups based on where they grow, such as just underneath the lining of the uterus, between the muscles of the uterus, or on the outside of the uterus. Most fibroids grow within the wall of the uterus, and some grow on stalks (called *peduncles*) that grow out from the surface of the uterus or into the cavity of the uterus.

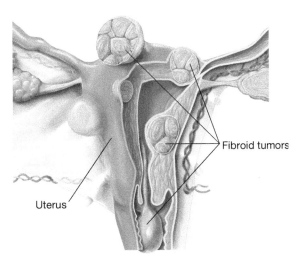

Fibroid tumors

Uterus

FIGURE 16.28 Types of uterine fibroid tumors.

fyi Types of surgery used to treat uterine fibroids include:

- *Dilation and curettage (D&C)* is a procedure that involves enlarging the cervix (dilation) and then scraping (curettage) out portions of the lining of the uterus. It is considered to be minor surgery performed in a hospital, ambulatory surgery center, or clinic.
- *Myomectomy* is a surgery to remove fibroids without taking out the healthy tissue of the uterus. It can be major surgery (with an abdominal incision) or minor surgery. The type, size, and location of the fibroids determine what type of procedure is done.
- *Hysterectomy* is a surgery to remove the uterus and is the only sure way to cure uterine fibroids. This surgery is used when a woman's fibroids are large or if she has heavy bleeding and is either near or past menopause and/or does not want to become pregnant in the future.

vaginitis (văj˝ ĭn-ī´ tĭs)	**vagin** **-itis**	vagina inflammation	Inflammation of the vagina

Study *and* Review II

Word Parts

Prefixes Give the definitions of the following prefixes.

1. a- _____

2. contra- _____

3. dys- _____

4. ec- _____

5. endo- _____

6. intra- _____

7. oligo- _____

8. peri- _____

9. post- _____

10. retro- _____

11. pre- _____

Combining Forms Give the definitions of the following combining forms.

1. abort/o _____

2. cervic/o _____

3. coit/o _____

4. colp/o _____

5. culd/o _____

6. cyst/o _____

7. fibr/o _____

8. gynec/o _____

9. hyster/o _____

10. mamm/o _____

11. mast/o _____

12. men/o _____

13. metr/o _____

14. my/o _____

15. o/o _____

16. oophor/o _____

17. pareun/o _____

18. rect/o _____

19. salping/o _____

20. uter/o _____

21. vagin/o _____

22. vers/o _____

Suffixes Give the definitions of the following suffixes.

1. -al _____

2. -arche _____

3. -cele _____

4. -centesis _____

5. -ectomy _____

6. -genesis _____

7. -ia _____

8. -ine _____

9. -ion _____

10. -ist _____

11. -itis _____

12. -oma _____

13. -osis _____

14. -plasty _____

15. -rrhagia _____

16. -rrhea _____

17. -scope _____

18. -oid _____

Identifying Medical Terms

In the spaces provided, write the medical terms for the following meanings.

1. _____ Inflammation of the uterine cervix

2. _____ Difficult or painful monthly flow

3. _____ Fibrous tissue tumor

4. _____ Study of the female

5. _____ Surgical excision of the hymen

6. _____ Surgical repair of the breast

7. _____ Normal monthly flow

8. _____ Formation of the ovum

9. _____ Difficult or painful sexual intercourse

10. _____ Male or female reproductive organs

Matching

Select the appropriate lettered meaning for each of the following words.

_____ 1. laser ablation

_____ 2. lumpectomy

_____ 3. menarche

_____ 4. mittelschmerz

_____ 5. ovulation

_____ 6. gynecologist

_____ 7. contraception

_____ 8. perimenopause

_____ 9. hysterotomy

_____ 10. rectovaginal

a. Beginning of the first monthly flow (menses, menstruation)

b. Surgical removal of a tumor from the breast

c. Abdominal pain that occurs midway between the menstrual periods at ovulation

d. Process in which an ovum is discharged from the cortex of the ovary

e. Procedure that uses a laser to destroy the uterine lining

f. Pertaining to the rectum and vagina

g. Period of gradual changes that lead into menopause

h. Physician who specializes in the study of the female

i. Incision into the uterus

j. Process of preventing conception

Medical Case Snapshots

This learning activity provides an opportunity to relate the medical terminology you are learning to sample patient case presentations. In the spaces provided, write in your answers.

Case 1

A pregnant 36-year-old woman calls her obstetrician's office, stating, "I am passing bright-red blood and I am cramping. Please tell me what to do. I don't want to lose my baby." The woman was advised to immediately come to the doctor's office. A threatened abortion is one with _____ bleeding or spotting accompanied by _____ or low-back pain. The _____ is not dilated.

Case 2

A 21-year-old female is seen in the emergency room. She has missed her last two periods and feels sick. An ultrasound is ordered stat (immediately). The ultrasound confirmed an _____ pregnancy or tubal _____. A(n) _____ or physician specializing in the care of women during pregnancy, childbirth, and the postpartum period is notified of this patient's condition.

Case 3

A 52-year-old female complains of irregular periods (menses), hot flashes, insomnia, difficult or painful sexual intercourse, and moodiness. The medical term for painful sexual intercourse is _____. Her condition is known as _____ (or period of gradual changes that lead into menopause).

Drug Highlights

Classification of Drug	Description and Examples
female hormones	
estrogens	Natural female sex hormone secreted by the ovarian follicles. Used for a variety of conditions including amenorrhea, dysfunctional uterine bleeding (DUB), and hirsutism as well as in palliative therapy for breast cancer in women and prostatic cancer in men. They are also used as hormone therapy (HT) in the treatment of uncomfortable symptoms that are related to menopause. EXAMPLES: Premarin (conjugated estrogens), estradiol, Ogen (estropipate), and Menest (esterified estrogens)
progestogens/ progestins	The class of steroid hormones that activate the progesterone receptor. Progesterone is the natural female steroid hormone secreted by the corpus luteum. When produced synthetically, progesterone can be used to prevent uterine bleeding; combined with estrogen they can be used for treatment of amenorrhea. They may be used in cases of infertility and threatened or habitual miscarriage. Progesterone is responsible for changes in the uterine endometrium during the second half of the menstrual cycle, development of maternal placenta after implantation, and development of mammary glands. EXAMPLES: Provera (medroxyprogesterone acetate), norethindrone acetate, and Prometrium (natural progesterone)
contraceptives	
combined oral contraceptives (COCs)	Oral contraceptives (also called *birth control pills*) containing mixtures of estrogen and progestin in various levels of strength that are nearly 100% effective when used as directed. See Figure 16.29. The estrogen in the pill inhibits ovulation, and the progestin inhibits pituitary secretion of luteinizing hormone, causes changes in the cervical mucus that renders it unfavorable to penetration by sperm, and alters the nature of the endometrium. EXAMPLES: Micronor, Brevicon, Lo/Ovral, and Nor-QD

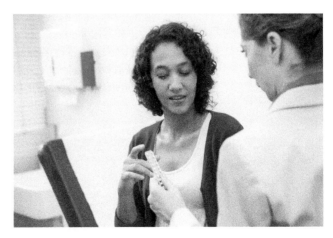

FIGURE 16.29 Physician showing her patient combined oral contraceptives (COCs).
Source: Image Point Fr/Shutterstock

minipill	Another oral contraceptive is the minipill, which contains only progestin. It is taken daily and continuously. It acts by interfering with sperm and ovum transport and by adversely affecting the suitability of the endometrium for ovum implant. EXAMPLE: Nexplanon

Classification of Drug	Description and Examples
birth control patch	Ortho Evra is the first transdermal birth control patch that continuously delivers two synthetic hormones, progestin (norelgestromin) and estrogen (ethinyl estradiol). The patch impedes pregnancy by preventing the ovaries from releasing eggs (ovulation) and thickening the cervical mucus. The patch is applied directly to the skin (buttocks, abdomen, upper torso, or upper outer arm) and has an effectiveness rate of 95%. See Figure 16.30.

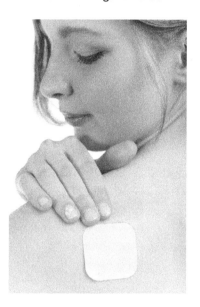

FIGURE 16.30 Birth control patch.
Source: Tomasz Trojanowski/Shutterstock

Classification of Drug	Description and Examples
injectable	Depo-Provera is an injectable contraceptive that is given four times a year. It contains medroxyprogesterone acetate, a synthetic drug that is similar to progesterone. Depo-Provera prevents pregnancy by stopping the ovaries from releasing eggs (ovulation) and thickens the cervical mucus. When used correctly, it can prevent pregnancy over 99% of the time.
intrauterine device (IUD)	Small device that is placed within the uterus to prevent pregnancy. See Figure 16.31. It is usually made of soft, flexible, ultralight plastic and is 99.2–99.9% effective as birth control. Two types are available: ParaGard and Mirena. ParaGard uses copper around the plastic. Anyone allergic to copper should not use it. Mirena releases small amounts of a synthetic progesterone over time and can be left in place for up to 5 years. IUDs do not protect against sexually transmitted infections (STIs) or the human immunodeficiency virus (HIV).

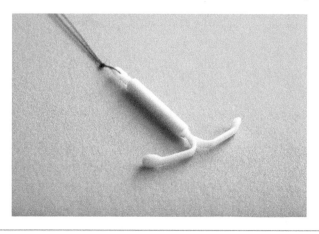

FIGURE 16.31 Example of intrauterine device (IUD).
Source: Image Point Fr/Shutterstock

Diagnostic *and* Laboratory Tests

Test	Description
amniocentesis (ăm″ nē-ō-sĕn-tē′ sĭs)	Surgical puncture of the amniotic sac to obtain a sample of amniotic fluid containing fetal cells that are examined. It can be determined whether the fetus has Down syndrome, neural tube defects, Tay-Sachs disease, or other genetic defects. Determines chromosomal abnormalities and biochemical disorders. See Figure 16.32.

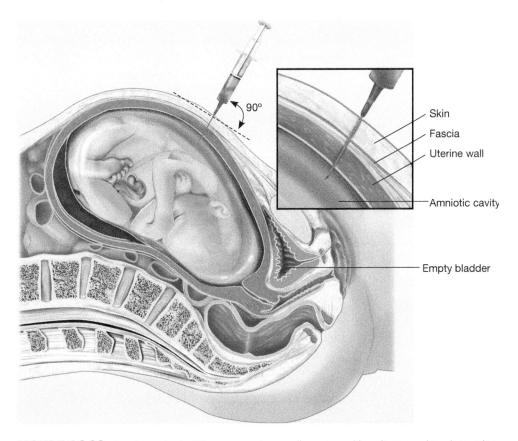

FIGURE 16.32 Amniocentesis. The woman is usually scanned by ultrasound to determine the placental site and to locate a pocket of fluid. As the needle is inserted, three levels of resistance are felt when the needle penetrates the skin, fascia, and uterine wall. When the needle is placed within the amniotic cavity, amniotic fluid is withdrawn.

blood grouping (A, B, AB, and O)	Determines blood type.
breast examination	Visual inspection and manual examination of the breast for changes in contour, symmetry, dimpling of skin, retraction of the nipple, and the presence of lumps.
chorionic villus sampling (CVS) (kō″ rē-ŏn′ ĭk vĭl′ ŭs)	Removal of a small sample of the placenta to determine chromosomal abnormalities and biochemical disorders (Down syndrome, Tay-Sachs disease, and cystic fibrosis). Unlike amniocentesis, CVS does not test for neural tube defects.

Test	Description
colposcopy (kŏl-pŏs´ kō-pē)	Visual examination of the vagina and cervix via a colposcope. Abnormal results can indicate cervical or vaginal erosion, tumors, and dysplasia.
complete blood count	Check for anemia, infection, and cell abnormalities.
cordocentesis (kor-dō-sĕn-tē´ sĭs)	Examine blood from the fetus to detect fetal abnormalities (Down syndrome and fetal blood disorders); also known as fetal blood sampling, percutaneous umbilical blood sampling (PUBS), and umbilical vein sampling.
culdoscopy (kŭl-dŏs´ kō-pē)	Direct visual examination of the viscera of the female pelvis through a culdoscope. The instrument is introduced into the pelvic cavity through the posterior vaginal fornix. Can be used to diagnose ectopic pregnancy and to determine the cause of pelvic pain and to check for pelvic masses.
estrogen (es´ trō-jĕn)	Test done on urine or blood serum to determine the level of estrone, estradiol, and estriol.
group B streptococcus (GBS) screening (strĕp˝ tō-kŏk´ ŭs)	Screen for vaginal strep B infection. It is to be performed between the 35th and 37th week of pregnancy. Any time other than this will not be significant to show if the expectant mother is carrying GBS during her time of delivery. *Note:* When the expectant mother tests positive, intravenous antibiotics are recommended during delivery to reduce the chance of the baby becoming infected with GBS.
hematocrit (hē-măt´ ō-krĭt)	Check for anemia during pregnancy.
hemoglobin (hē´ mŏ-glō˝ bĭn)	Check for anemia during pregnancy.
hepatitis B screen (hĕp˝ ă-tī´ tĭs)	Identify carriers of hepatitis.
human chorionic gonadotropin (hCG) (kō˝ rē-ŏn-ĭk gō-năd´ ō-trō´ pĭn)	Determine the presence of hCG, which is secreted by the placenta. A positive result usually indicates pregnancy.
human immunodeficiency virus (HIV) screen (ĭm˝ ū-nō-dĕ-fĭsh´ ĕn-sē)	Identify HIV infection.
hysterosalpingography (HSG) (hĭs˝ tĕr-ō-săl˝ pĭn-gŏg´ ră-fē)	X-ray of the uterus and fallopian tubes after the injection of a radiopaque substance. Size and structure of the uterus and fallopian tubes can be evaluated. Uterine tumors, fibroids, tubal pregnancy, and tubal occlusion can be observed. Also used for treatment of an occluded fallopian tube.
laparoscopy (lăp-ăr-ŏs´ kō-pē)	Visual examination of the abdominal cavity. A flexible, lighted instrument (laparoscope) is inserted through a periumbilical incision to examine the ovaries and fallopian tubes.

Test	Description
mammography (măm-ŏg´ ră-fē)	Specific type of imaging that uses a low-dose x-ray system for examination of the breasts. See Figure 16.33. A mammography exam is called a *mammogram*. The two types of mammograms are *screening*, which is generally used to detect breast cancer or other changes in the breast tissue in women who do not have symptoms, and *diagnostic*, which can be ordered when a screening mammogram shows something abnormal in the breast. It is the most effective means of detecting early breast cancers. See Figure 16.34.

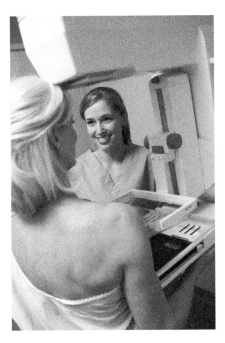

FIGURE 16.33 Recommended position for mammography.
Source: Shutterstock

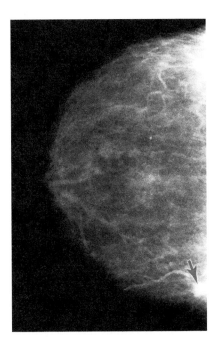

FIGURE 16.34 Mammogram with cancer indicated by arrow.
Source: Dr. Dwight Kaufman/National Cancer Institute

Test	Description
maternal blood glucose	Screen for gestational diabetes. If the level of glucose is moderately elevated, a more conclusive glucose tolerance test (GTT) may be ordered.
nonstress test (NST)	Identify fetal compromise in conditions with poor placenta function, such as hypertension, diabetes mellitus, or postterm gestation (pregnancy lasting beyond 42 weeks).

Test	Description
Papanicolaou (Pap) smear (păp″ ă-nē′ kă-lŏw″)	Screening technique to aid in the detection of cervical cancer. Both false-positive and false-negative results have been experienced with Pap smears. See Figure 16.35. Pap smear results are generally reported as within normal limits (WNL), atypical squamous cells of undetermined significance (ASCUS), mild dysplasia (CIN [cervical intraepithelial neoplasia] I), moderate dysplasia (CIN II), and severe dysplasia and/or carcinoma in situ (CIN III).

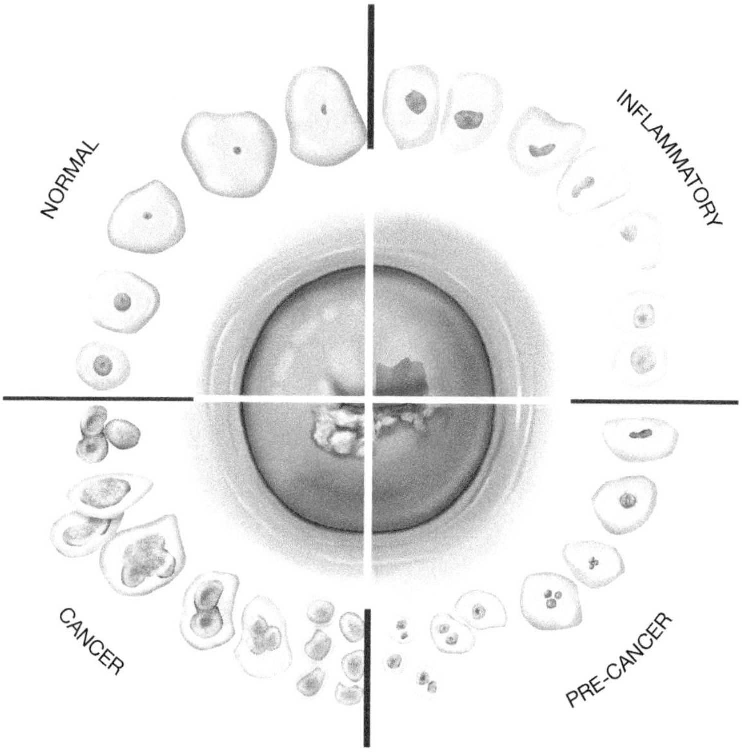

FIGURE 16.35 The Papanicolaou (Pap) smear is a screening technique to aid in the detection of cervical cancer. Note the drawn appearance of the cervix (in the center), starting with normal (left upper portion), inflammatory condition (right upper portion), pre-cancer (right lower portion), and cancer (left lower portion).

Test	Description
pregnanediol (prĕg″ năn-dī′ ŏl)	Urine test to determine menstrual disorders or possible abortion.
quad marker screen (AFP, hCG, UE, and inhibin-A)	Measures high and low levels of alpha-fetoprotein (AFP; a protein produced by the baby's liver) and abnormal levels of human chorionic gonadotropin (hCG; a hormone produced by the placenta), unconjugated estriol (UE; a hormone produced in the placenta and in the baby's liver), and inhibin-A (a hormone produced by the placenta) to assess probabilities of potential genetic disorders.
Rh factor (positive or negative)	Determine risk for maternal–fetal blood incompatibility.
rubella (German measles) titer (roo-bĕl′ lă tī′ tĕr)	Determine immunity to rubella.

Test	Description

GOOD TO KNOW ▶

Up to 80% of babies born to mothers who had rubella during the first 12 weeks of pregnancy develop congenital rubella syndrome. This syndrome can cause one or more problems, including:

- Growth retardation
- Cataracts

- Deafness
- Congenital heart defects
- Defects in other organs
- Intellectual disabilities

Test	Description
TORCH panel (tōrch)	Screen for toxoplasmosis, rubella, cytomegalovirus (CMV), and herpes simplex virus (HSV).
toxoplasmosis screen (tŏks-ō-plăs-mō′ sĭs)	Determine toxoplasmosis infection.
ultrasound (ŭl′ tră-sownd)	Uses during pregnancy include the following: • Confirming viable pregnancy • Confirming fetal heartbeat (FHB) • Measuring the crown–rump length or gestational age of the fetus • Confirming ectopic pregnancy • Confirming molar pregnancy (hydatidiform mole or hydatid mole) • Assessing abnormal gestation • Diagnosing fetal malformation and structural abnormalities • Confirming multiple fetuses • Determining sex of the baby • Identifying placenta location • Confirming intrauterine death • Observing fetal presentation and movements • Identifying uterine and pelvic abnormalities of the mother during pregnancy See Figures 16.36 and 16.37.

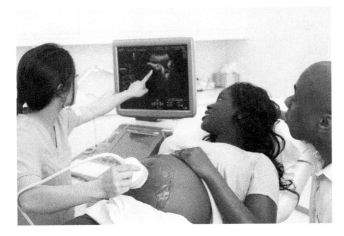

FIGURE 16.36 Ultrasound screening permits visualization of the fetus in utero.
Source: Shutterstock

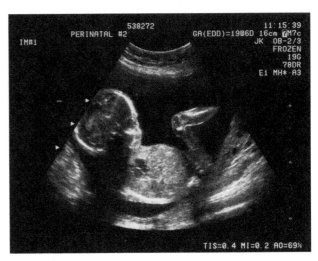

FIGURE 16.37 Ultrasound image of a fetus at 20 weeks gestation.
Source: Suzanne Tucker/Shutterstock

Test	Description
urinalysis (ū″ rĭ-năl′ ĭ-sĭs)	Check for infection, renal disease, or diabetes.
wet mount or wet prep	Examination of vaginal discharge for the presence of bacteria and yeast. Vaginal smear is placed on a microscopic slide, wet with normal saline, and then viewed under a microscope by the physician.

Abbreviations *and* Acronyms

Abbreviation/ Acronym	Meaning	Abbreviation/ Acronym	Meaning
AB	abortion	**HT**	hormone therapy
AFP	alpha-fetoprotein	**IUD**	intrauterine device
AROM	artificial rupture of membranes	**LH**	luteinizing hormone
ASCUS	atypical squamous cells of undetermined significance	**LMP**	last menstrual period
		NSSC	normal size, shape, and consistency
CIN	cervical intraepithelial neoplasia	**NST**	nonstress test
cm	centimeter	**OB**	obstetrics
CMV	cytomegalovirus	**OTC**	over-the-counter
COCs	combined oral contraceptives	**oz**	ounce
CS, C-section	cesarean section	**Pap**	Papanicolaou (smear)
CVS	chorionic villus sampling	**PID**	pelvic inflammatory disease
D&C	dilation and curettage	**PIH**	pregnancy-induced hypertension
DUB	dysfunctional uterine bleeding	**PMS**	premenstrual syndrome
FHB	fetal heartbeat	**PUBS**	percutaneous umbilical blood sampling
FSH	follicle-stimulating hormone	**RM**	recurrent miscarriage
g	gram	**STIs**	sexually transmitted infections
GBS	group B streptococcus	**TAH-BSO**	total abdominal hysterectomy with bilateral salpingo-oophorectomy
GTT	glucose tolerance test		
GYN	gynecology	**TORCH**	toxoplasmosis, rubella, cytomegalovirus, herpes simplex virus
hCG	human chorionic gonadotropin		
HIV	human immunodeficiency virus	**TSS**	toxic shock syndrome
HSG	hysterosalpingography	**UE**	unconjugated estriol
HSV	herpes simplex virus	**WNL**	within normal limits

Study *and* Review III

Building Medical Terms

Using the following word parts, fill in the blanks to build the correct medical terms.

bartholin	mast	salping	-centesis	-genesis
hyster	men/o	-al	-ectomy	-pause

Definition

Medical Term

1. Inflammation of the Bartholin glands

_____itis

2. Surgical puncture of the cul-de-sac for removal of fluid

culdo_____

3. Surgical excision of the uterus

_____ectomy

4. Surgical removal of a tumor from the breast

lump_____

5. Surgical excision of the breast

_____ectomy

6. Cessation of the monthly flow

meno_____

7. Normal monthly flow (menses, menstruation)

_____rrhea

8. Formation of the ovum

oo_____

9. Inflammation of a fallopian tube

_____itis

10. Pertaining to after sexual intercourse

postcoit_____

Combining Form Challenge

Using the combining forms provided, write the medical term correctly.

gynec/o	cyst/o	genital/o
colp/o	fibr/o	cervic/o

1. Inflammation of the uterine cervix: _____itis

2. Medical instrument used to examine the vagina and cervix: _____scope

3. Hernia of the bladder that protrudes into the vagina: _____cele

4. Fibrous tissue tumor: _____oma

5. Male or female reproductive organs: _____ia

6. Study of the female, especially the diseases of the female reproductive organs and the breast: _____logy

Select the Right Term

Select the correct answer, and write it on the line provided.

1. Accessory parts of a structure are _____.

    abortion   incomplete   adnexa   estrogens

2. Difficult or painful monthly flow (menses or menstruation) is _____.

    amenorrhea   dysmenorrhea   dyspareunia   eclampsia

3. A term that refers to any pregnancy, regardless of duration, including the present one is _____.

    gravida   nulligravida   primigravida   multigravida

4. Vaginal discharge occurring after childbirth is _____.

    menarche   mittelschmerz   lochiamenorrhagia

5. Serious complication of pregnancy characterized by increasing hypertension, proteinuria, and edema is _____.

    eclampsia   preeclampsia   placenta previa   endometriosis

6. Process of being turned backward is _____.

    rectovaginal   toxic shock   retroversion   retroverion

Drug Highlights

Match the appropriate lettered description or examples of drug(s) with the class of drug.

_____ **1.** estrogen

_____ **2.** progestogen/progestin

_____ **3.** combined oral contraceptives

_____ **4.** minipill

_____ **5.** transdermal birth control patch

a. Birth control pills

b. Ortho Evra

c. Depo-Provera

d. Natural female sex hormone secreted by the ovarian follicles

e. Small device that is placed within the uterus to prevent pregnancy

_____ **6.** birth control injectable

_____ **7.** intrauterine device

f. Oral contraceptive that contains only progestin

g. Female sex hormone responsible for changes in the uterine endometrium during the second half of the menstrual cycle

Diagnostic and Laboratory Tests

Select the best answer to each multiple-choice question. Circle the letter of your choice.

1. X-ray of the uterus and fallopian tubes after the injection of a radiopaque substance.

a. hysterosalpingography

b. laparoscopy

c. culdoscopy

d. mammography

2. Used to examine the ovaries and fallopian tubes.

a. colposcopy

b. culdoscopy

c. laparoscopy

d. mammography

3. Process of obtaining pictures of the breast by use of x-rays.

a. colposcopy

b. culdoscopy

c. laparoscopy

d. mammography

4. Screening technique to aid in the detection of cervical/uterine cancer and cancer precursors.

a. colposcopy

b. Papanicolaou (Pap) smear

c. estrogens

d. mammography

5. Urine test that determines menstrual disorders or possible abortion.

a. wet mount or wet prep

b. culdoscopy

c. Pap smear

d. pregnanediol

Abbreviations and Acronyms

Write the correct word, phrase, or abbreviation/acronym in the space provided.

1. AB _____

2. FHB _____

3. combined oral contraceptives _____

4. intrauterine device _____

5. pelvic inflammatory disease _____

6. cervical intraepithelial neoplasia _____

7. DUB _____

8. PMS _____

9. dilation and curettage _____

10. toxic shock syndrome _____

Practical Application

SOAP: Chart Note Analysis

This exercise will make you aware of information, abbreviations/acronyms, and medical terminology typically found in a gynecology patient's chart note. The names and any personal information have been created by the author. Read and study each form or case study and then answer the questions that follow. You may refer to Appendix III, *Abbreviations, Acronyms, and Symbols*.

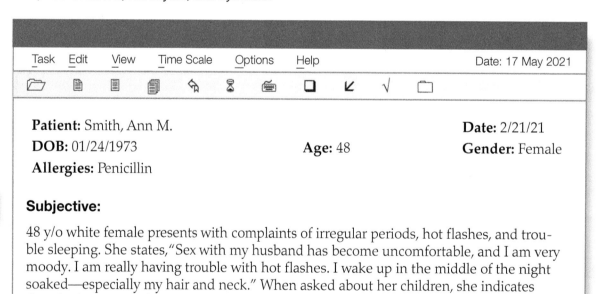

| Task | Edit | View | Time Scale | Options | Help | | | | | Date: 17 May 2021 |

Patient: Smith, Ann M.   **Date:** 2/21/21
DOB: 01/24/1973   **Age:** 48   **Gender:** Female
Allergies: Penicillin

S **Subjective:**

48 y/o white female presents with complaints of irregular periods, hot flashes, and trouble sleeping. She states, "Sex with my husband has become uncomfortable, and I am very moody. I am really having trouble with hot flashes. I wake up in the middle of the night soaked—especially my hair and neck." When asked about her children, she indicates that she has two children, one daughter who is an English teacher and one son who is a pharmacist. She also states that she has never had an abortion. Her LMP (last menstrual period) was 11/21/20.

Objective:

Vital Signs: T: 98.8 F; **P:** 70; **R:** 16; **BP:** 120/78

Ht: 5´ 3˝

Wt: 135 lb

General Appearance: Attractive, well groomed, and pleasant. Noted a slight nervousness and concern during initial interview.

GYN:

Breasts: Symmetrical, no palpable masses or tenderness, no dimpling or skin changes

External genitalia: No lesions or inflammation, normal hair distribution with thinning

Cervix: Pink, smooth, no cervical motion tenderness; Pap smear performed

Adnexa uteri: Nontender, no masses

Uterus: NSSC (normal size, shape, and consistency), noted retroversion position, firm, slightly enlarged, with possible uterine fibroid tumor

Rectal exam: No fissures, hemorrhoids, or skin lesions in perianal area. Sphincter tone good, no prolapse. No masses or tenderness.

Pregnancies: gravida 2 para 2 abortions 0

Assessment:

Perimenopause

Plan:

Patient elected the nonprescription treatment for 6 months. To be reevaluated August 2021.

1. Schedule mammogram ASAP. If WNL, then annually.

2. Advised to use over-the-counter (OTC) water-soluble vaginal lubricant for intercourse and moisturizer for vaginal dryness.

3. Advised to go to the laboratory for CBC, cholesterol, triglycerides, and glucose. Check TSH, FSH, and estradiol levels to rule out (R/O) thyroid disorder and obtain hormone baseline levels.

4. Recommended she take a multivitamin and mineral complex that contains 400 mcg of folic acid. Also, take 1500 mg of calcium with vitamin D daily and an antioxidant.

5. Schedule a pelvic ultrasound to R/O uterine fibroid tumor, ASAP.

6. Recommend a bone density study before reevaluation in August.

Chart Note Questions

Write the correct answer in the space provided.

1. What is the abbreviation for gynecology? _____

2. What does the statement, "I wake up in the middle of the night soaked—especially my hair and neck," indicate?

_____

3. What is the medical word for difficult or painful sexual intercourse? _____

4. What does gravida 2 indicate? _____

5. Why is a pelvic ultrasound recommended? _____

MyLab Medical Terminology™

MyLab Medical Terminology is a premium online homework management system that includes a host of features to help you study. Registered users will find:

- A multitude of quizzes and activities built within the MyLab platform

- Powerful tools that track and analyze your results—allowing you to create a personalized learning experience

- Videos and audio pronunciations to help enrich your progress

- Streaming lesson presentations (guided lectures) and self-paced learning modules

- A space where you and your instructor can check your progress and manage your assignments

Male Reproductive System

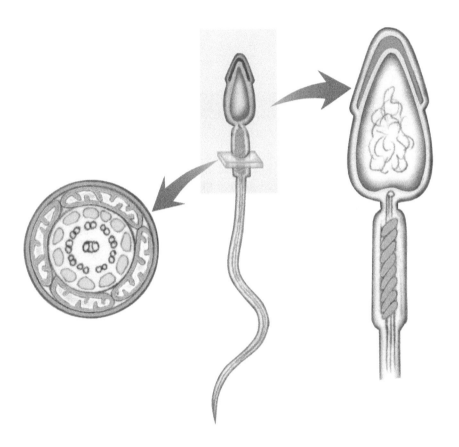

 Learning Outcomes

On completion of this chapter, you will be able to:

1. Identify the organs and structures of the male reproductive system.
2. Describe the primary functions of the organs and structures of the male reproductive system.
3. Analyze, build, spell, and pronounce medical words.
4. Explain the causes, symptoms, and treatments of selected sexually transmitted infections.
5. Describe the drugs highlighted in this chapter.
6. Provide the description of diagnostic and laboratory tests related to the male reproductive system.
7. Identify and define selected abbreviations and acronyms.

Anatomy and Physiology

The male reproductive system consists of the testes, epididymis, vas deferens, urethra, and the following accessory glands: bulbourethral, prostate, and the seminal vesicles. The supporting structures and accessory sex organs are the scrotum and the penis. The male reproductive system has two primary functions: (1) producing spermatozoa, the male reproductive cells, and (2) making testosterone, the male hormone. Table 17.1 provides an at-a-glance look at the male reproductive system. See Figure 17.1.

TABLE 17.1 Male Reproductive System at-a-Glance

Organ/Structure	Primary Functions/Description
Scrotum	Acts as a natural climate control center for the testicles in order to maintain viability of sperm. The temperature in the scrotum is a degree or two lower than the usual body temperature of 98.6°F, which would kill sperm.
Penis	Acts as male organ of copulation and urination; site of the orifice for the elimination of urine and semen from the body. **Semen** is the fluid-transporting medium for spermatozoa discharged during ejaculation.
Testes (also called *testicles*)	Provide the male sex hormone, testosterone, produced by cells within them; contain seminiferous tubules that are the site of sperm formation and development
Epididymis	Acts as site for the maturation of sperm
Vas deferens	Acts as excretory duct of the testis
Seminal vesicles	Produce a slightly alkaline fluid that becomes a part of the seminal fluid or semen
Prostate gland	Secretes an alkaline fluid that aids in maintaining the viability of spermatozoa
Bulbourethral or Cowper glands	Produce a mucous secretion before ejaculation that becomes a part of the semen
Urethra	Transmits urine and semen out of the body

External Organs

In the male, the scrotum, the testes, and the penis are the external organs of reproduction. See Figure 17.2 and refer to Figure 17.1.

Scrotum

The **scrotum** is a pouchlike structure located behind and below the penis. It is suspended from the perineal region and is divided by a septum into two sacs, each containing one of the testes along with a long, coiled tube called the **epididymis**. Within the tissues of the scrotum are fibers of smooth muscle that contract in the absence of sufficient heat, giving the scrotum a wrinkled appearance. This contractile action brings the testes closer to the perineum where they can absorb sufficient body heat to maintain the viability of the **spermatozoa**. These changes in the scrotum illustrate its primary function, which is to act as a natural climate control center for the testicles.

The temperature in the scrotum is a degree or two lower than the usual body temperature of 98.6°F. The testicles need this lower temperature in order to carry out their

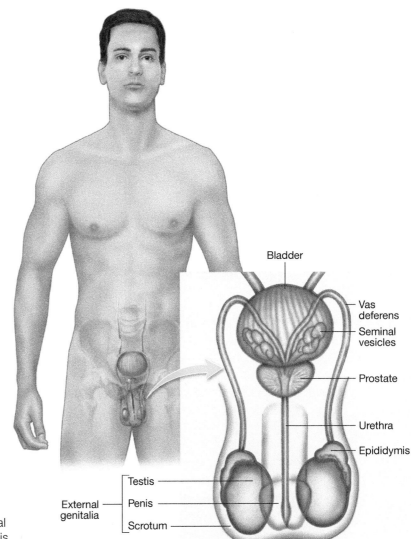

FIGURE 17.1 Male reproductive system: seminal vesicles, prostate, urethra, vas deferens, epididymis, and external genitalia.

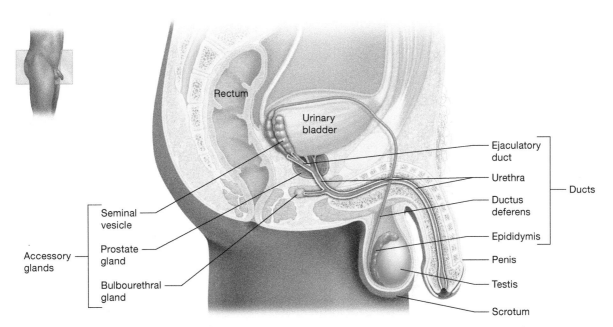

FIGURE 17.2 Sagittal section of the male pelvis, showing the organs, glands, supporting structures, and accessory sex organs (scrotum and penis) of the reproductive system.

Source: AMERMAN, ERIN C., HUMAN ANATOMY & PHYSIOLOGY, 2nd Ed., ©2019. Reprinted and Electronically reproduced by permission of Pearson Education, Inc., New York, NY.

job of producing viable sperm. If the testicles are kept at body temperature or higher for a prolonged period, infertility or sterility can result. The scrotum continually monitors the environment for temperature changes and responds automatically in the way that is best for the production of healthy sperm.

Under normal conditions, the walls of the scrotum are generally free of wrinkles, and it hangs loosely between the thighs (refer to Figure 17.1).

Testes

The male has two ovoid-shaped organs, the **testes**, located within the scrotum. See Figure 17.3. The interior of each testis is divided into about 250 wedge-shaped lobes by fibrous tissues. Coiled within each lobe are one to three small tubes called the **seminiferous tubules**, which are the site of the development of male reproductive cells, the **spermatozoa**. Cells within the testes also produce the male sex hormone, **testosterone**, which is responsible for the development of secondary male sexual characteristics during puberty and maintaining them through adulthood.

fyi **Puberty** is defined as a period of rapid change in the lives of boys and girls during which time the reproductive organs mature and become functionally capable of reproduction. In the male, puberty generally begins around 12 years of age when the genitals start to increase in size and the shoulders broaden and become muscular. As testosterone is released, secondary sexual characteristics develop, such as pubic and axillary hair, increase in size of the penis and testes, voice changes (deepening), facial hair, erections, and nocturnal emissions.

Testosterone is essential for normal growth and development of the male accessory sex organs. It plays a vital role in the erection process of the penis and thus is necessary for the reproductive act, or copulation. Additionally, testosterone affects the growth of hair on the face, muscular development, and vocal timbre. The *seminiferous tubules* form a plexus or network called the *rete testis* from which 15–20 small ducts, the efferent ductules, leave the testis and open into the epididymis (refer to Figure 17.3).

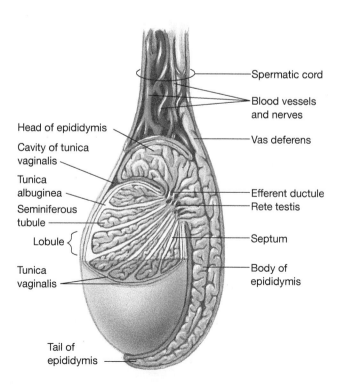

FIGURE 17.3 Sagittal view of a testis showing interior anatomy.

Penis

The **penis** is the external male sex organ and is composed of erectile tissue covered with skin. The penis has three longitudinal columns of erectile tissue that are capable of significant enlargement when engorged with blood, as is the case during sexual stimulation. Two of these columns, located side by side, form the greater part of the penis. These columns are known as the *corpora cavernosa penis*. The third longitudinal column, the *corpus spongiosum*, has the same function as the first two columns but contains the penile portion of the urethra and tends to be more elastic when in an erectile state. The *corpus spongiosum*, at its distal end, expands to form the *glans penis*, the cone-shaped head of the penis, and is the site of the urethral orifice. It is covered with loose skinfolds called the **foreskin** or *prepuce*. The foreskin contains glands that secrete a lubricating fluid called *smegma*. The foreskin can be removed by a surgical procedure known as **circumcision**. Refer to Figure 17.9.

The erectile state in the penis results when sexual stimulation causes large quantities of blood from dilated arteries supplying the penis to fill the cavernous spaces in the erectile tissue. When the arteries constrict, the pressure on the veins in the area is reduced, thus allowing more blood to leave the penis than enters, and the penis returns to its normal state. The functions of the penis are to serve as the male organ of **copulation** (sexual intercourse) and as the site of the orifice for the elimination of urine and semen from the body.

fyi At birth it is normal for the scrotum of the male newborn to appear large. Some abnormal conditions, however, can be noted. For example, one or both testes can fail to descend into the scrotum, causing a condition called **cryptorchidism**. The foreskin of the penis can be too tight at birth, causing **phimosis**, a condition of narrowing of the opening of the prepuce wherein the foreskin cannot be drawn back over the glans penis. **Paraphimosis** is a condition that only affects uncircumcised males. It develops when the foreskin can no longer be pulled forward over the tip of the penis. This causes the foreskin to become swollen and stuck, which may slow or stop the flow of blood to the tip of the penis. Congenital defects can be present, such as **epispadias** (urethra opens on the dorsal surface (top) of the penis) and **hypospadias** (urethra opens on the ventral surface (underside) of the penis). Refer to Figure 17.12.

Internal Organs

In the male, the epididymis, the vas deferens, the seminal vesicles, the prostate gland, the bulbourethral glands, and the urethra are the internal organs of reproduction.

Epididymis

Each testis is connected by efferent ductules to an **epididymis**, which is a coiled tube lying on the posterior aspect of the testis. Each epididymis functions as a site for the maturation of **sperm** (Figure 17.4) and as the first part of the duct system through which sperm pass on their journey to the urethra (refer to Figures 17.1 and 17.2).

Vas Deferens

The **vas deferens**, also called the **ductus deferens**, is a slim muscular tube that is a continuation of the epididymis (refer to Figures 17.1 and 17.2). It conveys sperm from the epididymis to the ejaculatory duct. It has been described as the *excretory duct* of the testis and extends from a point adjacent to the testis to enter the abdomen through the inguinal canal. Between the testis and the part of the abdomen known as the *internal inguinal ring*, the vas deferens is contained within a structure known as the **spermatic cord** that also contains arteries, veins, lymphatic vessels, and nerves.

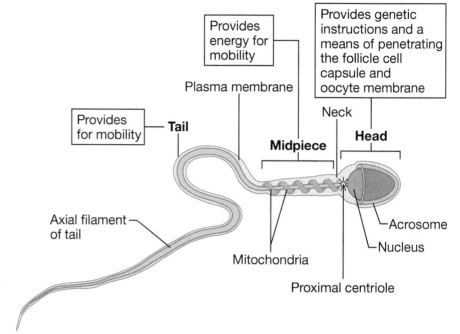

FIGURE 17.4 Basic structure of a spermatozoon (sperm).
Source: MARIEB, ELAINE N.; KELLER, SUZANNE M., ESSENTIALS OF HUMAN ANATOMY & PHYSIOLOGY, 12th Ed., ©2018. Reprinted and Electronically reproduced by permission of Pearson Education, Inc., New York, NY.

Seminal Vesicles

There are two **seminal vesicles**, each connected by a narrow duct to a vas deferens, which then forms a short tube, the **ejaculatory duct**, which penetrates the base of the prostate gland and opens into the prostatic portion of the urethra (see Figure 17.5 and refer to Figure 17.1). The seminal vesicles produce a slightly alkaline fluid that becomes a part of the seminal fluid or semen.

Prostate Gland

The **prostate gland** is about 4 cm wide and weighs approximately 20 g. It is composed of glandular, connective, and muscular tissue and lies behind the urinary bladder (refer to Figures 17.1 and 17.5). It surrounds the first 2.5 cm of the urethra and secretes an alkaline fluid that aids in maintaining the viability of spermatozoa. Enlargement of the prostate, called **benign prostatic hyperplasia (BPH)**, is a condition that can occur in older men. In this condition, the prostate obstructs the urethra and interferes with the normal passage of urine. When this occurs, a **prostatectomy** can be performed to remove a part of the gland. The prostate gland can also be a site of cancer in older men.

 With aging, the prostate gland enlarges and its glandular secretions decrease, the testes become smaller and firmer, the production of testosterone gradually decreases, and pubic hair becomes sparser and stiffer. In a healthy, normal male, **spermatogenesis** and the ability to have erections last a lifetime. However, sexual arousal can be slowed with a longer refractory period between erections. In men, a normal *refractory period* is the time span between orgasms during which time they are not physically able to have another orgasm. In older men the refractory time lengthens.

Bulbourethral Glands

The **bulbourethral glands**, or *Cowper glands*, are two small pea-sized glands located below the prostate and on either side of the urethra. A duct about 2.5 cm long connects them

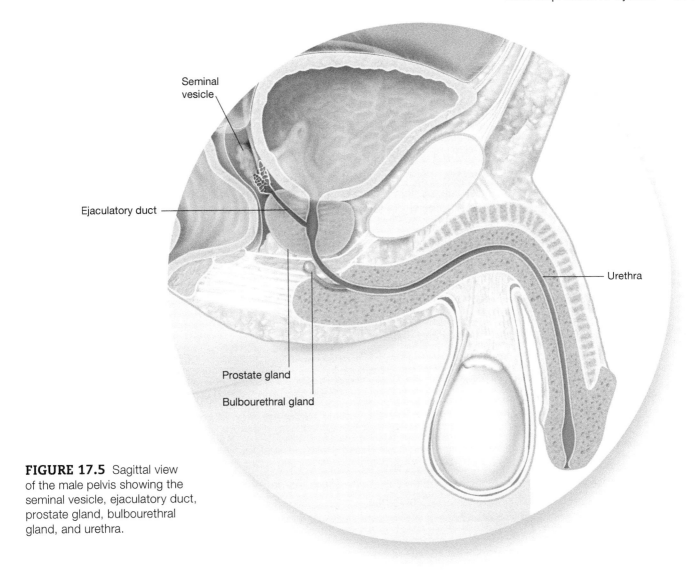

FIGURE 17.5 Sagittal view of the male pelvis showing the seminal vesicle, ejaculatory duct, prostate gland, bulbourethral gland, and urethra.

with the wall of the urethra. The bulbourethral glands produce a mucous secretion before ejaculation, which becomes a component of semen.

Urethra

The male **urethra** is divided into three sections: prostatic, membranous, and penile. It extends from the urinary bladder to the external urethral orifice at the head of the penis. It conducts urine from the urinary bladder out of the body and, during ejaculation, conducts semen from the ejaculatory ducts to the exterior of the body.

Sexually Transmitted Infections

Sexually transmitted infections (STIs) can occur in men, women, and children. They are passed from person to person through sexual contact or from mother to fetus or newborn. Table 17.2 is a summary of the most common sexually transmitted infections. Acquired immunodeficiency syndrome (AIDS) is the final stage of human immunodeficiency virus (HIV) disease. The virus attacks the immune system and leaves the body vulnerable to a variety of illnesses and cancers. While the virus can be transmitted sexually, it can also be transmitted through contact with infected blood and from mother to child during gestation or birth. See Chapter 9 for a more detailed discussion about HIV/AIDS.

TABLE 17.2 Sexually Transmitted Infections

Infection	Cause	Symptoms	Treatment
chlamydia (klă-mĭd´ ē-ă)	*Chlamydia trachomatis* (bacterium)	Can be asymptomatic or exhibit the following: **MALE:** Mucopurulent discharge from penis; burning, itching in genital area; dysuria; swollen testes; can cause nongonococcal urethritis (NGU) and sterility **FEMALE:** Mucopurulent discharge from vagina, cystitis, pelvic pain, cervicitis; can lead to pelvic inflammatory disease (PID) and sterility **NEWBORN:** Eye infection, pneumonia; can cause death	Antibiotics—Zithromax (azithromycin) and doxycycline, tetracycline, or erythromycin
genital warts (jĕn´ ĭ-tăl)	Human papillomavirus (HPV)	**MALE:** Cauliflower-like growths on the penis and perianal area (refer to Figure 17.10) **FEMALE:** Cauliflower-like growths around vagina and perianal area	Laser surgery, chemotherapy, cryosurgery, cauterization

fyi

According to the Centers for Disease Control and Prevention, every year about 14 million Americans become infected with the human papillomavirus (HPV); about 12,000 women are diagnosed with and about 4,000 women die from cervical cancer caused by certain HPV viruses. Additionally, HPV viruses are associated with several other forms of cancer affecting men and women.

Gardasil is the only HPV vaccine that helps protect against four types of HPV. In girls and young women ages 9–26, it helps protect against two types of HPV that cause about 75% of cervical cancer cases and two more types that cause 90% of genital warts cases. In boys and young men ages 9–26, Gardasil helps protect against 90% of genital warts cases. Gardasil also helps protect girls and young women ages 9–26 against 70% of vaginal cancer cases and up to 50% of vulvar cancer cases.

In 2018 the U.S. Food and Drug Administration approved a supplemental application for Gardasil 9 (Human Papillomavirus (HPV) 9-valent Vaccine, Recombinant), expanding the approved use of the vaccine to include women and men ages 27–45.

Infection	Cause	Symptoms	Treatment
gonorrhea (GC) (gŏn˝ ŏ-rē´ ă)	*Neisseria gonorrhoeae* (bacterium)	**MALE:** Purulent urethral discharge, dysuria, urinary frequency **FEMALE:** Purulent vaginal discharge, dysuria, urinary frequency, abnormal menstrual bleeding, abdominal tenderness; can lead to PID and sterility **NEWBORN:** Gonorrheal ophthalmia neonatorum, purulent eye discharge; can cause blindness	Antibiotics—ceftriaxone, cefixime, ciprofloxacin, ofloxacin
herpes genitalis (hĕr´ pēz jĕn-ĭ-tāl´ ĭs)	Herpes simplex virus–2 (HSV-2)	**ACTIVE PHASE** **MALE:** Fluid-filled vesicles (blisters) on penis; acute pain and itching **FEMALE:** Blisters in and around vagina **NEWBORN:** Can be infected during vaginal delivery; severe infection, physical and mental damage **GENERALIZED:** Flulike symptoms, fever, headache, malaise, anorexia, muscle pain	No cure; antiviral drugs Zovirax (acyclovir), Famvir (famciclovir), or Valtrex (valacyclovir hydrochloride) can be used to relieve symptoms during acute phase

(continued)

TABLE 17.2 Sexually Transmitted Infections *(continued)*

Infection	Cause	Symptoms	Treatment
syphilis (sĭf′ ĭ-lĭs)	*Treponema pallidum* (bacterium)	**PRIMARY STAGE:** Chancre at point of infection. See Figure 17.6. **MALE:** penis, anus, rectum **FEMALE:** vagina, cervix **BOTH:** lips, tongue, fingers, nipples	Antibiotics—penicillin, tetracycline, erythromycin

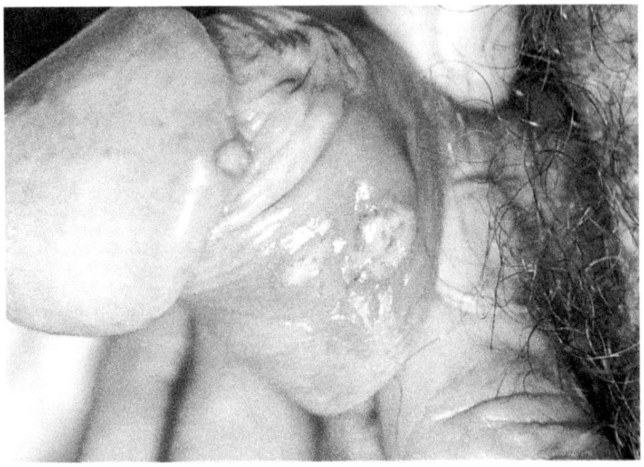

FIGURE 17.6 Chancre.
Source: Courtesy of Jason L. Smith, MD

SECONDARY STAGE: Flulike symptoms; skin rash that causes small, reddish-brown sores; fever; swollen lymph glands; moist warts in the groin; weight loss. See Figure 17.7.

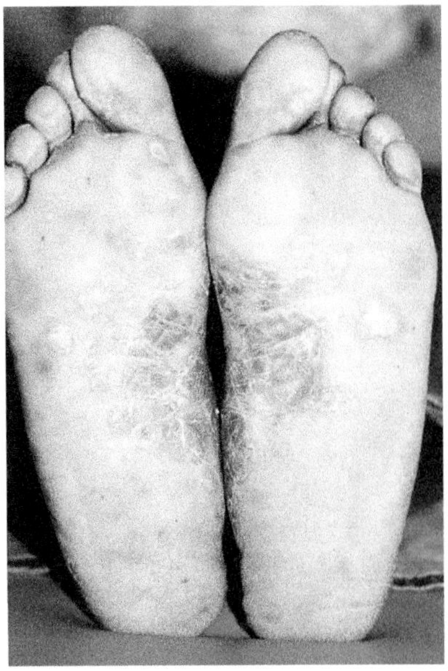

FIGURE 17.7 Secondary syphilis.
Source: Courtesy of Jason L. Smith, MD

LATE STAGE: Difficulty coordinating muscle movements, paralysis, numbness, gradual blindness, and dementia; this damage can be serious enough to cause death

NEWBORN: Congenital syphilis—heart defect, bone or other deformities

Infection	Cause	Symptoms	Treatment
trichomoniasis (trĭk″ ō-mō-nī′ ă-sĭs)	*Trichomonas* (parasitic protozoa)	**MALE:** Usually asymptomatic; can lead to cystitis, urethritis, prostatitis, and nongonococcal urethritis (NGU) **FEMALE:** White frothy vaginal discharge, burning and itching of vulva; can lead to cystitis, urethritis, vaginitis	Flagyl (metronidazole)

Study *and* Review I

Anatomy and Physiology

Write your answers to the following questions.

1. List the primary and accessory glands of the male reproductive system.

   a. _____   d. _____

   b. _____   e. _____

   c. _____   f. _____

2. Name the supporting structure and accessory sex organs of the male reproductive system.

   a. _____   b. _____

3. State two primary functions of the male reproductive system.

   a. _____   b. _____

4. The _____ is the cone-shaped head of the penis.

5. Define *prepuce*. _____

6. Define *smegma*. _____

7. State two functions of the penis.

   a. _____   b. _____

8. _____ is/are the site of the development of
   spermatozoa.

9. List five effects of testosterone regarding male development.

   a. _____   d. _____

   b. _____   e. _____

   c. _____

10. State two functions of the epididymis.

   a. _____   b. _____

11. The excretory duct of the testes is known by two names, _____

or _____.

12. State the function of the seminal vesicles. _____

13. Describe the prostate gland. _____

_____

14. Define the condition known as *benign prostatic hyperplasia*. _____

_____

15. The two small pea-sized glands located below the prostate and on either side of the urethra are known as

the _____ glands or as the _____ glands.

16. Name the three sections of the male urethra.

a. _____   **c.** _____

b. _____

17. State a function of the male urethra. _____

18. The male urethra is approximately _____ cm long.

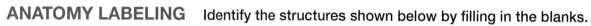

▶ **ANATOMY LABELING**   Identify the structures shown below by filling in the blanks.

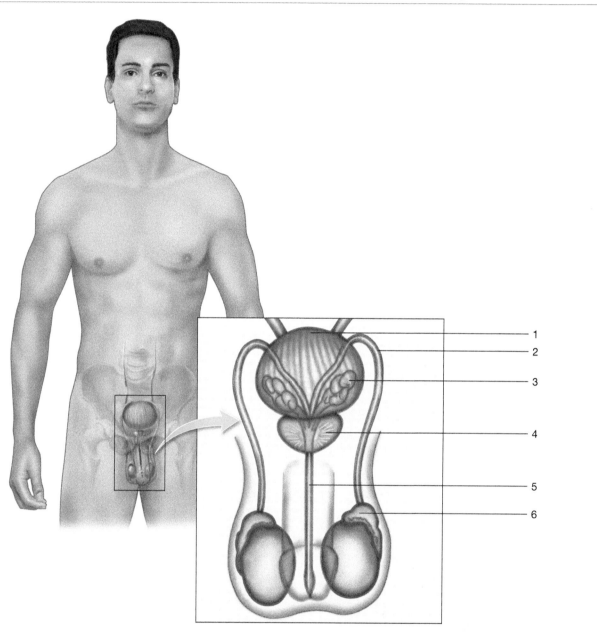

1

2

3

4

5

6

Building Your Medical Vocabulary

This section provides the foundation for learning medical terminology. Review the alphabetized list of medical terms in the following pages. Note how common prefixes and suffixes are repeatedly applied to word roots and combining forms to create different meanings. A combining form is a word root plus a vowel. The chart below lists the combining forms and word roots used in this chapter and can help to strengthen your understanding of how medical words are built and spelled.

You will find that some terms have not been divided into word parts. These are common words or specialized terms that are included to enhance your medical vocabulary.

Combining Forms

balan/o	glans penis		**orchid/o**	testicle
cis/o	to cut		**prostat/o**	prostate
crypt/o	hidden		**sperm/o, sperm/i**	seed, sperm
didym/o	testis		**spermat/o**	seed, sperm
ejaculat/o	to throw out		**testicul/o**	testicle
gon/o	genitals		**varic/o**	twisted vein
gynec/o	female		**vas/o**	vessel
mast/o	breast		**vesicul/o**	seminal vesicle
mit/o	thread		**zo/o**	animal
orch/o	testicle			

Word Roots

castr	to prune		**sexu**	sex
enchyma	to pour		**spadias**	a rent, an opening
phim	muzzle		**zoon**	life

Medical Word	Word Parts		Definition
	Part	**Meaning**	
anorchism (ăn-ōr´ kĭzm)	**an-**	lack of	Condition in which there is a lack of one or both testes
	orch	testicle	
	-ism	condition	
artificial insemination (ăr´ tĭ-fĭsh´ ăl ĭn-sĕm˝ ĭn-ā´ shŭn)			Process of artificially placing semen into the vagina so that conception can take place. *Artificial insemination homologous (AIH)* means using the husband's or mate's semen and *artificial insemination heterologous* refers to using sperm from a donor other than the husband or mate.
aspermia (ā-spĕr´ mē-ă)	**a-**	lack of	Condition involving lack of sperm or failure to ejaculate sperm
	sperm	seed	
	-ia	condition	
azoospermia (ā-zō˝ ŏ-spĕr´ mē-ă)	**a-**	lack of	Condition in which the semen lacks spermatozoa
	zo/o	animal	
	sperm	seed	
	-ia	condition	
balanitis (băl´ ă-nī´ tĭs)	**balan**	glans penis	Inflammation of the glans penis
	-itis	inflammation	
benign prostatic hyperplasia (BPH) (bē-nīn´ prŏs-tăt´ ĭk hī˝ pĕr-plā´ zhē-ă)			Enlargement of the prostate gland. As the prostate enlarges, it compresses the urethra, thereby restricting the normal flow of urine. See Figure 17.8. This restriction generally causes a number of symptoms and can be referred to as *prostatism*. **Prostatism** is any condition of the prostate gland that interferes with the flow of urine from the bladder. Symptoms usually include weak or difficult-to-start urine stream; feeling that the bladder is not empty; need to urinate often, especially at night (nocturia); feeling of *urgency* (a sudden need to urinate); abdominal straining; decrease in size and force of the urinary stream; and interruption of the stream.

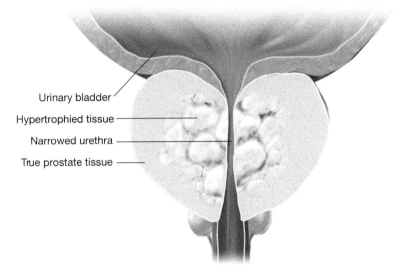

Urinary bladder
Hypertrophied tissue
Narrowed urethra
True prostate tissue

FIGURE 17.8 Benign prostatic hyperplasia showing an enlarged prostate compressing the urethra.

fyi By age 60, four out of five men have an enlarged prostate. A normal prostate is about 4 cm and weighs about 20 g (about the size of a whole walnut). To determine the size of the prostate gland, the physician will perform a digital rectal exam (DRE). Refer to Figure 17.15. In checking for abnormalities, the physician uses a gloved, lubricated finger to feel the back portion of the prostate gland for enlargement and any irregular or firm areas. Treatment for benign prostatic hyperplasia includes drug therapy (see Drug Highlights section), nonsurgical procedures, and/or surgery.

Nonsurgical treatments for benign prostatic hyperplasia include:

- **Transurethral microwave thermotherapy (TUMT)**. A treatment that employs microwaves to heat and destroy excess prostate tissue, sending computer-regulated microwaves through an antenna to heat selected portions of the prostate to at least 111°F. A cooling system protects the urinary tract during the procedure.
- **Transurethral needle ablation (TUNA)**. A minimally invasive treatment that delivers low-level radiofrequency energy through twin needles to burn away a well-defined region of the enlarged prostate. Shields protect the urethra from heat damage. Improves urine flow and relieves symptoms with fewer side effects when compared with transurethral resection of the prostate (TURP).

Types of surgery used for benign prostatic hyperplasia include:

- **Transurethral resection of the prostate (TURP or TUR)**. During this procedure, the most common form of surgery used for this condition, an endoscopic instrument that has ocular and surgical capabilities is introduced directly through the urethra to the prostate and small pieces of the prostate gland are removed by using an electrical cutting loop.
- **Transurethral incision of the prostate (TUIP)**. Used to widen the urethra by making a few small cuts in the bladder neck where the urethra joins the bladder and in the prostate gland itself.
- **Open surgery**. Used when a transurethral procedure cannot be done: when the gland is greatly enlarged, when there are complicating factors, or when the bladder has been damaged and needs to be repaired.

Medical Word	Word Parts		Definition
	Part	Meaning	
castrate (kăs′ trāt)	**castr** **-ate**	to prune use	Removal of the testicles in a man or ovaries in a woman
circumcision (sĕr″ kŭm-sī″ shŭn)	**circum-** **cis** **-ion**	around to cut process	Surgical procedure of removing the foreskin (prepuce) of the penis. See Figure 17.9.

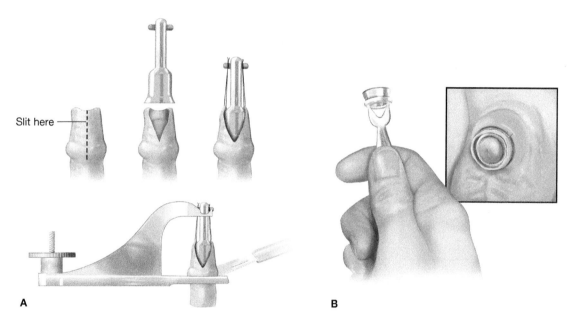

Slit here

A

B

FIGURE 17.9 Circumcision using the Plastibell. **A** The bell is fitted over the glans. A suture is tied around the bell's rim, and then the excess prepuce is cut away. **B** The plastic rim remains in place for 3–4 days until healing occurs. The bell may be allowed to fall off; it is removed if still in place after 8 days.

coitus (kō′ ĭ-tŭs)			Sexual intercourse between a man and a woman; *copulation*
condom (kŏn′ dŭm)			Thin, flexible protective sheath, usually rubber (latex), worn over the penis during copulation to help prevent impregnation (block the passage of sperm) or sexually transmitted infections (STIs)

Medical Word	Word Parts		Definition
	Part	Meaning	
condyloma (kŏn″ dĭ-lō′ mă)			Wartlike growth on the skin, most often seen on the external genitalia; either viral or syphilitic in origin. See Figure 17.10.

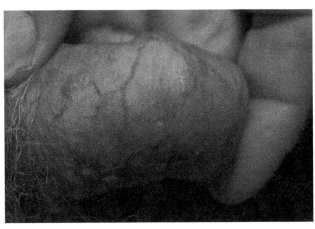

FIGURE 17.10 Genital warts.
Source: Courtesy of Jason L. Smith, MD

Medical Word	Word Parts		Definition
cryptorchidism (krĭpt-ōr′ kĭd-ĭzm)	crypt orchid -ism	hidden testicle condition	Condition in which one or both testes fail to descend into the scrotum. See Figure 17.11.

Undescended testes

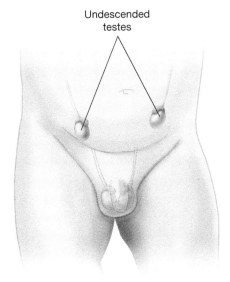

A

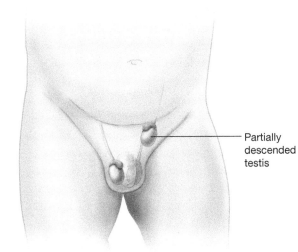

Partially descended testis

B

FIGURE 17.11 Cryptorchidism showing **A** undescended testes and **B** a partially descended testis.

Medical Word	Word Parts		Definition
ejaculation (ē-jăk″ ū-lā′ shŭn)	ejaculat -ion	to throw out process	Process of expulsion of seminal fluid and sperm from the male urethra
epididymitis (ĕp″ ĭ-dĭd″ ĭ-mī′ tĭs)	epi- didym -itis	upon testis inflammation	Inflammation of the epididymis

Medical Word	Word Parts		Definition
	Part	Meaning	
epispadias (ĕp″ ĭ-spā′ dē-ăs)	epi- spadias	upon a rent, an opening	Congenital defect in which the urethra opens on the dorsum of the penis. See Figure 17.12A.

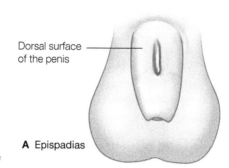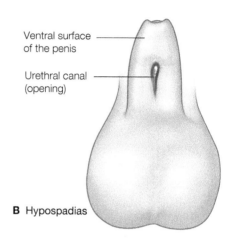

Ventral surface of the penis

Urethral canal (opening)

Dorsal surface of the penis

FIGURE 17.12 Epispadias and hypospadias. **A** In epispadias the canal is open on the dorsal surface. **B** In hypospadias the urethral canal is open on the ventral surface of the penis.

A Epispadias   **B** Hypospadias

erectile dysfunction (ED) (ĕ-rĕk′ tīl dĭs-fŭnk′ shŭn)			Inability to achieve and maintain penile erection sufficient to complete satisfactory intercourse. Many treatment options for ED are available today. These include the vacuum constriction device (VCD); oral medications; medication patches and gels; urethral and penile injection therapies; and surgical therapies including penile prostheses (implants). See the Drug Highlights section for examples of drugs used for this condition.

fyi Physical causes of erectile dysfunction include:

- *Vascular diseases:* arteriosclerosis, hypertension, high cholesterol, and other conditions can cause obstruction of blood flow to the penis
- *Diabetes:* can alter nerve function and blood flow to the penis
- *Prescription drugs:* certain antihypertensive and cardiac medications, antihistamines, psychiatric medications, and other prescription drugs can cause ED
- *Substance abuse:* excessive smoking, alcohol consumption, and illegal drugs constrict blood vessels, limiting blood flow to the penis
- *Neurological diseases:* multiple sclerosis, Parkinson disease, and other diseases can interrupt nerve impulses to the penis
- *Surgery:* prostate, colon, bladder, and other types of pelvic surgery can damage nerves and blood vessels
- *Spinal injury:* interruptions of nerve impulses from the spinal cord to the penis can cause ED
- *Other:* hormonal imbalance, kidney failure, dialysis, and reduced testosterone levels can contribute to ED

Medical Word	Word Parts		Definition
	Part	Meaning	
gamete (găm´ ēt)			Mature reproductive cell of the male or female; a *spermatozoon* or *ovum*
gonorrhea (GC) (gŏn˝ ŏ-rē´ ă)	gon/o -rrhea	genitals flow	Highly contagious sexually transmitted infection of the genital mucous membrane of either sex; the infection is transmitted by the gonococcus *Neisseria gonorrhoeae*.
gynecomastia (gī˝ nĕ-kō-măs´ tē-ă)	gynec/o mast -ia	female breast condition	Pathological condition of excessive development of the mammary glands in the male
heterosexual (hĕt˝ ĕr-ō-sĕk´ shoo-ăl)	hetero- sexu -al	different sex pertaining to	Pertaining to the opposite sex; refers to an individual who has a sexual preference and relationship with the opposite sex
homosexual (hŏ˝ mō-sĕk´ shoo-ăl)	homo- sexu -al	similar, same sex pertaining to	Pertaining to the same sex; refers to an individual who has a sexual preference and relationship with the same sex
hydrocele (hī´ drō-sēl)	hydro- -cele	water hernia, swelling, tumor	Accumulation of fluid in a saclike cavity. One that occurs during prenatal development is caused by a failure of the closure of the canal between the peritoneal cavity and the scrotum. See Figure 17.13A.

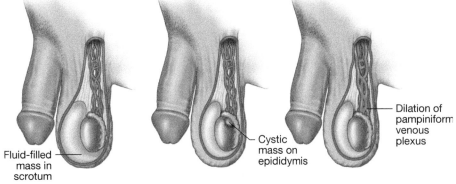

FIGURE 17.13 Common disorders of the scrotum. **A** and **B** Hydroceles and spermatoceles do not usually require treatment unless they become large and cause pain. **C** Varicoceles are usually treated to prevent infertility.

Fluid-filled mass in scrotum

A Hydrocele

Cystic mass on epididymis

B Spermatocele

Dilation of pampiniform venous plexus

C Varicocele

Medical Word	Word Parts		Definition
	Part	Meaning	
hypospadias (hī″ pō-spā′ dē-ăs)	hypo- spadias	under a rent, an opening	Congenital defect in which the urethra opens on the underside of the penis. Symptoms depend on the severity of the defect. An abnormal direction of urine spray is common. Circumcision is not recommended, as the foreskin should be kept for use in a surgical repair. Urologists usually recommend repair before the child is 18 months old. During the surgery, the penis is straightened and the opening is corrected using tissue grafts from the foreskin. The repair may require multiple surgeries. See Figure 17.12B.
infertility (ĭn″ fĕr-tĭl′ ĭ-tē)			Inability of a heterosexual couple to produce a viable offspring
mitosis (mī-tō′ sĭs)	mit -osis	thread condition	Ordinary condition of cell division
oligospermia (ŏl″ ĭ-gō-spĕr′ mē-ă)	oligo- sperm -ia	scanty seed condition	Condition in which there is insufficient (scanty) amount of spermatozoa in the semen
orchidectomy (or″ kĭ-dĕk′ tō-mē)	orchid -ectomy	testicle surgical excision	Surgical excision of a testicle; also called *orchiectomy*
orchiditis (or″ kĭ-dī′ tĭs)	orchid -itis	testicle inflammation	Inflammation of a testicle; also called *orchitis*
orchidotomy (or″ kĭ-dŏt′ ō-mē)	orchid/o -tomy	testicle incision	Incision into a testicle
parenchyma (păr-ĕn′ kĭ-mă)	par- enchyma	beside to pour	Essential cells of a gland or organ that are involved with its function
phimosis (fī-mō′ sĭs)	phim -osis	muzzle condition	A condition that can be present at birth in which there is narrowing of the opening of the prepuce and the foreskin cannot be drawn back over the glans penis. When this condition occurs later in life, it can be an emergency if blood flow is blocked to the penis.

Medical Word	Word Parts		Definition
	Part	Meaning	
prostate cancer (prŏs´ tāt)			Malignant tumor of the prostate gland. See Figure 17.14. Diagnosis of prostate cancer can be confirmed with a medical history; physical examination, including a digital rectal exam (DRE) to assess the size and condition (firm, soft, hard) of the prostate gland (see Figure 17.15); and results of a PSA blood test.

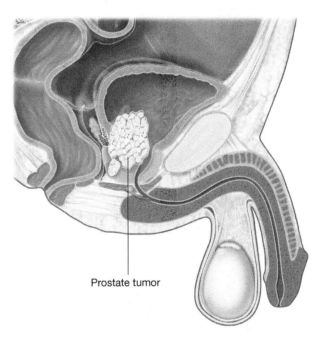

Prostate tumor

FIGURE 17.14 Prostate cancer showing metastasis to the urinary bladder. Note the large tumor mass.

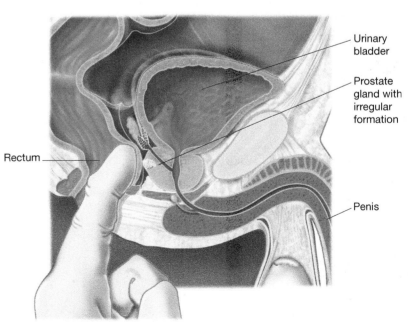

Urinary bladder

Prostate gland with irregular formation

Rectum

Penis

FIGURE 17.15 Digital rectal exam showing palpitation of the prostate gland.

Medical Word	Word Parts		Definition
	Part	Meaning	

 fyi Prostate cancer is the most common type of cancer found in American men, and by age 50, up to one in four men have some cancerous cells in the prostate gland. It is the second leading cause of cancer death in men, exceeded only by lung cancer. While one man in seven will have prostate cancer during his lifetime, only one man in 39 will die of this disease. A man is more likely to die *with* prostate cancer than to die *from* prostate cancer.

Medical Word	Word Parts		Definition
	Part	Meaning	
prostatectomy (prŏs″ tă-tĕk′ tō-mē)	**prostat** **-ectomy**	prostate surgical excision	Surgical excision of the prostate
prostatitis (prŏs″ tă-tī′ tĭs)	**prostat** **-itis**	prostate inflammation	Inflammation of the prostate
puberty (pū′ ber-tē)			Stage of development in the male and female when secondary sex characteristics begin to develop and the individual becomes functionally capable of reproduction
spermatid (spĕr′ mă-tĭd)			Sperm germ cell; also called *spermatoblast*, *spermoblast*
spermatocele (spĕr-măt′ ō-sēl)	**spermat/o** **-cele**	seed, sperm hernia, swelling, tumor	Cystic swelling of the epididymis that contains spermatozoa; mobile, usually painless, and requires no treatment. See Figure 17.13B.
spermatogenesis (spĕr″ măt-ō-jĕn′ ĕ-sĭs)	**spermat/o** **-genesis**	seed, sperm formation, produce	Formation of spermatozoa
spermatozoon (spĕr″ măt-ō-zō′ ŏn)	**spermat/o** **zoon**	seed, sperm life	Male sex cell; plural form is *spermatozoa*

> **! ALERT!**
>
> How many words can you build using the combining form **spermat/o**?

Medical Word	Word Parts		Definition
spermicide (spĕr′ mĭ-sīd)	**sperm/i** **-cide**	seed, sperm to kill	Agent that kills sperm
testicular (tĕs-tĭk′ ū-lar)	**testicul** **-ar**	testicle pertaining to	Pertaining to a testicle

Medical Word	Word Parts		Definition
	Part	Meaning	
varicocele (văr´ ĭ-kō-sēl)	varic/o -cele	twisted vein hernia, swelling, tumor	Enlargement and twisting of the veins of the spermatic cord. See Figure 17.13C.
vasectomy (vă-sĕk´ tō-mē)	vas -ectomy	vessel surgical excision	Surgical procedure in which both of the vas deferens are cut, then tied or sealed to prevent the transport of sperm out of the testes. See Figure 17.16.

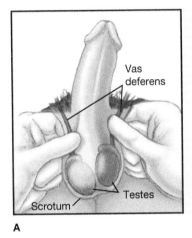 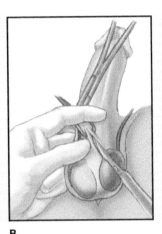 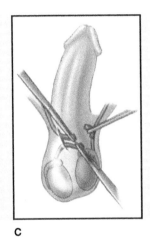 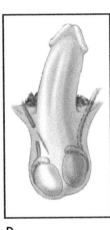

A B C D

FIGURE 17.16 Vasectomy. **A** The spermatic cords are located as they ascend from the scrotum. **B** Both of the vas deferens are severed. **C** A 1 cm section is removed. **D** The cut ends cannot reconnect, thereby preventing the passage of sperm cells and providing surgical sterilization.

fyi A vasectomy does not affect a man's ability to achieve orgasm, ejaculate, or achieve erections. After 4–6 weeks, sperm are no longer present in the semen. A semen specimen must be examined and found to be totally free of sperm a month or more after vasectomy before the patient can rely on the vasectomy for birth control.

| vesiculitis (vĕ-sĭk´ ū-lī´ tĭs) | vesicul -itis | seminal vesicle inflammation | Inflammation of a seminal vesicle |

Study *and* Review II

Word Parts

Prefixes   Give the definitions of the following prefixes.

1. a- _____   **7.** oligo- _____

2. an- _____   **8.** par- _____

3. circum- _____   **9.** in- _____

4. epi- _____   **10.** hetero- _____

5. hydro- _____   **11.** homo- _____

6. hypo- _____

Combining Forms   Give the definitions of the following combining forms.

1. balan/o _____   **11.** orchid/o _____

2. cis/o _____   **12.** prostat/o _____

3. crypt/o _____   **13.** sperm/o _____

4. didym/o _____   **14.** spermat/o _____

5. ejaculat/o _____   **15.** testicul/o _____

6. gon/o _____   **16.** varic/o _____

7. gynec/o _____   **17.** vas/o _____

8. mast/o _____   **18.** vesicul/o _____

9. mit/o _____   **19.** zo/o _____

10. orch/o _____

Suffixes   Give the definitions of the following suffixes.

1. -al _____   **6.** -genesis _____

2. -ar _____   **7.** -ia _____

3. -cele _____   **8.** -ion _____

4. -cide _____   **9.** -ism _____

5. -ectomy _____   **10.** -itis _____

11. -ate _____   **13.** -rrhea _____

12. -osis _____   **14.** -tomy _____

Identifying Medical Terms

In the spaces provided, write the medical terms for the following meanings.

1. _____ Inflammation of the glans penis

2. _____ Surgical excision of the epididymis

3. _____ Surgical excision of a testicle

4. _____ Foreskin (prepuce) over the glans penis

5. _____ Accumulation of fluid in a saclike cavity

6. _____ Wartlike growth on the skin

7. _____ Sperm germ cell

8. _____ Male sex cell

9. _____ Agent that kills sperm

10. _____ Pertaining to a testicle

Matching

Select the appropriate lettered meaning for each of the following words.

_____ **1.** circumcision

_____ **2.** coitus

_____ **3.** condom

_____ **4.** gamete

_____ **5.** orchiditis

_____ **6.** gonorrhea

_____ **7.** infertility

_____ **8.** prepuce

_____ **9.** spermicide

_____ **10.** parenchyma

a. Agent that kills sperm

b. Mature reproductive cell of the male or female

c. Sexual intercourse between a man and a woman

d. Essential cells of a gland or organ that are involved with its function

e. Surgical procedure of removing the foreskin of the penis

f. Thin, flexible protective sheath worn over the penis during copulation to help prevent impregnation or sexually transmitted infection

g. Inflammation of a testicle

h. Inability to produce a viable offspring

i. Causes purulent urethral discharge in the male and purulent vaginal discharge in the female

j. The foreskin over the glans penis in the male

Medical Case Snapshots

This learning activity provides an opportunity to relate the medical terminology you are learning to sample patient case presentations. In the spaces provided, write in your answers.

Case 1

A 45-year-old male presents with an inability to achieve and maintain penile erection sufficient to complete satisfactory intercourse. This condition is known as _____ _____. There are many treatment options for ED, with the most popular being drug therapy.

Case 2

During the assessment of the newborn male, it was noted that the urethra opened on the underside of the penis. This condition is referred to as _____ and an abnormal direction of urine spray is common. In this case, _____ is not recommended for the baby as the foreskin should be kept for use in a surgical repair. Urologists usually recommend repair before the child is _____ months of age.

Case 3

A 60-year-old male complains of difficulty with urinating, "I tend to urinate more frequently, especially at night." This is called _____. "I feel this sudden need to urinate." This is known as _____. "Then I have trouble starting my stream." After a complete physical and a digital rectal exam (DRE), the diagnosis was confirmed to be BPH, also known as benign _____ _____. BPH can also be referred to as having _____, (which is any condition of the prostate gland that interferes with the flow of urine from the bladder).

Drug Highlights

Classification of Drug	Description and Examples
testosterone (male hormone)	Responsible for growth, development, and maintenance of the male reproductive system and secondary sex characteristics.
therapeutic use	As replacement therapy in primary hypogonadism and to stimulate puberty in carefully selected males. It can be used to relieve symptoms of the male climacteric due to androgen deficiency and to help stimulate sperm production in oligospermia and impotence due to androgen deficiency. It can also be used with advanced inoperable metastatic breast cancer in women who are 1–5 years postmenopausal. In 2015, the Food and Drug Administration required labeling changes for testosterone products that clarifies the approved uses of these medications and includes information about a possible increased risk of heart attacks and strokes in aging patients taking testosterone. EXAMPLES: AndroGel (testosterone), Depo-Testosterone (testosterone cypionate [in oil]), and Androderm (testosterone transdermal systems)
patient teaching	Educate the patient to be aware of possible adverse reactions and report any of the following to the physician. *All patients:* nausea, vomiting, jaundice, edema. *Males:* frequent or persistent erection of the penis. *Females:* hoarseness, acne, changes in menstrual periods, growth of hair on face and/or body.
special considerations	Testosterone can decrease blood glucose and insulin requirements in diabetic patients. It can also decrease the anticoagulant requirements of patients receiving oral anticoagulants. These patients require close monitoring when testosterone therapy is begun and then when it is stopped. Individuals who seek to increase muscle mass, strength, and overall athletic ability can abuse anabolic steroids (testosterone). This form is illegal; signs of abuse include flulike symptoms; headaches; muscle aches; dizziness; bruises; needle marks; increased bleeding (nosebleeds, petechiae, gums, conjunctiva); enlarged spleen, liver, and/or prostate; edema; and in the female increased facial hair, menstrual irregularities, and enlarged clitoris.
drugs used to treat benign prostatic hyperplasia (BPH)	5α-reductase inhibitor that lowers the levels of dihydrotestosterone (DHT), the major factor in enlargement of the prostate. Shrinkage of the enlarged prostate usually occurs in 6–12 months with medication therapy. *Note:* Proscar (5 mg) is one brand of finasteride that is prescribed for BPH, while Propecia (1 mg) is another brand of finasteride that is prescribed for male-pattern baldness. EXAMPLES: Other medications used in the treatment of BPH include Cardura (doxazosin) and Flomax (tamsulosin) *Note:* Both drugs act by relaxing the smooth muscle of the prostate and bladder neck to improve urine flow and to reduce bladder outlet obstruction.
drugs used to treat erectile dysfunction (ED)	These drugs increase the body's ability to achieve and maintain an erection during sexual stimulation. They do not protect one from getting sexually transmitted infections, including HIV. They are contraindicated in patients who use nitrates, and they should not be used in men for whom sexual activity is inadvisable because of their underlying cardiovascular status. EXAMPLES: Viagra (sildenafil), Levitra (vardenafil), and Cialis (tadalafil)

Diagnostic *and* Laboratory Tests

Test	Description
fluorescent treponemal antibody absorption (FTA-ABS) (floo-ō-rĕs´ ĕnt trĕp˝ō-nē´ măl ăn´ tĭ-bŏd˝ ē ab-sorp´ shŭn)	Test performed on blood serum to determine the presence of *Treponema pallidum* to detect syphilis.
paternity (pă-tĕr´ nĭ-tē)	Test to determine whether a certain man is the father of a specific child. The most common and accurate test used is the DNA test, which compares a child's DNA pattern with that of the alleged father to check for evidence of inheritance. Result is either exclusion (not the father) or inclusion (is the father). The mother's participation helps exclude half of the child's DNA, leaving the other half for comparison with the alleged father's DNA. A buccal (cheek) sample is taken from each participating person. Most states have laws that allow the unmarried parents of a child to fill out an Acknowledgment of Paternity (AOP) form to legally establish the identity of the father.
prostate-specific antigen (PSA) immunoassay (prŏs´ tāt-spĕ-sĭf´ ĭk ăn´ tĭ-jĕn ĭm˝ ū-nō-ăs´ sā)	Blood test that measures concentrations of a special type of protein known as *prostate-specific antigen*. An increased level indicates prostate disease or possibly prostate cancer.
rapid plasma reagin (RPR) (rē-ā´ jĭn)	Blood test used to screen for syphilis; it works by detecting the nonspecific antibodies that the body produces while fighting the infection
semen (sē´ mĕn)	Test performed on semen that looks at the volume, pH, sperm count, sperm motility, and morphology to evaluate infertility in men.
venereal disease research laboratory (VDRL) (vĕ-nē´ rē-ăl)	Test performed on blood serum to determine the presence of *Treponema pallidum* to detect syphilis.

Abbreviations *and* Acronyms

Abbreviation/ Acronym	Meaning	Abbreviation/ Acronym	Meaning
AIH	artificial insemination homologous	**FTA-ABS**	fluorescent treponemal antibody absorption
AOP	acknowledgment of paternity		
BPH	benign prostatic hyperplasia (also denotes benign prostatic hypertrophy)	**GC**	gonorrhea
		HPV	human papillomavirus
DHT	dihydrotestosterone	**HSV-2**	herpes simplex virus–2
DRE	digital rectal exam	**NGU**	nongonococcal urethritis
ED	erectile dysfunction	**PID**	pelvic inflammatory disease

Abbreviation/ Acronym	Meaning	Abbreviation/ Acronym	Meaning
PSA	prostate-specific antigen	TUNA	transurethral needle ablation
RPR	rapid plasma reagin	TUR	transurethral resection
STIs	sexually transmitted infections	TURP	transurethral resection of the prostate
TUIP	transurethral incision of the prostate	VCD	vacuum constriction device
TUMT	transurethral microwave thermotherapy	VDRL	venereal disease research laboratory

Study *and* Review III

Building Medical Terms

Using the following word parts, fill in the blanks to build the correct medical terms.

hydro-	prostat	testicul	-cide	-itis
par-	spermat/o	-ate	-cele	-genesis

Definition	Medical Term
1. Removal of the testicles in a man or ovaries in a woman	castr_____
2. Accumulation of fluid in a saclike cavity	_____cele
3. Inflammation of a testicle	orchid_____
4. Essential cells of a gland that are involved with its function	_____enchyma
5. Inflammation of the prostate	_____itis
6. Formation of spermatozoa	spermato_____
7. Male sex cell	_____zoon
8. Agent that kills sperm	spermi_____
9. Pertaining to a testicle	_____ar
10. Enlargement and twisting of the veins of the spermatic cord	varico_____

Combining Form Challenge

Using the combining forms provided, write the medical term correctly.

balan/o   orchid/o   prostat/o

gon/o   mit/o   vesicul/o

1. Inflammation of the glans penis: _____itis

2. Highly contagious sexually transmitted infection of the genital mucous membrane: _____rrhea

3. Incision into a testicle: _____tomy

4. Ordinary condition of cell division: _____osis

5. Surgical excision of the prostate: _____ectomy

6. Inflammation of a seminal vesicle: _____itis

Select the Right Term

Select the correct answer, and write it on the line provided.

1. Condition in which there is a lack of one or both testes is _____.

    aspermia   anorchism   azoospermia   testicular

2. Surgical procedure of removing the foreskin of the penis is _____.

    condyloma   coitus   circumcision   castrate

3. Condition in which one or both testes fail to descend into the scrotum is _____.

    cryptorchidism   epispadias   hydrocele   cryptochidism

4. Pertains to the same sex is _____.

    eugenics   gamete   homosexual   phimosis

5. Surgical procedure in which both of the vas deferens are cut, then tied or sealed to prevent the transport of sperm out of the testes, is _____.

    vasectomy   vasotomy   vesiculitis   orchidectomy

6. Sexually transmitted infection caused by *Treponema pallidum* is _____.

    herpes   chlamydia   gonorrhea   syphilis

Drug Highlights

In this chapter of the male reproductive system, you learned about testosterone and its therapeutic use, patient teaching, and special considerations. Also included were drugs to treat benign prostatic hyperplasia and drugs used to treat erectile dysfunction. Referring to this information, write in the answers for the following questions.

1. Testosterone is responsible for _____, development, and maintenance of the male reproductive system and secondary sex characteristics.

2. Therapeutic use of testosterone is used as replacement therapy for primary _____ and to stimulate puberty in carefully selected males.

3. Give three other reasons that testosterone can be used.

   a. _____

   b. _____

   c. _____

4. It is important to educate the male patient about possible adverse reactions to testosterone and report the following to the physician: frequent or _____ erection of the penis.

5. It is important to educate the female patient about possible adverse reactions to testosterone and report any of the following to the physician: hoarseness, acne, changes in _____, and growth of hair on face and/or body.

6. Proscar (5 mg) is a medication used to help _____ an enlarged prostate.

7. Viagra and Cialis are drugs that increase the male body's ability to _____ and to _____ an erection.

Diagnostic and Laboratory Tests

Select the best answer to each multiple-choice question. Circle the letter of your choice.

1. Test performed on blood serum to detect syphilis.

   a. paternity

   b. semen

   c. FTA-ABS

   d. HSV-2

2. Test to determine whether a certain man is the father of a specific child.

   a. paternity

   b. semen

   c. FTA-ABS

   d. HSV-2

3. Increased level indicates prostate disease or possibly prostate cancer.

    a. fluorescent treponemal antibody   **c.** semen

    b. prostate-specific antigen   **d.** VDRL

4. Used to determine infertility in men.

    a. paternity   **c.** semen

    b. prostate-specific antigen   **d.** VDRL

5. Increased level can indicate benign prostatic hyperplasia.

    a. fluorescent treponemal antibody   **c.** VDRL

    b. prostate-specific antigen   **d.** semen test

Abbreviations and Acronyms

Place the correct word, phrase, or abbreviation/acronym in the space provided.

1. benign prostatic hyperplasia _____

2. GC _____

3. human papillomavirus _____

4. HSV-2 _____

5. STIs _____

6. erectile dysfunction _____

7. TURP _____

8. NGU _____

9. venereal disease research laboratory _____

10. prostate-specific antigen _____

Practical Application

SOAP: Chart Note Analysis

This exercise will make you aware of the information, abbreviations/acronyms, and medical terminology typically found in a male patient's chart. Refer to Appendix III, *Abbreviations, Acronyms, and Symbols*.

Read the chart note and answer the questions that follow.

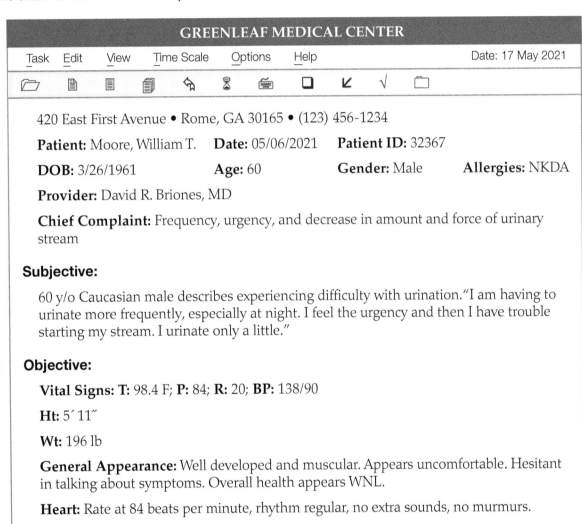

GREENLEAF MEDICAL CENTER

Task   Edit   View   Time Scale   Options   Help   Date: 17 May 2021

420 East First Avenue • Rome, GA 30165 • (123) 456-1234

Patient: Moore, William T.   **Date:** 05/06/2021   **Patient ID:** 32367

DOB: 3/26/1961   **Age:** 60   **Gender:** Male   **Allergies:** NKDA

Provider: David R. Briones, MD

Chief Complaint: Frequency, urgency, and decrease in amount and force of urinary stream

S

Subjective:

60 y/o Caucasian male describes experiencing difficulty with urination. "I am having to urinate more frequently, especially at night. I feel the urgency and then I have trouble starting my stream. I urinate only a little."

O

Objective:

Vital Signs: T: 98.4 F; **P:** 84; **R:** 20; **BP:** 138/90

Ht: 5´ 11˝

Wt: 196 lb

General Appearance: Well developed and muscular. Appears uncomfortable. Hesitant in talking about symptoms. Overall health appears WNL.

Heart: Rate at 84 beats per minute, rhythm regular, no extra sounds, no murmurs.

Lungs: CTA

Abd: Bowel sounds all four quadrants, no masses or tenderness.

Prostate: DRE revealed enlarged prostate, approximately 5.5 cm, projecting 1.5 cm into the rectum.

A

Assessment: Benign prostatic hyperplasia (BPH)

Plan:

1. Advised to go to the laboratory for a complete urinalysis and a PSA test.

2. Prescribed Proscar (finasteride) 5 mg PO once a day for 6 months.

3. Instructed to limit fluid intake during the PM hours, especially alcohol and caffeine, to reduce the need for nighttime urination.

4. Educate that side effects of Proscar can include impotence and decreased sexual desire.

5. Schedule follow-up visit for 6 months.

Chart Note Questions

Write the correct answer in the space provided.

1. Signs and symptoms of BPH include increased frequency, _____, and decrease in amount and force of urinary stream.

2. *DRE* is an abbreviation for _____ _____ _____.

3. The medication of choice for an enlarged prostate is _____ 5 mg.

4. Limiting PM fluids, especially alcohol and caffeine, should help _____ the need for nighttime urination.

5. To evaluate the effectiveness of drug therapy, a follow-up visit is recommended in _____ months.

MyLab Medical Terminology™

MyLab Medical Terminology is a premium online homework management system that includes a host of features to help you study. Registered users will find:

- A multitude of quizzes and activities built within the MyLab platform

- Powerful tools that track and analyze your results—allowing you to create a personalized learning experience

- Videos and audio pronunciations to help enrich your progress

- Streaming lesson presentations (guided lectures) and self-paced learning modules

- A space where you and your instructor can check your progress and manage your assignments

Mental Health

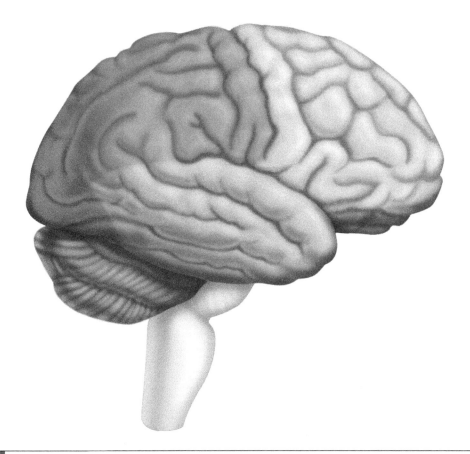

 Learning Outcomes

On completion of this chapter, you will be able to:

1. Define mental health.
2. Describe mental disorders and several possible contributing factors.
3. Identify general symptoms (according to age group) that can suggest a mental disorder.
4. Explain how the diagnosis of mental disorders may be obtained.
5. Describe three basic forms of treatment that can be employed.
6. Analyze, build, spell, and pronounce medical words.
7. Classify the drugs highlighted in this chapter.
8. Identify and define selected abbreviations and acronyms.

Mental Health and Mental Disorders

Please note that much of the information on mental disorders has been adapted from the National Institute of Mental Health (NIMH), which is a component of the National Institutes of Health (NIH), a part of the U.S. Department of Health and Human Services (HHS), and the Diagnostic and Statistical Manual of Mental Disorders, *Fifth Edition (DSM-5).*

The World Health Organization (WHO) defines **health** as a state of complete physical, mental, and social well-being, not merely the absence of disease or infirmity. It defines **mental health** as a state of well-being in which an individual realizes his or her own abilities, can cope with the normal stresses of life, can work productively and fruitfully, and is able to make a contribution to his or her community.

A **mental disorder** is an abnormal condition of the brain or mind. It affects the way a person thinks, feels, behaves, and relates to others and to his or her surroundings. In most cases, the exact cause of a mental disorder is not known. Possible contributing factors include genetics, the environment, chemical changes occurring in the brain, use of certain drugs, and psychological, social, and cultural conditions. See Figure 18.1.

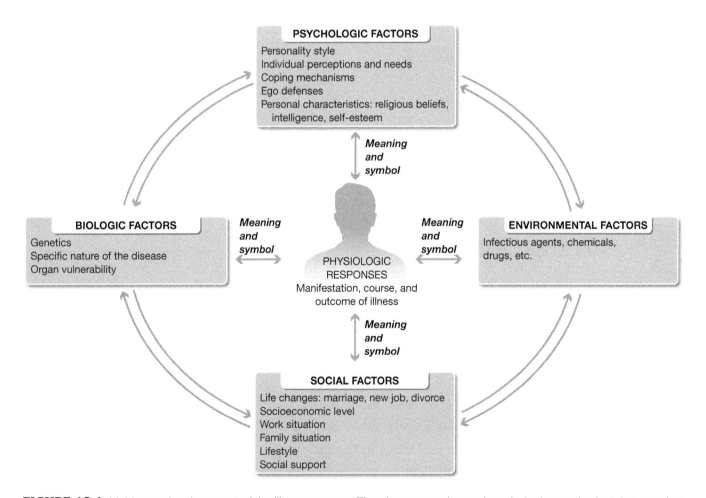

FIGURE 18.1 Multicausational concept of the illness process. The phrase *meaning and symbol* refers to the fact that a patient interprets all experiences in a highly individual manner according to his or her specific meaning and the broader meaning in the patient's culture.

Source: PEARSON EDUCATION; SERVICES, PEARSON; PEARSON EDUCATION, . ., NURSING: A CONCEPT-BASED APPROACH TO LEARNING, VOLUME I, 1st Ed., ©2019. Reprinted and Electronically reproduced by permission of Pearson Education, Inc., New York, NY.

fyi Science has identified six ingredients that can boost one's mood. These ingredients are contained in what is being called "superfoods." Some examples are described as follows.

- *Tomatoes* contain carotenoids, antioxidants that counteract the damage caused by free radicals, which can destroy mood-protecting fats in the brain.
- *Whole grains* promote the release of insulin, a hormone produced by the pancreas, which can stimulate serotonin, a neurotransmitter, vasoconstrictor, and smooth muscle stimulant. Serotonin plays an important role in the regulation of learning, mood, sleep, and vasoconstriction. It also might have a role in anxiety, migraine, vomiting, and appetite. Changes in serotonin levels in the brain may affect mood. Some antidepressant medications affect the action of serotonin and can be used to treat depression.
- *Fatty fish* such as salmon and mackerel contain omega-3 fats DHA and EPA. These fats are necessary for brain health and seem to be crucial to mood.
- *Dark chocolate* is believed to increase the brain's serotonin levels. This may increase mental alertness.
- *Spinach* contains folate, a B vitamin used by the brain to make mood-regulating chemicals: serotonin, dopamine, and norepinephrine. Folate may be effective in treating depression.
- *Red meat* is a good source of iron, which the brain uses to make mood-regulating dopamine. People who are iron deficient may become more depressed than those who have higher levels of iron.

According to NIMH, nearly one in five U.S. adults live with a mental illness (46.6 million in 2017). Mental illnesses include many different conditions that vary in degree of severity. Two broad categories can be used to describe these conditions: any mental illness (AMI) and serious mental illness (SMI). AMI encompasses all recognized mental illnesses (mental, behavioral, or emotional) and can vary in impact, ranging from no impairment to mild, moderate, or severe impairment. SMI is a smaller and more severe subset of AMI and results in serious functional impairment that substantially interferes with or limits one or more major life activities.

Many different conditions are classified as mental disorders. Examples include bipolar disorders, depressive disorders, anxiety disorders, attention-deficit/hyperactivity disorder, trauma- and stressor-related disorders, feeding and eating disorders, schizophrenia, obsessive–compulsive disorders, and autism spectrum disorder. Major depression, bipolar disorder, and schizophrenia are among the top 10 leading causes of disability in the United States. Other types of mental disorders are adjustment disorder, dissociative disorders, factitious disorders, sexual and gender disorders, somatic symptom disorders, and tic disorders. Various sleep-related problems and some forms of dementia, including Alzheimer disease, can be classified as mental disorders because they involve the brain. (See Chapter 13 for in-depth discussions of dementia and Alzheimer disease.)

Symptoms of a Mental Disorder

Symptoms of a mental disorder vary according to the type and severity of the condition and the age of the individual. The following are some general symptoms (according to age group) that can suggest a mental disorder:

In an adult:

- Confused thinking
- Long-lasting sadness or irritability
- Extreme highs and lows in mood
- Excessive fear, worry, or anxiety
- Social withdrawal

- Dramatic changes in eating or sleeping patterns
- Strong feelings of anger
- Delusion or hallucinations
- Increasing inability to cope with daily problems and activities
- Thoughts of suicide
- Denial of obvious problems
- Many unexplained physical problems
- Abuse of drugs and/or alcohol

In an adolescent:

- Abuse of drugs and/or alcohol
- Inability to cope with daily problems and activities
- Changes in eating or sleeping patterns
- Excessive complaints of physical problems
- Defying authority, skipping school, stealing, or damaging property
- Intense fear of gaining weight
- Long-lasting negative mood
- Thoughts of death
- Frequent outbursts of anger

In younger children:

- Changes in school performance
- Poor grades despite strong efforts
- Excessive worry or anxiety
- Hyperactivity
- Persistent nightmares
- Continual disobedience and/or aggressive behavior
- Frequent temper tantrums

Diagnosis of Mental Disorders

The standard manual used by experts for the diagnosis of recognized mental disorders in the United States is the *Diagnostic and Statistical Manual of Mental Disorders*, Fifth Edition (DSM-5).

This official manual of mental health disorders is compiled by the American Psychiatric Association (APA) and identifies categories of mental disorders. Psychiatrists, psychologists, social workers, and other healthcare providers use it to understand and diagnose mental health disorders. Insurance companies and healthcare providers also use it to classify and then code mental health disorders, as per the International Classification of Diseases, Tenth Revision, Clinical Modification (ICD-10-CM), for reimbursement of services rendered.

Psychiatry is the branch of medicine that deals with the study, diagnosis, and treatment of mental disorders. A person who specializes in this field of medicine is a **psychiatrist**, who is a medical doctor (MD) with specialized training in **psychotherapy** and drug therapy. Psychiatrists can further specialize in the treatment of children (child psychiatry) or in the legal aspects of psychiatry, such as the determination of mental competence in criminal cases (forensic psychiatry). **Psychoanalysts** are psychiatrists with specialized training in **psychoanalysis**, a method of obtaining a detailed account of past and present mental and emotional experiences and repressions.

Psychology is the study of the mind. A **psychologist** is a person who is not a medical doctor but has a master's degree or doctor of philosophy (PhD) degree in a specific field of psychology, such as clinical, experimental, or social.

Clinical psychologists are patient-oriented and can use various methods of psychotherapy to treat patients but cannot prescribe medications or electroconvulsive therapy (ECT). They are trained in the use of tests to evaluate various aspects of a patient's mental health and intelligence. Examples are **intelligence quotient (IQ)** tests such as the **Stanford–Binet Intelligence Scale** and the **Wechsler Adult Intelligence Scale–Revised (WAIS-R)**. Other tests used are the **Rorschach Inkblot Test** and the **Thematic Apperception Test (TAT)**, in which pictures are used as stimuli for the patient to create stories. The **Minnesota Multiphasic Personality Inventory–2 (MMPI-2)** consists of true–false questions that can reveal aspects of personality, such as dominance, sense of duty or responsibility, and ability to relate to others; it is used as an objective measure of psychological disorders in adolescents and adults. A patient's responses to the questions can be compared with responses made by individuals with diagnoses of schizophrenia, depression, and many other mental disorders.

Psychiatrists and psychologists also use specially designed interview and assessment tools to evaluate a person for a mental disorder. The therapist bases the diagnosis on the person's report of symptoms, including any social or functional problems caused by the symptoms. The therapist then determines whether the person's symptoms and degree of disability indicate a diagnosis of a specific disorder.

Treatments for Mental Disorders

The three basic forms of treatment for mental disorders are **drug therapy, psychotherapy,** and **electroconvulsive therapy**.

DRUG THERAPY

Drugs that are generally used to treat mental disorders include antianxiety agents, antidepressant agents, antimanic agents, and antipsychotic agents. Drugs used for attention-deficit/hyperactivity disorder (ADHD) include stimulants. See the Drug Highlights section for more information on drug therapy for mental disorders.

PSYCHOTHERAPY

Psychotherapy is a method of treating mental disorders using psychological techniques instead of physical methods. It involves talking, interpreting, listening, rewarding, and role-playing. Psychotherapy should be performed by a trained mental health professional, such as a psychiatrist, psychologist, social worker, or counselor. See Figure 18.2.

Types of psychotherapy include cognitive-behavioral therapy, family therapy, group therapy, play therapy, art therapy, hypnosis, and psychoanalysis.

- **Cognitive-behavioral therapy (CBT)** has two components. The cognitive component helps people change thinking patterns that keep them from overcoming their fears. The behavioral component seeks to change people's reactions to anxiety-provoking situations. A key element of this component is exposure, in which people confront the things they fear. Research has shown that CBT is an effective form of psychotherapy for several anxiety disorders, particularly panic disorder and social phobia.

- **Family therapy** involves an entire family. The focus is on resolving and understanding conflicts and problems as a *family* situation, not just as an individual member's problem.

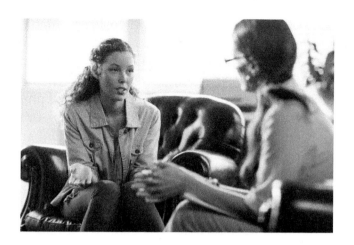

FIGURE 18.2 Young woman in a counseling session with her psychologist.
Source: wavebreakmedia/Shutterstock

- **Group therapy** involves small groups of people with similar problems attending meetings together. There are discussions and interactions between group participants; a therapist helps to focus and guide the therapy sessions. See Figure 18.3.

- **Play therapy** involves a child using toys, such as dolls and puppets, to express thoughts, feelings, fantasies, and conflicts. Because most emotionally disturbed children will not talk about their problems, play therapy provides an alternative method to encourage children to open up about what is troubling them. Children reveal themselves when they play with toys provided by the therapist and often act out their problems. See Figure 18.4.

- **Art therapy** can be used to encourage a child to portray his or her feelings in drawings. When asked to draw the family or a picture of him- or herself, information about the child, the family, and their interactions can be revealed.

- **Hypnosis** is a state of altered consciousness, usually artificially induced, used in treating mental disorders by lessening the mind's unconscious defenses and allowing some patients to be able to recall and even re-experience important childhood events that

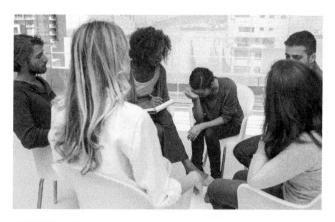

FIGURE 18.3 Therapist counseling a distraught woman in a group therapy session.
Source: wavebreakmedia/Shutterstock

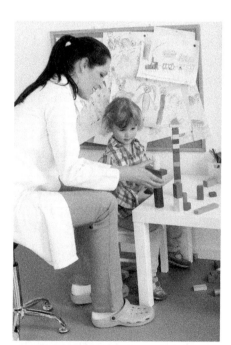

FIGURE 18.4 The therapist is using toys to encourage Kelly to talk about what is troubling her.
Source: CandyBox Images/Fotolia

have long been forgotten or repressed. Historically, Dr. Sigmund Freud, a noted Austrian neurologist and psychoanalyst, developed the theory of the unconscious as a result of his experiments with a hypnotized patient.

- **Psychoanalysis** is a method of obtaining a detailed account of past and present mental and emotional experiences and repressions. It was also developed by Dr. Freud. Psychoanalysis attempts, through free association and dream interpretation, to reveal and resolve the unconscious conflicts that are considered to be at the root of some mental disorders. It is believed that these conflicts have been repressed since childhood and after being brought to the conscious level can be resolved.

ELECTROCONVULSIVE THERAPY

Electroconvulsive therapy (ECT) is the use of an electric shock to produce convulsions. It is useful for individuals whose depression is severe or life-threatening, particularly for those who cannot take antidepressant medication. In recent years, ECT has been much improved. A muscle relaxant is given to the patient before treatment, which is performed under brief anesthesia. Electrodes are placed at precise locations on the head to deliver electrical impulses. The stimulation causes a brief (about 30 seconds) seizure within the brain. The person receiving ECT does not consciously experience the electrical stimulus. For full therapeutic benefit, at least several sessions of ECT, typically given at the rate of three per week, are required.

Study *and* Review I

Overview: Mental Health and Mental Disorders

Write your answers to the following questions.

1. A _____ is an abnormal condition of the brain or mind.

2. List the three mental disorders that are listed among the top 10 causes of disability in the United States.

   a. _____   c. _____

   b. _____

3. _____ is the branch of medicine that deals with the study, diagnosis, and treatment of mental disorders.

4. Give the three basic forms of treatment for mental disorders.

   a. _____   c. _____

   b. _____

5. _____ is a method of obtaining a detailed account of past and present mental and emotional experiences and repressions.

Building Your Medical Vocabulary

This section provides the foundation for learning medical terminology. Review the alphabetized list of medical terms in the following pages. Note how common prefixes and suffixes are repeatedly applied to word roots and combining forms to create different meanings. A combining form is a word root plus a vowel. The chart below lists the combining forms and word roots used in this chapter and can help to strengthen your understanding of how medical words are built and spelled.

You will find that some terms have not been divided into word parts. These are common words or specialized terms that are included to enhance your medical vocabulary.

Combining Forms

agor/a	marketplace	**path/o**	disease
aut/o	self	**phob/o**	fear
centr/o	center	**phren/o**	mind
compuls/o	compel, drive	**psych/o**	mind
cycl/o	circle, cycle	**schiz/o**	to divide
delus/o	to cheat	**somat/o**	body
eg/o	I, self	**thym/o**	mind, emotion
neur/o	nerve	**trop/o**	turning
obsess/o	besieged by thoughts		

Word Roots

hallucinat	to wander in mind	**iatr**	treatment

Medical Word	Word Parts		Definition
	Part	**Meaning**	
affect (ăf´ fĕkt)			In psychology, observable evidence of an individual's emotional reaction associated with an experience
affective disorder (ăf-fĕk´ tĭv)			Characterized by a disturbance of mood accompanied by a manic or depressive syndrome; this syndrome is not caused by any other physical or mental disorder
agoraphobia (ăg˝ ŏ-ră-fō´ bē-ă)	**agor/a** -**phobia**	marketplace fear	An anxiety disorder; agoraphobia involves intense fear and anxiety in any place or situation where escape might be difficult, leading to avoidance of being alone outside of the home; traveling in a car, bus, or airplane; or being in a crowded area
anorexia nervosa (ăn-ō-rĕk´ sē-ă nĕr-vō´ să)	**an-** -**orexia**	lack of, without appetite	Complex psychological disorder in which the individual refuses to eat or has an abnormally limited eating pattern. People with eating disorders may engage in self-induced vomiting and abuse of laxatives, diuretics, or prolonged exercise to control their weight. The condition could lead them to become excessively thin or even emaciated. In severe cases, this condition can be life-threatening.

Medical Word	Word Parts		Definition
	Part	Meaning	
anxiety (ăng-zī´ ĕ-tē)			Feeling of uneasiness, apprehension, worry, or dread; involuntary or reflex reaction of the body to stress. Anxiety can be a normal reaction to stress and can help us deal with a tense situation, study harder for an exam, or keep focused on an important speech. In general, it can help us cope.
anxiety disorders			Mental disorders that can affect adults and children and are chronic, growing progressively worse if not treated. These disorders appear to be caused by an interaction of biopsychosocial factors, including genetic vulnerability, which interact with situations, stress, or trauma to produce clinically significant syndromes. Symptoms, which may begin in childhood or adolescence, include excessive, irrational fear or dread. Examples include obsessive–compulsive disorder, posttraumatic stress disorder, social phobia, specific phobia, and generalized anxiety disorder. See Figure 18.5 for physiological responses in anxiety disorders.

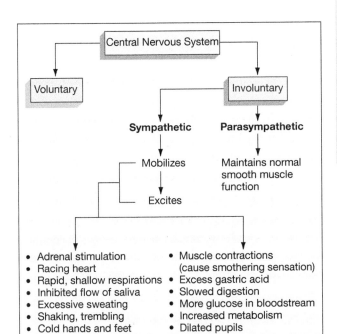

FIGURE 18.5 Physiological responses in anxiety disorders.

 fyi A form of anxiety disorder, **panic disorder** (often called *panic attacks*) causes feelings of terror that strike suddenly and repeatedly with no warning. People with this disorder cannot predict when an attack will occur, and many develop intense anxiety between episodes, worrying about when and where the next one will strike.

When having a panic attack, a person feels sweaty, flushed or chilled, weak, faint, or dizzy. The hands can tingle or feel numb. There can be nausea, chest pain or a smothering sensation, a sense of unreality, or fear of impending doom or loss of control. The individual can genuinely believe that he or she is having a heart attack, losing his or her mind, or on the verge of death.

| **apathy**
(ăp´ ă-thē) | **a-**
-pathy | without, lack of
emotion | Condition in which a person lacks feelings and emotions and is indifferent |

Medical Word	Word Parts		Definition
	Part	Meaning	
apperception (ăp˝ ĕr-sĕp´ shŭn)			Comprehension or assimilation of the meaning and significance of a particular sensory stimulus as modified by an individual's own experiences, knowledge, thoughts, and emotions
attention-deficit/ hyperactivity disorder (ADHD)			One of the most common childhood disorders, ADHD can continue through adolescence and adulthood. Symptoms include difficulty staying focused and paying attention, difficulty controlling behavior, and hyperactivity.

fyi ADHD has three subtypes:

- *Predominantly hyperactive-impulsive:* Child can't sit still; walks, runs, or climbs when others are seated; talks when others are talking.
- *Predominantly inattentive:* Child daydreams or seems to be in another world; is sidetracked by what is going on around him or her.
- *Combined hyperactive-impulsive and inattentive:* Six or more symptoms of inattention and six or more symptoms of hyperactivity-impulsivity are present in the child.

Most children have the combined type of ADHD.

Medical Word	Word Parts		Definition
autism spectrum disorder (ASD) (aw´ tĭzm)	aut -ism	self condition	A DSM-5 term that reflects a scientific consensus that four previously separate disorders are actually a single condition with different levels of symptom severity. Some children are mildly impaired by their symptoms, but others are severely disabled. DSM-5 currently defines four disorders: • Autistic disorder (autism) • Asperger disorder (Asperger syndrome) • Childhood disintegrative disorder (CDD) • Pervasive developmental disorder not otherwise specified (PDD-NOS) See Figure 18.6.

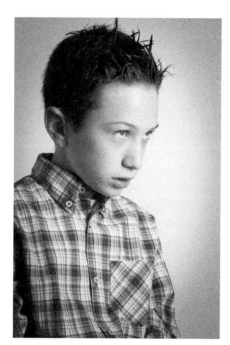

FIGURE 18.6 A child with autism may be self-absorbed, inaccessible, and unable to relate to others.
Source: UMB-O/Shutterstock

Medical Word	Word Parts		Definition
	Part	Meaning	
bipolar disorder (bī-pōl′ ăr)			Brain disorder also known as *manic-depressive illness* that causes unusual shifts in a person's mood, energy, and ability to carry out day-to-day tasks. Bipolar disorder is characterized by cycling mood changes: mania or hypomania (a less severe form of mania) and severe lows (depression). In DSM-5, a specifier, *with mixed features*, can be applied to episodes of mania/hypomania and depression that occur simultaneously.
compulsion (kŏm-pŭl′ shŭn)	**compuls** **-ion**	compel, drive process	Uncontrollable, recurrent, and distressing urge to perform an act in order to relieve fear connected with obsession. Common compulsions involve excessive handwashing, touching objects, and continual counting and checking.
cyclothymic disorder (sī-klō-thī′ mĭk)	**cycl/o** **thym** **-ic**	circle, cycle mind, emotion pertaining to	Mood disorder characterized by alternating moods of elation and depression, similar to bipolar disorder but of milder intensity
delirium (dĕ-lĭr′ ē-ŭm)			State of mental confusion marked by illusions, hallucinations, excitement, restlessness, delusions, and speech incoherence
delusion (dĕ-loo′ zhŭn)	**delus** **-ion**	to cheat process	Characterized by bizarre thoughts that have no basis in reality; a fixed, false belief or abnormal perception held by a person despite evidence to the contrary
dementia (di-men′ chă)			Problem in the brain that makes it difficult for a person to remember, learn, and communicate and eventually to take care of him- or herself; can also affect a person's mood and personality. Dementia of the Alzheimer type is the most common form.

Medical Word	Word Parts		Definition
	Part	Meaning	
depression (dĕ-prĕsh´ ŭn)			Mental disorder marked by altered mood and loss of interest in things that are usually pleasurable such as food, sex, work, friends, hobbies, or entertainment. See Figure 18.7. A less severe type of depression, *dysthymia*, involves long-term, chronic symptoms that do not disable but keep an individual from functioning well or feeling good. Many people with dysthymia also experience major depressive episodes at some time in their lives.

Mood depressed; Memory problems
Anxious; Apathetic; Appetite changes
"**J**ust no fun"
  Occupational impairment
  Restlessness; Ruminative

    Doubts self; Difficulty making decisions
    Empty feeling
      Pessimistic; Persistent sadness; Psychomotor retardation
      Report vague pains
      Energy gone
        Suicidal thoughts and impulses
        Sleep disturbances
          Irritability; Inability to concentrate
          Oppressive guilt
            "**N**othing can help" (Hopelessness)

FIGURE 18.7 Characteristics of major depression.

Medical Word	Word Parts		Definition
	Part	Meaning	

fyi The depressed child can pretend to be sick, refuse to go to school, cling to a parent, or worry that the parent could die. Older children sulk; get into trouble at school; and are negative, grouchy, and feel misunderstood. Because normal behaviors vary from one childhood stage to another, it can be difficult to tell whether a child is just going through a temporary phase or suffering from depression. Symptoms of depression in the child:

Toddlers. Sadness, inactivity, complaints of stomachaches, and, in rare cases, self-destructive behavior.

Elementary school–age children. Unhappiness, poor school performance, irritability, refusal to take part in activities he or she used to enjoy, and occasional thoughts of suicide.

Adolescents. Sadness, withdrawal, feelings of hopelessness or guilt, changes in sleeping or eating habits, and frequent thoughts of suicide.

A child does not understand feelings of stress, anxiety, or depression and does not know how to ask for help, so when a child exhibits dramatic mood or behavior shifts, a physician should be consulted immediately. The physician could recommend psychotherapy or prescribe an antidepressant for children who are at least 5 years of age or older.

| dissociation (dĭs-sō″ sē-ā′ shŭn) | | | Defense mechanism in which a group of mental processes become separated from normal consciousness and, thus separated, function as a unitary whole. In *dissociative disorder* there is a severe disturbance or trauma that causes changes in memory, consciousness, identity, and general awareness of oneself and one's environment. There are four primary types of dissociative disorders: *psychogenic amnesia, psychogenic fugue, dissociative identity disorder (DID),* and *depersonalization disorder.* |
| eating disorders | | | Disorders that cause serious disturbances to an individual's everyday diet, such as eating extremely small amounts of food or severely overeating; *anorexia nervosa, bulimia nervosa,* and *binge-eating disorder* are the most common types |

fyi **Bulimia nervosa** is a potentially life-threatening eating disorder. Preoccupied with weight and body shape, people with bulimia may judge themselves severely and secretly binge—eating excessive amounts of food—and then purge, trying to get rid of the extra calories in an unhealthy way, such as forcing vomiting, taking laxatives, or exercising excessively. Effective treatment can help a person with bulimia feel better about his or her self-image, adopt healthier eating patterns, and reverse serious complications.

Binge-eating disorder is a serious eating disorder characterized by uncontrollable, excessive eating, followed by feelings of shame and guilt. Unlike those with bulimia, the person with binge-eating disorder does not purge. However, a person with bulimia may also binge-eat.

Medical Word	Word Parts		Definition
	Part	Meaning	
egocentric (ē″ gō-sĕn′ trĭk)	**eg/o** **centr** **-ic**	I, self center pertaining to	Pertaining to being self-centered
factitious disorder (făk-tĭsh′ ŭs)			Disorder that is not real, genuine, or natural. The physical and psychological symptoms are produced by the person to place him- or herself or another in the role of a patient or someone in need of help. These patients have a severe personality disturbance. *Munchausen syndrome* is a chronic factitious disorder in which a healthy person habitually seeks medical treatment; in the rare *Munchausen-by-proxy syndrome (MBPS)*, a parent (usually the mother) or other caregiver is the deliberate cause of a child's illness (by poisoning, for instance) to gain sympathy or attention.
fugue (fūg)			Dissociative disorder in which amnesia is accompanied by physical flight from customary surroundings. In psychogenic fugue, there is sudden, unexpected travel away from an individual's home or place of work with inability to recall the past. The individual can assume a partial or completely new identity. This condition is usually of short duration but can last for months. Following recovery, the person does not recall anything that happened during the fugue.
generalized anxiety disorder (GAD)			Characterized by much higher levels of anxiety than people normally experience day to day. It is chronic and fills a person's day with exaggerated worry and tension. Having this disorder means always anticipating disaster, often worrying excessively about health, money, family, or work.
hallucination (hă-loo-sĭ-nā′ shŭn)	**hallucinat** **-ion**	to wander in mind process	Process of experiencing sensations that have no source. Some examples of hallucinations include hearing nonexistent voices, seeing nonexistent things, and experiencing burning or pain sensations with no physical cause.
hypomania (hī′ pō-mā′ nē-ă)	**hypo-** **-mania**	deficient, below madness	Abnormal mood of mild mania characterized by hyperactivity, inflated self-esteem, talkativeness, heightened sexual interest, quickness to anger, irritability, and a decreased need for sleep
impulse control disorder			Mental condition in which the person is unable to resist urges or impulses to perform acts that could be harmful to him- or herself or others. *Pyromania* (starting fires), *kleptomania* (stealing), and compulsive gambling are examples of impulse control disorders.

Medical Word	Word Parts		Definition
	Part	Meaning	
mania (mā´ nē-ă)			Mental disorder characterized by excessive excitement; literally means *madness*. See Figure 18.8.

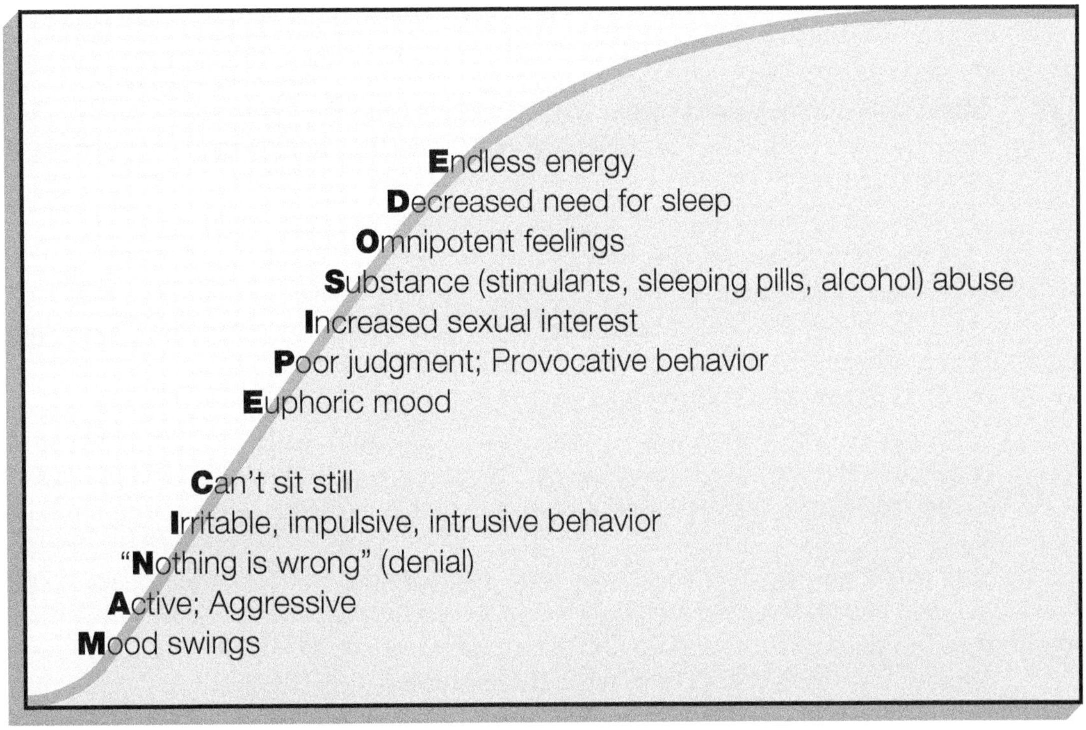

Endless energy
Decreased need for sleep
Omnipotent feelings
Substance (stimulants, sleeping pills, alcohol) abuse
Increased sexual interest
Poor judgment; Provocative behavior
Euphoric mood

Can't sit still
Irritable, impulsive, intrusive behavior
"Nothing is wrong" (denial)
Active; Aggressive
Mood swings

FIGURE 18.8 Characteristics of a manic episode.

mood			Pervasive and sustained emotion that plays a key role in an individual's perception of the world. Examples include depression, joy, elation, anger, and anxiety.
neurotic (noor-ŏt´ ĭk)	neur/o -tic	nerve pertaining to	Pertaining to one who has an abnormal emotional or mental disorder
norepinephrine (nor-ĕp˝ ĭ-nĕf´ rĭn)			Hormone produced by the adrenal medulla that acts as a neurotransmitter. It is believed that disturbances in its metabolism at important brain sites can be implicated in affective disorders.

Medical Word	Word Parts		Definition
	Part	**Meaning**	
obsession (ob-sesh´ ŏn)	**obsess**	besieged by thoughts	Neurotic state in which an individual has a recurrent, persistent thought, image, or impulse that is unwanted and distressing and comes involuntarily to mind despite attempts to resist
	-ion	process	

fyi

Obsessive–compulsive disorder (OCD) involves persistent, unwelcome thoughts or images or the urgent need to engage in certain rituals that the person cannot control. For example, individuals can exhibit the following:

- Obsession with germs or dirt, thus they repeatedly wash their hands
- Doubt and the need to check things repeatedly
- Frequent thoughts of violence and the fear that they will harm someone close to them
- Long periods of touching or counting things or being preoccupied with order or symmetry
- Persistent thoughts of performing repulsive sexual acts
- Thoughts against their religious beliefs

The disturbing thoughts or images are called *obsessions*, and the rituals performed to try to prevent or get rid of them are called *compulsions*. The person experiences only temporary *relief*, not pleasure, in carrying out the rituals, caused by the *anxiety* that increases when they are not performed. See Figure 18.9. DSM-5 includes four new obsessive–compulsive disorders: (1) excoriation (skin-picking) disorder, (2) hoarding disorder, (3) substance- or medication-induced obsessive–compulsive and related disorder, and (4) obsessive–compulsive and related disorder due to another medical condition. Other specified obsessive–compulsive and related disorders can include body-focused repetitive behavior disorder, such as nail biting, lip biting, and cheek chewing.

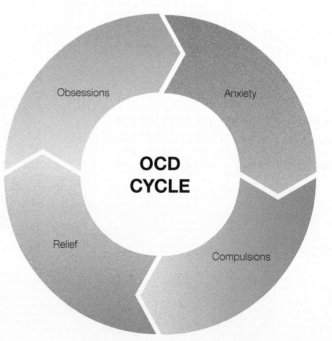

FIGURE 18.9 The cycle of obsessive–compulsive disorder.
Source: PEARSON EDUCATION; SERVICES, PEARSON; PEARSON EDUCATION, . ., NURSING: A CONCEPT-BASED APPROACH TO LEARNING, VOLUME I, 1st Ed., ©2019. Reprinted and Electronically reproduced by permission of Pearson Education, Inc., New York, NY.

Medical Word	Word Parts		Definition
	Part	Meaning	
paranoia (păr″ ă-noy′ ă)	**para-** **-noia**	beside, abnormal mind	Mental disorder characterized by highly exaggerated or unwarranted mistrust or suspiciousness; generally classified into three categories: *paranoid personality disorder, delusional (paranoid) disorder*, and *paranoid schizophrenia*. Delusional (paranoid) disorder is characterized by persistent delusions of persecution or grandeur or a combination of the two.
personality disorder (PD)			Mental disorder characterized by inflexible and maladaptive personality traits that are exhibited across many contexts and deviate markedly from those accepted by the individual's culture; often causes problems in work, school, or social relationships. See Figure 18.10.

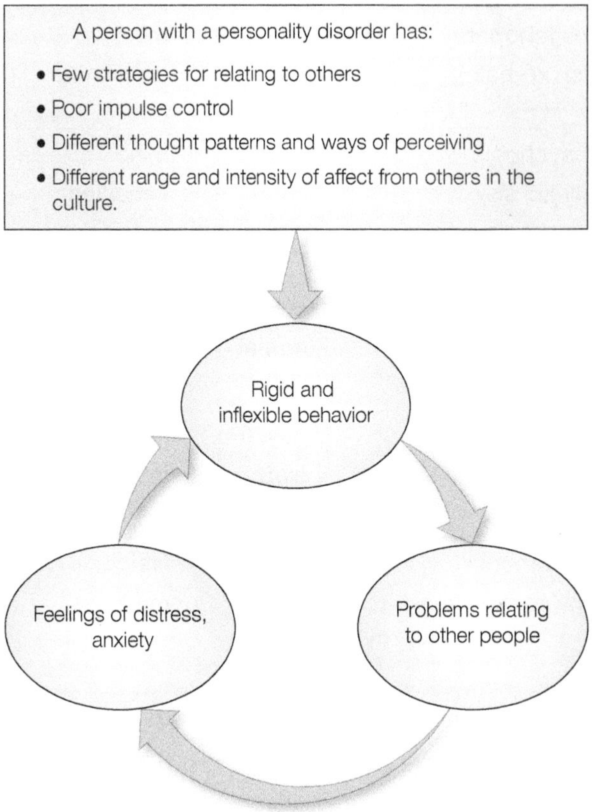

A person with a personality disorder has:

• Few strategies for relating to others
• Poor impulse control
• Different thought patterns and ways of perceiving
• Different range and intensity of affect from others in the culture.

Rigid and inflexible behavior

Feelings of distress, anxiety

Problems relating to other people

FIGURE 18.10 Persistent cycle of personality disorders.
Source: PEARSON EDUCATION; SERVICES, PEARSON; PEARSON EDUCATION, . ., NURSING: A CONCEPT-BASED APPROACH TO LEARNING, VOLUME I, 1st Ed., ©2019. Reprinted and Electronically reproduced by permission of Pearson Education, Inc., New York, NY.

Medical Word	Word Parts		Definition
phobia (fō′ bē-ă)	**phob** **-ia**	fear condition	Morbid and persistent fear of a specific object, activity, or situation that results in a compelling desire to avoid the feared stimulus. Examples include *claustrophobia* (fear of enclosed places), *acrophobia* (fear of heights), *photophobia* (fear of light), *arachnophobia* (fear of spiders), *nyctophobia* (fear of darkness/night), and *hematophobia* or *hemophobia* (fear of blood/bleeding).

Medical Word	Word Parts		Definition
	Part	Meaning	
posttraumatic stress disorder (PTSD)			Debilitating anxiety disorder that can develop following a terrifying event. It was brought to public attention by war veterans. In DSM-5, the diagnostic thresholds have been lowered for children and adolescents and separate criteria have been added for children age 6 years or younger. PTSD can result from any number of traumatic incidents, such as a mugging, rape, or torture; being kidnapped or held captive; child abuse; serious accidents; and natural disasters.
psychiatrist (sī-kī´ ă-trĭst)	**psych** **iatr** **-ist**	mind treatment one who specializes	Physician who specializes in the study and treatment of mental disorders
psychopath (sī´ kō-păth)	**psych/o** **path**	mind disease	Mentally ill individual with an antisocial personality disorder; also called *sociopath*. *Note:* Path is the root for the combining form path/o.
psychosis (sī-kō´ sĭs)	**psych** **-osis**	mind condition	Serious, abnormal mental condition in which the individual's mental capacity to recognize reality and communicate with and relate to others is impaired; the person can experience delusions and hallucinations
psychosomatic (sī˝ kō-sō-mặt´ ĭk)	**psych/o** **somat** **-ic**	mind body pertaining to	Pertaining to the interrelationship of the mind and the body; a manifestation of physical disease that has a mental origin
psychotropic (sī˝ kō-trō´ pĭk)	**psych/o** **trop** **-ic**	mind turning pertaining to	Drug that affects psychic function, behavior, or experience
pyromania (pī˝ rō-mā´ nē-ă)	**pyro-** **-mania**	fire madness	Impulsive disorder consisting of a compulsion to set fires or to watch fires; literally means *a madness for fire*; person suffering from this disorder (pyromaniac) receives pleasure and emotional relief from these activities
schizophrenia (skĭt˝ sō-frē´ nē-ă)	**schiz/o** **phren** **-ia**	to divide mind condition	Mental disorder characterized by *positive* and *negative* symptoms. Positive (psychotic) symptoms include delusions, hallucinations, and disorganized speech. Negative symptoms include social withdrawal, extreme apathy, diminished motivation, and blunted emotional expression.

Medical Word	Word Parts		Definition
	Part	Meaning	
seasonal affective disorder (SAD)			Form of depression that appears related to fluctuations in a person's exposure to natural light; usually strikes during autumn and often continues through the winter when natural light is reduced. Researchers have found that people who have SAD can be helped if they spend blocks of time bathed in light from a special full-spectrum light source called a *light therapy box*. See Figure 18.11.

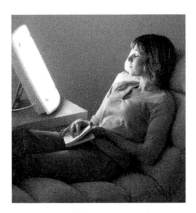

FIGURE 18.11 Woman using seasonal affective disorder light therapy box.
Source: Image Point Fr/Shutterstock

Medical Word	Word Parts		Definition
serotonin (sĕr″ ŏ-tō´ nĭn)			Chemical present in gastrointestinal mucosa, platelets, mast cells, and carcinoid tumors; a vasoconstrictor and a neurotransmitter in the central nervous system (CNS); affects sleep and sensory perception
sexual disorders			Disorders that affect sexual desire, performance, and behavior. *Sexual dysfunction, gender dysphoria* (characterized by a persistent discomfort concerning one's anatomical sexual makeup and the desire to live as a member of the opposite sex), and *paraphilias* are examples. In paraphilia, sexual arousal requires unusual or bizarre fantasies or acts involving nonhuman objects, sexual activity with humans in which real or simulated suffering or humiliation occurs, or sexual activity with nonconsenting partners. Included in this disorder are *bestiality, fetishism, transvestism, zoophilia, pedophilia, exhibitionism, voyeurism, sexual masochism*, and *sexual sadism*.

Medical Word	Word Parts		Definition
	Part	Meaning	
somatic symptom disorder (SSD) (sō-măt′ ĭk)	somat -ic	body pertaining to	Mental disorder in which the person experiences the physical symptoms of an illness that are not explained by a medical condition or a medication. SSD is characterized by somatic symptoms that are either very distressing or result in significant disruption of functioning, as well as excessive and disproportionate thoughts, feelings, and behaviors regarding those symptoms. To be diagnosed with SSD, the individual must be persistently symptomatic (typically at least for 6 months).
substance abuse			Misuse of medications, alcohol, or illegal substances
suicide			Willfully ending one's own life. In the United States, suicide is the seventh leading cause of death for males, the 14th for females, and the third for young people 15–24 years of age. Research shows that the risk for suicide is associated with changes in brain chemicals called *neurotransmitters*, including serotonin. Decreased levels of serotonin have been found in people with depression, impulsive disorders, and a history of suicide attempts and in the brains of suicide victims.

fyi According to NIMH, older Americans are disproportionately likely to die by suicide.

Depression, which can lead to suicide, is a serious problem in the older adult. Depressive symptoms are *not* a normal part of aging. Persistent sadness or grief or loss of interest in food, sex, work, family, friends, and hobbies should be noted in an older person. See Figure 18.12.

Depression often co-occurs with other serious conditions such as heart disease, stroke, diabetes, cancer, and Parkinson disease. Because many older adults face these conditions as well as various social and economic difficulties, healthcare professionals often mistakenly conclude that depression is a normal consequence of these problems—an attitude often shared by patients themselves. These factors together contribute to the underdiagnosis and undertreatment of depressive disorders in older people. See Figure 18.13.

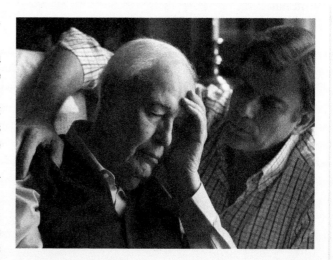

FIGURE 18.12 An elderly man suffering from depression being comforted by a family member.
Source: Christian Martinez Kempin/123RF

Medical Word	Word Parts		Definition
	Part	Meaning	

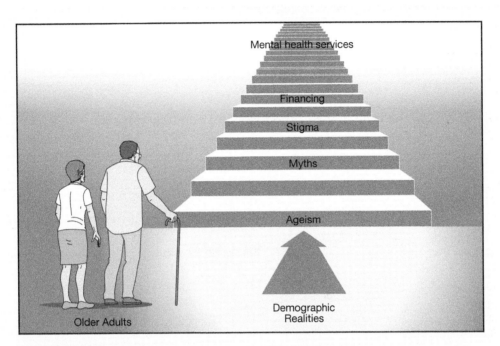

FIGURE 18.13 Roadblocks to mental health services for older adults.

| tic disorder | | | Characterized by spasmodic muscular contractions most commonly involving the face, mouth, eyes, head, neck, or shoulder muscles. People with tic disorders make sounds or display body movements that are repetitive, quick, sudden, and/or uncontrollable. In general, tics are of psychological or neurological origin. |

Tourette syndrome (TS) is a neurological disorder characterized by repetitive, stereotyped, involuntary movements and vocalizations called *tics*. The early symptoms of TS are typically noticed first in childhood, with the average onset between the ages of 3 and 9 years. TS occurs in people from all ethnic groups; males are affected about three to four times more often than females. It is estimated that 200,000 Americans have the most severe form of TS, and as many as one in 100 exhibit milder and less complex symptoms such as chronic motor or vocal tics.

Study *and* Review II

Word Parts

Prefixes   Give the definitions of the following prefixes.

1. an-   _____
2. hypo-   _____
3. para-   _____
4. pyro-   _____

Combining Forms   Give the definitions of the following combining forms.

1. agor/a   _____
2. centr/o   _____
3. cycl/o   _____
4. delus/o   _____
5. neur/o   _____
6. path/o   _____
7. phren/o   _____
8. psych/o   _____
9. schiz/o   _____
10. somat/o   _____
11. thym/o   _____

Suffixes   Give the definitions of the following suffixes.

1. -form   _____
2. -ia   _____
3. -ic   _____
4. -ion   _____
5. -ism   _____
6. -ist   _____
7. -mania   _____
8. -noia   _____
9. -orexia   _____
10. -osis   _____
11. -phobia   _____
12. -therapy   _____
13. -tic   _____

Identifying Medical Terms

In the spaces provided, write the medical terms for the following meanings.

1. _____ Intense fear and anxiety of any place or situation where escape might be difficult, leading to avoidance of such situations

2. _____ Condition in which a person lacks feelings and emotions

3. _____ Fixed, false belief or abnormal perception

4. _____ Mental disorder marked by altered mood and loss of interest in things that are usually pleasurable

5. _____ Pertaining to being self-centered

6. _____ Mental disorder characterized by excessive excitement; literally means *madness*

7. _____ Morbid and persistent fear of a specific object, activity, or situation that results in a compelling desire to avoid the feared stimulus

8. _____ Physician who specializes in the study and treatment of mental disorders

9. _____ Method of treating mental disorders by using psychological techniques instead of physical methods

10. _____ Literally means *a madness for fire*

Matching

Select the appropriate lettered meaning for each of the following words.

_____ 1. dysthymia

_____ 2. seasonal affective disorder

_____ 3. bipolar disorder

_____ 4. schizophrenia

_____ 5. delusion

_____ 6. hallucination

_____ 7. obsessive–compulsive disorder

_____ 8. posttraumatic stress disorder

_____ 9. generalized anxiety disorder

_____ 10. attention-deficit/ hyperactivity disorder

a. Mental disorder characterized by positive, negative, and cognitive symptoms

b. Process of experiencing sensations that have no source

c. Brain disorder also known as *manic-depressive illness* that causes unusual shifts in a person's mood, energy, and ability to function

d. Less severe type of depression involving long-term, chronic symptoms that do not disable but keep the person from functioning well or from feeling good

e. Debilitating anxiety disorder that can develop following a terrifying event

f. Characterized by bizarre thoughts that have no basis in reality

g. Form of depression that appears related to fluctuations in a person's exposure to natural light

h. Characterized by much higher levels of anxiety than people normally experience day to day

i. Involves persistent, unwelcome thoughts or images or the urgent need to engage in certain rituals that the person cannot control

j. One of the most common childhood disorders and can continue through adolescence and adulthood

Medical Case Snapshot

This learning activity provides an opportunity to relate the medical terminology you are learning to a sample patient case presentation. In the spaces provided, write in your answers.

A 67-year-old female complains of sadness. She describes loss of interest in eating and social activities. After

careful evaluation and examination, it was determined that this patient was experiencing depression. This is a

_____ _____ marked by altered _____

and loss of interest in things that are usually pleasurable. A less severe type of this condition known as

_____ involves long-term, chronic symptoms.

Drug Highlights

Classification of Drug	Description and Examples
antianxiety agents	Chemical substances that relieve anxiety and muscle tension are indicated when anxiety interferes with a person's ability to function properly.
benzodiazepines	The *benzodiazepines* are a group of drugs with similar chemical structures and pharmaceutical activities. They are the most widely prescribed drugs for the treatment of anxiety.
	EXAMPLES: Xanax (alprazolam), Klonopin (clonazepam), Tranxene (clorazepate), Librium (chlordiazepoxide HCl), Valium (diazepam), and Ativan (lorazepam).
nonbenzodiazepines	Serotonin receptor agonists that increase action at serotonin receptors in the brain, which helps to alleviate anxiety.
	EXAMPLE: BuSpar (buspirone)
antidepressant agents	Chemical substances that relieve the symptoms of depression are indicated when depression interferes with a person's ability to function properly. Antidepressant agents can be grouped as SSRIs, SNRIs, TCAs, or MAOIs.
selective serotonin reuptake inhibitors (SSRIs)	Drugs in this group specifically block reabsorption of serotonin.
	EXAMPLES: Prozac (fluoxetine), Zoloft (sertraline), Paxil (paroxetine), and Luvox (fluvoxamine)
serotonin-norepinephrine reuptake inhibitors (SNRIs)	Drugs in this group are used to treat depression, anxiety disorders, and long-time chronic pain. They increase the level of serotonin and norepinephrine in the brain, which helps improve mood.
	EXAMPLES: Pristiq, Khedezla (desvenlafaxine), Cymbalta (duloxetine), Effexor XR (venlafaxine)

Classification of Drug	Description and Examples
tricyclic antidepressants (TCAs)	Drugs in this group raise the level of norepinephrine and serotonin in the brain by slowing the rate at which they are reabsorbed by nerve cells. EXAMPLES: Tofranil (imipramine HC1), Pamelor (nortriptyline HC1), and amoxapine
monoamine oxidase inhibitors (MAOIs)	Drugs in this group work by blocking the breakdown of two potent neurotransmitters—norepinephrine and serotonin—allowing them to bathe the nerve endings for an extended length of time. EXAMPLES: Nardil (phenelzine sulfate) and Parnate (tranylcypromine sulfate)
additional drugs	There are a number of additional drugs used to treat depression. Some of these drugs are used for other conditions and are being tested for treating depression; others do not fit into any of the described groups. EXAMPLES: Mirapex (pramipexole dihydrochloride), nefazodone HC1, Wellbutrin (bupropion HC1), and Remeron (mirtazapine)
antimanic agent	Although not a group of drugs, various lithium medications control mood disorders by directly affecting internal nerve cell processes in all of the neurotransmitter systems. Lithium is best known as an antimanic drug used in the treatment of bipolar disorder. EXAMPLE: Carbolith (lithium carbonate)
antipsychotic agents	Also called *neuroleptics*, these agents modify psychotic behavior. Many antipsychotic agents are derivatives of phenothiazine (an organic compound used in the manufacture of certain of these drugs). These agents are used in the treatment of acute and chronic schizophrenia, organic psychoses, the manic phase of bipolar disorder, and psychotic disorders. EXAMPLE: chlorpromazine HCl Some antipsychotic agents are not actually phenothiazines but resemble them in action. Others resemble tricyclic antidepressants, while some are miscellaneous compounds. EXAMPLES: Clozaril (clozapine), Zyprexa (olanzapine), Orap (pimozide), and loxapine
atypical antipsychotics	Drugs in this group affect serotonin and dopamine. EXAMPLES: Risperdal (risperidone), Clozaril (clozapine), and Zyprexa (olanzapine)
stimulants	These drugs stimulate the central nervous system (CNS) and are generally prescribed for attention-deficit/hyperactivity disorder. Patients using these drugs must take care to avoid abuse and excessive CNS stimulation by overdose. Many of these drugs are Schedule II agents with a very high potential for abuse. EXAMPLES: Dexedrine (dextroamphetamine sulfate), Ritalin (methylphenidate HCl), and Adderall, which is a combination of amphetamine salts

Abbreviations *and* Acronyms

Abbreviation/Acronym	Meaning	Abbreviation/Acronym	Meaning
ADHD	attention-deficit/hyperactivity disorder	NIH	National Institutes of Health
AMI	any mental illness	NIMH	National Institute of Mental Health
APA	American Psychiatric Association	OCD	obsessive–compulsive disorder
ASD	autism spectrum disorder	PD	personality disorder
CBT	cognitive-behavioral therapy	PDD-NOS	pervasive developmental disorder not otherwise specified
CDD	childhood disintegrative disorder		
CNS	central nervous system	PTSD	posttraumatic stress disorder
DID	dissociative identity disorder	SAD	seasonal affective disorder
DSM-5	*Diagnostic and Statistical Manual of Mental Disorders*, Fifth Edition	SMI	serious mental illness
		SNRIs	serotonin-norepinephrine reuptake inhibitors
ECT	electroconvulsive therapy		
GAD	generalized anxiety disorder	SSD	somatic symptom disorder
HHS	Department of Health and Human Services	SSRIs	selective serotonin reuptake inhibitors
		TAT	Thematic Apperception Test
IQ	intelligence quotient	TCAs	tricyclic antidepressants
MAOIs	monoamine oxidase inhibitors	TS	Tourette syndrome
MBPS	Munchausen-by-proxy syndrome	WAIS-R	Wechsler Adult Intelligence Scale–Revised
MD	medical doctor	WHO	World Health Organization
MMPI-2	Minnesota Multiphasic Personality Inventory-2		

Study *and* Review III

Drug Highlights

Match the appropriate lettered description or examples of drug(s) with the class of drug.

_____ 1. nonbenzodiapines

_____ 2. tricyclic antidepressants (TCAs)

_____ 3. antimanic agents

a. Act on the central nervous system and are generally prescribed for attention-deficit/hyperactivity disorder

b. Drugs in this group, such as Risperdal (risperidone), affect serotonin and dopamine

_____ 4. antipsychotic agents

_____ 5. atypical antipsychotics

_____ 6. stimulants

_____ 7. benzodiazepines

_____ 8. examples of selective serotonin reuptake inhibitors (SSRIs)

_____ 9. monoamine oxidase inhibitors (MAOIs)

_____ 10. antidepressant agents

c. Used in the treatment of acute and chronic schizophrenia, organic psychoses, the manic phase of bipolar disorder, and psychotic disorders

d. Lithium medications that control mood disorders by directly affecting internal nerve cell processes in all of the neurotransmitter systems

e. Prozac (fluoxetine), Zoloft (sertraline), and Paxil (paroxetine)

f. Serotonin receptor agonists that increase action at serotonin receptors in the brain, which helps to alleviate anxiety

g. The most widely prescribed drugs for the treatment of anxiety

h. Raise the level of norepinephrine and serotonin in the brain by slowing the rate at which they are reabsorbed by nerve cells

i. Chemical agents that are grouped into these categories: SSRIs, SNRIs, TCAs, or MAOIs

j. Block the breakdown of two potent neurotransmitters— norepinephrine and serotonin—and allow them to bathe the nerve endings for an extended length of time

Abbreviations and Acronyms

Write the correct word, phrase, or abbreviation/acronym in the space provided.

1. cognitive-behavioral therapy _____

2. *Diagnostic and Statistical Manual of Mental Disorders*, Fifth Edition _____

3. ECT _____

4. MMPI-2 _____

5. National Institute of Mental Health _____

6. OCD _____

7. posttraumatic stress disorder _____

8. SAD _____

9. TAT _____

10. World Health Organization _____

Practical Application

Medical Record Analysis

This exercise contains information, abbreviations/acronyms, and medical terminology from an actual medical record or case study that has been adapted for this text. The names and any personal information have been created by the author. Read and study each form or case study and then answer the questions that follow. You may refer to Appendix III, *Abbreviations, Acronyms, and Symbols*.

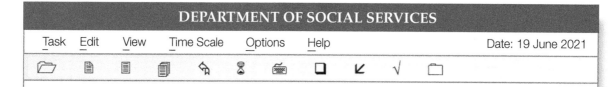

DEPARTMENT OF SOCIAL SERVICES

| Task | Edit | View | Time Scale | Options | Help | | Date: 19 June 2021 |

Disability Evaluation Division
1888 Golden Gate Blvd., Suite 10
San Francisco, CA 94132
Re: Rotha, Maly # 123-45-6789

Dear Staff:

Thank you for referring to me the case of Ms. Rotha for psychiatric evaluation. She was examined in psychiatric consultation on June 17, 2021. No physical exam was performed. No psychological testing was given. Medical records provided were reviewed. The patient was a clean, neatly dressed, well-groomed Asian female. She understood English and responded to questions. There was no evidence of any ambulation difficulties or speech impediments. Energy level was described as poor, with description of fatigue with minimal exertion.

History of Present Illness

Ms. Rotha is a 42-year-old Cambodian female. She lives in an apartment with her husband and three children. She describes feeling sick all the time and too weak and tired, dizzy and depressed to do anything except "rest." Currently, she is taking a combination of five different medications under the care of two different physicians. She takes Proventil inhaler for relief of asthmatic symptoms, analgesics, decongestants, and two different forms of tricyclic antidepressants. She feels that the medications are helping her. She is not receiving any formal psychiatric treatment with or without medication.

Mental Examination

There is no evidence or history of alcoholism or illicit drug use. She is oriented to time, place, persons, and events. There is no evidence of delusion or hallucinations at the present time and no history of such in the past. There is no evidence of paranoia such as feelings of being persecuted or plotted against. Thought content is generally well organized, coherent, and relevant without flight of ideas or loose associations.

Depression is manifested by occasional crying, usually occurring every other day. There is fitful sleep. There are occasional nightmares. There is no suicidal ideation or history of any suicide attempts.

Memory for recent and remote events, she feels, is impaired. She cannot recall her Social Security number. She can recall her address and phone number. She can do simple arithmetic.

Medical Opinion

It is my medical opinion that at Ms. Rotha's current level of daily functioning, she has minimal difficulty in relating to others. In appearance she seems to have the ability to care for her personal needs. How much her interest, habits, and daily activities are constricted as a result of mental impairments is difficult to assess because it is my medical opinion that this represents a factitious disorder, although posttraumatic stress disorder should not be ruled out.

Very truly yours,

Hana Eun Kim, MD

Medical Record Questions

Write the correct answer in the space provided.

1. What are the symptoms Ms. Rotha described? _____

2. What medications does this patient take? _____

3. What is a delusion? _____

4. Define *hallucination*. _____

5. Define *factitious disorder*. _____

MyLab Medical Terminology™

MyLab Medical Terminology is a premium online homework management system that includes a host of features to help you study. Registered users will find:

- A multitude of quizzes and activities built within the MyLab platform
- Powerful tools that track and analyze your results—allowing you to create a personalized learning experience
- Videos and audio pronunciations to help enrich your progress
- Streaming lesson presentations (guided lectures) and self-paced learning modules
- A space where you and your instructor can check your progress and manage your assignments

Appendix I

ANSWER KEY

Chapter 1

Study *and* Review I
Word Parts

Prefixes
1. anti-
2. endo-
3. per-
4. inter-
5. hypo-

Suffixes
1. -poiesis
2. -rrhaphy
3. -scopy
4. -tomy
5. -trophy

Formation of Plural Endings
1. bursae
2. thoraces or thoraxes
3. foramina
4. crises
5. irides
6. femora
7. appendices
8. phalanges
9. spermatozoa
10. ova

Study *and* Review II
Word Parts

Prefixes
1. without
2. away from
3. against
4. bad
5. one hundred, one-hundredth
6. through
7. apart
8. upon
9. out
10. different

11. in, into
12. bad
13. small
14. one-thousandth
15. many, much
16. beside
17. before
18. together

Roots and Combining Forms
1. stuck to
2. armpit
3. chemical
4. shaping
5. formation, produce
6. a thousand
7. large
8. death
9. rule
10. tumor
11. organ
12. fever
13. heat, fire
14. ray, x-ray
15. to examine
16. putrefaction
17. hot, heat
18. cough
19. to infect
20. people
21. cause
22. to cut
23. bad kind
24. greatest
25. least
26. palm
27. guarding

Suffixes
1. pertaining to
2. pertaining to
3. pertaining to
4. surgical puncture

5. that which runs together
6. shape
7. formation, produce
8. knowledge
9. a step
10. a weight
11. condition
12. pertaining to
13. process
14. condition
15. nature of, quality of
16. liter
17. study of
18. instrument to measure
19. condition
20. pertaining to
21. to carry
22. instrument for examining
23. decay
24. treatment

Identifying Medical Terms
1. adhesion
2. asepsis
3. axillary
4. chemotherapy
5. heterogeneous
6. malformation
7. microscope
8. multiform
9. oncology

Using Component Parts to Build Medical Words
1. anti-
   pyret
   -ic
2. epi-
   dem
   -ic
3. ex-
   cis
   -ion

4. eti/o

-logy

5. onc/o

-logy

Matching

1. f	**6.** h
2. d	**7.** b
3. j	**8.** i
4. g	**9.** c
5. a	**10.** e

Study *and* Review III
Abbreviations and Acronyms

1. chief complaint	**6.** Ht
2. axillary	**7.** mL
3. Bx	**8.** g
4. Wt	**9.** Dx
5. AD	**10.** PE

Medical Case Snapshot

A Acknowledge: "Hello, Ms. Styles."

I Introduce: "I am Sally Jones, your caregiver for this morning."

D Duration: "The lab technician will be here before breakfast. I will be back to check on you in a little while."

E Explanation: "I want to check your name band and then check your vital signs. What is your full name? Now, let's check your temperature, pulse, respirations, and blood pressure."

T Thank you: "You have been very helpful this morning, and I thank you."

Practical Application

1. SOAP

2. subjective

3. objective

4. AIDET

5. acknowledge

6. explanation

7. thank you

8. SBAR

9. diagnosis; dosages

10. assessment

Chapter 2
Study *and* Review I
General-Use Suffixes

1. To signify that they are to be linked to the end of a root, combining form, or, in some cases, a prefix.

2. -algesia; condition of pain

3. neurocyte

4. hematuria

5. hematocrit

Matching

1. c	**6.** d
2. e	**7.** j
3. a	**8.** f
4. b	**9.** h
5. i	**10.** g

Study *and* Review II
Suffixes That Pertain to Pathological Conditions

1. b	**4.** a
2. d	**5.** d
3. c	

Suffixes That Pertain to Surgical and Diagnostic Procedures

1. True

2. False

3. False

4. True

5. True

Study *and* Review III
General-Use Prefixes

1. c	**4.** b
2. b	**5.** c
3. d	

Prefixes That Have More Than One Meaning

1. f	**6.** i
2. g	**7.** b
3. h	**8.** j
4. a	**9.** d
5. c	**10.** e

Study *and* Review IV
Prefixes That Pertain to Position or Placement

1. c	**6.** d
2. i	**7.** g
3. e	**8.** j
4. b	**9.** f
5. a	**10.** h

Prefixes That Pertain to Numbers and Amounts

1. b	**4.** a
2. d	**5.** c
3. c	

Study *and* Review V
Using Suffixes to Build Medical Words

1. hyperhidrosis

2. muscular

3. macula

4. alopecia

5. ventricle

6. decubitus

7. integumentary

8. penile

9. congenital

10. anterior

Using Prefixes to Build Medical Words

1. apnea	**5.** hyperpnea
2. tachypnea	**6.** bradypnea
3. eupnea	**7.** hypopnea
4. dyspnea	

Identifying Medical Terms—Suffixes

1. abrasion
2. anesthetize
3. arousal
4. asymmetrical
5. infection
6. comatose
7. turgor
8. grandiose
9. gynecoid
10. palpate

Identifying Medical Terms—Prefixes

1. bilateral
2. hyperactive
3. hypoplasia
4. insomnia
5. intravenous
6. pericardial
7. polydactyly
8. premenstrual
9. superinfection
10. unconscious

Chapter 3

Study *and* Review I
Anatomy and Physiology

1. body...cells...sustain
2. cell membrane
3. cell membrane...cytoplasm... nucleus
4. metabolism...growth... reproduction
5. embryonic cell
6. a. protection   d. excretion
   b. absorption   e. sensation
   c. secretion   f. diffusion
7. Connective
8. a. striated (voluntary)
   b. cardiac
   c. smooth (involuntary)

9. excitability...conductivity
10. tissue serving a common purpose
11. group of organs functioning together for a common purpose

Matching

1. f   6. h
2. d   7. b
3. j   8. i
4. g   9. c
5. a   10. e

Anatomical Locations and Positions

1. a. above, in an upward direction
   b. in front of, before
   c. toward the back
   d. pertaining to the head
   e. nearest the midline or middle
   f. to the side, away from the middle
   g. nearest the point of attachment
   h. away from the point of attachment
2. midsagittal plane
3. transverse or horizontal
4. coronal or frontal
5. a. thoracic
   b. abdominal
   c. pelvic
6. a. cranial
   b. spinal
7. abdominopelvic
8. nine
9. four
10. trunk or torso

Anatomy Labeling

1. posterior
2. anterior
3. cranial cavity
4. spinal cavity
5. thoracic cavity
6. diaphragm
7. abdominal cavity

8. pelvic cavity
9. pericardial membranes
10. heart

Study *and* Review II
The Body in Health and Disease

1. Health
2. pathogenic
3. pertussis
4. directly or indirectly, from one person to another
5. West Nile virus, dengue, Zika

Study *and* Review III
Word Parts

Prefixes

1. both
2. up, apart
3. two
4. color
5. down, away from
6. apart
7. outside
8. within
9. similar, same
10. middle
11. through
12. first
13. one

Combining Forms

1. fat
2. man
3. toward the front
4. life
5. tail
6. cell
7. away from the point of origin
8. backward
9. tissue
10. water
11. below
12. groin
13. cell's nucleus

14. side
15. toward the middle
16. organ
17. disease
18. to show
19. nature
20. behind, toward the back, back
21. near the point of origin
22. body
23. near or on the belly side of the body
24. body organs

Suffixes

1. pertaining to
2. use, action
3. formation, produce
4. pertaining to
5. process
6. study of
7. form, shape
8. resemble
9. pertaining to
10. a thing formed, plasma
11. body
12. control, stop, stand still
13. incision
14. type

Identifying Medical Terms

1. android
2. bilateral
3. cytology
4. ectomorph
5. karyogenesis
6. somatotrophic
7. unilateral

Matching

1. c
2. d
3. e
4. f
5. a
6. i
7. g
8. h
9. j
10. b

Study *and* Review IV
Building Medical Terms

1. bilateral
2. biology
3. distal
4. inguinal
5. lateral
6. pathology
7. physiology
8. systemic
9. unilateral
10. visceral

Combining Form Challenge

1. adipose
2. android
3. histology
4. karyogenesis
5. phenotype
6. somatotrophic

Select the Right Term

1. anatomy
2. anterior
3. mesomorph
4. base
5. proximal
6. horizontal

Drug Highlights

1. h
2. e
3. j
4. c
5. b
6. i
7. d
8. f
9. g
10. a

Abbreviations and Acronyms

1. abdomen
2. anatomy and physiology
3. deoxyribonucleic acid
4. BMI
5. GI
6. water
7. left lower quadrant
8. O_2

9. OTC
10. right upper quadrant

Practical Application

1. *Bordetella pertussis bacterium*
2. can cause them to stop breathing
3. ventilator
4. too young to be protected by their own vaccination
5. DTaP (diphtheria, tetanus, and pertussis)

Chapter 4

Study *and* Review I
Anatomy and Physiology

1. skin
2. a. hair
   b. nails
   c. sebaceous glands
   d. sweat glands
3. a. protection
   b. regulation
   c. sensory reception
   d. secretion
4. epidermis…dermis
5. a. stratum basale
   b. stratum spinosum
   c. stratum granulosum
   d. stratum lucidum
   e. stratum corneum
6. Keratin
7. Melanin
8. dermis
9. a. papillary layer
   b. reticular layer
10. lunula

Anatomy Labeling

1. epidermis
2. dermis
3. subcutaneous layer
4. sweat gland
5. sebaceous gland

6. hair
7. nerve
8. artery
9. vein

Study *and* Review II
Word Parts

Prefixes

1. without, lack of
2. self
3. out
4. down
5. out
6. excessive
7. under
8. within
9. around
10. below

Combining Forms

1. white
2. burn, burning
3. skin
4. skin
5. red
6. sweat
7. jaundice
8. tumor
9. horn
10. white
11. black
12. nail
13. thick
14. a louse
15. plate
16. itching
17. wrinkle
18. hard, hardening
19. oil
20. hot, heat
21. hair
22. to pull

23. yellow
24. dry

Suffixes

1. pertaining to
2. pain
3. pertaining to
4. pertaining to
5. skin
6. pertaining to
7. sensation
8. pencil, grafting knife
9. condition
10. pertaining to
11. process
12. condition
13. one who specializes
14. inflammation
15. study of
16. dilatation
17. resemble
18. tumor
19. condition
20. pertaining to
21. surgical repair
22. flow, discharge
23. instrument to cut

Identifying Medical Terms

1. actinic dermatitis
2. cutaneous
3. dermatitis
4. dermatology
5. pruritus
6. hyperhidrosis
7. hypodermic
8. icteric
9. onychitis
10. pachyderma

Matching

1. d   **4.** h
2. f   **5.** j
3. e   **6.** i

7. b   **9.** a
8. g   **10.** c

Medical Case Snapshot

Case 1: alopecia
Case 2: dermabrasion, rhytidoplasty
Case 3: a lying down

Study *and* Review III
Building Medical Terms

1. decubitus
2. dermatology
3. icteric
4. melanoma
5. onychitis
6. pachyderma
7. seborrhea
8. xanthoderma
9. xanthoma
10. xerosis

Combining Form Challenge

1. albinism
2. causalgia
3. cutaneous
4. dermatitis
5. erythroderma
6. integumentary

Select the Right Term

1. acne   **4.** eschar
2. alopecia   **5.** lentigo
3. cicatrix   **6.** roseola

Drug Highlights

1. c   **6.** b
2. f   **7.** a
3. j   **8.** d
4. g   **9.** i
5. h   **10.** e

Diagnostic and Laboratory Tests

1. c   **4.** b
2. d   **5.** a
3. a

Abbreviations and Acronyms

1. BCC
2. biopsy
3. decubitus
4. intradermal
5. squamous cell carcinoma
6. purified protein derivative
7. SG
8. staphylococcus
9. streptococcus
10. TIMs

Practical Application

1. Dx
2. basal cell carcinoma
3. telangiectasia
4. actinic keratosis
5. mid back

Chapter 5

Study *and* Review I
Anatomy and Physiology

1. 206
2. **a.** axial
   b. appendicular
3. **a.** flat…ribs, scapula, parts of the pelvic girdle, bones of the skull
   b. long…tibia, femur, humerus, radius
   c. short…carpal, tarsal
   d. irregular…vertebrae, ossicles of the ear
   e. sesamoid…patella
   *Optional answer to question 3:
   f. sutural or wormian…between the flat bones of the skull
4. **a.** Provide shape, support, and the framework of the body
   b. Provide protection for internal organs
   c. Serve as a storage place for mineral salts, calcium, and phosphorus

d. Play an important role in the formation of blood cells (hematopoiesis)
e. Provide areas for the attachment of skeletal muscles
f. Help make movement possible through articulation
5. **a.** ends of a developing bone
   b. narrow portion of a long bone between the epiphysis and the diaphysis
   c. shaft of a long bone
   d. membrane that forms the covering of bones except at their articular surfaces
   e. dense, hard layer of bone tissue
   f. narrow space or cavity throughout the length of the diaphysis
   g. tough connective tissue membrane lining the medullary canal and containing the bone marrow
   h. reticular tissue that makes up most of the volume of bone
6. 1. f   6. j
   2. e   7. i
   3. d   8. c
   4. b   9. a
   5. h   10. g
7. **a.** synarthrosis
   b. amphiarthrosis
   c. diarthrosis
8. Abduction
9. moving a body part toward the midline
10. Circumduction
11. bending a body part backward
12. Eversion
13. straightening a flexed limb
14. Flexion
15. turning inward
16. Pronation
17. moving a body part forward
18. Retraction

19. moving a body part around a central axis
20. Supination

Anatomy Labeling

1. cranium   6. humerus
2. mandible   7. ulna
3. clavicle   8. radius
4. scapula   9. femur
5. sternum   10. tibia

Study *and* Review II
Word Parts

Prefixes
1. without
2. apart
3. water
4. between
5. beyond
6. many, much
7. under, beneath
8. together
9. back

Combining Forms
1. extremity
2. stiffening, crooked
3. joint
4. a pouch
5. heel bone
6. wrist
7. cartilage
8. coccyx, tailbone
9. rib
10. skull
11. finger or toe
12. ischium, hip
13. a hump
14. bending, curve, swayback
15. loin, lower back
16. bone
17. kneecap
18. foot
19. sacrum
20. curvature

21. spine
22. sternum, breastbone
23. ulna, elbow
24. sword

Suffixes

1. pertaining to
2. pertaining to
3. pain
4. pertaining to
5. pertaining to
6. immature cell, germ cell
7. surgical puncture
8. process
9. pain
10. excision
11. swelling
12. formation, produce
13. formation, produce
14. mark, record
15. instrument for recording
16. pertaining to
17. inflammation
18. nature of
19. instrument for examining
20. softening
21. structure
22. resemble
23. tumor
24. condition
25. deficiency
26. growth
27. formation, produce
28. surgical repair
29. formation
30. instrument to cut
31. incision
32. structure, tissue

Identifying Medical Terms

1. acroarthritis
2. ankylosis
3. arthritis
4. calcaneal
5. chondral
6. coccygodynia
7. chondrocostal
8. craniectomy
9. dactylic
10. osteotome

Matching

1. i
2. j
3. e
4. c
5. b
6. h
7. g
8. a
9. d
10. f

Medical Case Snapshot

Case 1: osteopenia, osteoporosis

Case 2: scoliosis, asymmetry, scapula

Case 3: rheumatoid arthritis

Study *and* Review III

Building Medical Terms

1. coccygodynia
2. dactylic
3. lordosis
4. metacarpals
5. myelopoiesis
6. osteomalacia
7. patellar
8. phalangeal
9. scoliosis
10. xiphoid

Combining Form Challenge

1. arthroplasty
2. bursitis
3. carpal
4. chondral
5. chondrocostal
6. dactylogram

Select the Right Term

1. ankylosis
2. craniectomy
3. ischialgia
4. mandibular
5. osteosarcoma
6. spondylodesis

Drug Highlights

1. f
2. e
3. j
4. h
5. b
6. i

7. d
8. c
9. g
10. a

Diagnostic and Laboratory Tests

1. c
2. d
3. c
4. b
5. b

Abbreviations and Acronyms

1. ANA
2. Fx
3. bone mineral density
4. osteoarthritis
5. P
6. rheumatoid arthritis
7. ROM
8. thoracic vertebra, first
9. ligament
10. Tx

Practical Application

1. dual-energy x-ray absorptiometry scan
2. deficiency of bone tissue
3. oste/o bone
   -penia deficiency
4. standard deviations; BMD
5. 18–24 months

Chapter 6

Study *and* Review I

Anatomy and Physiology

1. **a.** skeletal
   b. smooth
   c. cardiac
2. 42
3. **a.** nutrition
   b. oxygen
4. **a.** origin
   b. insertion
5. voluntary or striated

6. aponeurosis
7. **a.** body
   b. origin
   c. insertion
8. **a.** muscle that counteracts the action of another muscle; when one contracts the other relaxes
   b. muscle that is primary in a given movement produced by its contraction
   c. muscle that acts with another muscle to produce movement
9. involuntary, visceral, or unstriated
10. **a.** digestive tract
    b. respiratory tract
    c. urinary tract
    d. eye
    e. skin
11. Cardiac
12. **a.** movement
    b. maintain posture
    c. produce heat

Anatomy Labeling

Anterior View

1. trapezius
2. deltoid
3. rectus femoris
4. pectoralis major
5. biceps brachii

Posterior View

6. gluteus maximus
7. biceps femoris
8. gastrocnemius
9. latissimus dorsi
10. triceps
11. Achilles tendon

Study *and* Review II
Word Parts

Prefixes

1. lack of
2. away from
3. toward
4. against
5. two
6. slow
7. with
8. through
9. difficult
10. into
11. within
12. water
13. four
14. with, together
15. three

Combining Forms

1. agony, a contest
2. to cut through
3. arm
4. clavicle
5. to lead
6. a band
7. fiber
8. equal
9. to measure
10. muscle
11. muscle
12. nerve
13. disease
14. an addition
15. rod
16. to turn
17. flesh
18. synovial
19. tendon
20. tone, tension
21. twisted
22. nourishment, development
23. will

Suffixes

1. pain
2. pertaining to
3. pertaining to
4. weakness
5. immature cell, germ cell
6. head
7. binding
8. pain
9. chemical
10. treatment
11. instrument for recording
12. condition
13. pertaining to
14. process
15. agent
16. inflammation
17. condition
18. motion
19. motion
20. study of
21. process
22. softening
23. resemble
24. tumor
25. a doer
26. condition
27. weakness
28. disease
29. a fence
30. surgical repair
31. stroke, paralysis
32. suture
33. pertaining to
34. tension, spasm
35. order
36. instrument to cut
37. incision
38. nourishment, development
39. condition
40. condition

Identifying Medical Terms

1. atonic
2. bradykinesia
3. dactylospasm
4. dystrophy
5. intramuscular

6. levator
7. myasthenia gravis
8. myoparesis
9. myoplasty
10. myosarcoma

Matching

1. d
2. i
3. g
4. e
5. j
6. a
7. h
8. c
9. b
10. f

Medical Case Snapshot

Case 1: fibromyalgia syndrome, myalgia
Case 2: muscle spasm
Case 3: body erect, forward, palms

Study *and* Review III
Building Medical Terms

1. amputation
2. ataxia
3. biceps
4. levator
5. myograph
6. polyplegia
7. rhabdomyoma
8. sarcolemma
9. tenodynia
10. voluntary

Combining Form Challenge

1. brachialgia
2. dactylospasm
3. fasciitis
4. isometric
5. myoparesis
6. tenodynia

Select the Right Term

1. antagonist
2. contraction
3. flaccid
4. myoplasty
5. synergism
6. torticollis

Drug Highlights

1. skeletal muscle relaxants
2. sprains, spasticity
3. involuntary
4. Muscle spasticity
5. muscle relaxant, cyclobenzaprine HCl
6. sedative
7. drive, operate equipment

Diagnostic and Laboratory Tests

1. b
2. d
3. b
4. c
5. a

Abbreviations and Acronyms

1. above elbow
2. aspartate aminotransferase
3. Ca
4. EMG
5. full range of motion
6. musculoskeletal
7. ROM
8. myasthenia gravis
9. muscular dystrophy
10. fibromyalgia syndrome

Practical Application

1. waddling
2. electromyography
3. a. minimize deformities
   b. preserve mobility
4. Test to measure electrical activity across muscle membranes by means of electrodes attached to a needle that is inserted into the muscle
5. Surgical removal of a small piece of muscle tissue for examination

Chapter 7

Study *and* Review I
Anatomy and Physiology

1. a. mouth
   b. pharynx
   c. esophagus
   d. stomach
   e. small intestine
   f. large intestine
2. a. salivary glands
   b. liver
   c. gallbladder
   d. pancreas
3. a. digestion
   b. absorption
   c. elimination
4. soft mass of chewed food ready to be swallowed
5. series of wavelike muscular contractions that are involuntary
6. hydrochloric acid and gastric juices
7. duodenum
8. chyme
9. circulatory system
10. cecum, colon, rectum, and anal canal
11. liver
12. stores and concentrates bile
13. produces digestive enzymes
14. a. plays an important role in metabolism
    b. manufactures bile
    c. stores iron and vitamins B_{12}, A, D, E, and K
15. small intestine
16. parotid, sublingual, submandibular
17. a. insulin
    b. glucagon

Anatomy Labeling

1. right lobe of liver
2. gallbladder
3. appendix
4. parotid gland
5. pharynx
6. esophagus
7. spleen
8. body of stomach
9. pancreas
10. small intestine

Study *and* Review II
Word Parts

Prefixes

1. lack of
2. difficult
3. above

4. excessive, above
5. deficient, below
6. bad
7. around
8. after
9. through
10. below

Combining Forms

1. starch
2. appendix
3. gall, bile
4. cheek
5. abdomen, belly
6. gall, bile
7. orange-yellow
8. colon
9. tooth
10. intestine
11. esophagus
12. stomach
13. gums
14. tongue
15. liver
16. ileum
17. lip
18. abdomen
19. tongue
20. tooth
21. meal
22. anus and rectum
23. rectum
24. mouth

Suffixes

1. pertaining to
2. pertaining to
3. pain, ache
4. pertaining to
5. enzyme
6. hernia
7. resemble
8. condition
9. surgical excision
10. vomiting

11. shape
12. formation, produce
13. pertaining to
14. process
15. condition
16. one who specializes
17. inflammation
18. nature of, quality of
19. study of
20. enlargement, large
21. appetite
22. condition
23. flow
24. to digest
25. pertaining to
26. to eat, to swallow
27. instrument for examining
28. visual examination, to view, examine
29. contraction
30. new opening
31. incision
32. pertaining to
33. suture

Identifying Medical Terms

1. amylase
2. anabolism
3. anorexia
4. appendectomy
5. appendicitis
6. biliary
7. celiac
8. dysphagia
9. hepatitis
10. herniorrhaphy

Matching

1. e
2. f
3. d
4. b
5. i
6. h
7. j
8. a
9. g
10. c

Medical Case Snapshot

Case 1: colonoscopy, colostomy
Case 2: constipation, hemorrhoid
Case 3: *Helicobacter pylori*, antibiotics

Study *and* Review III
Building Medical Terms

1. appendectomy
2. buccal
3. cirrhosis
4. colostomy
5. diverticulitis
6. dyspepsia
7. gingivitis
8. laparotomy
9. lingual
10. rectocele

Combining Form Challenge

1. absorption
2. stomatitis
3. biliary
4. esophageal
5. glossectomy
6. hepatitis

Select the Right Term

1. cholecystitis
2. ascites
3. colostomy
4. gastroesophageal
5. gavage
6. mastication

Drug Highlights

1. f
2. e
3. a
4. h
5. b
6. d
7. c
8. g

Diagnostic and Laboratory Tests

1. a
2. c
3. d
4. c
5. c

Abbreviations and Acronyms

1. Ba
2. carbohydrate

3. hepatitis C virus
4. HCl
5. GB
6. HAV
7. nasogastric
8. IBS
9. PP
10. PPIs

Practical Application

1. October 17, 2021, 8:45 A.M.
2. Seymour Butts, MD
   Endoscopy Center
   14 Maddox Drive
   Rome, GA 30165
3. Screening colonoscopy
4. Bring a driver, all current medications, driver's license, and proof of insurance
5. Angel De'Crohn, MD
   09/28/21
   (706) 235-7765
   (706) 235-6676

Chapter 8

Study *and* Review I
Anatomy and Physiology

1. blood, blood vessels
2. a. endocardium
   b. myocardium
   c. pericardium
3. 300
4. atria, interatrial
5. ventricles, interventricular
6. electrocardiogram
7. autonomic
8. sinoatrial node
9. Purkinje network
10. a. radial, on the radial side of the wrist
    b. brachial, in the antecubital space of the elbow
    c. carotid, in the neck

11. a. pressure exerted by the blood on the walls of the vessels
    b. difference between the systolic and diastolic readings
12. person's fist, 60, 100
13. 140, 90
14. transport blood from the right and left ventricles of the heart to all body parts; transports blood away from the heart
15. transport blood from peripheral tissues back to the heart

Anatomy Labeling

1. superior vena cava
2. aorta
3. right atrium
4. tricuspid valve
5. right ventricle
6. inferior vena cava
7. mitral valve
8. endocardium
9. myocardium
10. pericardium

Study *and* Review II
Word Parts

Prefixes

1. lack of
2. two
3. slow
4. together
5. within
6. within
7. outside
8. excessive, above
9. deficient, below
10. around
11. difficult, abnormal
12. half
13. rapid
14. three

Combining Forms

1. vessel
2. artery
3. fatty substance
4. heart
5. dark blue
6. to widen
7. a throwing in
8. blood
9. to hold back
10. fat
11. moon
12. thin
13. mitral valve
14. to close up
15. oxygen
16. vein
17. hardening
18. a curve
19. chest
20. clot
21. vessel

Suffixes

1. pertaining to
2. pertaining to
3. pertaining to
4. surgical puncture
5. measurement
6. dilatation
7. surgical excision
8. blood condition
9. relating to
10. formation, produce
11. recording
12. condition
13. pertaining to
14. having a particular quality
15. process
16. condition
17. one who specializes
18. inflammation
19. nature of, quality of
20. study of

21. softening
22. enlargement, large
23. instrument to measure
24. tumor
25. one who
26. condition
27. disease
28. surgical repair
29. instrument for examining
30. contraction, spasm
31. incision
32. tissue

Identifying Medical Terms

1. angioma
2. angioplasty
3. angiostenosis
4. arrhythmia
5. arteritis
6. bicuspid
7. cardiologist
8. cardiomegaly
9. cardiopulmonary
10. constriction

Matching

1. d	6. c
2. e	7. a
3. f	8. i
4. g	9. j
5. b	10. h

Medical Case Snapshot

Case 1: angina pectoris, neck, jaw
Case 2: auscultation, arteriosclerosis, atherosclerosis
Case 3: angina pectoris, coronary artery

Study *and* Review III
Building Medical Terms

1. bicuspid
2. claudication
3. occlusion
4. oxygen
5. palpitation
6. septum

7. stethoscope
8. tricuspid
9. valvuloplasty
10. venipuncture

Combining Form Challenge

1. angioplasty
2. arterial
3. atheroma
4. cardiomegaly
5. cyanosis
6. phlebitis

Select the Right Term

1. bradycardia
2. hyperlipidemia
3. pericardial
4. semilunar
5. triglyceride
6. ischemia

Drug Highlights

1. g	6. a
2. e	7. c
3. i	
4. b	8. f
5. d	9. h

Diagnostic and Laboratory Tests

1. c	4. c
2. a	
3. b	5. b

Abbreviations and Acronyms

1. AMI
2. AV
3. blood pressure
4. coronary artery disease
5. DVT
6. electrocardiogram
7. high-density lipoprotein
8. H & L
9. myocardial infarction
10. tissue plasminogen activator

Practical Application

1. dyspnea
2. blood enzyme
3. oxygenated

4. electrocardiogram
5. vasodilator

Chapter 9
Study *and* Review I
Anatomy and Physiology— Blood

1. circulates
2. a. erythrocytes
   b. thrombocytes
   c. leukocytes
3. oxygen
4. clotting
5. Coagulation
6. Leukocytes
7. ABO
8. Rh
9. plasma
10. a. albumin
    b. globulin
    c. fibrinogen
    d. prothrombin

Matching

1. f	5. a
2. d	6. h
3. c	7. b
4. e	8. g

Study *and* Review II
Anatomy and Physiology— Lymphatic and Immune Systems

1. False
2. False
3. Lymph
4. MALT
5. a. digestive tract
   b. genitourinary tract
   c. respiratory tract
6. small intestine
7. antigens

8. **a.** spleen
   b. tonsils
   c. thymus
9. tonsils
10. thymus

Matching

1. f	**6.** h
2. d	**7.** b
3. j	**8.** g
4. i	**9.** c
5. a	**10.** e

Anatomy Labeling

1. tonsil
2. lymphatic vessel
3. thymus gland
4. thoracic duct
5. spleen
6. lymph nodes

Study *and* Review III
Word Parts

Prefixes

1. lack of
2. against
3. self
4. up
5. beyond
6. excessive
7. deficient
8. one
9. all
10. many
11. before
12. across
13. deficient

Combining Forms

1. gland
2. unequal
3. clots, to clot
4. cell
5. red
6. sweet, sugar

7. blood
8. blood
9. immunity
10. white
11. lymph
12. large
13. plasma
14. putrefying
15. iron
16. spleen
17. thymus
18. small vessel

Suffixes

1. capable
2. forming
3. removal
4. immature cell, germ cell
5. body
6. swelling
7. cell
8. surgical excision
9. blood condition
10. work
11. formation, produce
12. protection
13. globe, protein
14. chemical
15. process
16. one who specializes
17. inflammation
18. study of
19. destruction
20. enlargement
21. mass, fluid collection, tumor
22. condition
23. lack of
24. attraction
25. formation
26. bursting forth
27. control, stop, stand still
28. condition
29. oxygen

Identifying Medical Terms

1. agglutination
2. allergy
3. antibody
4. anticoagulant
5. antigen
6. autotransfusion
7. coagulable
8. creatinemia
9. embolus
10. granulocyte

Matching

1. h	**6.** c
2. d	**7.** b
3. e	**8.** a
4. g	**9.** j
5. f	**10.** i

Medical Case Snapshot

Case 1: human immunodeficiency, T4
Case 2: SOB, hypoxia
Case 3: hemoglobin, hematocrit

Study *and* Review IV
Building Medical Terms

1. erythropoiesis
2. globulin
3. hemolysis
4. septicemia
5. lymphoma
6. erythrocyte
7. seroculture
8. sideropenia
9. splenomegaly
10. thrombosis

Combining Form Challenge

1. hemolysis
2. coagulable
3. erythroblast
4. hematology
5. leukemia
6. lymphedema

Select the Right Term

1. allergy
2. antibody
3. hemophilia
4. thalassemia
5. embolus
6. thromboplastin

Drug Highlights

1. b
2. c
3. a
4. g

5. f
6. e
7. d

Diagnostic and Laboratory Tests

1. d
2. c
3. c

4. b
5. a

Abbreviations and Acronyms

1. AIDS
2. ALL
3. chronic myeloid leukemia
4. Hb, Hgb
5. hematocrit
6. HIV
7. *Pneumocystis jiroveci* pneumonia
8. prothrombin time
9. red blood cell (count)
10. deep vein thrombosis

Practical Application

1. e
2. d
3. a

4. b
5. c

Chapter 10

Study *and* Review I
Anatomy and Physiology

1. a. nose
   b. pharynx
   c. larynx
   d. trachea
   e. bronchi
   f. lungs

2. to furnish oxygen for use by individual cells and to take away their gaseous waste product, carbon dioxide

3. process in which the lungs are ventilated and oxygen and carbon dioxide are exchanged between the air in the lungs and the blood within capillaries of the alveoli

4. process in which oxygen and carbon dioxide are exchanged between the bloodstream and the cells of the body

5. a. serves as an air passageway
   b. warms and moistens inhaled air
   c. its cilia and mucous membrane trap dust, pollen, bacteria, and foreign matter
   d. contains special smell receptor cells (nerve cells), which assist in distinguishing various smells
   e. contributes to phonation and the quality of voice

6. a. serves as a passageway for air
   b. serves as a passageway for food
   c. contributes to phonation as a chamber where the sound is able to resonate

7. acts as a lid to prevent aspiration of food into the trachea

8. narrow slit at the opening between the true vocal folds

9. production of vocal sounds

10. serves as a passageway for air

11. provide a passageway for air to and from the lungs

12. conical-shaped, spongy organs of respiration lying on both sides of the heart

13. serous membrane composed of several layers

14. diaphragm

15. mediastinum
16. 3...2
17. alveoli
18. to bring air into intimate contact with blood so that oxygen and carbon dioxide can be exchanged in the alveoli
19. temperature, pulse, respiration, and blood pressure
20. a. amount of air in a single inspiration and expiration
    b. amount of air remaining in the lungs after maximal expiration
    c. volume of air that can be exhaled after maximal inspiration
21. medulla oblongata...pons
22. 30–60
23. 16–20

Anatomy Labeling

1. nasopharynx
2. hard palate
3. soft palate
4. oropharynx
5. laryngopharynx
6. epiglottis
7. trachea
8. thyroid cartilage
9. cricoid cartilage

Study *and* Review II
Word Parts

Prefixes

1. lack of
2. upon
3. difficult
4. within
5. good
6. out
7. below, deficient
8. excessive
9. in
10. rapid

Combining Forms

1. small, hollow air sac
2. coal
3. imperfect
4. bronchi
5. dust
6. breathe
7. larynx, voice box
8. nose
9. smell
10. straight
11. chest
12. pharynx, throat
13. pleura
14. air
15. pus
16. nose
17. snore
18. breath
19. chest
20. tonsil, almond
21. trachea
22. a little swelling

Suffixes

1. pertaining to
2. surgical puncture
3. pain
4. dilation
5. surgical excision
6. pertaining to
7. condition
8. process
9. inflammation
10. instrument to measure
11. condition
12. tumor
13. dripping
14. surgical repair
15. a doer
16. breathing
17. to spit
18. flow, discharge
19. instrument for examining
20. new opening
21. incision
22. pertaining to

Identifying Medical Terms

1. alveolus
2. bronchiectasis
3. bronchitis
4. dysphonia
5. eupnea
6. hemoptysis
7. inhalation
8. laryngitis
9. pneumothorax
10. rhinoplasty

Matching

1. h
2. i
3. j
4. f
5. c
6. b
7. d
8. a
9. e
10. g

Medical Case Snapshot

Case 1: asthma, orthopnea
Case 2: dyspnea, shortness of breath, spirometer, chronic obstructive pulmonary disease
Case 3: tuberculosis, sputum

Study *and* Review III
Building Medical Terms

1. atelectasis
2. dyspnea
3. epistaxis
4. hyperpnea
5. pharyngitis
6. pneumonectomy
7. rhinoplasty
8. tachypnea
9. thoracotomy
10. tuberculosis

Combining Form Challenge

1. anthracosis
2. bronchoscope
3. hemoptysis
4. laryngoscope
5. olfaction
6. orthopnea

Select the Right Term

1. asthma
2. croup
3. hypoxia
4. pertussis
5. rale
6. rhinovirus

Drug Highlights

1. f
2. h
3. a
4. e
5. g
6. i
7. c
8. d
9. b
10. j

Diagnostic and Laboratory Tests

1. b
2. c
3. c
4. d
5. a

Abbreviations and Acronyms

1. AFB
2. cystic fibrosis
3. total lung capacity
4. COPD
5. endotracheal
6. HMD
7. R
8. severe acute respiratory syndrome
9. SOB
10. tuberculosis

Practical Application

1. e
2. d
3. b
4. a
5. c

Chapter 11

Study *and* Review I
Anatomy and Physiology

1. **a.** kidneys
   b. ureters
   c. bladder
   d. urethra
2. extraction of certain wastes from the bloodstream, conversion of these materials to urine, and transport of the urine from the kidney, via the ureters, to the bladder for elimination
3. a notch
4. saclike collecting portion of the kidney
5. inner
6. structural and functional unit of the kidney
7. renal corpuscle, tubule
8. glomerulus, glomerular (Bowman) capsule
9. reabsorption
10. 1000–1500
11. narrow, muscular tubes that transport urine from the kidneys to the bladder
12. muscular, membranous sac that serves as a reservoir for urine
13. urinary meatus
14. laboratory test that evaluates the physical, chemical, and microscopic properties of urine
15. **a.** yellow to amber
    b. clear
    c. 4.6–8.0 pH
    d. 1.003–1.030
    e. aromatic
    f. 1000–1500 mL/day
16. diabetes mellitus
17. renal disease, acute glomerulonephritis, pyelonephritis

Anatomy Labeling

1. kidney
2. ureter
3. bladder
4. urethra

Study *and* Review II
Word Parts

Prefixes

1. without
2. against
3. complete, through
4. difficult, painful
5. within
6. water
7. outside, beyond
8. not
9. scanty
10. through
11. beyond
12. excessive

Combining Forms

1. protein
2. bacteria
3. calcium
4. body
5. bladder
6. glomerulus, little ball
7. glucose, sugar
8. blood
9. ketone
10. stone
11. passage
12. kidney
13. night
14. perineum
15. peritoneum
16. renal pelvis
17. kidney
18. sound
19. urine, urinate, urination
20. ureter
21. urethra
22. urine

Suffixes

1. pertaining to
2. pertaining to
3. hernia
4. pertaining to
5. pertaining to
6. surgical excision
7. blood condition
8. mark, record
9. pertaining to
10. chemical
11. process
12. one who specializes
13. inflammation
14. stone
15. study of
16. separation
17. crushing
18. process
19. tumor
20. condition
21. disease
22. surgical repair
23. instrument for examining
24. condition
25. new opening
26. incision
27. urine

Identifying Medical Terms

1. antidiuretic
2. cystectomy
3. cystitis
4. dysuria
5. glomerulitis
6. hypercalciuria
7. urination
8. nephrolithiasis
9. periurethral
10. pyuria

Matching

1. d
2. e
3. b
4. f

5. a   8. c
6. g   9. h
7. j   10. i

Medical Case Snapshot

Case 1: dysuria, nocturia, hematuria

Case 2: urinalysis, blood, urinary tract infection, bacteriuria, cystitis

Case 3: nephrolithiasis, extracorporeal shock wave, ultrasonic

Study *and* Review III
Building Medical Terms

1. albuminuria   6. nephrolithiasis
2. cystogram   7. oliguria
3. incontinence   8. polyuria
4. meatotomy   9. renal
5. dysuria   10. urination

Combining Form Challenge

1. cystocele   4. nephroma
2. glycosuria   5. nocturia
3. lithotripsy   6. ureteropathy

Select the Right Term

1. calciuria
2. edema
3. hematuria
4. nephrosclerosis
5. pyelonephritis
6. renal colic

Drug Highlights

1. g   5. b
2. e   6. c
3. a   7. d
4. h   8. f

Diagnostic and Laboratory Tests

1. c   4. c
2. c   5. b
3. b

Abbreviations and Acronyms

1. AGN
2. blood urea nitrogen
3. CKD
4. cystoscopy
5. genitourinary
6. hemodialysis
7. IVP
8. peritoneal dialysis
9. hydrogen ion concentration
10. UA

Practical Application

1. yellow to amber
2. weight of a substance compared with an equal amount of water; urine has a specific gravity of 1.003–1.030
3. higher
4. yes
5. diabetes mellitus

Chapter 12

Study *and* Review I
Anatomy and Physiology

1. **a.** pituitary
   b. pineal
   c. thyroid
   d. parathyroid
   e. islets of Langerhans
   f. adrenals
   g. ovaries (female)
   h. testes (male)
2. involves the production and regulation of chemical substances (hormones) that play an essential role in maintaining homeostasis
3. chemical transmitter that is released in small amounts and transported via the bloodstream to a targeted organ or other cells

4. synthesizes and secretes releasing hormones, releasing factors, release-inhibiting hormones, and release-inhibiting factors
5. because of its regulatory effects on the other endocrine glands
6. **a.** growth hormone (GH)
   b. adrenocorticotropin hormone (ACTH)
   c. thyroid-stimulating hormone (TSH)
   d. follicle-stimulating hormone (FSH)
   e. luteinizing hormone (LH)
   f. prolactin (PRL)
   g. melanocyte-stimulating hormone (MSH)
7. **a.** antidiuretic hormone (ADH)
   b. oxytocin
8. melatonin…serotonin
9. plays a vital role in metabolism and regulates the body's metabolic processes
10. **a.** thyroxine (T4)
    b. triiodothyronine (T3)
    c. calcitonin
11. serum calcium…phosphorus
12. blood sugar
13. glucocorticoids, mineralocorticoids, and the androgens
14. **a.** regulates carbohydrate, protein, and fat metabolism
    b. stimulates output of glucose from the liver (gluconeogenesis)
    c. increases the blood sugar level
    d. regulates other physiological body processes
    *Optional answers to question 14:
    e. promotes the transport of amino acids into extracellular tissue

f. influences the effectiveness of catecholamines such as dopamine, epinephrine, and norepinephrine

g. has an anti-inflammatory effect

h. helps the body cope during times of stress

15. a. use of carbohydrates

b. absorption of glucose

c. gluconeogenesis

d. potassium and sodium metabolism

16. Aldosterone

17. substance or hormone that promotes the development of male characteristics

18. a. dopamine   **b.** epinephrine

c. norepinephrine

19. a. elevates the systolic blood pressure

b. increases the heart rate and cardiac output

c. Increases glycogenolysis, thereby hastening release of glucose from the liver; this action elevates the blood sugar level and provides the body with a spurt of energy

*Optional answers to question 19:

d. dilates the bronchial tubes

e. dilates the pupils

20. estrogen…progesterone

21. testosterone

22. a. thymosin

b. thymopoietin

23. a. gastrin

b. secretin

c. cholecystokinin (pancreozymin)

d. enterogastrone

Anatomy Labeling

1. pineal gland
2. pituitary gland
3. thyroid gland
4. parathyroid gland
5. thymus
6. adrenal gland
7. pancreas
8. ovary (female)
9. testis (male)

Study *and* Review II

Word Parts

Prefixes

1. through
2. within
3. good, normal
4. out, away from
5. out, away from
6. excessive
7. deficient, under
8. beside
9. before
10. upon

Combining Forms

1. acid
2. extremity, point
3. gland
4. adrenal gland
5. man
6. cortex
7. to secrete
8. female
9. old age
10. giant
11. sweet, sugar
12. seed
13. hairy
14. insulin
15. potassium (K)
16. mucus
17. pancreas
18. testicle
19. thymus
20. thyroid, shield
21. poison
22. masculine

Suffixes

1. pertaining to
2. formation, produce
3. pertaining to
4. to go
5. surgical excision
6. swelling
7. blood condition
8. formation, produce
9. condition
10. pertaining to
11. condition
12. one who specializes
13. inflammation
14. study of
15. hormone
16. enlargement, large
17. resemble
18. tumor
19. condition
20. disease
21. substance
22. growth
23. chemical
24. pertaining to

Identifying Medical Terms

1. adenoma
2. congenital hypothyroidism
3. diabetes
4. endocrinology
5. euthyroid
6. exocrine
7. gigantism
8. glucocorticoid
9. hyperkalemia
10. hypogonadism

Matching

1. e	6. i
2. f	7. c
3. b	8. j
4. g	9. d
5. h	10. a

Medical Case Snapshot

Case 1: Cushing, buffalo hump

Case 2: polydipsia, polyphagia, polyuria

Case 3: exophthalmic, Graves, swollen, light, blurring

Study *and* Review III
Building Medical Terms

1. adrenal
2. cortisone
3. dwarfism
4. gigantism
5. hirsutism
6. hypophysis
7. insulin
8. lethargic
9. myxedema
10. pineal

Combining Form Challenge

1. adenosis
2. androgen
3. estrogen
4. insulinogenic
5. thymectomy
6. thyroid

Select the Right Term

1. acromegaly
2. diabetes
3. epinephrine
4. hypothyroidism
5. progeria
6. virilism

Drug Highlights

1. f
2. d
3. e
4. a
5. b
6. c

Diagnostic and Laboratory Tests

1. a
2. c
3. c
4. b
5. c

Abbreviations and Acronyms

1. BMR
2. DM
3. fasting blood sugar
4. glucose tolerance tests
5. PBI
6. parathyroid hormone
7. body mass index
8. STH
9. thyroid-stimulating hormone
10. vasopressin

Practical Application

1. because his dad and grandfather both take insulin
2. Hb A1C and FBS
3. thirsty (polydipsia), hungry (polyphagia), and urinating a lot (polyuria)
4. fasting blood sugar
5. 25
6. Hb A1C

Chapter 13

Study *and* Review I
Anatomy and Physiology

1. **a.** central
   b. peripheral
2. Neurons
3. process that can generate and conduct action potentials
4. resembles the branches of a tree and has short processes that transmit impulses to the cell body
5. sensory nerves transmit impulses to the central nervous system
6. **a.** single elongated process
   b. bundle of nerve fibers
   c. groups of nerve fibers
7. brain…spinal cord
8. **a.** dura mater
   b. arachnoid
   c. pia mater
9. **a.** cerebrum
   b. cerebellum
   c. diencephalon
   d. brainstem
10. frontal lobe
11. somesthetic area
12. auditory…language
13. vision
14. **a.** relay center for all sensory impulses
    b. relays motor impulses from the cerebellum to the cortex
15. **a.** is a regulator
    b. produces neurosecretions
    c. produces hormones
16. sensory perception and motor output
17. **a.** regulates and controls breathing
    b. regulates and controls swallowing
    c. regulates and controls coughing
    d. regulates and controls sneezing
    e. regulates and controls vomiting
18. **a.** conducts sensory impulses
    b. conducts motor impulses
    c. is a reflex center
19. 120…150
20. **a.** controls sweating
    b. controls the secretions of glands
    c. controls arterial blood pressure
    d. controls smooth muscle tissue
21. **a.** sympathetic
    b. parasympathetic

Anatomy Labeling

1. cerebrum
2. frontal lobe
3. parietal lobe
4. occipital lobe
5. cerebellum
6. spinal cord
7. medulla oblongata
8. pons
9. temporal lobe
10. lateral fissure

Study *and* Review II
Word Parts
Prefixes

1. lack of
2. lack of
3. star-shaped
4. slow
5. down
6. difficult
7. upon
8. half
9. water
10. excessive
11. within
12. small
13. little
14. beside
15. beside
16. many
17. four
18. below

Combining Forms

1. head
2. little brain
3. cerebrum
4. skull
5. tree
6. disk
7. dura, hard
8. electricity
9. brain
10. feeling
11. sleep
12. thin plate
13. membrane, meninges
14. bone marrow, spinal cord
15. numbness, sleep, stupor
16. nerve
17. globus pallidus
18. gray
19. sleep
20. spine
21. vertebra
22. vagus, wandering
23. ventricle

Suffixes

1. pertaining to
2. condition of pain
3. pain
4. pertaining to
5. weakness

6. germ cell
7. hernia
8. binding
9. surgical excision
10. swelling
11. feeling
12. glue
13. mark, record
14. recording
15. condition
16. pertaining to
17. process
18. condition
19. one who specializes
20. inflammation
21. motion, movement
22. motion
23. seizure
24. diction, word, phrase
25. study of
26. nourishment, development
27. visual examination, to view, examine
28. tumor
29. condition
30. weakness
31. disease
32. to eat, swallow
33. to speak, speech
34. action
35. strength
36. order, coordination
37. incision
38. pertaining to
39. condition

Identifying Medical Terms

1. amnesia
2. analgesia
3. aphagia
4. ataxia
5. cephalalgia

6. cerebellar
7. craniectomy
8. dyslexia
9. encephalitis
10. epidural

Matching

1. g
2. d
3. c
4. b
5. e
6. h
7. j
8. f
9. a
10. i

Medical Case Snapshot

Case 1: epilepsy, idiopathic
Case 2: herpes zoster, chickenpox, shingles
Case 3: bradykinesia, akinesia, pallidotomy

Study *and* Review III
Building Medical Terms

1. analgesia
2. bradykinesia
3. concussion
4. encephalitis
5. laminectomy
6. neuralgia
7. papilledema
8. paresthesia
9. quadriplegia
10. vagotomy

Combining Form Challenge

1. cephalalgia
2. craniectomy
3. encephalopathy
4. hypnosis
5. meningitis
6. neuroglia

Select the Right Term

1. akathisia
2. anesthesia
3. coma
4. dementia
5. hyperkinesis
6. stroke

Drug Highlights

1. d   **6.** c
2. g   **7.** i
3. a   **8.** e
4. h   **9.** j
5. b   **10.** f

Diagnostic and Laboratory Tests

1. a   **4.** d
2. b   **5.** c
3. c

Abbreviations and Acronyms

1. AD
2. ALS
3. central nervous system
4. cerebral palsy
5. CT
6. HDS
7. intracranial pressure
8. lumbar puncture
9. multiple sclerosis
10. PET

Practical Application

1. cognition
2. tremor
3. difficult articulation of speech
4. antiparkinsonism
5. used for palliative relief from such major symptoms of Parkinson disease as bradykinesia, rigidity, tremor, and disorder of equilibrium and posture

Chapter 14

Study *and* Review I
Anatomy and Physiology

1. hearing...balance
2. external...middle...inner
3. auricle or pinna and the external acoustic meatus

4. auricle
5. a. to lubricate the ear
   b. to protect the ear
6. a. malleus (hammer)
   b. incus (anvil)
   c. stapes (stirrup)
7. mechanically transmit sound vibrations from the tympanic membrane to the oval window
8. a. transmits sound vibrations from the tympanic membrane to the cochlea
   b. equalizes external/internal air pressure on the tympanic membrane
9. cochlea, vestibule, and the semicircular canals
10. a. cochlear duct
   b. semicircular ducts
   c. utricle and saccule
11. organ of Corti
12. vestibule
13. acoustic or eighth cranial nerve
14. motion sickness
15. a. endolymph
   b. perilymph

Anatomy Labeling

1. external auditory canal
2. auricle
3. malleus
4. incus
5. stapes
6. cochlea
7. eustachian tube
8. round window
9. tympanic membrane

Study *and* Review II
Word Parts

Prefixes

1. within   **4.** twice
2. within   **5.** one
3. around

Combining Forms

1. to hear
2. ear
3. gall, bile
4. land snail
5. electricity
6. maze, inner ear
7. larynx, voice box
8. mastoid process, breast-shaped
9. eardrum, tympanic membrane
10. nerve
11. ear
12. pharynx
13. old
14. pus
15. hardening
16. stapes, stirrup
17. fat
18. eardrum, tympanic membrane

Suffixes

1. pertaining to
2. pain
3. hearing
4. surgical excision
5. mark, record
6. recording
7. pertaining to
8. one who specializes
9. inflammation
10. stone
11. study of
12. serum, clear fluid
13. instrument to measure
14. resemble
15. tumor
16. condition
17. surgical repair
18. flow
19. instrument for examining
20. instrument to cut
21. incision
22. pertaining to
23. small

24. process
25. condition

Identifying Medical Terms

1. audiologist
2. audiometry
3. auditory
4. endaural
5. labyrinthitis
6. myringoplasty
7. myringotome
8. otalgia
9. otolaryngology
10. otopharyngeal

Matching

1. h
2. e
3. i
4. a
5. g
6. b
7. j
8. c
9. d
10. f

Medical Case Snapshot

Case 1: otitis media
Case 2: tinnitus, organ of Corti
Case 3: audiologist, audiometer, deafness

Study *and* Review III
Building Medical Terms

1. acoustic
2. aural
3. endolymph
4. myringotome
5. otitis
6. otoplasty
7. perilymph
8. stapedectomy
9. tympanic
10. tympanoplasty

Combining Form Challenge

1. audiometer
2. auricle

3. labyrinthectomy
4. myringoplasty
5. otalgia
6. presbycusis

Select the Right Term

1. audiogram
2. equilibrium
3. fenestration
4. malleus
5. tinnitus
6. monaural

Drug Highlights

1. h
2. d
3. f
4. b
5. g
6. a
7. e
8. c

Diagnostic and Laboratory Tests

1. a
2. b
3. d
4. b
5. a

Abbreviations and Acronyms

1. AC
2. BC
3. decibel
4. ENG
5. ear, nose, throat
6. HD
7. OM

Practical Application

1. 102.2°F, pulling
2. otoscopy
3. analgesic/antipyretic, pain, fever
4. antibiotic, infection
5. acid, antibiotic

Chapter 15

Study *and* Review I
Anatomy and Physiology

1. orbit, muscles, eyelids, conjunctiva, and the lacrimal apparatus
2. fatty tissue

3. optic nerve...ophthalmic artery
4. a. support
   b. rotary movement
5. intense light, foreign particles... impact
6. mucous membrane that acts as a protective covering for the exposed surface of the eyeball
7. structures that produce, store, and remove the tears that cleanse and lubricate the eye
8. eyeball, its structures, and the nerve fibers
9. vision
10. optic disk
11. process of sharpening the focus of light on the retina
12. 1. c   6. d
    2. e   7. h
    3. b   8. i
    4. a   9. j
    5. f   10. g

Anatomy Labeling

1. iris
2. lens
3. pupil
4. cornea
5. aqueous humor
6. retina
7. choroid
8. sclera
9. optic nerve

Study *and* Review II
Word Parts

Prefixes

1. lack of, without
2. two
3. in
4. in
5. inward
6. beyond

7. within
8. three
9. out
10. half
11. lack of
12. behind

Combining Forms

1. dull
2. unequal
3. eyelid
4. choroid
5. to join together, conjunctiva
6. pupil
7. cornea
8. cold
9. ciliary body
10. tear, lacrimal duct, tear duct
11. double
12. iris
13. cornea
14. tear, lacrimal duct, tear duct
15. lens
16. less, small
17. eye
18. eye
19. straight
20. lens
21. light
22. retina
23. foreign material
24. dry

Suffixes

1. pertaining to
2. pertaining to
3. pertaining to
4. germ cell
5. condition
6. surgical excision
7. mark, record
8. recording
9. condition
10. pertaining to
11. specialist

12. process
13. condition
14. one who specializes
15. inflammation
16. study of
17. destruction, to separate
18. formation
19. instrument to measure
20. tumor
21. sight, vision
22. condition
23. disease
24. fear
25. surgical repair
26. stroke, paralysis
27. prolapse, drooping
28. instrument for examining
29. pertaining to
30. incision
31. structure

Identifying Medical Terms

1. amblyopia
2. bifocal
3. blepharoptosis
4. corneal
5. dacryoma
6. diplopia
7. emmetropia
8. intraocular
9. keratitis
10. keratoplasty

Matching

1. e   6. d
2. f   7. g
3. j   8. b
4. h   9. a
5. c   10. i

Medical Case Snapshot

Case 1: cataract, phacoemulsification

Case 2: conjunctivitis, redness, yellow, blurred

Case 3: glaucoma, vision loss

Study *and* Review III

Building Medical Terms

1. diplopia
2. iridectomy
3. lacrimal
4. miotic
5. nyctalopia
6. ophthalmology
7. photophobia
8. retinopathy
9. trichiasis
10. uveal

Combining Form Challenge

1. amblyopia
2. blepharoptosis
3. cycloplegia
4. dacryoma
5. gonioscope
6. keratitis

Select the Right Term

1. accommodation
2. cataract
3. entropion
4. glaucoma
5. hyperopia
6. sty(e)

Drug Highlights

1. e   6. j
2. c   7. a
3. g   8. d
4. b   9. i
5. h   10. f

Diagnostic and Laboratory Tests

1. c   4. d
2. b   5. d
3. c

Abbreviations and Acronyms

1. Acc
2. emmetropia
3. hyperopia

4. IOL
5. ET
6. myopia
7. visual acuity
8. intraocular pressure
9. RLF
10. exotropia

Practical Application

1. antibiotic to prevent/treat bacterial infection
2. antibiotic to prevent/treat bacterial infection
3. yes
4. any time before the day of surgery
5. Tylenol regular-strength (325 mg) acetaminophen

Chapter 16
Study *and* Review I
Anatomy and Physiology

1. a. ovaries
   b. fallopian tubes
   c. uterus
   d. vagina
   e. vulva
   f. breasts
2. anteflexion
3. rounded portion of the uterine body superior to the attachment of the fallopian tube
4. a. perimetrium
   b. myometrium
   c. endometrium
5. a. provides a place for the nourishment and development of the fetus during pregnancy
   b. contracts rhythmically and powerfully to help push out the fetus during the process of birthing
6. a. bent backward at an angle with the cervix usually unchanged from its normal position
   b. fundus forward toward the pubis with the cervix tilted up toward the sacrum
   c. bent backward with the cervix pointing forward toward the symphysis pubis
7. uterine tubes or oviducts
8. fertilization
9. a. production of ova
   b. production of hormones
10. a. female organ of copulation
    b. passageway for discharge of menstruation
    c. passageway for birth of the fetus
11. mammary glands
12. areola...nipple
13. thin yellowish secretion containing mainly serum and white blood cells; the "first milk"
14. a. follicular phase
    b. ovulation
    c. luteal phase

Overview of Obstetrics

1. Obstetrics
2. Fertilization
3. zygote
4. yolk sac and amniotic cavity
5. a. time period from conception to onset of labor
   b. last phase of pregnancy to the time of delivery
   c. act of giving birth, also known as *childbirth* or *delivery*
   d. the 6 weeks following childbirth and expulsion of the placenta
6. a. begins from the onset of true labor and lasts until the cervix is fully dilated to 10 cm
   b. continues after the cervix is dilated to 10 cm until the delivery of the baby
   c. delivery of the placenta

Anatomy Labeling

1. uterus
2. cervix
3. vagina
4. fallopian tube
5. ovary
6. symphysis pubis
7. labia majora
8. labia minora

Study *and* Review II
Word Parts
Prefixes

1. lack of
2. against
3. difficult, painful
4. out
5. within
6. within
7. scanty
8. around
9. after
10. backward
11. before

Combining Forms

1. to miscarry
2. cervix, neck
3. a coming together
4. vagina
5. cul-de-sac
6. bladder
7. fibrous tissue
8. female
9. womb, uterus
10. breast
11. breast
12. month, menses, menstruation
13. womb, uterus
14. muscle
15. ovum, egg
16. ovary
17. lying beside, sexual intercourse

18. rectum
19. fallopian tube
20. uterus
21. vagina
22. turning

Suffixes

1. pertaining to
2. beginning
3. hernia
4. surgical puncture
5. surgical excision
6. formation, produce
7. condition
8. pertaining to
9. process
10. one who specializes
11. inflammation
12. tumor
13. condition
14. surgical repair
15. to burst forth
16. flow
17. instrument for examining
18. resemble

Identifying Medical Terms

1. cervicitis   6. mammoplasty
2. dysmenorrhea   7. menorrhea
3. fibroma   8. oogenesis
4. gynecology   9. dyspareunia
5. hymenectomy   10. genitalia

Matching

1. e   6. h
2. b   7. j
3. a   8. g
4. c   9. i
5. d   10. f

Medical Case Snapshot

Case 1: uterine, cramping, cervix
Case 2: ectopic, pregnancy,
            obstetrician
Case 3: dyspareunia, perimenopause

Study *and* Review III
Building Medical Terms

1. bartholinitis   6. menopause
2. culdocentesis   7. menorrhea
3. hysterectomy   8. oogenesis
4. lumpectomy   9. salpingitis
5. mastectomy   10. postcoital

Combining Form Challenge

1. cervicitis   4. fibroma
2. colposcope   5. genitalia
3. cystocele   6. gynecology

Select the Right Term

1. adnexa   4. lochia
2. dysmenorrhea 5. preeclampsia
3. gravida   6. retroversion

Drug Highlights

1. d   5. b
2. g   6. c
3. a   7. e
4. f

Diagnostic and Laboratory Tests

1. a   4. b
2. c   5. d
3. d

Abbreviations and Acronyms

1. abortion
2. fetal heartbeat
3. COCs
4. IUD
5. PID
6. CIN
7. dysfunctional uterine bleeding
8. premenstrual syndrome
9. D&C
10. TSS

Practical Application

1. GYN
2. hot flashes
3. dyspareunia

4. two pregnancies
5. rule out uterine fibroid tumor

Chapter 17

Study *and* Review I
Anatomy and Physiology

1. **a.** testes
   b. various ducts
   c. urethra
   d. bulbourethral gland
   e. prostate gland
   f. seminal vesicles
2. **a.** scrotum
   b. penis
3. **a.** producing spermatozoa
      (sperm), the male reproductive
      cells,
   b. making testosterone, the male
      hormone
4. glans penis
5. loose skinfolds that cover the penis
6. lubricating fluid
7. **a.** male organ of copulation
   b. site of the orifice for the
      elimination of urine and semen
      from the body
8. seminiferous tubules
9. **a.** responsible for the devel-
      opment of secondary male
      characteristics during puberty
   b. essential for normal growth
      and development of the male
      accessory sex organs
   c. plays a vital role in the erection
      process of the penis
   d. affects the growth of hair
      on the face
   e. affects muscular development
      and vocal timbre
10. **a.** storage site for sperm
    b. duct for the passage of sperm
11. vas deferens or ductus deferens

12. production of a slightly alkaline fluid
13. about 4 cm wide and weighs about 20 g; composed of glandular, connective, and muscular tissues and lies behind the urinary bladder
14. enlargement of the prostate that can occur in older men
15. bulbourethral...Cowper
16. a. prostatic
    b. membranous
    c. penile
17. transmits urine and semen out of the body
18. 20

Anatomy Labeling

1. bladder
2. vas deferens
3. seminal vesicles
4. prostate
5. urethra
6. epididymis

Study *and* Review II
Word Parts

Prefixes

1. lack of
2. lack of
3. around
4. upon
5. water
6. under
7. scanty
8. beside
9. into
10. different
11. similar, same

Combining Forms

1. glans penis
2. to cut
3. hidden
4. testis
5. to throw out
6. genitals
7. female
8. breast
9. thread
10. testicle

11. testicle
12. prostate
13. seed, sperm
14. seed, sperm
15. testicle
16. twisted vein
17. vessel
18. seminal vesicle
19. animal

Suffixes

1. pertaining to
2. pertaining to
3. hernia, swelling, tumor
4. to kill
5. surgical excision
6. formation, produce
7. condition
8. process
9. condition
10. inflammation
11. use
12. condition
13. flow
14. incision

Identifying Medical Terms

1. balanitis
2. epididymectomy
3. orchidectomy
4. prepuce
5. hydrocele
6. condyloma
7. spermatid
8. spermatozoon
9. spermicide
10. testicular

Matching

1. e
2. c
3. f
4. b
5. g
6. i
7. h
8. j
9. a
10. d

Medical Case Snapshot

Case 1: erectile dysfunction, Viagra, Levitra, Cialis
Case 2: hypospadias, circumcision, 18
Case 3: nocturia, urgency, prostatic hypertrophy, prostatism

Study *and* Review III
Building Medical Terms

1. castrate
2. hydrocele
3. orchiditis
4. parenchyma
5. prostatitis
6. spermatoblast
7. spermatozoon
8. spermicide
9. testicular
10. varicocele

Combining Form Challenge

1. balanitis
2. gonorrhea
3. orchidotomy
4. mitosis
5. prostatectomy
6. vesiculitis

Select the Right Term

1. anorchism
2. circumcision
3. cryptorchidism
4. homosexual
5. vasectomy
6. syphilis

Drug Highlights

1. growth
2. hypogonadism
3. a. relieve symptoms of the male climacteric
   b. help stimulate sperm production
   c. treat inoperable metastatic breast cancer in women
4. persistent
5. menstrual periods
6. shrink
7. achieve, maintain

Diagnostic and Laboratory Tests

1. c
2. a
3. b
4. c
5. b

Abbreviations and Acronyms

1. BPH
2. gonorrhea
3. HPV
4. herpes simplex virus–2
5. sexually transmitted infections
6. ED
7. transurethral resection of the prostate
8. nongonococcal urethritis
9. VDRL
10. PSA

Practical Application

1. urgency
2. digital rectal examination
3. Proscar
4. reduce
5. 6

Chapter 18

Study *and* Review I
An Overview: Mental Health and Mental Disorders

1. mental disorder
2. **a.** major depression
   b. bipolar disorder
   c. schizophrenia
3. Psychiatry
4. **a.** drug therapy
   b. psychotherapy
   c. electroconvulsive therapy
5. Psychoanalysis

Study *and* Review II
Word Parts

Prefixes

1. lack of, without
2. deficient, below
3. beside, abnormal
4. fire

Combining Forms

1. marketplace
2. center
3. circle, cycle
4. to cheat
5. nerve
6. disease
7. mind
8. mind
9. to divide
10. body
11. mind, emotion

Suffixes

1. shape
2. condition
3. pertaining to
4. process
5. condition
6. one who specializes
7. madness
8. mind
9. appetite
10. condition
11. fear
12. treatment
13. pertaining to

Identifying Medical Terms

1. agoraphobia
2. apathy
3. delusion
4. depression
5. egocentric
6. mania
7. phobia
8. psychiatrist
9. psychotherapy
10. pyromania

Matching

1. d
2. g
3. c
4. a
5. f
6. b
7. i
8. e
9. h
10. j

Medical Case Snapshot

mental disorder, mood, dysthymia

Study *and* Review III
Drug Highlights

1. f
2. h
3. d
4. c
5. b
6. a
7. g
8. e
9. j
10. i

Abbreviations and Acronyms

1. CBT
2. DSM-5
3. electroconvulsive therapy
4. Minnesota Multiphasic Personality Inventory–2
5. NIMH
6. obsessive–compulsive disorder
7. PTSD
8. seasonal affective disorder
9. Thematic Apperception Test
10. WHO

Practical Application

1. feels sick all the time; too weak and tired, dizzy and depressed, to do anything except "rest"
2. Proventil inhaler for relief of asthmatic symptoms, analgesics, decongestants, and two different forms of tricyclic antidepressants
3. a fixed, false belief or abnormal perception held by a person despite evidence to the contrary
4. process of experiencing sensations that have no source
5. disorder that is not real, genuine, or natural; the physical and psychological symptoms are produced by the person to place him- or herself or another in the role of a patient or someone in need of help

Appendix II

GLOSSARY OF WORD PARTS

Prefixes

a-	no, not, without, lack of, apart	**em-**	in
ab-	away from	**en-**	in, within
ad-	toward, near	**end-**	within, inner
ambi-	both, both sides, around, about	**endo-**	within, inner
an-	no, not, without, lack of	**ep-**	upon, over, above
ana-	up, apart, backward, again, anew	**epi-**	upon, over, above
ant-	against	**erg-**	work
ante-	before, forward	**eso-**	inward
anti-	against	**eu-**	good, normal
apo-	separation	**ex-**	out, away from
astro-	star-shaped	**exo-**	out, away from
auto-	self	**extra-**	outside, beyond
bi-	two, double	**hemi-**	half
bin-	twice, two	**heter-**	different
brachy-	short	**hetero-**	different
brady-	slow	**homeo-**	similar, same, likeness, constant
cac-	bad	**homo-**	similar, same
centi-	one hundred, one hundredth	**hydr-**	water
chromo-	color	**hyp-**	below, deficient
circum-	around	**hyper-**	above, beyond, excessive
con-	with, together	**hypo-**	below, under, deficient
contra-	against, opposite	**in-**	in, into, not
de-	down, away from	**infer-**	below
deca-	ten	**inter-**	between
di-	two, double	**intra-**	within
dia-, di(a)-	through, between, complete	**ir-**	in
dif-	apart, free from, separate	**mal-**	bad
di(s)-	two, apart	**mega-**	large, great
dis-	apart	**meso-**	middle
dys-	bad, difficult, painful, abnormal	**meta-**	beyond, over, between, change
ec-	out, outside, outer	**micro-**	small
ecto-	out, outside, outer	**milli-**	one-thousandth

mon(o)-	one	**pseudo-**	false
mono-	one	**pyro-**	fire
multi-	many, much	**quadri-**	four
neo-	new	**re-**	back, backward, again
nulli-	none	**retro-**	backward
olig-	little, scanty	**semi-**	half
oligo-	little, scanty	**sub-**	below, under, beneath
pan-	all	**super-**	upper, above
par-	around, beside	**supra-**	above, beyond, superior
para-	beside, alongside, next to, abnormal	**sym-**	together, with
per-	through	**syn-**	with, together
peri-	around	**tachy-**	rapid, fast
poly-	many, much, excessive	**trans-**	across
post-	after, behind	**tri-**	three
pre-	before, in front of	**ultra-**	beyond
primi-	first	**un-**	back, reversal, not, annulment
pro-	before, in front of	**uni-**	one
proto-	first		

Word Roots/Combining Forms

abdomin, abdomin/o	abdomen	**agglutin/o**	clumping
abort, abort/o	to miscarry	**agglutinat**	clumping
absorpt, absorpt/o	to suck in	**agon, agon/o**	agony
acanth	thorn	**agor/a**	marketplace
acetabul, acetabul/o	acetabulum, hip socket	**albin, albin/o**	white
acid, acid/o	acid	**albumin, albumin/o**	protein
acoust	hearing	**aliment, aliment/o**	nourishment
acr, acr/o	extremity, point	**all, all/o**	other
act, act/o	acting, act	**alveol, alveol/o**	small, hollow air sac
actin	ray, light	**ambly, ambly/o**	dull
acute	sharp	**ambul**	to walk
aden, aden/o	gland	**amni/o**	amniotic fluid
adhes	stuck to	**ampere**	ampere
adip, adip/o	fat	**amputat, amputat/o**	to cut through
adren, adren/o	adrenal gland	**amyl, amyl/o**	starch

an/o	anus	**blast/o**	germ cell
anabol, anabol/o	building up	**blephar, blephar/o**	eyelid
anastom	opening	**brach/i, brachi/o**	arm
andr, andr/o	man	**bronch, bronch/o**	bronchus
angi, angi/o	vessel	**bronchi, bronchi/o**	bronchus
angin, angin/o	to choke	**bronchiol, bronchiol/o**	bronchiole
anis/o	unequal	**bucc, bucc/o**	cheek
ankyl, ankyl/o	stiffening, crooked	**burs, burs/o**	pouch
anter, anter/o	toward the front	**calc, calc/i, calc/o**	lime, calcium
anthrac, anthrac/o	coal	**calcan/e**	heel bone
aort, aort/o	aorta	**cancer, cancer/o**	crab, cancer
append, append/o	appendix	**capn**	smoke
appendic, appendic/o	appendix	**capsul, capsul/o**	little box
arachn	spider	**carcin, carcin/o**	cancer
arche	beginning	**cardi, cardi/o**	heart
arous	alertness, to rise	**carp, carp/o**	wrist, carpus
arter	artery	**cartil**	gristle
arteri, arteri/o	artery	**cartilagin/o**	cartilage
arthr, arthr/o	joint, to articulate	**castr**	to prune
aspirat, aspirat/o	to draw in	**catabol, catabol/o**	casting down
atel, atel/o	imperfect	**caud, caud/o**	tail
ather, ather/o	fatty substance	**caus, caus/o**	burn, burning
atri, atri/o	atrium	**cavit**	cavity
audi/o	to hear	**celi, celi/o**	abdomen, belly
auditor	hearing	**cellul, cellul/o**	little cell
aur, aur/i	ear	**centr, centr/i, centr/o**	center
auscultat, auscultat/o	listen to	**centrat**	center
aut	self	**cephal, cephal/o**	head
axill	armpit	**cept**	receive
bacteri/o	bacteria	**cerebell, cerebell/o**	little brain
balan, balan/o	glans penis	**cerebr/o**	cerebrum
bartholin	Bartholin glands	**cervic, cervic/o**	cervix, neck
bas/o	base	**cheil, cheil/o**	lip
bi/o	life	**chem/o**	chemical
bil, bil/i	bile	**chir/o**	hand

chlor/o	green	connect	to bind together
chol, chole, chol/e	gall, bile	consci	aware
choledoch/o	common bile duct	constipat	to press together
chondr, chondr/o	cartilage	contin	to hold
chord	cord	cor, cor/o	pupil
chori/o	chorion	cord/o	cord
choroid, choroid/o	choroid	coriat	corium
chrom/o	color	corne, corne/o	cornea
chromat, chromat/o	color	corpor, corpore/o, corpor/o	body
chym	juice		
cine	motion	cortic, cortic/o	cortex
cinemat/o	motion	cortis	cortex
circulat, circulat/o	circular	cost, cost/o	rib
cirrh, cirrh/o	orange-yellow	crani, cran/i, crani/o	skull
cis, cis/o	to cut	creat	flesh
claudicat, claudicat/o	to limp	creatin	flesh, creatine
clavicul, clavicul/o	clavicle, collar bone	crine, crin/o	to secrete
cleid/o	clavicle	crur	leg
coagul, coagul/o	to clot	cry/o	cold
coagulat	to clot	crypt, crypt/o	hidden
coccyg/e, coccyg/o	coccyx, tailbone	cubit	to lie
cochle/o	land snail	cubit/o	elbow
coit, coit/o	a coming-together	culd/o	cul-de-sac
col, col/o	colon	curie	curie
coll/a	glue	cutane, cutane/o	skin
collis	neck	cyan, cyan/o	dark blue
colon, colon/o	colon	cycl, cycl/o	ciliary body of eye, circle, cycle
colp/o	vagina	cyst, cyst/o	bladder, sac
comat	a deep sleep	cyt, cyt/o	cell
compensat	to make good	cyth	cell
compuls/o	compel, drive	dacry, dacry/o	tear, lacrimal duct, tear duct
coni/o	dust	dactyl, dactyl/o	finger or toe
concuss	shaken violently	defecat	to remove dregs
condyle	knuckle	delus, delus/o	to cheat
conjunctiv, conjunctiv/o	conjunctiva, to join together	dem	people
		dendr/o	tree

dent, dent/i, dent/o	tooth	esophag/o, esophage/o	esophagus
derm, derm/a, derm/o	skin	esthes	sensation
dermat, dermat/o	skin	esthesi/o	feeling, sensation
dextr/o	to the right	esthet	feeling, sensation
didym, didym/o	testis	estr/o	female
digit, digit/o	finger or toe	eti/o	cause
dilat, dilat/o	to widen	excret/o	sifted out
dipl/o	double	excretor	sifted out
disk, disk/o	disk	fasc	band (fascia)
dist, dist/o	away from the point of origin	fasci/o	band (fascia)
diverticul, diverticul/o	diverticula	febr	fever
dors, dors/i, dors/o	backward	femor, femor/o	femur, thigh bone
duct, duct/o	to lead	fenestrat	window
duoden, duoden/o	duodenum	fibr, fibr/o	fibrous tissue, fiber
dur, dur/o	dura, hard	fibrillat	fibrils (small fibers)
dwarf	small	fibrin/o	fiber
dynam, dynam/o	power	fibul, fibul/o	fibula
ech/o	echo, reflected sound	filtrat, filtrat/o	to strain through
ectop	displaced	fixat, fixat/o	fastened
eg/o	I, self	flex	to bend
ejaculat, ejaculat/o	to throw out	fluor/o	fluorescence, luminous
electr/o	electricity	foc, foc/o	focus
embol, embol/o	to cast, to throw	follicul, follicul/o	little bag
eme	to vomit	format	shaping
emulsificat	disintegrate	fungat	mushroom, fungus
encephal, encephal/o	brain	furc/o	forking, branching
enchyma	to pour	fus, fus/o	to pour
enter/o	intestines (usually small intestine)	ganglion	knot
enucleat	to remove the kernel of	gastr, gastr/o	stomach
eosin/o	rose-colored	gen, gene, genet	formation, produce
episi/o	vulva, pudenda	gen/o	kind
erg/o	work	genital	belonging to birth
erget	work	ger, ger/o	old age
erysi	red	gester	to bear
erythr/o	red		

gigant, gigant/o	giant	horizont	horizon
gingiv, gingiv/o	gums	humer, humer/o	humerus
glandul	little acorn	hydr, hydr/o	water
gli, gli/o	glue	hymen	hymen
glob, globul/o	globule, globe	hypn, hypn/o	sleep
globin	globule	hyster, hyster/o	womb, uterus
glomerul, glomerul/o	glomerulus, little ball	iatr	treatment
gloss/o	tongue	icter, icter/o	jaundice
gluc/o	sweet, sugar	ile, ile/o	ileum
glyc, glyc/o, glycos, glycos/o	glucose, sweet, sugar	ili, ili/o	ilium
		illus	foot
gnost	knowledge	immun/o	safe, immunity
gon/o	genitals	infarct, infarct/o	infarct (necrosis of an area)
gonad, gonad/o	seed	infect	to infect
goni/o	angle	infer, infer/o	below
grand/i	great	inguin, inguin/o	groin
granul/o	little grain, granular	insul, insulin/o	insulin
gravida, gravidar	pregnancy	integument, integument/o	covering
gravis	grave		
gryp	curve	intern	within
gurgitat	to flood	irid, irid/o	iris
gynec/o	female	is/o	equal
halat, halat/o	breathe	isch, isch/o	to hold back
halit/o	breath	ischi	ischium
hallucinat	to wander in mind	jaund/o	yellow
hallux	great (big) toe	kal, kal/i	potassium
hem, hem/o, hemat, hemat/o	blood	kary/o	cell's nucleus
		kel, kel/o	tumor
hemorrh, hemorrh/o	vein liable to bleed	kerat, kerat/o	horn, cornea
hepat, hepat/o	liver	keton, keton/o	ketone
herni/o	hernia	kil/o	one thousand
hidr, hidr/o	sweat	kinet	motion
hirsut, hirsut/o	hairy	kyph, kyph/o	hump
hist/o	tissue	labi, labi/o	lip
hol/o	whole	labyrinth, labyrinth/o	maze

lacrim, lacrim/o	tear, lacrimal duct, tear duct	masticat	to chew
lamin, lamin/o	lamina, thin plate	mat	to ripen
lamp(s)	to shine	maxill, maxill/o	upper jawbone
lapar/o	abdomen	maxilla	jaw
laryng, laryng/o	larynx, voice box	maxim	greatest
later, later/o	side	meat, meat/o	passage
laxat	to loosen	med	middle
lei/o	smooth	medi, medi/o	toward the middle
lent, lent/o	lens	medull, medull/o	marrow
lept	seizure	melan, melan/o	black
letharg	drowsiness	men, men/o	month, menses, menstruation
leuk, leuk/o	white	mening, meningi/o, mening/o	membrane, meninges
levat	lifter		
lingu, lingu/o	tongue	menisc, menisc/i, menisc/o	crescent-shaped
lip, lip/o	fat		
lipid, lipid/o	fat	menstru	to discharge the menses
lith, lith/o	stone	ment, ment/o	mind
lob, lob/o	lobe	mes, mes/o	middle
lobul	small lobe	mester	month
locat	to place	metr	to measure
log	study	metr/o	womb, uterus
log/o	word	metri/o	womb, uterus
lopec	fox mange	mi/o	less, smaller
lord, lord/o	bending, curve, swayback	miliar	millet (tiny)
lumb, lumb/o	loin, lower back	minim	least
lump	lump	mit, mit/o	thread
lun, lun/o	moon	mitr, mitr/o	mitral valve
lymph, lymph/o	lymph, clear fluid	mnes	memory
macr/o	large	morbid	sick
malign, malign/o	bad kind	mortal	human being
mamm/o	breast	mucos, mucos/o, mucus	mucus
man/o	thin		
mandibul, mandibul/o	lower jawbone	muscul, muscul/o	muscle
mast, mast/o	mastoid process, breast-shaped, breast	muta, mutat, mutat/o	to change
		my, my/o	muscle

my/o, my/o(s)	muscle	**orch, orch/o**	testicle
myc, myc/o	fungus	**orchid, orchid/o**	testicle
mydriat	dilate, widen	**organ, organ/o**	organ
myel, myel/o	bone marrow, spinal cord	**orth, orth/o**	straight
myring, myring/o	eardrum, tympanic membrane	**oscill, oscill/o**	to swing
myx, myx/o	mucus	**oste, oste/o**	bone
narc/o	numbness, sleep, stupor	**ot, ot/o**	ear
nas/o	nose	**ovar**	ovary
nat, nat/o	birth	**ovul, ovulat**	ovary
necr, necr/o	death	**ox/i**	oxygen
nephr, nephr/o	kidney	**oxy**	sour, sharp, acid
neur, neur/o	nerve	**pachy, pachy/o**	thick
neutr/o	neither	**palat/o**	palate
nid	nest	**palliat, palliat/o**	cloaked
noct, noct/o	night	**pallid/o**	globus pallidus
nom	law	**palm**	palm
norm	rule	**palp**	touch
nucl	nucleus	**palpitat, palpit/o**	throbbing
nucle	kernel, nucleus	**pancreat, pancreat/o**	pancreas
nyctal	night	**pannicul**	fat cells
o/o	ovum, egg	**papill, papill/o**	papilla
obsess, obsess/o	besieged by thoughts	**para**	to bear, bring forth
occlus, occlus/o	to close up	**paralyt**	to disable, paralysis
ocul, ocul/o	eye	**pareun, pareun/o**	lying beside, sexual intercourse
odont, odont/o	tooth	**partum**	labor
olecran, olecran/o	elbow	**parturit**	in labor
olfact/o	smell	**patell, patell/o**	kneecap, patella
omion	shoulder	**path, path/o**	disease
omphal/o	navel, umbilicus	**pause**	cessation
onc/o	tumor	**pector, pector/o, pector (at)**	chest
onych, onych/o	nail	**ped, ped/o, ped/i**	foot, child
oophor, oophor/o	ovary	**pedicul, pedicul/o**	louse
ophthalm, ophthalm/o	eye	**pelv/i**	pelvis
opt, opt/o	eye	**penile**	penis
or, or/o	mouth		

pept, pept/o	to digest		pod/o	foot
perine, perine/o	perineum		poiet	formation
peritone/o	peritoneum		poli/o	gray
phac, phac/o	lens		por	passage
phag, phag/o	to eat, engulf		porphyr	purple
phak, phak/o	lens		poster, poster/o	behind, toward the back, back
phalang/e, phalang/o	phalanges, finger/toe bones		prand/i	meal
pharyng, pharynge/o, pharyng/o	pharynx, throat		presby, presby/o	old
phas	speech		press	to press
phe/o	dusky		proct, proct/o	anus and rectum
phen/o	to show		prophylact	guarding
phim	muzzle		prostat, prostat/o	prostate
phleb, phleb/o	vein		prosth/e	an addition
phob, phob/o	fear		proxim, proxim/o	near the point of origin
phon, phon/o	voice, sound		prurit, prurit/o	itching
phor	carrying		psych, psych/o	mind
phos	light		pudend	external genitals
phot/o	light		pulm/o	lung
phragm	partition		pulmon/o	lung
phras	speech		pupill, pupill/o	pupil
phren, phren/o	mind		purpur	purple
physi/o	nature, function		py, py/o	pus
physic/o	nature		pyel, pyel/o	renal pelvis
pil/o	hair		pylor, pylor/o	pylorus, gatekeeper
pine	pine cone		pyr/o	heat, fire
pineal	pineal body		pyret	fever
pituitar	pituitary gland		rach, rachi/o	spinal column, vertebrae
plak, plak/o	plate		radi/o	ray, x-ray
plasma, plasm/o	plasma		radiat	radiant
plast	developing		radic/o	spinal nerve root
pleur, pleur/o	pleura		radicul	spinal nerve root
plicat	to fold		ras	to scrape off
pneum/o	air		rect/o	rectum
pneumon, pneumon/o	lung		regul	rule
			relaxat	to loosen

remiss, remiss/o	remit	**sial, sial/o**	saliva, salivary
ren, ren/o	kidney	**sider/o**	iron
respirat, respirat/o	breathing	**sigmoid, sigmoid/o**	sigmoid
reticul/o	net	**sin/o**	curve
retin, retin/o	retina	**sinus**	curve, hollow
rhabd/o	rod	**situ**	place
rheumat, rheumat/o	discharge	**som, somat, somat/o**	body
rhin/o	nose	**somn, somn/o**	sleep
rhonch, rhonch/o	snore	**son, son/o**	sound
rhytid/o	wrinkle	**spadias**	rent, opening
roent	roentgen	**spastic**	convulsive
rotat, rotat/o	to turn	**sperm, sperm/i, sperm/o**	seed (sperm)
rrhyth, rrhythm, rrhythm/o	rhythm	**spermat, spermat/o**	seed (sperm)
rube/o	red	**sphygm/o**	pulse
sacr, sacr/o	sacrum	**sphyxis, sphyx**	pulse
salping, salping/o,	tube, fallopian	**spin, spin/o**	spine, thorn
salpinx	tube	**spir/o**	breathe
sarc, sarc/o	flesh	**splen/o**	spleen
scapul, scapul/o	shoulder blade	**spondyl, spondyl/o**	vertebra
schiz/o	to divide	**staped, staped/o**	stapes, stirrup
scler, scler/o	hard, hardening, sclera	**steat, steat/o**	fat
scoli, scoli/o	curvature	**sten, sten/o**	narrowing
scop	to examine	**ster**	solid
seb/o	oil	**stern, stern/o**	sternum, breastbone
secund	second	**sterol**	solid (fat)
semin, semin/o	seed, semen	**steth, steth/o**	chest
seminat	seed, semen	**stigmat, stigmat/o**	point
senil, senile	old	**stom, stom/o**	mouth
sept	putrefaction	**stomat, stomat/o**	mouth
sept/o	a partition	**strabism**	squinting
septic, septic/o	putrefying	**strict**	to draw, to bind
ser(a), ser/o	whey, serum	**suppress, suppress/o**	suppress
sert	to gain	**surg/o**	surgery
sexu	sex	**surrog**	substitute

symmetric	symmetry	toxic, toxic/o	poison
sympath	sympathy	trache/o	trachea
synov, synov/o	synovial membrane	tract, tract/o	to draw
system/o	composite, whole	trephinat	bore
systol	contraction	trich, trich/o	hair
systole	contraction	trism	grating
tars/o	ankle, tarsus	trop, trop/o	turning
tel	end, distant	troph, troph/o	nourishment, development
tele	distant	tuber	bulge
tempor	temples	tubercul, tubercul/o	little swelling, nodule
ten/o	tendon	turg	swelling
tend/o	tendon	tuss	cough
tendin, tendin/o	tendon	tympan, tympan/o	eardrum, drum
tendon, tendon/o	tendon	uln, uln/o	ulna
tenos	tendon	umbilic	navel
tens	tension	ungu/o	nail
tentori	tentorium, tent	ur, ur/o	urinate, urination
terat, terat/o	monster	urea	urea
test/o	testicle	uret	urine
testicul, testicul/o	testicle	ureter, ureter/o	ureter
thalass	sea	urethr, urethr/o	urethra
therm, therm/o	hot, heat	urinat/o	urine
thorac, thorac/o	chest	uter, uter/o	uterus
thromb, thromb/o	clot	uve, uve/o	uvea
thym, thym/o	thymus, mind, emotion	vag/o	vagus, wandering
thyr, thyr/o	thyroid, shield	vagin, vagin/o	vagina
tibi, tibi/o	tibia	valvul/o	valve
toc, toc/o	labor, birth	varic/o	twisted vein
tom/o	to cut	vas, vas/o	vessel
ton, ton/o	tone, tension	vascul, vascul/o	small vessel
tonsill, tonsill/o	tonsil, almond	vector	carrier
topic, top/o	place	ven/o	vein
tors, tors/o	twisted	venere, venere/o	sexual intercourse
tort/i	twisted	ventilat, ventilat/o	to air
tox, tox/o	poison	ventr, ventr/o	near or on the belly side of the body

ventricul, ventricul/o	ventricle, little belly	**volunt, volunt/o**	will
vermin, verm/i	worm	**volvul**	to roll
vers, vers/o	turning	**vuls, vuls/o**	to pull
vertebr, vertebr/o	vertebra	**watt**	watt
vesic	bladder	**xanth/o**	yellow
vesicul, vesicul/o	seminal vesicle	**xen, xen/o**	foreign material
vir, vir/o	virus (poison)	**xer, xer/o**	dry
viril, viril/o	masculine	**xiph, xiph/o**	sword
viscer, viscer/o	body organs	**zo/o**	animal
volt	volt	**zoon**	life

Suffixes

-able	capable	**-clasia**	a breaking
-ac	pertaining to	**-clasis**	crushing, breaking up
-act	to act	**-clysis**	injection
-ad	pertaining to	**-cope**	strike
-age	related to	**-crine**	to secrete
-al	pertaining to	**-crit**	to separate
-algesia	condition of pain	**-culture**	cultivation
-algia	pain, ache	**-cusis**	hearing
-ant	forming	**-cuspid**	point
-apheresis	removal, remove	**-cyesis**	pregnancy
-ar, -ary	pertaining to	**-cyst**	bladder, sac
-arche	beginning	**-cyte**	cell
-ase	enzyme	**-derma**	skin
-asthenia	weakness	**-dermis**	skin
-ate, -ate(d)	use, action, having the form of, possessing	**-desis**	binding
		-drome	course
-betes	to go	**-dynia**	pain, ache
-blast	immature cell, germ cell, embryonic cell	**-eal**	pertaining to
		-ectasia	dilatation
-body	body	**-ectasis**	dilatation, dilation, stretching, expansion
-cele	hernia, tumor, swelling		
-centesis	surgical puncture	**-ectasy**	dilation
-ceps	head	**-ectomy**	surgical excision, surgical removal, resection
-cide	to kill		

-edema	swelling	-ion	process
-emesis	vomiting	-ior	pertaining to
-emia	blood condition	-is	pertaining to
-ence	state	-ism	condition
-er	relating to, one who	-ist	one who specializes, agent
-ergy	work	-itis	inflammation
-esis	condition	-ity	condition
-esthesia	feeling	-ive	nature of, quality of
-form	shape	-ize	to make, to treat or combine with
-fuge	to flee	-kinesia	motion, movement
-gen	formation, produce	-kinesis	motion, movement
-genes	produce	-lalia	to talk
-genesis	formation, produce	-lemma	sheath, rind
-genic	formation, produce	-lepsy	seizure
-glia	glue	-lexia	diction, word, phrase
-globin	protein	-liter	liter
-gnosis	knowledge	-lith	stone
-grade	step	-logy	study of
-graft	pencil, grafting knife	-lucent	to shine
-gram	weight, mark, record	-lymph	clear fluid, serum, pale fluid
-graph	to write, record, instrument for recording	-lysis	destruction, separation, breakdown, loosening, dissolution
-graphy	recording	-malacia	softening
-hexia	condition	-mania	madness
-ia	condition	-megaly	enlargement, large
-iasis	condition	-meter	instrument to measure
-iatrics	treatment	-metry	measurement
-iatry	treatment	-mnesia	memory
-ic	pertaining to	-morph	form, shape
-ician	specialist, physician	-noia	mind
-icle	small, minute	-oid	resemble, like, similar
-ide	having a particular quality	-ole	opening, small
-ile	pertaining to	-oma	tumor, mass, fluid collection
-in	substance	-on	pertaining to
-ine	pertaining to, substance	-one	hormone
-ing	quality of	-opaque	dark, nontransparent

-opia	sight, vision	-rrhage	to burst forth, bursting forth
-opsia	sight, vision	-rrhagia	to burst forth, bursting forth
-opsy	to view	-rrhaphy	suture
-or	one who, a doer	-rrhea	flow, discharge
-orexia	appetite	-rrhexis	rupture
-ose	pertaining to	-scope	instrument for examining
-osis	condition	-scopy	to view, examine, visual examination
-ous	pertaining to	-sepsis	decay
-oxia	oxygen	-sis	state of, condition
-paresis	weakness	-some	body
-pathy	disease, emotion	-sound	sound
-penia	lack of, deficiency, abnormal reduction	-spasm	tension, spasm, contraction
		-stalsis	contraction
-pepsia	to digest, digestion	-stasis	control, stop, stand still
-pexy	surgical fixation	-staxis	dripping, trickling
-phagia	to eat, to swallow	-sthenia	strength
-phasia	to speak, speech	-stomy	new opening
-phil	attraction	-systole	contraction
-philia	attraction	-taxia	order, coordination
-phobia	fear	-therapy	treatment
-phoresis	to carry	-thermy	heat
-phragm	fence, partition	-thorax	chest
-phraxis	to obstruct	-tic	pertaining to
-phylaxis	protection	-tome	instrument to cut
-physis	growth	-tomy	incision
-plakia	plaque	-tone	tension
-plasia	formation, produce	-tripsy	crushing
-plasm	thing formed, plasma	-troph(y)	nourishment, development
-plasty	surgical repair	-trophy	nourishment, development
-plegia	stroke, paralysis, palsy	-type	type
-pnea	breathing	-um	tissue, structure
-poiesis	formation	-ure	process
-praxia	action	-uria	urination, condition of urine
-ptosis	prolapse, drooping, sagging, falling down	-us	pertaining to, structure
		-y	condition, process, pertaining to
-ptysis	spitting, coughing up		

Appendix III

ABBREVIATIONS, ACRONYMS, AND SYMBOLS

Abbreviations and Acronyms

17-KS	17-ketosteroids
17-OHCS	17-hydroxycorticosteroids
A	
A&P	anatomy and physiology
AAP	American Academy of Pediatrics
AB	abortion
Abd, abd	abdomen
ABGs	arterial blood gases
ABO	blood groups
AC	air conduction
ac	before meals (ante cibum)
ACA	adenocarcinoma
Acc	accommodation
ACE	angiotensin-converting enzyme
ACG	angiocardiography
ACh	acetylcholine
ACIP	Advisory Committee of Immunization Practices
ACR	American College of Rheumatology
ACS	American Cancer Society
ACTH	adrenocorticotropic hormone
AD	Alzheimer disease; advance directive
ADE	adverse drug effect
ADH	antidiuretic hormone
ADHD	attention-deficit/hyperactivity disorder
ADL	activities of daily living
ADR	adverse drug reaction
AE	above elbow
AED	automated external defibrillator
AF or AFib	atrial fibrillation

AFB	acid-fast bacilli
AFP	alpha-fetoprotein
AGN	acute glomerulonephritis
AIDET	Acknowledge, Introduce, Duration, Explanation, Thank you
AIDS	acquired immunodeficiency syndrome
AIH	artificial insemination homologous
AK	above knee
ALD	aldolase
ALL	acute lymphocytic leukemia
ALS	amyotrophic lateral sclerosis
ALT	argon laser trabeculoplasty; alanine aminotransferase
AMD	age-related macular degeneration
AMI	acute myocardial infarction; any mental illness
AML	acute myeloid leukemia
ANA	antinuclear antibodies
ANS	autonomic nervous system; acute nephritic syndrome
AOM	acute otitis media
AOP	acknowledgment of paternity
APA	American Psychiatric Association
ARBs	ANG-II receptor blockers
ARD	acute respiratory disease
ARDS	acute respiratory distress syndrome
AROM	artificial rupture of membranes
ASAP	as soon as possible
ASCUS	atypical squamous cells of undetermined significance
ASD	autism spectrum disorder

ASHD	arteriosclerotic heart disease
ASO	antistreptolysin O
ASPD	advanced sleep phase disorder
AST	aspartate aminotransferase
ATC	Anatomical Therapeutic Chemical Classification System
AT/RT	atypical teratoid rhabdoid tumor
AV	atrioventricular
ax	axillary

B

Ba	barium
BAC	blood alcohol concentration
baso	basophil
BC	bone conduction
BCC	basal cell carcinoma
BCG	bacille Calmette–Guérin
BE	Barrett esophagus; below elbow; barium enema
BG	blood glucose
BK	below knee
BM	bowel movement
BMD	bone mineral density (test)
BMI	body mass index
BMR	basal metabolic rate
Botox®	Botulinum toxin type A
BP	blood pressure
BPH	benign prostatic hyperplasia (hypertrophy)
BUN	blood urea nitrogen
Bx	biopsy

C

C	centigrade; Celsius
C1, C2, etc.	first cervical vertebra; second cervical vertebra
$C_6H_{12}O_6$	glucose

CA	cancer
Ca	calcium
CA-125	cancer antigen 125
CABG	coronary artery bypass graft
CAD	coronary artery disease
CaO	calcium oxide
CAPD	continuous ambulatory peritoneal dialysis
CAT	computerized axial tomography
CBC	complete blood count
CBT	cognitive-behavioral therapy
CC	chief complaint; clean catch (urine)
CD	Crohn disease
CDC	Centers for Disease Control and Prevention
CEA	carcinoembryonic antigen
CF	cystic fibrosis
CGN	chronic glomerulonephritis
CHD	coronary heart disease
chemo	chemotherapy
CHF	congestive heart failure
CHO	carbohydrate
chol	cholesterol
Ci	curie
CIN	cervical intraepithelial neoplasia
CK	creatine kinase
CKD	chronic kidney disease
CLI	critical limb ischemia
CLIA	clinical laboratory improvement amendments
CLL	chronic lymphocytic leukemia
cm	centimeter
CML	chronic myeloid leukemia
CMP	cardiomyopathy; comprehensive metabolic panel

CMV	cytomegalovirus		DHT	dihydrotestosterone
CNS	central nervous system		DI	diabetes insipidus
c/o	complains of		diff	differential count (white blood cells)
CO	cardiac output		DM	diabetes mellitus
CO_2	carbon dioxide		DMARDs	disease-modifying antirheumatic drugs
COCs	combined oral contraceptives		DMD	Duchenne muscular dystrophy
COPD	chronic obstructive pulmonary disease		DNA	deoxyribonucleic acid; does not apply
CP	cerebral palsy		DOB	date of birth
CRF	corticotropin-releasing factor		Dr.	doctor
CRP	C-reactive protein blood test		DRE	digital rectal examination
CS, C-section	cesarean section		DSM-5	*Diagnostic and Statistical Manual of Mental Disorders*, Fifth Edition
CSF	cerebrospinal fluid			
CT	computed tomography		DSPS	delayed sleep phase syndrome
CT KUB	computed tomography of kidneys, ureters, bladder		DTaP	diphtheria, tetanus, and pertussis
			DUB	dysfunctional uterine bleeding
CTA	clear to auscultation		DVT	deep vein thrombosis
CTE	chronic traumatic encephalopathy		Dx	diagnosis
CV	cardiovascular		DXA	dual-energy X-ray absorptiometry scan
CVA	cerebrovascular accident (stroke)		**E**	
CVD	cardiovascular disease		ECC	extracorporeal circulation
CVS	chorionic villus sampling; computer vision syndrome		ECG, EKG	electrocardiogram
			ECHO	echocardiogram
CXR	chest x-ray		ECT	electroconvulsive therapy
cysto	cystoscopic examination; cystoscopy		ED	erectile dysfunction
			EE	erosive esophagitis
D			EEG	electroencephalogram
DALK	deep anterior lamellar keratoplasty		EF	ejection fraction
D&C	dilation (dilatation) and curettage		EGD	esophagogastroduodenoscopy
db, Db	decibel		EHR	electronic health record
DBS	deep brain stimulation		EHT	estrogen hormone therapy
DCIS	ductal carcinoma in situ		EK	endothelial keratoplasty
DEA	Drug Enforcement Administration		ELISA	enzyme-linked immunosorbent assay
decub	decubitus		EM	emmetropia
Derm	dermatology			

EMG	electromyography		FTLD	frontotemporal lobar degeneration
ENG	electronystagmography		F-V loop	flow volume loop
ENT	ear, nose, throat (otorhinolaryngology)		Fx	fracture
eos, eosin	eosinophil		**G**	
EPS	electrophysiology study (intracardiac)		g	gram
ER	emergency room; endoplasmic reticulum		GAD	generalized anxiety disorder
ERCP	endoscopic retrograde cholangiopancreatography		GB	gallbladder
			GBS	group B streptococcus
ERT	external radiation therapy		GC	gonorrhea
ERV	expiratory reserve volume		GCS	Glasgow Coma Scale
ESR, sed rate	erythrocyte sedimentation rate		GERD	gastroesophageal reflux disease
ESRD	end-stage renal disease		GFR	glomerular filtration rate
ESWL	extracorporeal shockwave lithotripsy		GGT	gamma-glutamyl transferase
ET	esotropia; endotracheal		GH	growth hormone
ETS	environmental tobacco smoke		GHRF	growth hormone–releasing factor
Ex	examination		GI	gastrointestinal
F			GnRF	gonadotropin-releasing factor
F	Fahrenheit; female		grav I	pregnancy one
FBG	fasting blood glucose		GTT	glucose tolerance test
FBS	fasting blood sugar		GU	genitourinary
FDA	Food and Drug Administration		GYN	gynecology
FFA	free fatty acids		**H**	
FH	family history		H_2O	water
FHB	fetal heartbeat		H&E	hematoxylin and eosin
FIV	forced inspiratory volume		H&L	heart & lungs
FMS	fibromyalgia syndrome		HAART	highly active antiretroviral therapy
FNA	fine-needle aspiration		HAV	hepatitis A virus
FP	family practice		HBIG	hepatitis B immune globulin
FRC	forced residual capacity		HBP	high blood pressure
FROM	full range of motion		HBSAg	hepatitis B surface antigen
FSH	follicle-stimulating hormone		HBV	hepatitis B virus
FTA-ABS	fluorescent treponemal antibody absorption		hCG	human chorionic gonadotropin
FTD	frontotemporal dementia		HCl	hydrochloric acid

HCO$_3$	bicarbonate
Hct, HCT	hematocrit
HCV	hepatitis C virus
HD	hearing distance; Hodgkin disease; hemodialysis
HDL	high-density lipoprotein
HDS	herniated disk syndrome
HDV	hepatitis D virus
heart cath	cardiac catheterization
HER-2/neu	human epidermal growth factor receptor–2
HEV	hepatitis E virus
HF	heart failure
Hg	mercury
Hgb, HGB, Hb	hemoglobin
HHS	Health and Human Services (Department of)
HI-ART	highly integrated adaptive radiotherapy
HIPAA	Health Insurance Portability and Accountability Act
HIV	human immunodeficiency virus
HMD	hyaline membrane disease
HNP	herniated nucleus pulposus
HPV	human papillomavirus
HSG	hysterosalpingography
HSV	herpes simplex virus
HSV-2	herpes simplex virus–2
HT	hormone therapy
Ht	height
HTLV	human T-cell leukemia-lymphoma virus
HTN	hypertension
Hx	history
Hy	hyperopia
Hz	cycles/seconds

I

IBD	inflammatory bowel disease
IBS	irritable bowel syndrome
IC	interstitial cystitis; inspiratory capacity
ICP	intracranial pressure
ID	intradermal
IDDM	insulin-dependent diabetes mellitus
Ig	immunoglobulin
IGRA	interferon-gamma (IFN-γ) release assay
IM	intramuscular
IMRT	intensity-modulated radiation therapy
IOL	intraocular lens
IOP	intraocular pressure
IPD	intermittent peritoneal dialysis
IPL	intense pulsed light
IQ	intelligence quotient
IR	interventional radiology
IRDS	infant respiratory distress syndrome
IRT	internal radiation therapy
IRV	inspiratory reserve volume
ISMP	Institute for Safe Medication Practices
IUD	intrauterine device
IV	intravenous
IVP	intravenous pyelogram

J

jt	joint

K

K	potassium
kg	kilogram
KS	Kaposi sarcoma

L

L	liter
L1, L2, etc.	first lumbar vertebra, second lumbar vertebra, etc.

LA	left atrium
LASIK	laser-assisted in situ keratomileusis
LAT, lat	lateral
LATE	limbic-predominant age-related TDP-43 encephalopathy
LBD	Lewy body dementia
LCIS	lobular carcinoma in situ
LD, LDH	lactate dehydrogenase
LDL	low-density lipoprotein
LES	lower esophageal sphincter
LH	luteinizing hormone
lig	ligament
LLQ	left lower quadrant
LMP	last menstrual period
LP	lumbar puncture
LPI	laser peripheral iridotomy
LTBI	latent TB infection
LTH	lactogenic hormone
LUQ	left upper quadrant
LV	left ventricle
LVEF	left-ventricular ejection fraction
lymphs	lymphocytes

M

MALT	mucosa-associated lymphoid tissue (lymphoma)
MAOIs	monoamine oxidase inhibitors
MBPS	Munchausen-by-proxy syndrome
mcg	microgram
mCi	millicurie
MD	medical doctor; muscular dystrophy
MG	myasthenia gravis
mg	milligram (0.001 gram)
MGD	meibomian gland dysfunction
MHI	mild head injury

MHT	minor head trauma
MI	myocardial infarction
MIF	melanocyte-stimulating hormone release-inhibiting factor
mL	milliliter (0.001 liter)
mm	millimeter (0.001 meter; 0.039 inch)
MMPI-2	Minnesota Multiphasic Personality Inventory–2
MMR	measles, mumps, and rubella
MPD	mammary Paget disease
MRAs	mineralocorticoid receptor antagonists
MRF	melanocyte-stimulating hormone–releasing factor
MRI	magnetic resonance imaging
MS	mitral stenosis; multiple sclerosis; musculoskeletal
MSG	monosodium glutamate
MSH	melanocyte-stimulating hormone
MTBI	mild traumatic brain injury
MV	mitral valve
MVP	mitral valve prolapse
MVV	maximal voluntary ventilation
My	myopia

N

Na	sodium
NaCl	sodium chloride
N&V	nausea and vomiting
NCI	National Cancer Institute
Neuro	neurology
ng	nanogram
NG	nasogastric (tube)
NGU	nongonococcal urethritis
NH3	ammonia
NHL	non-Hodgkin lymphoma
NIDDM	non-insulin-dependent diabetes mellitus

NIH	National Institutes of Health
NIMH	National Institute of Mental Health
NK	natural killer (cells)
NKDA	no known drug allergies
NPO, npo	nothing by mouth (*nil per os*)
NRDS	neonatal respiratory distress syndrome
NREM	no rapid eye movement (sleep)
NSAIDs	nonsteroidal anti-inflammatory drugs
NSCLC	non–small cell lung cancer
NSSC	normal size, shape, and consistency
NST	nonstress test
NSTEMI	non-ST-segment elevation myocardial infarction

O

O, O₂	oxygen
O₃	ozone
O&P	ova and parasites
OA	osteoarthritis
OB	obstetrics
OCD	obsessive–compulsive disorder
OD	doctor of optometry, optometrist
OIC	opioid-induced constipation
OM	otitis media
OP	outpatient
OPCAB	off-pump coronary artery bypass surgery
OR	operating room
Orth, ortho	orthopedics; orthopaedics
OTC	over-the-counter
OV	office visit
oz	ounce

P

P	pulse; phosphorus
PA	posteroanterior
PAD	peripheral artery disease
Pap	Papanicolaou (smear)
Path	pathology
Pb	lead
PBI	protein-bound iodine
PCV13	pneumococcal conjugate vaccine
PD	Parkinson disease
PDD-NOS	pervasive developmental disorder not otherwise specified
PDT	photodynamic therapy
PE	physical examination; pulmonary embolism
Peds	pediatrics
PET	positron emission tomography
pH	hydrogen ion concentration
PHN	postherpetic neuralgia
PID	pelvic inflammatory disease
PIF	prolactin release-inhibiting factor
PIH	pregnancy-induced hypertension
PJP	*Pneumocystis jiroveci* pneumonia
PK	penetrating keratoplasty
PMS	premenstrual syndrome
PNS	peripheral nervous system
PO	orally, by mouth
PP	postprandial (after meals)
PPD	purified protein derivative (TB test)
PPIs	proton pump inhibitors
PPSV23	pneumococcal polysaccharide vaccine
PrEP	pre-exposure prophylaxis
PRF	prolactin-releasing factor
PRL	prolactin hormone
PRN, prn	as necessary; as required; when necessary; as needed
PSA	prostate-specific antigen
Psych	psychiatry; psychology

PT	prothrombin time
PTCA	percutaneous transluminal coronary angioplasty
PTH	parathyroid hormone (parathormone)
PTSD	posttraumatic stress disorder
PTT	partial thromboplastin time
PUBS	percutaneous umbilical blood sampling
PUD	peptic ulcer disease
PUL	percutaneous ultrasonic lithotripsy

Q

q	every (quaque)
q2h	every 2 hours
q4h	every 4 hours
QFT	QuantiFERON-TB Gold
qh	every hour
qid	four times a day
qm	every morning (quaque mane)
qns	quantity not sufficient
qs	quantity sufficient
qt	quart

R

R	respiration
R, rt	right
RA	right atrium; rheumatoid arthritis
Ra	radium
rad	radiation absorbed dose
RAIU	radioactive iodine uptake
RBC(s)	red blood cell(s); red blood cell (count)
RD	respiratory disease
RDS	respiratory distress syndrome
REM	rapid eye movement (sleep)
RF	rheumatoid factor
Rh	Rhesus blood factor (Rh+ or Rh−)
RLF	retrolental fibroplasia

RLQ	right lower quadrant
RM	recurrent miscarriage
RNA	ribonucleic acid
R/O	rule out
ROM	range of motion
RP	retrograde pyelography
RPE	retinal pigment epithelium
RPR	rapid plasma reagin
RSV	respiratory syncytial virus
RUQ	right upper quadrant
RV	right ventricle; residual volume
RVEF	right-ventricular ejection fraction
Rx	take thou; prescribe; treatment; therapy

S

SA	sinoatrial (node)
SAD	seasonal affective disorder
SARS	severe acute respiratory syndrome
SBAR	Situation, Background, Assessment, Recommendation
SCA	sudden cardiac arrest
SCC	squamous cell carcinoma
SCD	sudden cardiac death
SDs	standard deviations
SG	skin graft
SLT	selective laser trabeculoplasty
SMI	serious mental illness
SNRI	serotonin-norepinephrine reuptake inhibitor
SOAP	subjective, objective, assessment, plan
SOB	shortness of breath
sp. gr	specific gravity
SSD	somatic symptom disorder
SSRIs	selective serotonin reuptake inhibitors
St	stage (of disease)

staph	staphylococcus		TM	tympanic membrane
STEMI	ST-segment elevation myocardial infarction		TNF	tumor necrosis factor
			TOF	tetralogy of Fallot
STH	somatotropin hormone		TORCH	toxoplasmosis, rubella, cytomegalovirus, herpes simplex virus
STIs	sexually transmitted infections			
strep	streptococcus		TPA, tPA	tissue plasminogen activator
			TPR	temperature, pulse, respiration
T			TRH	thyrotropin-releasing hormone
T	temperature		TSE	testicular self-exam
T1, T2, etc.	thoracic vertebrae first, thoracic vertebrae second, etc.		TSH	thyroid-stimulating hormone
			TSS	toxic shock syndrome
T3	triiodothyronine		TST	tuberculin skin test
T3U	triiodothyronine uptake		TUIP	transurethral incision of the prostate
T4	thyroxine		TUMT	transurethral microwave thermotherapy
TAH-BSO	total abdominal hysterectomy with bilateral salpingo-oophorectomy		TUNA	transurethral needle ablation
			TUR	transurethral resection
TAT	Thematic Apperception Test		TURP	transurethral resection of the prostate
TB	tuberculosis		TV	tidal volume
TBSA	total body surface area		Tx	traction
TC	testicular cancer			
TCAs	tricyclic antidepressants		**U**	
Tdap	tetanus, diphtheria, and pertussis		UA	urinalysis
TDP-43	transactive response DNA binding protein 43 kDa		UC	ulcerative colitis
			UE	unconjugated estriol
TENS	transcutaneous electrical nerve stimulation		UG	urogenital
			UGI	upper gastrointestinal
TH	thyroid hormone		URI	upper respiratory infection
TJA	total joint arthroplasty		US	ultrasound
TJC	The Joint Commission		UTI	urinary tract infection
TIA	transient ischemic attacks		UV	ultraviolet
tid	three times a day			
TIMs	topical immunomodulators		**V**	
TIPS	transjugular intrahepatic portosystemic shunt		VA	visual acuity
			VAD	vacuum-assisted needle biopsy device
TIS	tumor in situ		VC	vital capacity
TLC	tender loving care; total lung capacity			

VCD	vacuum constriction device	**WHOCC**	World Health Organization Collaborating Centre
VD	venereal disease	**WNL**	within normal limits
VDRL	Venereal Disease Research Laboratory (syphilis test)	**WNV**	West Nile virus
VLDL	very low-density lipoprotein	**Wt**	weight
VLNT	vascularized lymph node transfer		
VP	vasopressin	**X**	
VS, V/S	vital signs	**XR**	x-ray
VSD	ventricular septal defect	**XT**	exotropia
W		**Y**	
WAIS-R	Wechsler Adult Intelligence Scale–Revised	**y/o**	year(s) old
WBC	white blood cell; white blood (cell) count	**YOB**	year of birth
WHO	World Health Organization	**yr**	year

Symbols

•	times; power	%	percent
–	negative	#	number; pound
+	positive	=	equal
+/–	positive or negative	?	question
<	less than	™	trademark
>	more than	©	copyright
*	birth	®	registered
†	death	¶	paragraph

Index

Page numbers followed by *f* indicate figures and those followed by *t* indicate tables.

17-hydroxycorticosteroids (17-OHCS), 500
17-ketosteroids (17-KS), 500
20-20-20 rule, 614

A

Abate, 5, 11
Abbreviations
  acronyms as, 8
  blood and lymphatic system, 372–373
  cardiovascular system, 327–328
  definition, 7
  digestive system, 266–267
  ear, 586
  endocrine system, 501
  eye, 625
  female reproductive system, 678
  human body organization, 89
  initialism, 8
  integumentary system, 132–133
  male reproductive system, 712–713
  medical terminology, 7–8, 28–29
  mental health, 744
  muscular system, 216
  nervous system, 555
  respiratory system, 417–418
  skeletal system, 179–180
  unapproved, 7
  urinary system, 457–458
  use of, 7
ABCDEs Rule, 115
Abdomen, 72
Abdomen quadrants, 72–73, 73*f*
Abdominal cavity, 71*f*, 72
Abdominal thrusts, 401, 401*f*
Abdominopelvic cavity, 72, 73*f*
Abdominoplasty, 117
Abducens nerve, 520*f*, 521*t*
Abduction, 147*f*
Abductor, 196
ABGs (arterial blood gases), 415
Ablative laser, 126
Abnormal, 11, 43
ABO system, 339–340, 340*t*, 371
Abortion, 652–653, 653*f*
Abrasion, 51, 51*f*
Abscess, 12
Absorption, 224
  defined, 239
  function of epithelial tissue, 67
  in small intestine, 231

Accent marks, 88
Accessory nerve, 520*f*, 521*t*
Accessory organs
  of digestive system, 233–235
  of lymphatic system, 344–345
Accessory structures of skin, 98–100, 99*f*
Accommodation (Acc), 598, 602
Accommodative intraocular lens, 613
ACE inhibitors, 322
Acetabulum, 156
Acetylcholine, 527
ACG (angiocardiography), 323
Achondroplasia, 156
Acid-fast bacilli (AFB), 415
Acidosis, 482
Acknowledge, in AIDET communication, 28
Acne, 103, 103*f*
Acne fulminans, 103, 103*f*
Acoustic, 571
Acquired immunodeficiency syndrome (AIDS), 352, 363, 370, 691
Acroarthritis, 156
Acrochordon, 103
Acromegaly, 482, 482*f*
Acromion, 156
Acronyms
  blood and lymphatic system, 372–373
  cardiovascular system, 327–328
  definition, 8
  digestive system, 266–267
  ear, 586
  endocrine system, 501
  eye, 625
  female reproductive system, 678
  human body organization, 89
  integumentary system, 132–133
  male reproductive system, 712–713
  medical terminology, 7–8, 28–29
  mental health, 744
  muscular system, 216
  nervous system, 555
  respiratory system, 417–418
  skeletal system, 179–180
  urinary system, 457–458
  use of, 8
Acrophobia, 735
ACTH (adrenocorticotropin hormone), 467*t*

Actinic dermatitis, 104
Active exercise, 200
Active immunity, 345
Acute, 12
Acute angle-closure glaucoma, 607
Acute febrile polynephritis, 535
Acute idiopathic polynephritis, 535
Acute lymphocytic leukemia (ALL), 361
Acute myeloid leukemia (AML), 361
Acute nephritic syndrome (ANS), 441
Acute respiratory distress syndrome (ARDS), 394
Adam's apple, 385
Adaptive (specific defense mechanisms), 346*f*
Addison disease, 483
Adduction, 147*f*
Adductor, 196
Adenectomy, 483
Adenohypophysis. *See* Pituitary gland anterior lobe (adenohypophysis)
Adenoids, 344, 383
Adenoma, 483
ADH (antidiuretic hormone), 467*t*, 495
ADHD (attention-deficit/hyperactivity disorder), 728
Adhesion, 4–5, 12
Adipose, 82
Adjective suffixes, 37*t*
Adnexa, 654
Adrenal cortex, 465*t*, 468*t*, 473, 474–475, 474*f*, 483
Adrenal glands (suprarenals), 465*t*, 466*f*, 468*t*, 474–475, 474*f*, 483
Adrenal insufficiency, 483
Adrenal medulla, 465*t*, 468*t*, 473, 474*f*, 475
Adrenalectomy, 483
Adrenaline, 468*t*, 475, 487
Adrenocorticotropin hormone (ACTH), 467*t*
Advanced sleep-phase syndrome (ASPD), 545
Adverse drug event (ADE), 88
Adverse drug reaction (ADR), 88
Aerobic exercise, 200
Affect, 726
Affective disorder, 726

Afferent nerves, 511, 512
Afterbirth, 647
Age-related macular degeneration (AMD), 610
Agglutination, 340, 353
Aging
  Alzheimer disease (AD), 527
  arteriosclerosis, 294
  atrophy of pharynx and larynx muscle, 385
  autoimmune disease, 356
  bone density, 140
  bone growth, 145
  dementia, 532
  depression, 738, 738*f*
  digestive system, 225
  ear, 568
  hair, 98
  heart muscle, 192
  hormone production, 661
  immune response, 348
  joints and, 146
  male reproductive system, 690
  menopause, 661
  muscle, 192
  osteoarthritis, 163
  osteoporosis, 165, 165*f*
  prostate cancer, 706
  prostate gland, 690
  respiratory rate, 389
  respiratory system, 387
  roadblocks to mental health services for older adults, 739*f*
  skin, 98, 126
  stroke, 546
  thymus, 348
  urinary system, 431
  voice change, 385
Agonist skeletal muscle, 191
Agoraphobia, 726
AIDET, 28
AIDS (acquired immunodeficiency syndrome), 352, 363, 370, 691
AIDS dementia complex, 533
Akathisia, 527
Akinesia, 527, 544
Alanine aminotransferase (ALT), 216, 324
Albinism, 104
Albumin, 340, 353, 441
Albuminuria, 437
Alcohol toxicology, 264
Aldolase (ALD) blood test, 216
Aldosterone, 468*t*, 474

Alimentary canal, 224

Alkaline phosphatase blood test, 179

ALL (acute lymphocytic leukemia), 361

Allergic rhinitis, 353, 353*f*

Allergy, 353

Allograft, 105

All-or-none principle, 512

Alopecia, 104, 104*f*

Alopecia areata, 104, 104*f*

Alpha adrenergic antagonist, 622

Alpha cells, 472, 472*f*

Alpha-synuclein, 532

ALS (amyotrophic lateral sclerosis), 527

ALT (alanine aminotransferase), 216

Alveoli, 380, 386, 387*f*, 388

Alveolus, 228, 394

Alzheimer, Alois, 8

Alzheimer disease (AD), 8, 515, 527, 532

drugs used to treat, 552

Ambilateral, 82

Amblyopia, 602

Ambulatory, 12, 12*f*

AMD (age-related macular degeneration), 610

Amenorrhea, 654

AML (acute myeloid leukemia), 361

Amnesia, 527

Amniocentesis, 673, 673*f*

Amniotic cavity, 638

Amounts, prefixes pertaining to, 48, 48*t*

Amphiarthrosis, 146

Ampulla
ear, 568
fallopian tube, 635*f*, 637

Amputation, 196, 196*f*

Amylase, 239

Amyotrophic lateral sclerosis (ALS), 527

ANA (antinuclear antibodies), 179, 371

Anabolism, 234, 239

Anal canal, 232, 232*f*

Analgesia, 527

Analgesics, 215
for ear, 582
narcotic, 175, 551
for nervous system, 551
non-narcotic, 175, 551
for skeletal system, 175

Analgesics-antipyretics, 551

Anaphylaxis, 354, 354*f*

Anastomosis, 292

Anatomic patient position, 206*t*

Anatomical locations and positions, 68–74
abdomen quadrants, 72–73, 73*f*
body area terminology, 74*t*
cavities, 68, 69, 71*f*, 72
direction, 69, 70*f*, 70*t*–71*t*
planes, 69, 69*f*
positional terms, 70*t*–71*t*
trunk, 73–74

Anatomical position, 68

Anatomical Therapeutic Chemical Classification System (ATC), 87

Anatomy, defined, 82

Anatomy and physiology
blood and lymphatic system, 336–345, 336*t*
body organization levels, 60–67, 61*f*
cardiovascular system, 275–288, 275*t*, 276*f*
digestive system, 224–225, 224*t*, 225*f*
ear, 563–568, 563*t*, 564*f*
endocrine system, 465, 465*t*, 466*f*
eye, 593–599, 593*t*, 594*f*
female reproductive system, 633–644, 633*t*, 634*f*–635*f*
integumentary system, 95, 95*t*, 96*f*
male reproductive system, 686–691, 686*t*, 687*f*
muscular system, 187–192, 187*t*
nervous system, 509–523, 509*t*, 510*f*
respiratory system, 380–390, 380*t*, 381*f*
skeletal system, 140–150, 140*t*, 141*f*
urinary system, 425–431, 425*t*, 426*f*

Ancillary/miscellaneous reports, 25

Androgenic alopecia, 104, 104*f*

Androgens, 475, 483

Android, 82

Androsterone, 468*t*, 475

Anemia, 35

Anesthesia, 527

Anesthesiologist, 527

Anesthesiology report, 26

Anesthetics, 551

Anesthetize, 52, 52*f*

Aneurysm, 292, 292*f*

Angina, 292, 309
unstable, 301

Angina pectoris, 292

Angiocardiography (ACG), 323

Angiography, 323

Angioma, 293, 293*f*

Angioplasty, 293

Angiostenosis, 293

Angiotensin-receptor blockers (ARBs), 322

Anhidrosis, 105, 113

Anisocoria, 602

Anisocytosis, 356

Ankylosis, 156

Anomaloscope, 623

Anorchism, 698

Anorexia, 239

Anorexia nervosa, 726, 731

ANS (acute nephritic syndrome), 441

ANS (autonomic nervous system), 522–523, 522*f*

Antacid mixtures, 262

Antacids
nonsystemic, 262
systemic, 262

Antagonist, 197

Antagonist skeletal muscle, 191, 191*f*

Anteflexion position of uterus, 634, 635*f*

Anterior (directional term), 69, 70*f*, 70*t*

Anterior cavity, 69, 594*f*, 597

Anterior nares, 381

Anteversion position of the uterus, 636, 636*f*

Anthracosis, 394, 405

Antianemic agents, 370

Antianxiety drugs, 742

Antiarrhythmic agents, 321

Antibacterials, for urinary tract, 455

Antibiotics
for ear, 582–583
for eyes, 623
for integumentary system, 130

Antibodies, 340, 347, 356
classes of, 347*t*

Anticholinergics, 622

Anticoagulants, 323, 356, 359, 370

Anticonvulsants, 552

Antidepressant agents, 742

Antidiarrheal agents, 263

Antidiuretic, 437

Antidiuretic hormone (ADH), 467*t*, 495

Antidote, 12

Antiemetics, 263

Antifungal agents, 130
for eyes, 623

Antigens, 340, 356

Antihistamines, 130, 414

Antihyperlipidemic agents, 322

Antihypertensive agents, 322

Anti-inflammatory agents, 130, 174, 215

Antimanic agent, 743

Antinuclear antibodies (ANA), 179, 371

Antiparkinsonism drugs, 551

Antiplatelet drugs, 322

Antipruritic agents, 130

Antipsychotic agents, 743

Antipyretics, 12
for ear, 582

Antiresorptive agents, 175

Antiretroviral agents, 370

Antiseptic agents, 13, 13*f*, 130
urinary tract, 455

Antistreptolysin O (ASO titer), 415

Antithyroid hormones, 498

Antituberculosis agents, 415

Antitussives, 13

Antiviral agents, 130, 370
for eyes, 623

Antrum, stomach, 230, 230*f*

Anuria, 437

Anxiety, 727

Anxiety disorders, 727, 727*f*

Aortic (semilunar) valve, 280, 280*f*, 281*f*, 282

Apathy, 13, 727

Apex
definition, 82
lung, 387, 388*f*

Apgar, Virginia, 648–649

Apgar score, 648–649, 649*t*

Aphagia, 527

Aphakia, 602

Aphasia, 528

Apical foramen, 227

Apnea, 394

Apocrine sweat glands, 99

Aponeurosis, 189, 197

Apoptosis, 606

Appendectomy, 239, 239*f*

Appendicitis, 240, 240*f*

Appendicular skeleton, 140

Appendix, 232, 232*f*

Apperception, 728

Appetite, 230

Apraxia, 528
Aqueous humor, 594f, 597
Arachnoid, 513, 513f
Arachnophobia, 735
ARBs (angiotensin-receptor blockers), 322
ARDS (acute respiratory distress syndrome), 394
Areola, 641
Argon laser trabeculoplasty (ALT), 609
AROM (artificial rupture of membranes), 647
Arrector pili muscle, 98
Arrhythmia, 293, 302
Art therapy, 724
Arterial, 293
Arterial blood gases (ABGs), 415
Arteries, 284–285, 284f
    primary functions/description, 275t
Arterioles, 287, 287f
Arteriosclerosis, 294, 300f
Arteritis, 294, 294f
Arthralgia, 156
Arthritis, 156
Arthrocentesis, 157
Arthrodesis, 157
Arthrography, 176
Arthroplasty, 157
Arthropods, 79
Arthroscope, 157
Arthroscopy, 176, 176f
Articulation, 140
Artificial insemination, 698
Artificial insemination heterologous, 698
Artificial insemination homologous, 698
Artificial pacemaker, 295, 295f
Arytenoid cartilage, 384, 385f
Asbestosis, 405
Ascites, 240
ASD (autism spectrum disorder), 728, 728f
Asepsis, 13
Aspartate aminotransferase (AST), 216, 324
Aspergillus niger, 241
Aspermia, 698
Asphyxia, 394
Aspiration, 394
Assessment
    in SBAR technique, 28
    in SOAP chart note, 27
Assistive exercise, 200
Associative neurons, 512

AST (aspartate aminotransferase), 216, 324
Asthenia, 528
Asthma, 395–396, 395f–396f
Astigmatism, 599, 602
Astrocytoma, 528
Asymmetrical, 52
Ataxia, 197, 528
ATC (Anatomical Therapeutic Chemical Classification System), 87
Atelectasis, 397
Atheroma, 295
Atherosclerosis, 294, 295, 300, 300f, 301f, 546
Atherosclerotic heart disease (ASHD), 294
Atoms, 60
Atonic, 197
Atria, 278–280, 279f, 280f
Atrial fibrillation (AF, AFib), 303
Atrioventricular bundle, 282, 283f
Atrioventricular node (AV node), 282, 283f
Atrophy, 197
    of digestive tract mucosal lining, 225
Attention-deficit/hyperactivity disorder (ADHD), 728
Attic (epitympanic recess), 564
Atypical antipsychotics, 743
Atypical muscle fibers, 282
Audiogram, 571
Audiologist, 572
Audiology, 572
Audiometer, 572
Auditory, 572
Auditory-evoked response, 583
Aural, 572
Auricle (pinna), 563t, 564, 564t, 572
Auscultation, 285, 296, 296f
Autism spectrum disorder (ASD), 728, 728f
Autograft, 105
Autoimmune disease, 356
Automated external defibrillator (AED), 296
Autonomic nervous system (ANS), 522–523, 522f
Autotransfusion, 356
AV node (atrioventricular node), 282, 283f
Avulsion, 105
Avulsion fracture, 150f
Axial skeleton, 140
Axillary (ax), 13

Axons, 511, 511f
Azoospermia, 698

B

B lymphocytes (B cells), 346, 347–348, 347t
Baby teeth, 227
Background, in SBAR technique, 28
Bacteria, 78, 78f
Bacteriuria, 437
Balanced suspension traction, 170f
Balanitis, 698
Balloon angioplasty, 310f
Barbiturates, 551
Barrett esophagus, 248
Bartholinitis, 654
Basal cell carcinoma (BCC), 105, 105f
Base, 82
Base, lung, 387, 388f
Basilar membrane, 566
Basophils, 337t, 338f, 339
BCC (basal cell carcinoma), 105, 105f
Bedsore, 109
Bell palsy, 529, 529f
Benign, 19
Benign prostatic hyperplasia (BPH), 431, 690, 698–699, 699f
    drugs used to treat, 711
Benzodiazepines, 742
Bestiality, 737
Beta blockers, 622
Beta cells, 472, 472f
Biceps, 197
Biceps band, 191
Bicuspid, 296
    teeth, 227, 228f
    (mitral) valve, 280, 280f, 281, 281f
Bifocal, 602
Bilateral, 52, 82
Bilateral salpingo-oophorectomy (BSO), 657
Bilateral seizures, 534
Bile, 234, 235, 337
Biliary, 240
Bilirubin, 240
Binaural, 572
Binge-eating disorder, 731
Biologics, 175
Biology, 82
Biopsy (Bx), 14, 14f, 132
    muscle, 216
    needle, 216

open, 216
    specimens for Helicobacter pylori, 265
Bipolar disorder, 729
Birth control patch, 672, 672f
Birth control pills, 671
Bite, 106, 160f
Black hairy tongue, 241, 241f
Black lung, 394
Blastocyst, 638, 638f
Blasts, 364
Bleb, 107
Blepharitis, 602
Blepharoplasty, 602
Blepharoptosis, 603
Blind spot, 598
Blood, 336–340, 336t, 337t, 338f–339f
    formed elements, 336–339, 337t, 338f
    functions, 336
    primary functions/description, 275t
Blood alcohol concentration (BAC), 264
Blood and lymphatic system, 335–378
    abbreviations and acronyms, 372–373
    anatomy and physiology, 336–345, 336t
        blood, 336–340, 336t, 337t, 338f–339f
        lymphatic system, 336t, 342–344, 342f–339f
        spleen, 336t, 344
        thymus, 336t, 344–345
        tonsils, 336t, 344, 345f
    diagnostic and laboratory tests, 371–372
    drug highlights, 370
    immune system, 345–348, 346f, 347t
    medical vocabulary, 351–366
        combining forms, 351
        medical word list, 352–366
        word roots, 351
    Practical Application, 377–378
Blood clot, stationary, 316
Blood grouping test, 673
Blood groups, 339–340, 340t, 371, 371f
Blood pressure, 287–288, 288f
    classifications, 288t
    measurement, 287, 288f
    pulse pressure, 288
Blood proteins, 234
Blood transfusion, 339–340, 340t

Blood typing, 371, 371*f*
Blood urea nitrogen (BUN), 455
Blood vessels, 283–288, 284*f*–287*f*
Bloody show, 647
BMD (bone mineral density), 177, 179
BMI (body mass index), 82, 477
Body
  muscle, 189
  stomach, 230, 230*f*
  tongue, 226
Body area terminology, 74*t*
Body mass index (BMI), 82, 477
Body organization. *See* Human body organization
Boil, 106
Bolus, 224, 227, 227*f*
Bone density, aging and, 140
Bone markings, 144, 145*t*
Bone marrow aspiration, 371
Bone marrow transplant, 157
Bone mineral density (BMD), 177, 179
Bones, 140–145, 140*t*, 142*t*, 143*f*–145*f*
  classification of, 142, 142*f*, 142*t*
  formation of, 140
  fractures, 150, 150*f*–151*f*
  growth at epiphyseal plate, 145, 145*f*
  markings of, 144, 145*t*
  osteoporosis, 164, 165*f*
  structure of long, 143, 144*f*
Bordetella pertussis, 92, 404
Borrelia burgdorferi, 106
Botulinum toxin type A (Botox®), 126, 131
Bowel, 241
Bowleg, 160, 160*f*
Bowman capsule, 427
BPH. *See* Benign prostatic hyperplasia
Brachial pulse checkpoint, 285*f*, 285*t*
Brachialgia, 197
Bradycardia, 296, 302
Bradykinesia, 197, 528, 544
Brain, 509*t*, 510*f*, 513–517, 513*f*–514*f*, 514*t*–515*t*, 516*f*
  anatomy, 513–517, 513*f*–514*f*, 516*f*
    brainstem, 514*f*, 515*t*, 517
    cerebellum, 514*f*, 514*t*, 516, 516*f*
    cerebrum, 513, 514*f*, 514*t*, 515, 516*f*
    diencephalon, 514*f*, 514*t*–515*t*, 516–517

epithalamus, 514*f*, 514*t*, 516
hypothalamus, 514*f*, 515*t*, 517
lobes, 515, 516*f*
medulla oblongata, 514*f*, 515*t*, 517
meninges, 513, 513*f*
midbrain, 514*f*, 515*t*, 517
pons, 514*f*, 515*t*, 517
thalamus, 514*f*, 514*t*, 517
Brain abscess, 164, 164*f*
Brain attack, 545
Brainstem, 514*f*, 515*t*, 517
Brand name, 88
Braxton Hicks contractions, 647
Breast examination, 673
Breastfeeding, 642
Breasts, 633*t*, 641–642, 641*f*–642*f*
Breathing machine, 410
Broken heart syndrome, 309
Bronchi, 380*t*, 381*f*, 386, 387*f*
Bronchiectasis, 397
Bronchiole, 395*f*
Bronchiolitis, 397
Bronchitis, 397
Bronchodilators, 415
Bronchopneumonia, 405*f*
Bronchoscope, 397, 397*f*
Bronchoscopy, 416, 416*f*
Brown recluse spider bite, 160*f*
Bruit, 296
BSO (bilateral salpingo-oophorectomy), 657
Buccal, 241
Bulbourethral (Cowper) glands, 686*t*, 687*f*, 690–691, 691*f*
Bulimia nervosa, 731
Bulla, 107, 107*f*
BUN (blood urea nitrogen), 455
Bundle of His, 282, 283*f*
Burn, 107, 107*f*
  depth of injury, 107*f*
Bursa, 157
Bursitis, 157

C

CABG (coronary artery bypass graft), 299, 299*f*
Cachexia, 14
Caculi, 444, 444*f*
CAD (coronary artery disease), 292, 300, 300*f*, 307
Calcaneal, 157
Calcitonin, 468*t*
Calcium, total, 500
Calcium blood test, 157, 179, 216

Calciuria, 437
Calculus, 437, 437*f*
Cancellous bone, 143, 144*f*
Candida albicans, 108, 241
Candidiasis, 108, 108*f*
Canine teeth, 227, 228*f*
Canthus, 594
Capillaries, 287, 287*f*
  lymphatic, 342, 342*f*
  primary functions/description, 275*t*
Carbon dioxide (CO₂), 397
Carbonic anhydrase inhibitors, 454, 622
Carbuncle, 108, 108*f*
Carcinoembryonic antigen (CEA), 264
Carcinoma, 105, 105*f*
Cardiac, 296
Cardiac ablation, 293
Cardiac arrest, 296
Cardiac catheterization (heart cath), 324, 324*f*
Cardiac depression, 387
Cardiac enzymes, 324
Cardiac muscle, 67, 187*t*, 188*f*, 192
Cardiac sphincter, 229
Cardiac troponin, 30, 324
Cardiologist, 296
Cardiology, 6, 296
Cardiomegaly, 297
Cardiometabolic syndrome (CMS), 297
Cardiomyopathy (CMP), 297, 297*f*
Cardiopulmonary bypass, 299
Cardiotonic, 298
Cardiovascular, 298
Cardiovascular system, 274–334
  abbreviations and acronyms, 327–328
  anatomy and physiology, 275–288, 275*t*, 276*f*
    blood pressure, 287–288, 288*f*
    blood vessels, 283–288, 284*f*–287*f*
    circulation of blood through the chambers of the heart, 278–281, 280*f*
    conduction system of the heart, 282–283, 283*f*
    heart, 275*t*, 276–283, 277*f*–283*f*
    heart valves, 280*f*, 281–282, 281*f*
    vascular system of the heart, 282, 282*f*

diagnostic and laboratory tests, 323–327
drug highlights, 321–323
medical vocabulary, 291–317
  combining forms, 291
  medical word list, 292–317
  word roots, 291
Practical Application, 333–334
Cardioversion, 298
Cardioverter, 302, 302*f*
Cardiopulmonary, 298
Carotid pulse checkpoint, 285*f*, 285*t*
Carpal, 157
Carpal tunnel syndrome, 158, 158*f*
Cartilage, 140, 140*t*
Cartilages of the larynx, 384–385, 385*f*
Cartilaginous joint, 146
Cast, 158, 158*f*
Castrate, 700
CAT scan, 324
Catabolism, 234, 241
Cataract, 603, 603*f*
Catecholamines test, 499
Catheter, 438, 438*f*
Catheterization, urinary, 432
Cauda equina, 518, 521*f*
Caudal (directional term), 70*f*, 71*t*
Causalgia, 108
Cavities, 68, 69, 71*f*, 72
CBC (complete blood count), 371, 674
CBT (cognitive-behavioral therapy), 723
CD4 cell count, 371
CD4 cells, 364
CEA (carcinoembryonic antigen), 264
Cecum, 232, 232*f*
Celiac, 241
Celiac disease, 241
Cell membrane, 62, 63*t*, 64
Cell-mediated immunity, 345, 347–348
Cells, 60, 62, 62*f*, 63*f*, 63*t*, 64–65. *See also specific cell types*
  components, 62, 63*f*, 63*t*, 64
  stem, 65, 364
Cellulitis, 108, 108*f*
Cementum, 228, 229*f*
Center, 82
Centigrade (C), 4, 14
Centimeter (cm), 4, 14
Central adiposity, 297
Central apnea, 394

Central nervous system (CNS), 509, 509t, 510f, 512–519, 513f–514f, 514t–515t, 516f, 518f
Central neurons, 512
Centrioles, 63f, 63t
Cephalagia, 528
Cephalic (directional term), 71t
Cephalosporins, 583
Cerebellar, 528
Cerebellum, 514f, 514t, 516, 516f
Cerebral angiography, 554
Cerebral cortex, 514f, 515
Cerebral palsy (CP), 528, 529f
Cerebrospinal, 530
Cerebrospinal fluid (CSF), 519
Cerebrospinal fluid (CSF) analysis, 554
Cerebrovascular accident (CVA), 545, 546f
Cerebrum, 513, 514f, 514t, 515, 516f
Cerumen, 564
Cervical curve, 148, 148f
Cervical spinal nerves, 519, 521f
Cervical vertebrae, 148, 148f
Cervicitis, 654
Cesarean section (CS, C-section), 654, 654f
CF (cystic fibrosis), 132, 399, 399f
Chalazion(s), 595, 603
Chalicosis, 405
Chambers of the heart, 278–281, 280f
Cheiloplasty, 382
Cheilosis, 242
Chemical elements, 60
Chemical name, 88
Chemical peels, 126
Chemotherapy, 3, 14
Cheyne–Stokes respiration, 398
CHF (congestive heart failure), 304
Chickenpox, 125, 125f
Chief complaint, 27
Childbirth, 646
Children. See also Newborns
    acromegaly, 482
    bone growth, 145
    breastfeeding, 642
    cerebral palsy (CP), 528, 529f
    cochlear implant, 566, 566f
    congenital heart defects, 281
    depression, 731
    diabetes mellitus (DM), 472
    earlobes, 565
    with high cholesterol, 298
    HIV infection, 353

male reproductive system, 689
mental disorder symptoms, 722
obesity, 472
otitis media in, 576, 576f
pulse, blood pressure, and respirations, 287
scoliosis, 168, 168f
sex determination, 638
spinal curves, 149, 149f
urinary system, 429
urinary tract infections (UTIs), 431
visual acuity, 596
Chlamydia, 692t
Cholangiography, 264
Cholecystectomy, 242
Cholecystitis, 242
Cholecystography, 264
Cholecystokinin, 469t, 476
Choledochotomy, 242
Cholelithiasis, 242, 242f
Cholesteatoma, 572
Cholesterol (chol), 298, 324
Cholinergics, 622
Cholinesterase, 622
Cholinesterase inhibitors, 552
Chondral, 159
Chondrocostal, 159
Chondrocytes, 145
Chorea, 530
Chorionic gonadotropin hormone, 476
Chorionic villus sampling (CVS), 673
Choroid, 593t, 594f, 597
Choroid plexuses, 519
Choroiditis, 603
Chromosomes, 64, 64f, 82
Chronic, 14
Chronic kidney disease (CKD), 438
    glomerular filtration rate (GFR) classification of, 456
Chronic lymphocytic leukemia (CLL), 361
Chronic myeloid leukemia (CML), 361
Chronic obstructive pulmonary disease (COPD), 400
Chronic traumatic encephalopathy (CTE), 530
Chyme, 230, 231
Cicatrix, 109
Cilia, 63t
    nasal smell receptor cells, 382
    tracheal, 386, 387
Ciliary body, 593t, 594f, 597

Circadian rhythm disorders, 545
Circadian rhythms, 545
Circulation
    of blood through the chambers of the heart, 278–281, 280f
    definition, 298
    fetal, 337
Circulatory system, 275
Circumcision, 689, 700, 700f
Circumduction, 147f
Cirrhosis, 243, 243f
CK (creatine kinase), 216, 324
CKD. See Chronic kidney disease (CKD)
Claudication, 298
    intermittent, 311
Claustrophobia, 735
Clavicular, 159
Cleft palate, 382
CLI (critical limb ischemia), 311
Clinical résumé, 26
Clinical summary, 26
Clitoris, 640, 640f
CLL (chronic lymphocytic leukemia), 361
Closed (simple) fracture, 150f
Clotting, 338–339, 339f
Clotting factors, 338, 339f
CML (chronic myeloid leukemia), 361
CMP (cardiomyopathy), 297, 297f
CMP (comprehensive metabolic panel), 264
CMS (cardiometabolic syndrome), 297
CNS. See Central nervous system (CNS)
Coagulable, 356
Coagulation, 338–339, 339f
Coagulation factors. See Clotting factors
Coccygeal, 159
Coccygeal spinal nerves, 519, 521f
Coccygodynia, 159
Coccyx, 148, 148f
Cochlea, 563t, 564t, 565–566, 573
Cochlear duct, 566
Cochlear implant, 566, 566f
COCs (combined oral contraceptives), 671, 671f
Cognitive-behavioral therapy (CBT), 723
Coitus, 700
Cold

cryotherapy, 202
    sensation of, 97
Cold sore, 112
Colectomy, 243
Colitis, 257
Collagen, 159
Collapsed lung, 397
Colon, 232, 232f
Colon cancer, 243, 243f
Colonoscope, 244, 244f
Colonoscopy, 244, 244f, 264, 264f
Color blindness, 623, 623f
Color vision tests, 623, 623f
Colostomy, 245, 245f
Colostrum, 642
Colposcope, 654
Colposcopy, 674
Coma, 530
Comatose, 52
Combined hyperactive-impulsive and inattentive ADHD, 728
Combined oral contraceptives (COCs), 671, 671f
Combining forms, 2
    blood and lymphatic system, 351
    cardiovascular system, 291
    definition, 3
    digestive system, 238
    of directional and positional terms, 70t–71t
    ear, 571
    endocrine system, 481
    eye, 601
    female reproductive system, 652
    human body organization, 81
    integumentary system, 102
    male reproductive system, 697
    medical terminology, 11
    muscular system, 195
    nervous system, 526
    respiratory system, 393
    skeletal system, 155
    suffixes and prefixes, 51
    urinary system, 436
Comedo, 109
Comminuted fracture, 150f
Communication, tools for effective, 28
Community immunity, 346
Compact bone, 143, 144f
Complement system, 347t
Complete (spontaneous abortion type), 653
Complete blood count (CBC), 371, 674

Complete fracture, 150f
Component parts, principles of, 4–5
Comprehensive metabolic panel (CMP), 264
Compression, 202
Compression fracture, 151f
Compulsion, 729, 734
Computed tomography (CT), 176, 176f, 324
  of kidneys, ureters, bladder (CT KUB), 455
  nervous system, 554
Computer vision syndrome (CVS), 614
Concave border, kidney, 427
Conception, 637
Concussion, 530
Condom, 700
Conduction system of the heart, 282–283, 283f
Condyle (bone marking), 145
Condyloma, 701, 701f
Cones, 593, 597
Congenital heart defects, 281
Congenital hypothyroidism, 483
Congenital rubella syndrome, 677
Congestive heart failure (CHF), 304
Conjunctiva, 593t, 594f, 595
Conjunctivitis, 604, 604f
Connective, 159
Connective tissue, 66f, 67
Consent form, 25
Constipation, 245
Constriction, 299
Consultation reports, 25
Contraception, 655
Contraceptives, 671–672
Contractility, of skeletal muscle, 188
Contraction, 197
Contracture, 198, 198f, 203
Conus medullaris, 518
Convex border, kidney, 427
Convolution, 515
COPD (chronic obstructive pulmonary disease), 400
Copulation, 689, 700
Cordocentesis, 674
Corium, 98
Corn, 109
Cornea, 593t, 594f, 597
Corneal, 604
Corneal graft, 605
Corneal reshaping, 611
Corneal transplant, 605

Corniculate cartilage, 384, 385f
Coronal plane, 69, 69f
Coronary arteries, 282, 282f
Coronary artery bypass graft (CABG), 299, 299f
Coronary artery disease (CAD), 292, 300, 300f, 307
Coronary heart disease, 307
Corpora cavernosa penis, 689
Corpora quadrigemina, 517
Corpus, uterus, 634
Corpus callosum, 512, 515
Corpus luteum, 639
Corpus spongiosum, 689
Corpuscle, 356
Cortex
  adrenal, 473, 474–475, 474f
  cerebral, 514f, 515
  ovary, 639
  renal, 427, 428f
Corticosteroids, 174
Corticosterone, 468t, 474
Corticotropin test, 499
Corticotropin-releasing factor (CRF), 467
Corticotropin-releasing factor (CRF) test, 499
Cortisol, 468t, 474
Cortisone, 484
Coryza, 407
Costosternal, 159
Cough, 398
Cowper glands, 686t, 690–691.
  See also Bulbourethral (Cowper) glands
COX (cyclooxygenase), 175
COX-2 inhibitors, 175
CP (cerebral palsy), 528, 529f
Cranial (directional term), 70f
Cranial cavity, 71f, 72
Cranial nerves, 509t, 519, 520f, 521t
Cranial suture, 146
Craniectomy, 159, 530
Craniotomy, 159, 531, 531f
Craving, 230
C-reactive protein (CRP), 179
Creatine kinase (CK), 216, 324
Creatine kinase isoenzymes, 324
Creatinemia, 356
Creatinine clearance, 456
Crest (bone marking), 145
Cretinism, 483
CRF. See Corticotropin-releasing factor (CRF)
Cricoid cartilage, 384, 385, 385f
Critical limb ischemia (CLI), 311
Crohn disease, 246, 246f, 252

Croup, 398, 398f
Crown, tooth, 227, 229f
CRP (C-reactive protein), 179
Cryoabaltion, 293
Cryosurgery, 109, 605
Cryotherapy, 202
Cryptolipolysis, 117
Cryptorchidism, 689, 701, 701f
CSF (cerebrospinal fluid), 519
CT. See Computed tomography (CT)
CTE (chronic traumatic encephalopathy), 530
Culdocentesis, 655
Culdoscopy, 674
Culture
  sputum, 416
  stool, 266
  throat, 416
  urine, 456
Cuneiform cartilage, 384, 385f
Curative use, of drugs, 88
Cushing disease, 474, 484, 484f
Cuspid teeth, 227, 228f
Cutaneous, 109
Cuticle, 99, 99f
CVA (cerebrovascular accident), 545, 546f
CVS (chorionic villus sampling), 673
CVS (computer vision syndrome), 614
Cyanosis, 301, 398
Cyclooxygenase (COX), 175
Cycloplegia, 605
Cyclothymic disorder, 729
Cyst, 109, 439
Cystectomy, 438
Cystic fibrosis (CF), 132, 399, 399f
Cystitis, 438
  interstitial, 438, 443
Cysto. See Cystoscopy
Cystocele, 439, 655
Cystogram, 439
Cystolith, 439
Cystoscope, 439
Cystoscopy, 456
Cytology, 82
Cytoplasm, 63f, 63t, 64

D

Dacryoma, 605
Dactylic, 159
Dactylogram, 159
Dactylospasm, 198
DALK (deep anterior lamellar keratoplasty), 605

Dark chocolate, mood boost from, 721
DBS (deep brain stimulation), 531
D&C (dilation and curettage), 667
DEA (Drug Enforcement Administration), 87
Deafness, 572–573, 572f
Debridement, 109
Deciduous (primary) teeth, 227, 228f
Decongestants, 414
Decubitus ulcer, 109
Deep (directional term), 70f
Deep anterior lamellar keratoplasty (DALK), 605
Deep brain stimulation (DBS), 531
Deep vein thrombosis (DVT), 365, 365f
Defecation, 232
Defense mechanisms, 346f
Defibrillator, 302, 302f
Dehiscence, 109, 109f
Dehydrate, 83
Delayed sleep-phase syndrome (DSPS), 545
Delirium, 729
Delivery, 646, 647–648
Delta cells, 472
Delusion, 729
Delusional (paranoid) disorder, 735
Dementia, 532, 729
Dendrites, 511, 511f
Dentalgia, 246
Dentin, 228, 229f
Dentition, 246
Deoxyribonucleic acid (DNA), 64, 64f
Depersonalization disorder, 731
Depo-Provera, 672
Depression, 730–731, 730f, 738, 738f
Depression fracture, 151f
Dermabrasion, 109
Dermal fillers, 126
Dermatitis, 110, 110f
Dermatologist, 110
Dermatology, 110
Dermatome, 110
Dermatomycosis, 111
Dermatomyositis, 199, 199f
Dermatopolymyositis, 199
Dermis, 95t, 96f, 97f, 98
Dermomycosis, 111
Descending colon, 232, 232f

Detrusor muscle, 430
DI (diabetes insipidus), 439, 495
Diabetes, 484–485
    as erectile dysfunction cause, 702
Diabetes insipidus (DI), 439, 495
Diabetes mellitus (DM), 439, 472, 485
    multisystem effects of, 473f
    type 1, 472
    type 2, 472
Diabetic ketoacidosis, 473
Diabetic retinopathy, 616, 616f
Diacritics, 88
Diagnosis (Dx), 14
Diagnostic and laboratory tests
    blood and lymphatic system, 371–372
    cardiovascular system, 323–327
    digestive system, 264–266
    ear, 583–585
    endocrine system, 499–500
    eye, 623–625
    female reproductive system, 673–678
    integumentary system, 131–132
    male reproductive system, 712
    muscular system, 216
    nervous system, 554–555
    respiratory system, 415–417
    skeletal system, 176–179
    urinary system, 455–457
Diagnostic procedures, suffixes for, 40, 40t–41t
Diagnostic tests/laboratory reports, 25
Diagnostic use, of drugs, 88
Dialysis, 439
    hemodialysis, 439, 442, 442f
    peritoneal, 439, 447, 447f
Diaphoresis, 15
Diaphragm, 199, 199f, 387
Diaphysis, 143, 144f, 145
Diarrhea, 246
Diarthrosis, 146
Diastole, 302
Diastolic blood pressure, 287, 288t
Diastolic failure, 304
Diathermy, 200
Dichoptic therapy, 602
DID (dissociative identity disorder), 731
Diencephalon, 514f, 514t–515t, 516–517
Differential diagnosis, 27

Diffusion
    defined, 83
    function of epithelial tissue, 67
Digestion, 224
    beginning of, 227
    in small intestine, 231
    in stomach, 230
    waste product of, 232
Digestive system, 223–273
    abbreviations and acronyms, 266–267
    accessory organs, 233–235
    aging and, 225
    anatomy and physiology, 224–225, 224t, 225f
        esophagus, 224t, 225f, 227f, 229
        gall bladder, 224t, 225f, 234f, 235
        large intestine, 224t, 225f, 232, 232f
        liver, 224t, 225f, 233–234, 234f
        mouth, 224t, 225f, 226–227, 226f, 227f
        pancreas, 224t, 225f, 234f, 235
        pharynx, 224t, 225f, 226f, 229
        salivary glands, 224t, 225f, 227, 233, 233f
        small intestine, 224t, 225f, 231, 231f
        stomach, 224t, 225f, 230, 230f
        teeth, 224t, 227–229, 228f, 229f
    diagnostic and laboratory tests, 264–266
    drug highlights, 262–263
    functions of, 224
    medical vocabulary, 238–258
        combining forms, 238
        medical word list, 239–258
        word roots, 239
    of newborns, 234
    Practical Applications, 271–272
Digital rectal exam (DRE), 699, 705, 705f
Digitalis drugs, 321
Dilation and curettage (D&C), 667
Dilation stage of labor, 647, 648f
Diminutive suffixes, 38t
Diplopia, 605
Directional terms, 69, 70f, 70t–71t
Discharge abstract, 26
Discharge summary, 26

Disease, 15
    infectious, 78–79
    pathogenic organisms that cause, 78, 78f
    terms associated with causative agents, 79–80
Disease-modifying antirheumatic drugs (DMARDs), 175
Disinfectant, 15, 15f
Diskectomy, 532
Dislocation, 159
Displaced fracture, 150f
Dissection, 82
Dissociation, 731
Dissociative disorder, 731
Dissociative identity disorder (DID), 731
Distal (directional term), 70f, 71t
Diuresis, 439
Diuretics, 454
Diverticulitis, 247, 247f
DM. See Diabetes mellitus
DMARDs (disease-modifying antirheumatic drugs), 175
DNA (deoxyribonucleic acid), 64, 64f
DOB (date of birth), 8
Documentation, methods of, 26–28
Dopamine, 468t, 475, 544
Doppler ultrasound, 655, 655f
Dorsal (directional term), 69, 70f
Dorsal cavity, 69, 72
Dorsal pedis pulse checkpoint, 285f, 285t
Dorsal rami, 519
Dorsal recumbent patient position, 206t
Dorsal root, 518f, 519
Dorsiflexion, 147f
Dosage, 89
DRE (digital rectal exam), 699, 705, 705f
Dream sleep, 544
Drug(s). See also Drug Highlights
    defined, 87
    interactions, 88
    medical uses for, 88
    medication order and dosage, 89
    names, 88
    undesirable actions of, 88
Drug Enforcement Administration (DEA), 87
Drug Highlights
    blood and lymphatic system, 370
    cardiovascular system, 321–323

    digestive system, 262–263
    ear, 582–583
    endocrine system, 498–499
    eye, 622–623
    female reproductive system, 671–672
    human body organization, 87–89
    integumentary system, 130–131
    male reproductive system, 711
    mental health, 742–743
    muscular system, 215
    nervous system, 551–553
    respiratory system, 414–415
    skeletal system, 174–175
    urinary system, 454–455
Drug therapy for mental disorders, 723
DSPS (delayed sleep-phase syndrome), 545
DTaP vaccine, 53, 92, 404
Dual-energy x-ray absorptiometry (DXA) scan, 177
Duchenne muscular dystrophy, 200, 203
Ductus deferens, 689
Duncan mechanism of placental expulsion, 648
Duodenal, 247
Duodenum, 231, 231f
Dupuytren contracture, 198, 198f
Dura mater, 513, 513f
Duration, in AIDET communication, 28
DVT (deep vein thrombosis), 365, 365f
Dwarfism, 486, 486f
DXA (dual-energy x-ray absorptiometry) scan, 177
Dysentery, 247
Dysesthesia, 485
Dyslexia, 532
Dyslipidemia, 297
Dysmenorrhea, 655
Dyspareunia, 655
Dyspepsia, 247
Dysphagia, 247
Dysphasia, 533
Dysphonia, 399
Dyspnea, 45, 399
Dysrhythmia, 293, 302
Dysthymia, 730
Dystonia, 200

Dystrophin, 200
Dystrophy, 200
Dysuria, 439

E

Ear, 562–591
    abbreviations and acronyms,
        586
    anatomy and physiology,
        563–568, 563t, 564f
        external ear, 563t, 564,
            564f, 567f
        inner ear, 563t, 564f,
            565–568, 566f–567f
        middle ear, 563t, 564–565,
            564f, 565f, 567f
    diagnosis and laboratory tests,
        583–585
    drug highlights, 582–583
    hearing, process of, 567
    medical vocabulary, 571–579
        combining forms, 571
        medical word list, 572–579
        word roots, 571
    Practical Application, 591
Ear stones, 568, 577
Earlobes, 565
Earwax, 564
Eating disorders, 731
ECC (extracorporeal circulation),
    303
Ecchymosis, 111, 111f
Eccrine sweat glands, 99
ECG (electrocardiogram), 283,
    325, 325f
Echocardiography (ECHO), 325
Echoencephalography, 554
Eclampsia, 655
ECT (electroconvulsive therapy),
    725
Ectomorph, 83
Ectopic pregnancy, 656, 656f
Eczema, 111
ED. See Erectile dysfunction
Edema, 439
EEG (electroencephalography),
    554
EF (ejection fraction), 304
Efferent, 15
Efferent nerves, 512
Efferent processes, 510
EGD (esophagogastroduode-
    noscopy), 265
Egocentric, 732
EHR (electronic health record),
    24–26, 60
EHT (estrogen hormone
    therapy), 175

Ejaculation, 701
Ejaculatory duct, 690, 691f
Ejection fraction (EF), 304
EKG (electrocardiogram), 283,
    325, 325f
Elasticity, of skeletal muscle, 188
Electrocardiogram (ECG, EKG),
    283, 325, 325f
Electrocochleography, 573
Electroconvulsive therapy (ECT),
    725
Electroencephalography (EEG),
    554
Electromyography (EMG), 216,
    533
Electronic health record (EHR),
    24–26, 60
Electronystagmography, 583
Electrophysiology study (EPS)
    (intracardiac), 326
Electroretinogram, 605
Element, 60
Elevation, 202
Elimination, 224
ELISA (enzyme-linked
    immunosorbent assay), 371
Embolism, 302, 546, 546f
Embolus, 356
Embryo, 637–638
    blood development, 337
    sex differentiaton, 638
Embryonic stage, 644–645, 645f
Emesis, 247
Emetics, 263
EMG (electromyography), 216
Emmetropia (EM), 605
Emollients, 130
Empathy, 15
Emphysema, 400, 400f
Empyema, 400
Enamel, 228, 229f
Encephalitis, 533
Encephalopathy, 533
Endarterectomy, 302
Endaural, 573
Endemic goiter, 471, 491
Endocarditis, 302, 303f
Endocardium, 276, 279f, 282
Endochondral ossification, 140
Endocrine glands, 465t, 466f,
    467t–469t
    adrenal glands, 465t, 466f,
        468t, 474–475, 474f
    gastrointestinal mucosa, 469t,
        476
    ovaries, 465t, 466f, 468t, 475
    pancreas, 465t, 466f, 468t,
        472–473, 472f

parathyroid gland, 465t, 466f,
    468t, 471, 471f
pineal gland, 465t, 466f, 467t,
    469
pituitary gland (hypophysis),
    465t, 466f, 467t, 469, 470f
placenta, 476
testes, 465t, 466f, 468t, 476
thymus, 466f, 469t, 476, 476f
thyroid gland, 465t, 466f,
    467t–468t, 470, 471f
Endocrine system, 464–507
    abbreviations and acronyms,
        501
    anatomy and physiology, 465,
        465t, 466f
    diagnostic and laboratory
        tests, 499–500
    drug highlights, 498–499
    endocrine glands, 465t, 466f,
        467t–469t
    hormonal functions of,
        466–477, 467t–469t
    leptin and ghrelin hormones,
        477
    medical vocabulary, 481–495
        combining forms, 481
        medical word list, 482–495
        word roots, 481
    Practical Application, 506
Endocrinologist, 486
Endocrinology, 487
Endolymph, 565, 573
Endometrial ablation, 658
Endometriosis, 4, 656
Endometrium, 635f, 636
Endomorph, 83
Endoplasmic reticulum (ER), 63f,
    63t
Endorphins, 533
Endoscopic retrograde
    cholangiopancreatography
    (ERCP), 264
Endosteum, 143, 144f
Endothelial keratoplasty, 605
Endotracheal (ET), 400
Energy spurt (sign of impending
    labor), 647
ENT (ear, nose, throat), 577
Enteric, 247
Enteritis, 247
Enterogastrone, 469t, 476
Entropion, 605
Enucleation, 605
Enuresis, 439
Enzyme, 248
Enzyme-linked immunosorbent
    assay (ELISA), 371

Enzymes, digestive, 235
Eosinophils, 337t, 338f, 339
Epidemic, 15
Epidermis, 95t, 97f, 98
Epididymis, 686, 686t, 687f,
    688f, 689
Epididymitis, 701
Epidural, 533
Epiduroscopy, 533
Epigastric, 248
Epigastric region, 72, 73f
Epigastrium, 230
Epiglottis, 226f, 229, 384, 385,
    385f
Epilepsy, 534, 534f
Epinephrine, 467, 468t, 475,
    487
Epiphyseal plate, 143, 145, 145f
Epiphysis, 143, 144f, 145
Episiotomy, 641, 647
Epispadias, 689, 702, 702f
Epistaxis, 400
Epithalamus, 514f, 514t, 516
Epithelial tissue, 65–67, 66f
Epoetin alfa (EPO, Procrit), 370
Eponychium, 99, 99f
Eponym, 8
EPS (electrophysiology study)
    (intracardiac), 326
Equilibrium, 567, 573
ER (endoplasmic reticulum), 63f,
    63t
ERCP (endoscopic retrograde
    cholangiopancreatography),
    264
Erectile dysfunction (ED), 702
    drugs used to treat, 711
Erosion, 122f
Erosive esophagitis, 248
ERV (expiratory reserve volume),
    390, 417
Erythema, 111
Erythema infectiosum, 111,
    111f
Erythema migrans, 106
Erythroblast, 357
Erythrocyte, 357
Erythrocyte sedimentation rate
    (ESR, sed rate), 132, 371
Erythrocytes (red blood cells,
    RBCs), 337, 337t, 338f
    sickling, 355
Erythrocytosis, 357
Erythroderma, 112
Erythromycins, 583
Erythropoiesis, 357
Erythropoietin (EPO), 357, 427
Eschar, 112

Esophageal, 248
Esophagitis, erosive, 248
Esophagogastroduodenoscopy (EGD), 265
Esophagus, 224t, 225f, 227f, 229
  Barrett, 248
  primary functions/description, 224t
Esotropia (ET), 606
ESR (erythrocyte sedimentation rate), 132
Estradiol, 468t, 475
Estriol, 468t, 475
Estrogen hormone therapy (EHT), 175
Estrogen test, 674
Estrogens, 468t, 475–476, 487, 640, 671
Estrone, 468t, 475
ESWL (extracorporeal shock wave lithotripsy), 440, 440f, 445
Ethmoidal sinus, 382, 383f
Etiology, 16
Eupnea, 400
Eustachian tube, 546f, 565
Euthyroid, 487
Evaporation, 96
Eversion, 147f
Excision, 3, 16
Excitability, of skeletal muscle, 188
Excoriation, 112
Excretion, function of epithelial tissue, 67
Excretory, 440
Excretory duct, 689
Excretory system, 425
Exercise, 200
Exercise stress test, 327
Exercise test, 327
Exhalation, 389f, 400
Exhibitionism, 737
Exocrine, 487
Exophthalmic, 487
Exophthalmometry, 624
Expectorants, 415
Expectoration, 400
Expiratory reserve volume (ERV), 390, 417
Explanation, in AIDET communication, 28
Expulsion stage of labor, 647, 648f
Extensibility, of skeletal muscle, 188
Extension, 147f
External acoustic meatus (auditory canal), 563t, 564, 564t

External ear, 563t, 564, 564f, 567f
External organs, 686–689
External respiration, 380
External structures, 594–596, 594f–596f
Extracorporeal circulation (ECC), 303
Extracorporeal shock wave lithotripsy (ESWL), 440, 440f, 445
Extravasation, 357
Extropia (XT), 606
Exudate, 112
Exudative retinal detachment, 615
Eye, 592–631
  abbreviations and acronyms, 625
  anatomy and physiology, 593–599, 593t, 594f
    choroid, 593t, 594f, 597
    ciliary body, 593t, 594f, 597
    conjunctiva, 593t, 594f, 595
    cornea, 593t, 594f, 597
    external structures, 594–596, 594f–596f
    eyeball, 593t, 594, 594f, 597–598
    eyelids, 593t, 594–595, 594f
    internal structures, 594f, 597–598, 598f
    iris, 593t, 594f, 597
    lacrimal apparatus, 593t, 595–596, 596f
    lens, 593t, 594f, 598
    muscles of the eye, 593t, 594, 595f
    orbit, 593t, 594
    retina, 593t, 594f, 597, 598t
    sclera, 593t, 594f, 597
  development of, 596
  diagnostic and laboratory tests, 623–625
  drug highlights, 622–623
  how sight occurs, 598–599, 598f–599f
  medical vocabulary, 601–618
    combining forms, 601
    medical word list, 602–618
    word roots, 601
  meibomian gland dysfunction (MGD), 595
  Practical Application, 630
  visual acuity, 596
Eyeball, 593t, 594, 594f, 597–598

Eyelashes, 595
Eyelids, 593t, 594–595, 594f

F

Facial nerve, 520f, 521t, 529
Factitious disorder, 732
Fallopian canal, 529
Fallopian tubes, 633t, 634f–635f, 636–637
  anatomical features of, 637
False vocal cords, 384
Family therapy, 723
Farsightedness, 599, 608, 608f, 614
Fascia, 187, 187f, 200
Fasciitis, 200
FAST test, 546
Fasting blood glucose (FBG), 499
Fasting blood sugar (FBS), 499
Fatigue, 201
Fatty fish, mood boost from, 721
Faucial tonsils, 383
Febrile, 16
Feces, 248
Female hormones, 671
Female pelvis, 149f, 150
Female reproductive system, 632–684. See also Obstetrics
  abbreviation and acronyms, 678
  anatomy and physiology, 633–644, 633t, 634f–635f
    breasts, 633t, 641–642, 641f–642f
    fallopian tubes, 633t, 634f–635f, 636–637
    fertilization, 637–638, 637f–638f
    hormone production, 640
    menstrual cycle, 643–644, 643f
    ovaries, 633t, 634f–635f, 638f–639f, 639–640
    uterus, 633t, 634f–636f, 636, 638f
    vagina, 633t, 634f–635f
    vulva, 633t, 640, 640f
  diagnostic and laboratory tests, 673–678
  drug highlights, 671–672
  functions of, 633
  medical vocabulary, 652–667
    combining forms, 652
    medical word list, 652–667
    word roots, 652
  Practical Application, 682–683

Femoral, 160
Femoral pulse checkpoint, 285f, 285t
Fenestration, 573
Fertilization, 637–638, 637f–638f
Fetal heartbeat (FHB), 655, 655f
Fetal stage, 644–645, 645f
Fetishism, 737
Fetus, 645
  at 20 weeks, 645f
  blood development, 337
  bone development, 140
  earlobes, 565
  external genitals, 638
  eye development, 596
  lungs, 388
  microcephaly, 540
  nervous system, 513
  position in full-term pregnancy, 646f
  ultrasonography of, 638, 638f
  ultrasound, 677, 677f
  urine formation, 429, 431
  vernix caseosa, 97
Fever blister, 112
Fiberoptic colonscopy, 265
Fibers, muscle, 187, 187f, 192
Fibrillation, 303
Fibrin, 337, 338–339, 339f, 357
Fibrinogen, 234, 337, 338–339, 340, 357
Fibroid tumor, 656, 667, 667f
Fibroma, 656
Fibromyalgia syndrome (FMS), 201, 201f
Fibromyitis, 201
Fibromyositis, 201
Fibrosis, 198
Fibrous joint, 146
Fibular, 160
Fifth disease, 111
Fight-or-flight response, 523
Filtering microsurgery, 609
Filtration, 83, 431, 432f
Filum terminale, 518
Fimbriae, fallopian tube, 635f, 637
Fingernails, 99, 99f
First aid treatment, 202
First milk, 642
Fissure, 122f, 145
FIV (forced inspiratory volume), 417
Fixation, 160
Flaccid, 202
Flagella, 63t
Flatfoot, 160
Flatus, 248
Flea bite, 160f
Flexion, 147f

Flow volume loop (F-V loop), 417
Fluorescent treponemal antibody absorption (FTA-ABS), 712
Flutter, 304
FMS (fibromyalgia syndrome), 201, 201f
Focal seizures, 534
Follicle, hair, 98
Follicle-stimulating hormone (FSH), 467t, 639, 643, 643f
Follicular phase, 643f, 644
Folliculitis, 112, 112f
Foramen (bone marking), 145
Foramina, 594
Forced inspiratory volume (FIV), 417
Foreskin, 689
Formed elements, 336–339, 337t, 338f
Fossa (bone marking), 145
Fovea centralis, 597, 598f
Fowler patient position, 206t
Fractures, 150, 150f–151f
    traction for, 170
Framework of the body, 140
FRC (functional residual capacity), 390, 417
Free edge, nail, 99, 99f
Freely movable joint, 146
Frontal lobe, 515, 516f
Frontal plane, 69, 69f
Frontal sinus, 382, 383f
Frontotemporal dementia (FTD), 532
Frontotemporal lobar degeneration (FTLD), 532
FSH. See Follicle-stimulating hormone (FSH)
FTA-ABS (fluorescent treponemal antibody absorption), 712
FTD (frontotemporal dementia), 532
FTLD (frontotemporal lobar degeneration), 532
Fugue, 732
Functional residual capacity (FRC), 390, 417
Fundus
    stomach, 230, 230f
    uterus, 634
Furuncle, 106

G

GAD (generalized anxiety disorder), 732
Gallbladder, 224t, 225f, 234f, 235
    primary functions/description, 224t
    ultrasonography, 266

Gallstones, 242, 242f
Gamete, 703
Gamma-glutamyltransferase (GGT), 265
Ganglionectomy, 534
Gangrene, 112
Gardasil, 692t
Gastrectomy, 34, 248
Gastric, 34, 248
Gastric acid pump inhibitors, 262
Gastric analysis, 265
Gastrin, 469t, 476
Gastritis, 34
Gastroenteritis, 248
Gastroenterologist, 248
Gastroenterology, 6, 248
Gastroesophageal, 248
Gastroesophageal reflux disease (GERD), 249, 249f
Gastrointestinal mucosa, 469t, 476
Gastrointestinal (GI) series, 265
Gastrointestinal tract, 224
Gastrotomy, 34
Gavage, 249
Gender dysphoria, 737
General anesthetics, 551
Generalized anxiety disorder (GAD), 732
Generalized seizures, 534
Generic name, 88
Genes, 64, 64f, 83
Genital warts, 692t
Genitalia, 656
    of newborn, 647
Genitourinary (GU) system, 425
Genome, 64
Genu valgum, 160, 160f
Genu varum, 160, 160f
GERD (gastroesophageal reflux disease), 249, 249f
German measles, 120
Gestation period, 644
GFR (glomerular filtration rate), 456
GGT (gamma-glutamyltransferase), 265
GH (growth hormone), 467t, 482
Ghrelin, 477
GHRF (growth hormone-releasing factor), 467
Gigantism, 482, 487
Gingivae (gums), 226, 229
Gingival sulcus, 229
Gingivitis, 249
Glandular, 487
Glans penis, 689

Glaucoma, 606–607, 606f
    drugs used to treat, 622
Glioma, 535
Globulin, 340, 357
Glomerular, 441
Glomerular capsule, 427
Glomerular filtration, 429, 431, 432f
Glomerular filtration rate (GFR), 456
Glomerulitis, 441
Glomerulonephritis, 441
Glomerulus, 427–429, 428f–429f
Glossectomy, 249
Glossopharyngeal nerve, 520f, 521t
Glottis, 384
Glucagon, 235, 468t, 472
Glucocorticoids, 174, 474, 487
    inhalational, 415
Glucose tolerance test (GTT), 499
Gluten, 241
Glycogen, 233
Glycogenesis, 249
Glycosuria, 441
GnRH (gonadotropin-releasing hormone), 467
Goiter, 471, 491
    endemic, 471, 491
Golgi apparatus, 63f, 63t
Gomphosis, 228
Gonadotropic hormones, 639
Gonadotropin-releasing hormone (GnRH), 467
Goniometry, 177
Gonioscope, 607
Gonioscopy, 624
Gonorrhea, 692t, 703
Gout, 160
    agents to treat, 175
Gowers maneuver, 204, 204f
Graffian follicle, 639
Gram (g), 16
Grammatical suffixes, 37, 37t–38t
Granulocyte, 357
Graves disease, 470, 487, 488
Gravida, 657
Gray matter, 512–513, 523
Greenstick fracture, 150f
Group B streptococcus (GBS), 657
Group B streptococcus (GBS) screening, 674
Group therapy, 724, 724f
Growing follicle, 639
Growth hormone (GH), 467t, 482
Growth hormone-releasing

factor (GHRF), 467
Growth plate, 143, 145
GTT (glucose tolerance test), 499
Guillain-Barré syndrome, 535
Gynecoid, 52
Gynecoid pelvis, 150
Gynecologist, 657
Gynecology, 657
Gynecomastia, 703
Gyrus, 515

H

HAART (highly active antiretroviral therapy), 370
Hair, 95t, 98
    aging and, 98
    alopecia, 104, 104f
    lanugo, 97
Hair cells, 568
Hair papilla, 98
Halitosis, 249
Hallucination, 732
Hallux, 160
Hammertoe, 161, 161f
Harelip, 382
Hashimoto disease (Hashimoto thyroiditis), 470
Hay fever, 353
Hb A1C test, 499
hCG (human chorionic gonadotropin), 674
Hct (hematocrit), 372, 674
HD (hemodialysis), 439, 442, 442f
HDL (high-density lipoproteins), 308
HDL cholesterol, 326
HDS (herniated disk syndrome), 536, 536f
Head (bone marking), 145
Head-to-toe assessment, 74
Health, definition of, 78, 720
Health Insurance Portability and Accountability Act (HIPAA), 8, 25, 26
Hearing, process of, 567
Hearing impairment, 572, 572f
Hearing loss, 568, 573, 573f
Heart, 72, 275t, 276–283, 277f–283f
    anterior view of external, 277f
    circulation of blood through the chambers of the heart, 278–281, 280f
    conduction system of, 282–283, 283f

congenital defects, 281
location in chest, 278f
posterior view of external, 277f
primary functions/description, 275t
vascular system of, 282, 282f
Heart attack, 309
Heart failure, 304
multisystem effects of, 305f
Heart transplant, 306
Heart valves, 280f, 281–282, 281f
Heartbeat, 282, 283
Heartburn, 249
Heart-lung transplant, 306
Heat
sensation of, 97
therapy use of, 202
Heimlich maneuver, 401, 401f
Helicobacter pylori, 254, 265
Helminthiasis, 79
Helminths, 78f, 79
Hemangioma, 306, 306f
Hematemesis, 249
Hematocrit (Hct), 372, 674
Hematologist, 357
Hematology, 358
Hematoma, 358, 358f
Hematophobia, 735
Hematopoiesis, 140
Hematuria, 442, 442f
Hemianopia, 607
Hemiparesis, 535
Hemiplegia, 535, 535f
Hemochromatosis, 358
Hemodialysis (HD), 439, 442, 442f
Hemodynamic, 306
Hemoglobin (Hb, Hgb, HGB), 358, 372
Hemoglobin S, 355
Hemoglobin test, 674
Hemolysis, 358
Hemophilia, 358
Hemophobia, 735
Hemoptysis, 401
Hemorrhage, 338, 358
Hemorrhoid, 250, 250f
Hemostasis, 338, 359, 359f
Hemostatic agents, 370
Heparin, 234, 359
Hepatitis, 250
Hepatitis A (HAV), 250
Hepatitis B (HBV), 250
Hepatitis B screen, 674
Hepatitis C (HCV), 250
Hepatitis D (HDV), 250

Hepatitis E (HEV), 250
Hepatitis panel, 265
Herd immunity, 346
Hernia, 251, 251f
hiatal, 249, 251, 251f
inguinal, 251, 251f
umbilical, 251
Herniated disk syndrome (HDS), 536, 536f
Herniated intervertebral disk, 536, 536f
Herniated nucleus pulposus (HNP), 536
Herniorrhaphy, 252
Herpes genitalis, 692t
Herpes labialis, 112f
Herpes simplex, 112
Herpes zoster, 537, 537f
Heterogeneous, 16
Heterosexual, 703
Hiatal hernia, 249, 251, 251f
Hidradenitis, 112
High blood pressure, 287, 288t, 306
Highly active antiretroviral therapy (HAART), 370
Hilum
kidney, 427
lung, 386
HIPAA (Health Insurance Portability and Accountability Act), 8, 25, 26
Hippocampal sclerosis, 532
Hippocampus, 514f, 515
Hippocrates, 2
Hirsutism, 488, 488f
Histamine H₂-receptor antagonists, 262
Histology, 83
HIV. See Human immunodeficiency virus (HIV)
Hives, 113, 113f
HMD (hyaline membrane disease), 388
HNP (herniated nucleus pulposus), 536
Hoarseness, 399
Hodgkin disease, 363
Holter monitor, 326
Homeostasis, 60, 83
Homosexual, 703
Hordeolum, 617
Horizontal, 83
Horizontal plane, 69, 69f
Hormonal functions of endocrine system, 466–477, 467t–469t

Hormones, 465. See also Endocrine system; specific hormones
female, 671
of the hypothalamus, 467
ovarian production of, 640
HPV (human papilloma virus), 692t
HSG (hysterosalpingography), 674
HTN. See Hypertension
Human body organization, 60–67, 61f
abbreviations and acronyms, 89
atoms, 60
cells, 60, 62, 62f, 63f, 63t, 64–65
drug highlights, 87–89
medical vocabulary, 81–85
combining forms, 81
medical word list, 82–85
word roots, 81
molecules, 60
organs, 67
systems, 67, 68f
tissues, 65–67, 66f
Human chorionic gonadotropin (hCG), 674
Human genome, 83
Human immunodeficiency virus (HIV), 352–353, 352f, 363, 364, 691
Human immunodeficiency virus (HIV) screen, 674
Human papilloma virus (HPV), 692t
Humeral, 161
Humoral immunity, 345, 346–347
Humpback appearance, 162, 162f
Hunger, 230
Hyaline membrane disease (HMD), 388, 407
Hydrarthrosis, 161
Hydrocele, 703, 703f
Hydrocephalus, 538, 538f
Hydrocortisone, 488
Hydronephrosis, 443, 443f
Hydrotherapy, 202
Hymen, 640
Hymenectomy, 657
Hyperactive, 52
Hypercalcemia, 359, 471
Hypercalciuria, 443
Hyperemesis, 252
Hyperesthesia, 538
Hyperglycemia, 359, 472

Hyperglycemic agents, 499
Hypergonadism, 488
Hyperhidrosis, 113
Hyperhydrosis, 100
Hyperinsulinism, 472, 488
Hyperkalemia, 488
Hyperkinesis, 538
Hyperlipidemia, 306, 360
Hypernea, 401
Hyperopia, 608, 608f, 614
Hyperparathyroidism, 471
Hypertension (HTN), 287, 288t, 306
antihypertensive agents, 322
factors contributing to, 307t
Hyperthyroidism, 470, 488
Hyperventilation, 401
Hypnosis, 538, 724–725
Hypnotics, 551
Hypodermic, 113
Hypogastric, 252
Hypogastric region, 72, 73f
Hypoglossal nerve, 520f, 521t
Hypoglycemia, 360, 472
Hypogonadism, 489
Hypohidrosis, 100, 113
Hypohydrosis, 100
Hypomania, 732
Hypoparathyroidism, 471, 471f, 489
Hypophysis, 490. See also Pituitary gland (hypophysis)
Hypoplasia, 52
Hypospadias, 689, 702f, 704
Hypotension, 307
Hypothalamus, 466–467, 466f, 514f, 515t, 517
Hypothyroidism, 470, 490–491
congenital, 483
multisystem effects of, 490f
Hypoxemia, 401
Hypoxia, 35, 360, 394, 407
Hysterectomy, 657, 667
Hysterosalpingography (HSG), 674
Hysteroscope, 657
Hysterotomy, 658

I
IBD. See Inflammatory bowel disease (IBD)
IBS (irritable bowel syndrome), 253
IC (inspiratory capacity), 417
IC (interstitial cystitis), 438
Icteric, 113
Icterus, 114
ID (intradermal), 114

IgA, 347t
IgD, 347t
IgE, 347t
IgG, 347t
IgM, 347t
IGRAs (interferon-gamma release assays), 132
Ileostomy, 6, 252, 252f
Ileum, 231, 231f
Iliac, 161
Iliosacral, 161
Illness, 16
IM (intramuscular), 202
Imminent (spontaneous abortion type), 653, 653f
Immune response
    decline with age, 348
    phases of, 347–348
Immune system, 345–348, 346f, 347t
    overview of body's defenses, 346f
Immunity, 345
    active, 345
    cell-mediated, 345, 347–348
    community, 346
    herd, 346
    humoral, 345, 346–347
    passive, 345
Immunization, 115
Immunoglobulin (Ig), 347, 347t, 360, 372
Impacted fracture, 150f
Impetigo, 113, 113f
Impulse control disorder, 732
In vitro, 65
Incision, 16, 16f
Incisors, 227, 228f
Incomplete (spontaneous abortion type), 653, 653f
Incontinence, 443
Incus (anvil), 563t, 564t, 565, 565f
Indigestion, 247
Inevitable (spontaneous abortion type), 653, 653f
Infant respiratory distress syndrome (IRDS), 388
Infarction, 307
Infection, 52. See also specific infectious diseases
    opportunistic, 363
    prion, 79
    superinfection, 55
    urinary tract infections (UTIs), 431
Infectious diseases, 78–79
Infectious polyneuritis, 535

Inferior (directional term), 70f, 70t
Inferior colliculi, 517
Inferior palpebrae, 594
Infertility, 704
Inflammatory bowel disease (IBD), 252
    agents for, 263
Influenza, 401
Informed consent form, 25
Infundibulum
    fallopian tube, 635f, 637
    hypothalamus, 517
Inguinal, 83
Inguinal hernia, 251, 251f
Inhalation, 389f, 401
Inhalational glucocorticoids, 415
Initialism, 8
Innate (nonspecific) defense mechanisms, 346f
Inner ear, 563t, 564f, 565–568, 566f–567f
Insects, role in disease transmission, 79
Insertion, muscle, 189, 190f, 202
Insomnia, 53
Inspiratory capacity (IC), 417
Inspiratory reserve volume (IRV), 390
Institute for Safe Medication Practices (ISMP), 7
Insulin, 235, 468t, 472, 485, 491
    preparations for injection, 499
Insulin resistance syndrome, 493
Insulinogenic, 491
Integumentary, 114
Integumentary system, 94–138
    abbreviations and acronyms, 132–133
    accessory structures of skin, 98–100, 99f
    anatomy and physiology, 95, 95t, 96f
    diagnostic and laboratory tests, 131–132
    drug highlights, 130–131
    functions of skin, 95–97
    layers of skin, 97–98, 97f
    medical vocabulary, 102–126
        combining forms, 102
        medical word list, 103–126
        word roots, 102
    Practical Applications, 137–138
    skin rejuvenation and resurfacing treatment modalities, 126
Intelligence quotient (IQ), 723
Intense pulsed light (IPL), 126

Intercostal, 161
Interferon-gamma release assays (IGRAs), 132
Intermittent claudication, 311
Internal, 84
Internal inguinal ring, 689
Internal organs, 689–691
Internal respiration, 380
Internal structures, 594f, 597–598, 598f
Interneurons, 512
Interstitial cystitis (IC), 438, 443
Interstitial pneumonia, 405f
Intervertebral disk, herniated, 536, 536f
Intestinal villi, 231
Intracranial, 538
Intradermal (ID), 114
Intramuscular (IM), 202
Intraocular, 608
Intraocular lens (IOL), 613
Intrauterine, 658
Intrauterine device (IUD), 672, 672f
Intravenous, 53
Intravenous pyelography (pyelogram) (IVP), 456
Introduce, in AIDET communication, 28
Intussusception, 253
Inversion, 147f
Involuntary muscle, 67, 191–192. See also Cardiac muscle; Smooth muscle
Iodine, 491
IOL (intraocular lens), 613
IPL (intense pulsed light), 126
IQ (intelligence quotient), 723
IRDS (infant respiratory distress syndrome), 388
Iridectomy, 608
Iridocyclitis, 608
Iris, 593t, 594f, 597
Irons, 370
Irritable bowel syndrome (IBS), 253
IRV (inspiratory reserve volume), 390
Ischemia, 307
    silent, 307
Ischemic heart disease, 307
Ischemic time period, 644
Ischial, 161
Ischialgia, 162
Islets of Langerhans, 235, 468t, 472, 472f
ISMP (Institute for Safe Medication Practices), 7

Isometric, 202
Isometric exercise, 200
Isotonic, 202
Isthmus
    fallopian tube, 635f, 637
    uterus, 634
IUD (intrauterine device), 672, 672f
IVP (intravenous pyelography), 456

J
Jaundice, 114, 234
Jejunum, 231, 231f
Jet lag, 545
Joint (jt), 146, 146f
    age-realted changes, 146
    classification of, 146
    measurement of joint movements, 177
    movements, 146, 147f
    replacements, 156
The Joint Commission (TJC), 7

K
Kaposi sarcoma (KS), 352, 360, 360f
Karyogenesis, 84
Keloid, 114, 114f
Keratin, 95t
Keratinization, 95t
Keratitis, 608
Keratoconjunctivitis, 609
Keratoconus, 605
Keratolytics, 130
Keratome, 611
Keratometry, 624
Keratoplasty, 605, 609
Ketonuria, 443
Kidney failure, 448
Kidney stones, 444–445, 444f, 471
Kidney transplantation, 449, 449f
Kidneys, 425–429, 425t, 426f–429f
    external structure, 427, 428f
    internal structure, 427, 428f
    microscopic anatomy, 427–429, 428f–429f
    nephrons, 427–429, 428f–429f
    position of, 425, 427f
    primary functions, 425–426, 425t
Kilogram (kg), 17
Kissing disease, 362
Kleptomania, 732
Knee joint, 146f
Knee-chest patient position, 207t

Knock-knee, 160, 160*f*
KS (Kaposi sarcoma), 352
Kyphosis, 162, 162*f*

L

Labia majora, 640, 640*f*
Labia minora, 640, 640*f*
Labial, 253
Labor
    defined, 646
    signs of impending, 646–647
    stages of, 647, 648*f*
Laboratory tests. *See* Diagnostic and laboratory tests
Labyrinthectomy, 573
Labyrinthitis, 573
Labyrinthotomy, 573
Labyrinths, 565, 573
Lacrimal, 609
Lacrimal apparatus, 593*t*, 595–596, 596*f*
Lacrimal canaliculi, 596, 596*f*
Lacrimal gland, 596, 596*f*
Lacrimal sac, 596, 596*f*
Lactate dehydrogenase (LD or LDH), 326
Lactation, 641, 641*f*–642*f*
Lacteals, 231
Lactic dehydrogenase (LDH, LD), 216
Lactiferous glands, 641
Lactogenic hormone (LTH), 467*t*
Laminectomy, 162, 538
Landsteiner, Karl, 339
Lanugo hair, 97, 647
Laparoscopy, 674
Laparotomy, 253
Large intestine, 224*t*, 225*f*, 232, 232*f*
    primary functions/description, 224*t*
Laryngeal, 401
Laryngitis, 402, 402*f*
Laryngopharynx, 229, 383, 384*f*
Laryngoscope, 402
Laryngoscopy, 402, 416
Larynx, 229, 380*t*, 381*f*, 384–385, 385*f*
Laser, 609
Laser ablation, 658
Laser peripheral iridotomy (LPI), 609
LASIK (laser-assisted in situ keratomileusis), 611
LATE (limbic-predominant age-related TDP-43 encephalopathy), 532

Latent, 53
Lateral, 84
Lateral (directional term), 70*f*, 71*t*
Lateral humeral epicondylitis, 170
Lavage, 253
Laxative, 253, 263
Lazy eye, 602
LBD (Lewy body dementia), 532
LDL (low-density lipoproteins), 308
LDL cholesterol, 326
Left atrium, 279*f*, 280, 280*f*
Left bronchus, 386, 387*f*
Left hypochondriac region, 72, 73*f*
Left iliac (inguinal) region, 72, 73*f*
Left lower quadrant (LLQ), 73, 73*f*
Left lumbar region, 72, 73*f*
Left upper quadrant (LUQ), 73, 73*f*
Left ventricle, 279*f*, 280, 280*f*
Left-ventricular ejection fraction (LVEF), 304
Legionella pneumophilia, 402
Legionnaires disease, 402
Lens, 593*t*, 594*f*, 598
    artificial, 613, 613*f*
Lentigo, 114
Leptin, 477
LES (lower esophageal sphincter), 229
Lethargic, 491
Leukapheresis, 360
Leukemia, 361
Leukocytes (white blood cells, WBCs), 337*t*, 338*f*, 339
Leukocytopenia, 361
Leukoderma, 114
Leukoplakia, 114
Levator, 202
Lewy bodies, 532
Lewy body dementia (LBD), 532
LH. *See* Luteinizing hormone (LH)
Ligaments, 140, 140*t*
Light therapy box, 737, 737*f*
Lightening, 647
Limbic system, 514*f*, 515
Limbic-predominant age-related TDP-43 encephalopathy (LATE), 532
Linea nigra, 658, 658*f*
Linear fracture, 150*f*
Lingual frenulum, 226, 253
Lingual tonsils, 344, 383

Lipid profile, 326
Lipoprotein, 308
Liter (L), 17
Lithotomy patient position, 207*t*
Lithotripsy, 443
Liver, 224*t*, 225*f*, 233–234, 234*f*
    anatomy, 233, 234*f*
    fetal, 337
    functions, 233–234
    primary functions/description, 224*t*
    substances manufactured by, 234
    ultrasonography, 266, 266*f*
Liver biopsy, 265
Lobar pneumonia, 405*f*
Lobectomy, 403
Lobes
    brain, 515, 516*f*
    lung, 387, 388*f*
Lobotomy, 538
Lobule, lung lobe, 387
Local anesthetic agents, 130
Local anesthetics, 551
Lochia, 658
Lochia alba, 658
Lochia rubra, 658
Lochia serosa, 658
Loop diuretics, 454
Lordosis, 162, 162*f*
    lumbar, 149, 149*f*
Lou Gehrig disease, 527
Lower esophageal sphincter (LES), 229
LPI (laser peripheral iridotomy), 609
LTH (lactogenic hormone), 467*t*
Lumbar curve, 148, 148*f*, 162
Lumbar lordosis, 149, 149*f*
Lumbar puncture, 554, 554*f*
Lumbar spinal nerves, 519, 521*f*
Lumbar vertebrae, 148, 148*f*
Lumbodynia, 162
Lumen, 54
Lumpectomy, 659, 659*f*
Lung(s), 72, 380*t*, 381*f*, 387–388, 388*f*
    collapsed, 397
Lung cancer, 403, 403*f*
Lunula, 99, 99*f*
Lupus, 114
Lupus erythematosus, 114
Lupus vulgaris, 114
Luteal phase, 643*f*, 644
Luteinizing hormone (LH), 467*t*, 639, 643, 643*f*
LVEF (left-ventricular ejection fraction), 304

Lyme disease, 106
Lymph, 343
Lymph nodes, 342, 342*f*, 343*f*
    vascularized lymph node transfer (VLNT), 361
Lymphadenitis, 361
Lymphatic capillaries, 342, 342*f*
Lymphatic ducts, 342
Lymphatic system, 336, 336*t*, 342–344, 342*f*–339*f*
    conducting system, 344
    functions, 336, 342
    lymphoid tissue, 344
Lymphatic vessels, 342, 342*f*, 343*f*
Lymphedema, 361, 361*f*
Lymphocytes, 337*t*, 338*f*, 339
    in lymphoid tissue, 344
Lymphoid follicles, 344
Lymphoid neoplasm, 362*f*, 363
Lymphoma, 362*f*, 363
Lymphostasis, 362
Lysosomes, 63*f*, 63*t*

M

Macrocytosis, 362
Macrophages, 347–348
Macroscopic, 17
Macula lutea, 597, 598*f*
Maculae, 119, 568
Macular degeneration, 610, 610*f*
Macule, 122*f*
Maculopapular eruption, 115
Magnetic resonance imaging (MRI), 178, 178*f*
    cardiovascular system, 326
Major depression, 730*f*
Malabsorption, 253
Malaise, 17
Male pattern alopecia, 104, 104*f*
Male pelvis, 149, 149*f*, 687*f*
Male reproductive system, 685–718
    abbreviations and acronyms, 712–713
    anatomy and physiology, 686–691, 686*t*, 687*f*
        bulbourethral (Cowper) glands, 686*t*, 687*f*, 690–691, 691*f*
        epididymis, 686, 686*t*, 687*f*, 688*f*, 689
        external organs, 686–689
        internal organs, 689–691
        penis, 686*t*, 687*f*, 689
        scrotum, 686, 686*t*, 687*f*, 688
        seminal vesicles, 686*t*, 687*f*, 690, 691*f*
        testes, 686*t*, 687*f*, 688, 688*f*

Male reproductive system *(continued)*
urethra, 686*t*, 687*f*, 691, 691*f*
vas deferens, 686*t*, 687*f*, 688*f*, 689
diagnostic and laboratory tests, 712
drug highlights, 711
medical vocabulary, 697–707
combining forms, 697
medical word list, 698–707
word roots, 697
Practical Application, 717–718
sexually transmitted infections (STIs), 691, 692*t*–693*t*, 693*f*
Malformation, 3, 17
Malignant, 17, 19
Malleus (hammer), 563*t*, 564*t*, 565, 565*f*, 574
MALT (mucosa-associated lymphoid tissue), 344
Mammary glands, 41. *See also* Breasts
Mammography, 675, 675*f*
Mammoplasty, 659
Mandibular, 163
Mania, 733, 733*f*
Manic-depressive illness, 729
Mantoux tuberculin skin test, 131, 131*f*, 417
MAOIs (monoamine oxidase inhibitors), 743
Markings of bones, 144, 145*t*
Massage, 202
Mastectomy, 659, 659*f*
Master gland, pituitary gland as, 469
Mastication, 51, 253
Mastitis, 660, 660*f*
Mastoiditis, 565, 574
Maternal blood glucose, 675
Matrix, bone, 140
Mature follicle, 639
Maxillae, 382
Maxillary, 163
Maxillary sinus, 382, 383*f*
Maximal, 17
Maximal voluntary ventilation (MVV), 417
MBPS (Munchausen-by-proxy syndrome), 732
McBurney point, 240, 240*f*
Measles, 115
Meatotomy, 443
Meatus, 443
bone marking, 145
Mechanical ablations, 126
Meconium, 232

Medial, 84
Medial (directional term), 70*f*, 71*t*
Mediastinum, 387
Medical history (Hx), 24
Medical record analysis
blood and lymphatic system, 377–378
digestive system, 271–272
ear, 591
eyes, 630
integumentary system, 137–138
mental health, 746–747
muscular system, 221
nervous system, 560
respiratory system, 422
skeletal system, 184
urinary system, 462–463
Medical records, 24–26
Medical terminology
abbreviations and acronyms, 7–8, 28–29
component parts, principles of, 4–5
definition, 2
identification of medical words, 5
introduction to, 1–32
medical vocabulary, 11–20
plural endings, 7
pronunciation, 8
spelling, 5–7
vocabulary words, 5
word structure fundamentals, 2–4
Medical vocabulary, 11–20. *See also* Combining forms; Medical word list; Word roots
blood and lymphatic system, 351–366
cardiovascular system, 291–317
digestive system, 238–258
ear, 571–579
endocrine system, 481–495
eye, 601–618
female reproductive system, 652–667
human body organization, 81–85
integumentary system, 102–126
male reproductive system, 697–707
mental health, 726–729
muscular system, 195–211
nervous system, 526–547
respiratory system, 393–410

skeletal system, 155–171
suffixes and prefixes, 51–55
urinary system, 436–450
Medical words
building and spelling, 6–7
identification of, 5
Medication order, 89
Medulla
adrenal, 473, 474*f*, 475
ovary, 639
renal, 427, 428*f*
Medulla oblongata, 389, 514*f*, 515*t*, 517
Medullary canal, 143, 144*f*
Megakaryocytes, 339
Meibomian gland dysfunction (MGD), 595
Meibomian glands, 595
Melanin, 95*t*, 96*f*, 98
Melanocyte-stimulating hormone (MSH), 467*t*
Melanocyte-stimulating hormone-releasing factor (MRF), 467
Melanoma, 115, 115*f*
Melatonin, 467*t*, 469
Melena, 253
Membranous urethra, 430, 431*f*
Menarche, 643, 660
Ménière disease, 574
Meninges, 513, 513*f*
Meningioma, 539
Meningitis, 539
Meningocele, 539, 539*f*
Meningomyelocele, 540
Meniscus, 163
Menopause, 643, 661
surgical, 657
Menorrhagia, 661
Menorrhea, 661
Menstrual cycle, 643–644, 643*f*
Mental disorder
conditions classified as, 721
definition, 720
diagnosis of, 722–723
multicausational concept of illness process, 720*f*
severity, 721
symptoms of, 721–722
treatments for, 723–725, 724*f*
Mental health, 719–747
abbreviations and acronyms, 744
definition, 720
drug highlights, 742–743
medical vocabulary, 726–729

combining forms, 726
medical word list, 726–739
word roots, 726
Practical Application, 746–747
Mesenchymal, 65
Mesentery, 253
Mesomorph, 84
Mesothelioma, 404
Mesovaium, 639
Metabolic syndrome, 493
Metacarpals, 163
Metacarpectomy, 163
Metaphysis, 143, 144*f*
MG (myasthenia gravis), 205
MGD (meibomian gland dysfunction), 595
MI (myocardial infarction), 309
Microcephaly, 540, 540*f*
Microgram (mcg), 17
Microorganism, 17
Microscope, 18, 18*f*
Microwave, 5
Midbrain, 514*f*, 515*t*, 517
Middle ear, 563*t*, 564–565, 564*f*, 565*f*, 567*f*
Midline, 73
Midsagittal plane, 69, 69*f*
Mild brain injury, 530
Mild head injury (MHI), 530
Mild head trauma (MHT), 530
Mild traumatic brain injury (MTBI), 530
Miliaria, 116, 116*f*
Milk teeth, 227
Milligram (mg), 18
Milliliter (ml), 18
Mineralocorticoid receptor antagonists (MRAs), 322
Mineralocorticoids, 474–475
Minimally invasive ablative methods, 18, 126
Minipill, 671
Ministroke, 545
Minnesota Multiphasic Personality Inventory-2 (MMPI-2), 723
Miotic, 610
Miotic drugs, 622
Missed (spontaneous abortion type), 653
Mitochondria, 63*f*, 63*t*
Mitosis, 704
Mitral stenosis, 308
Mitral (bicuspid) valve, 280, 280*f*, 281, 281*f*
Mitral valve prolapse, 308
Mittelschmerz, 661

MMPI-2 (Minnesota Multiphasic Personality Inventory-2), 723
MMR (measles, mumps, rubella) vaccine, 115, 120
Modified radical mastectomy, 659, 659f
Molars, 227, 228f
Mole, 116, 116f
Molecules, 60
Monaural, 574
Monoamine oxidase inhibitors (MAOIs), 743
Monocytes, 337t, 338f, 339
Mononucleosis, 362, 362f
Mons pubis, 640, 640f
Mons veneris, 640
Mood, 733
    ingredients to boost, 721
Morbidity, 18
Mortality, 18
    leading causes of US in 2017, 18
Morula, 636f, 637
Mosquito, 79, 79f
Motor neurons, 510–511
Mound of Venus, 640
Mouth, 224t, 225f, 226–227, 226f, 227f
Movement
    joints and, 146, 146f–147f
    muscles and, 192
MRAs (mineralocorticoid receptor antagonists), 322
MRF (melanocyte-stimulating hormone-releasing factor), 467
MRI. See Magnetic resonance imaging (MRI)
MSH (melanocyte-stimulating hormone), 467t
Mucolytics, 415
Mucosa, fallopian tube, 637
Mucosa-associated lymphoid tissue (MALT), 344
Multifocal intraocular lens, 613
Multiform, 19
Multigravida, 657
Multipara, 662
Multiple sclerosis (MS), 541, 541f
    multisystem effects of, 541f
Multisystem effects
    of diabetes mellitus (DM), 473f
    of heart failure, 305f
    of hyperthyroidism, 489f
    of hypothyroidism, 490f

of multiple sclerosis (MS), 541f
of premenstrual syndrome (PMS), 665f
of shock, 313f
Munchausen syndrome, 732
Munchausen-by-proxy syndrome (MBPS), 732
Murmur, 308
Muscle(s), 187, 187f, 187t
    attachments, 189, 190f
    biopsy, 216
    bladder wall, 430
    cardiac, 187t, 188f, 192
    development in newborns, 189
    eye, 593t, 594, 595f
    functions of, 192
    parts of, 189
    skeletal, 187f, 187t, 188–189, 188f, 189t, 190f, 191
    smooth, 187t, 188f, 191
    tissue, 66f, 67
    types, 187t, 188–192, 188f
Muscle spasm, 203
Muscosal protective medications, 262
Muscular dystrophy, 203–204, 203f–204f
    Duchenne, 200, 203
    Gowers maneuver, 204, 204f
Muscular layer, fallopian tube, 636–637
Muscular system, 186–222
    abbreviations and acronyms, 216
    anatomy and physiology, 187–192, 187t
        cardiac muscle, 187t, 188f, 192
        skeletal muscle, 187f, 187t, 188–189, 188f, 189t, 190f, 191
        smooth muscle, 187t, 188f, 191
    diagnostic and laboratory tests, 216
    drug highlights, 215
    functions of muscles, 192
    medical vocabulary, 195–211
        combining forms, 195
        medical word list, 195–211
        word roots, 195
    Practical Applications, 221
MVV (maximal voluntary ventilation), 417
Myalgia, 201, 205
Myasthenia gravis (MG), 205
Mycobacterium tuberculosis, 410, 417

Mycoses, 79
Mydriatic, 610
Mydriatic drugs, 622
Myelinated fibers, 512
Myelitis, 163, 542
Myelodysplastic syndromes, 364
Myelogram, 554
Myeloma, 163
Myelopoiesis, 163
Myoblast, 205
Myocardial, 308
Myocardial infarction (MI), 309
Myocarditis, 309
Myocardium, 192, 276, 279f, 308
Myofibroma, 205
Myograph, 205
Myokinesis, 205
Myoma, 205
Myomalacia, 205
Myomectomy, 667
Myometritis, 661
Myometrium, 635f, 636
Myoparesis, 205
Myopathy, 205
Myopia (My), 611, 611f, 614
Myoplasty, 205
Myorrhaphy, 205
Myosarcoma, 205
Myosclerosis, 205
Myositis, 206
Myospasm, 206
Myotome, 206
Myotomy, 206
Myringectomy, 574
Myringoplasty, 574
Myringoscope, 574
Myringotome, 574
Myringotomy, 6, 574
Myxedema, 470, 492, 492f

N

Nail bed, 99, 99f
Nail body, 99, 99f
Nail root, 99, 99f
Nails, 95t, 99, 99f
    aging and, 98
Naloxone, 553
Narcolepsy, 542
Narcotic analgesics, 175, 551
Narcotic antitussives, 414
Nasolacrimal duct, 596, 596f
Nasopharyngitis, 404
Nasopharynx, 229, 383, 384f
Natural killer (NK) cells, 346, 347–348, 347t
Nausea, 253

Nearsightedness, 599, 611, 611f, 614
Neck, tooth, 227, 229f
Necrosis, 19
Needle biopsy, 216
Neonatal respiratory distress syndrome (NRDS), 388
Nephrectomy, 444
Nephritis, 444
Nephrolithiasis, 444, 444f
Nephrology, 445
Nephroma, 445
Nephrons, 427–429, 428f–429f, 445
Nephropathy, 445
Nephrosclerosis, 445
Nephrosis, 445
Nephrotic syndrome, 445
Nerve fibers and tracts, 509t, 512
Nerve impulse transmission, 512
Nerve tissue, 66f, 67
Nerves
    afferent, 511, 512
    cranial, 509t, 519, 520f, 521t
    defined, 512
    efferent, 512
    spinal, 509t, 518f, 519, 521t
Nervous system, 508–561
    abbreviations and acronyms, 555
    anatomy and physiology, 509–523, 509t, 510f
        autonomic nervous system (ANS), 522–523, 522f
        brain, 509t, 510f, 513–517, 513f–514f, 514t–515t, 516f
        central nervous system (CNS), 509, 509t, 510f, 512–519, 513f–514f, 514t–515t, 516f, 518f
        nerve fibers and tracts, 509t, 512
        nerve impulse transmission, 512
        neuroglia, 509t, 510, 511f
        neurons, 509t, 510–512, 510f–511f
        peripheral nervous system (PNS), 509, 509t, 510f, 519, 520f–521f, 521t
        spinal cord, 509t, 510f, 517–518, 518f
        tissues, 510–512
    diagnostic and laboratory tests, 554–555

Nervous system (continued)
drug highlights, 551–553
fetal, 513
medical vocabulary, 526–547
combining forms, 526
medical word list, 527–547
word roots, 526
Practical Application, 560
Nesting, 647
Neural tube development, 513
Neuralgia, 542
Neurasthenia, 542
Neurectomy, 542
Neurilemma, 512
Neuritis, 542
Neuroblast, 542
Neuroblastoma, 542
Neurofibroma, 542, 542f
Neuroglia, 67, 509t, 510, 511f, 543
Neurohypophysis. See Pituitary gland posterior lobe (neuroohypophysis)
Neuroleptics, 743
Neurological disease, as erectile dysfunction cause, 702
Neurological examination, 555
Neurologist, 543
Neurology (Neuro), 543
Neuroma, 543
Neuromuscular, 206
Neuromyopathic, 206
Neurons, 509t, 510–512, 510f–511f
interneurons, 512
motor, 510–511
sensory, 511
Neuropathy, 543
Neurotic, 733
Neurotransmitters, 512, 543, 738
Neutron, 60
Neutrophils, 337t, 338f, 339
Nevus, 116, 116f
Newborn assessment, 648–649, 649t
Newborns
appearance of, 647
digestive system, 234
immune response in, 345
lungs, 388
microcephaly, 540, 540f
muscle development, 189
pulse, blood pressure, and respirations, 287
respiratory rate, 389
skin, 97
visual acuity, 596
Night blindness, 611

NK (natural killer) cells, 346, 347–348, 347t
No rapid eye movement (NREM), 544
Nocturia, 445
Non-24-hour sleep-wake disorder, 545
Nondisplaced fracture, 150f
Non-narcotic analgesics, 175, 551
Non-narcotic antitussives, 414
Non-small-cell lung cancer (NSCLC), 403
Nonsteroidal anti-inflammatory drugs (NSAIDs), 174
Nonstress test (NST), 675
Non-ST-segment elevation myocardial infarction (NSTEMI), 301
Noradrenaline, 468t, 475
Norepinephrine, 467, 468t, 475, 492, 733
Nose, 380t, 381–382, 381f, 382f
Nostrils, 381
Noun suffixes, 37t
NRDS (neonatal respiratory distress syndrome), 388
NREM (no rapid eye movement), 544
NSAIDs (nonsteroidal anti-inflammatory drugs), 174
NSCLC (non-small-cell lung cancer), 403
NST (nonstress test), 675
NSTEMI (non-ST-segment elevation myocardial infarction), 301
Nucleus, 63f, 63t, 64
Nulligravida, 657
Nullipara, 662
Numbers, prefixes pertaining to, 48, 48t
Nurse's notes, 25
Nyctalopia, 611
Nyctophobia, 735
Nystagmus, 611

O

Obesity, 82
in children, 472
classified as a disease, 477
defined, 477
Objective, in SOAP chart note, 27
Oblique fracture, 150f
Oblique muscles of the eye, 594, 595f
Obsession, 734

Obsessive-compulsive disorder (OCD), 734, 734f
Obstetrician, 644
Obstetrics, 644–649
defined, 644
labor and delivery, 646–648, 648f
newborn assessment, 648–649, 649t
pregnancy, 644–646, 645f–646f
Obstructive apnea, 394
Occipital lobe, 515, 516f
Occlusion, 309
Occult blood, 265
OCD (obsessive-compulsive disorder), 734, 734f
Ocular, 611
Ocular fundus, 611
Ocular ultrasonography, 624
Oculomotor nerve, 520f, 521t
OD (optometrist), 612, 612f
Off-pump coronary bypass (OPCAB), 299
OIC (opioid-induced constipation), 245
Olecranal, 163
Olfaction, 404
Olfactory bulb, 382
Olfactory nerve, 520f, 521t
Olgiodendroglioma, 543
Oligomenorrhea, 661
Oligospermia, 704
Oliguria, 446
OM (otitis media), 565
Oncologist, 19
Oncology, 19
Onychia, 116
Onychomycosis, 116, 116f
Oocyte, 638f, 639
Oogenesis, 661
Oophorectomy, 661
O&P (ova and parasites), 265
OPCAB (off-pump coronary bypass), 299
Open biopsy, 216
Open (compound) fracture, 150f
Open surgery, for benign prostatic hyperplasia (BPH), 699
Open-angle glaucoma, 607
Operative report, 26
Ophthalmologist, 611
Ophthalmology, 612
Ophthalmoscope, 612, 624f
Ophthalmoscopy, 624
Opioid antagonist, 553

Opioid epidemic, 15, 553, 553f
Opioid-induced constipation (OIC), 245
Opportunistic infection, 363
Optic, 612
Optic disk, 597–598, 598f
Optic foramen, 594
Optic nerve, 520f, 521t
Optician, 612
Optometrist (OD), 612, 612f
Oral cavity, 226, 226f. See also Mouth
Oral hypoglycemic agents, 499
Orbit, 593t, 594
Orchidectomy, 704
Orchiditis, 704
Orchidotomy, 704
Organ of Corti, 563t, 566
Organelles, 64
Organic, 84
Organs, 67
Origin, muscle, 189, 190f
Oropharynx, 229, 383, 384f
Orthopedics, 163
Orthopedist, 163
Orthopnea, 404
Orthopneic patient position, 207t
Orthoptics, 612
Orthoses, 203
Osmotic diuretics, 454
Osseous tissue, 140
Ossicles, 563t, 565, 565f
Osteoarthritis, 156
Osteoarthrosis, 163
Osteoblasts, 140, 164
Osteochondritis, 164
Osteogenesis, 164
Osteomalacia, 164
Osteomyelitis, 164, 164f
Osteopenia, 164
Osteoporosis, 164, 165f, 471, 661
agents used to treat/prevent, 175
dual-energy x-ray absorptiometry (DXA) scan, 177
postmenopausal, 164, 175
Osteosarcoma, 166
Osteotome, 166
Ostium, fallopian tube, 637
Otalgia, 575
Otic, 575
Otitis, 575
Otitis media (OM), 565, 575–576, 575f–576f

Otoconia, 568
Otolaryngologist, 577
Otolaryngology, 577
Otolith organs, 568
Otolithic membrane, 568
Otoliths, 563t, 567, 568, 577
Otomycosis, 577
Otoneurology, 577
Otopharyngeal, 577
Otoplasty, 577
Otopyorrhea, 577
Otorhinolaryngology, 577
Otosclerosis, 577
Otoscope, 578, 578f
Otoscopy, 584, 584f
Ova and parasites (O&P), 265
Ovarian cycle, 662f
Ovaries, 465t, 466f, 468t, 475,
    633t, 634f–635f, 638f–639f,
    639–640
    functions of, 633t, 639–640
    hormone production by, 640
    microscopic anatomy, 639
    ova production by, 639
Overweight, 82, 477
Oviducts, 636. See also
    Fallopian tubes
Ovulation, 638f, 639, 662, 662f
Ovulatory phase, 644
Oximetry, 309, 309f
Oxygen (O₂), 310
Oxytocin, 467t, 642, 642f

P

Pacemaker, 282, 283f
    artificial, 295, 295f
Pacemaker cells, 192, 282
Pachyderma, 117
PAD. See Peripheral artery
    disease (PAD)
Pain, 97, 543
Palate, cleft, 382
Palatine bones, 382
Palatine tonsil, 226f, 227, 227f,
    344, 383
Palatopharyngoplasty, 404
Palatoplasty, 382
Pallidotomy, 543
Pallor, 19
Palmar, 19
Palpate, 54, 54f
Palpation, 25, 25f, 310
Palpebral fissure, 594
Pancreas, 224t, 225f, 234f,
    235, 465t, 466f, 468t, 472–473,
    472f
    primary functions/description,
    224t

Pancreatic, 492
Pancreatic islets, 468t, 472, 472t
Pancreatitis, 254
Pancytopenia, 363
Panhypopituitarism, 493
Panic attack, 727
Panic disorder, 727
Panniculectomy, 117
Papanicolaou (Pap) smear, 676,
    676f
Papillae, 95t, 98
Papillae, tongue, 226
Papillary layer, 98
Papilledema, 543
Papule, 122f
Paracentesis, 19
Paralysis agitans, 544
Paranasal sinus, 382, 383f, 402
Paranoia, 735
Paranoid personality disorder,
    735
Paranoid schizophrenia, 735
Paraphilias, 737
Paraphimosis, 689
Paraplegia, 535f, 543
Parasympathetic division, 522,
    522f, 523
Parathyroid gland, 465t, 466f,
    468t, 471, 471f
Parathyroid hormone (PTH)
    (parathormone), 468t, 471
Parenchyma, 704
Paresis, 543
Paresthesia, 544
Parietal lobe, 515, 516f
Parkinson disease, 475, 544
Paronychia, 117
Parotid salivary glands, 233,
    233f
Partial seizures, 534
Partial thromboplastin time
    (PTT), 372
Parturition, 646
Passive exercise, 200
Passive immunity, 345
Patechiae, 117
Patellar, 166
Patent, 54
Paternity test, 712
Pathogenic, 19, 78
Pathogenic microorganisms, 78,
    78f
Pathogens, 66
Pathologic fracture, 151f
Pathological conditions, suffixes
    for, 38, 38t–39t
Pathology, 84
Pathology report, 26

Patient data, 24
Patient positions, 206t–208t
PD (peritoneal dialysis), 439,
    447, 447f
PE (physical examination),
    24–25, 25f, 26f
PE (pulmonary embolism), 315
Pedal, 166
Pediculosis, 117, 117f
Pedophilia, 737
Pelvic cavity, 71f, 72
Pelvic inflammatory disease
    (PID), 662
Pelvis, 149
    female, 149f, 150
    gynecoid, 150
    male, 149, 149f, 687f
Penduncles, 667
Penetrating keratoplasty, 605
Penicillins, 583
Penile urethra, 430
Penis, 686t, 687f, 689
Peptic, 254
Peptic ulcer disease (PUD), 254,
    254f
Percussion, 25, 25f
Percutaneous transluminal
    coronary angioplasty (PTCA),
    310, 310f
Percutaneous ultrasonic
    lithotripsy (PUL), 445, 446,
    446f
Perfusion, 84
Pericardial, 54, 310
Pericardial cavity, 72
Pericardiocentesis, 311, 311f
Pericarditis, 311
Pericardium, 276, 279f
Perilymph, 565, 578
Perimenopause, 662
Perimetrium, 635f, 636
Perineum, 641
Periodontal, 255
Periodontal disease, 255
Periodontal ligament, 228, 229f
Periosteum, 143, 144f
Peripheral artery disease (PAD),
    298, 311
Peripheral nervous system
    (PNS), 509, 509t, 510f, 519,
    520f–521f, 521t
Peripheral processes, 511
Peristalsis, 229, 255
Peritoneal dialysis (PD), 439,
    447, 447f
Periurethral, 447
Personality disorder, 735, 735f
Perspiration, 97

Pertusis, 404
Pes planus, 160
PET. See Positron emission
    tomography (PET)
PET scan, 326
Peyer patches, 344
Phacoemulsification, 612–613,
    613f
Phacolysis, 614
Phagocytosis, 348, 363
Phalangeal, 166
Pharyngeal, 255
Pharyngeal tonsils, 344, 383
Pharyngitis, 404
Pharynx, 224t, 225f, 226f, 229,
    380t, 381f, 383, 384f
    primary functions/description,
    224t
Phenotype, 84
Phimosis, 689, 704
Phlebitis, 311
Phlebotomy, 312
PHN (postherpetic neuralgia),
    537
Phobia, 735
Phosphorus, 166
Phosphorus blood test, 179
Photocoagulation, 614
Photodermatitis, 104f
Photon absorptiometry, 178
Photophobia, 614, 735
Phylum, 79
Physical examination (PE),
    24–25, 25f, 26f
Physician's orders, 25
Physician's progress notes, 25
Physiology, 84
Physis, 145
Pia mater, 513, 513f
PID (pelvic inflammatory
    disease), 662
PIH (pregnancy-induced
    hypertension), 655
Pilonidal cyst, 255
Pimples, 103
Pineal, 492
Pineal gland, 465t, 466f, 467t,
    469
Pink eye, 604, 604f
Pituitarism, 492
Pituitary gland (hypophysis),
    465t, 466f, 467t, 469, 470f, 492
Pituitary gland anterior lobe
    (adenohypophysis), 465t, 467t,
    469
Pituitary gland posterior lobe
    (neuroohypophysis), 465t,
    467t, 469

PJP (*Pneumocystis jiroveci* pneumonia), 352
Placement, prefixes pertaining to, 47, 47*t*
Placenta, 476, 647–648
Placenta previa, 663, 663*f*
Placental stage of labor, 647, 648*f*
Plan, in SOAP chart note, 27
Planes, 68, 69, 69*f*
Plantar wart, 125, 125*f*
Plasma, 340
Plasma lymphocytes, 346
Plasma proteins, 340
Plasmapheresis, 363
Plastic surgeons, 65, 117, 126
Platelet count, 372
Platelets, 337–339, 337*t*, 338*f*
    clotting, 338–339, 339*f*
Play therapy, 724, 724*f*
Pleural cavities, 72, 387
Pleurisy, 404
Pleuritic chest pain, 404
Pleuritis, 404
Pleurodynia, 405
Plural endings, 7
PMS. *See* Premenstrual syndrome (PMS)
Pneumococcal disease, 406
Pneumococcal vaccine, 406
Pneumoconiosis, 405
Pneumocystis jiroveci pneumonia (PJP), 352, 363
Pneumonectomy, 405
Pneumonia, 405, 405*f*
Pneumonitis, 406
Pneumothorax, 406, 406*f*
PNS. *See* Peripheral nervous system (PNS)
Poison ivy, 110, 110*f*
Poliomyelitis, 544
Polyarthritis, 166
Polycythemia, 363
Polydactyly, 54
Polydipsia, 472, 495
Polyneuritis, 544
Polyneuropathy, 485
Polyphagia, 472
Polyplegia, 206
Polyuria, 447, 472, 495
Pons, 389, 514*f*, 515*t*, 517
Popliteal pulse checkpoint, 285*f*, 285*t*
Position, patient, 206*t*–208*t*
Position, prefixes pertaining to, 47, 47*t*
Positional terms, 70*t*–71*t*

Positron emission tomography (PET)
    cardiovascular system, 326
    nervous system, 555
Postcoital, 664
Posterior (directional term), 69, 70*f*, 70*t*
Posterior cavity, 69, 594*f*, 597
Postherpetic neuralgia (PHN), 537
Postmenopausal osteoporosis, 164, 175
Postpartum period, 646
Postprandial (PP), 255
Posttraumatic stress disorder (PTSD), 736
Potassium sparing diuretics, 454
PP (postprandial), 255
PPD (purified protein derivative), 131
PPIs (proton-pump inhibitors), 60, 262
Practical Application
    blood and lymphatic system, 377–378
    cardiovascular system, 333–334
    digestive system, 271–272
    ear, 591
    endocrine system, 506
    eye, 630
    female reproductive system, 682–683
    integumentary system, 137–138
    male reproductive system, 717–718
    mental health, 746–747
    methods of documentation and tools for effective communication, 31–32
    muscular system, 221
    nervous system, 560
    respiratory system, 422
    skeletal system, 184
    urinary system, 462–463
    whooping cough, 92–93
Prediabetes, 493
Predominantly hyperactive-impulsive ADHD, 728
Predominantly inattentive ADHD, 728
Preeclampsia, 664
Preembryonic stage, 644
Pre-exposure prophylaxis (PrEP), 370

Prefixes
    definition, 3
    frequently misspelled, 6
    general-use, 43, 44*t*
    medical vocabulary, 51–55
        combining forms, 51
        medical word list, 51–55
        word roots, 51
    with multiple meanings, 45, 45*t*
    for numbers or amounts, 48, 48*t*
    overview, 43
    for position or placement, 47, 47*t*
Pregnancy, 643, 644–646, 645*f*–646*f*
    ectopic, 656, 656*f*
    stages of, 646
Pregnancy-induced hypertension (PIH), 655, 664
Pregnanediol, 676
Premenstrual, 54
Premenstrual syndrome (PMS), 664
    multisystem effects of, 665*f*
Premenstrual time period, 644
Premolars, 227, 228*f*
Prenatal period, 646
PrEP (pre-exposure prophylaxis), 370
Prepuce, 689
Presbycusis, 568, 578
Presbyopia, 599, 614
Prescription drugs, as erectile dysfunction cause, 702
Pressure, sense of, 97
Pressure ulcer, 109
Preventive use, of drugs, 88
PRF (prolactin-releasing factor), 467
Prickly heat, 116
Primary follicle, 639
Primary homeostasis, 338
Prime mover skeletal muscle, 191
Primigravida, 657
Primipara, 662
Prion infections, 79
Privacy Rule, 26
PRL (prolactin hormone), 467*t*, 641–642
Probiotics, 255
Process (bone marking), 145
Proctitis, 257
Proctoscope, 255
Proctoscopy, 255

Progeria, 493
Progesterone, 468*t*, 475–476, 476, 493, 640
Progestins, 671
Progestogens, 671
Prognosis, 19
Prolactin hormone (PRL), 467*t*, 641–642
Prolactin-releasing factor (PRF), 467
Pronation, 147*f*
Prone patient position, 207*t*
Pronunciation, 8
Prophylactic, 19
Prophylactic use, of drugs, 88
Prostaglandin analogues, 622
Prostate cancer, 431, 705–706, 705*f*
Prostatectomy, 690, 706
Prostate-specific antigen (PSA) immunoassay, 712
Prostatic urethra, 430, 431*f*
Prostatism, 698
Prostatitis, 706
Prosthesis, 156, 209, 209*f*
Protection, function of epithelial tissue, 66
Protection, function of skin, 96
Protein-bound iodine (PBI), 500
Prothrombin, 234, 337, 340, 363
Prothrombin time (PT), 372
Proton-pump inhibitors (PPIs), 60, 262
Protoplasm, 84
Protozoal, 79
Protozoan pathogens, 78*f*
Protraction, 147*f*
Proximal (directional term), 70*f*, 71*t*
Pruritus, 117
PSA (prostate-specific antigen) immunoassay, 712
Psoriasis, 118, 118*f*
Psychiatrist, 722, 736
Psychiatry, 722–723
Psychoanalysis, 723, 725
Psychoanalysts, 723
Psychogenic amnesia, 731
Psychogenic fugue, 731
Psychologist, 723, 724*f*
Psychology, 723
Psychopath, 736
Psychosis, 736
Psychosomatic, 6, 736
Psychotherapy, 722, 723–725
Psychotropic, 736

PT (prothrombin time), 372
PTCA (percutaneous transluminal coronary angioplasty), 310, 310f
PTH (parathyroid hormone) (parathormone), 468t, 471
PTSD (posttraumatic stress disorder), 736
PTT (partial thromboplastin time), 372
Puberty, 643, 688, 706
PUD (peptic ulcer disease), 254, 254f
Puerperium, 644, 646
PUL (percutaneous ultrasonic lithotripsy), 445, 446, 446f
Pulmonary artery stenosis, 281
Pulmonary edema, 304
Pulmonary embolism (PE), 315
Pulmonary function test, 417, 417f
Pulmonary (semilunar) valve, 279, 280f, 281, 281f
Pulmonologist, 406
Pulmonology, 407
Pulp cavity, tooth, 227, 229f
Pulse, 283, 284–285, 287
apical, 285
checkpoints, 285f, 285t
Pulse oximetry, 309, 309f
Pulse pressure, 288
Pupil, 597
Pupillary, 614
Pure tone audiometry, 584, 584f
Purified protein derivative (PPD), 131
Purkinje fibers, 282, 283f
Purpura, 118, 118f
Pustule, 122f
Pyelitis, 447
Pyelogram, 456
Pyelolithotomy, 448
Pyelonephritis, 448, 448f
Pyloric, 256
Pyloric stenosis, 256f
Pyothorax, 407
Pyrogenic, 19
Pyromania, 732, 736
Pyuria, 448

Q
Quad marker screen (AFP, hCG, UE, and inhibin-A), 676
Quadriceps, 209
Quadriplegia, 535f, 544
QuantiFERON-TB Gold (QFT), 417

R
RAAS (renin angiotensin aldosterone systems), 322, 449
Radial, 166
Radial keratotomy, 614
Radial pulse checkpoint, 285f, 285t
Radiation, 96
Radioactive iodine uptake (RAIU), 500
Radiofrequency ablation, 293
Radiograph, 166
Radiology, 19
Radiotracer, 326
Rale, 407
Range of motion (ROM), 200
Rapid eye movement (REM), 544
Rapid plasma reagin (RPR), 712
Rapid time zone change syndrome, 545
Rapport, 19
Raynaud phenomenon, 312, 312f
RDS (respiratory distress syndrome) of the newborn, 388
Reabsorption, 428, 431, 432f
Recommendation, in SBAR technique, 28
Rectocele, 256
Rectovaginal, 666
Rectum, 232, 232f
Rectus muscles of the eye, 594, 595f
Recurrent miscarriage (RM) (spontaneous abortion type), 653
Red blood cells (RBCs). See Erythrocytes
Red blood count (RBC), 372
Red meat, mood boost from, 721
Reduction, 166
Refraction of light, 598–599
Refractory period, 690
Regenerative medicine, 65
Regulation, function of skin, 96
Reissner membrane, 566
Relaxants, skeletal muscle, 215
Relaxation, 209
Relief of tension, 200
REM, See Rapid eye movement
Renal, 448
Renal biopsy, 456
Renal calculi, 440
Renal colic, 448
Renal failure, 448
Renal pelvis, 427, 428f

Renal transplantation, 449, 449f
Renin angiotensin aldosterone systems (RAAS), 322, 449
Replacement use, of drugs, 88
Residual volume (RV), 387, 390, 417
Respiration, 287, 389–390, 389f
external, 380
internal, 380
Respiration (R), 380
Respirator, 410
Respiratory distress syndrome (RDS) of the newborn, 388, 407
Respiratory syncytial virus (RSV) infection, 407
Respiratory system, 379–423
abbreviations and acronyms, 417–418
anatomy and physiology, 380–390, 380t, 381f
bronchi, 380t, 381f, 386, 387f
larynx, 380t, 381f, 384–385, 385f
lungs, 380t, 381f, 387–388, 388f
nose, 380t, 381–382, 381f, 382f
pharynx, 380t, 381f, 383, 384f
sinuses, 382, 383f
trachea, 380t, 381f, 386, 386f
diagnostic and laboratory tests, 415–417
drug highlights, 414–415
medical vocabulary, 393–410
combining forms, 393
medical word list, 394–410
word roots, 393
Practical Application, 422
respiration, 389–390, 389f
Rete testis, 688, 688f
Reticular layer, 98
Reticulocyte, 363
Retina, 593, 593t, 594f, 597, 598f
Retin-A (tretinoin), 131
Retinal breaks, 615
Retinal detachment, 615, 615f
Retinal tears, 615
Retinitis, 615
Retinitis pigmentosa, 615
Retinoblastoma, 615
Retinopathy, 616, 616f
Retraction, 147f
Retroflexion position of the uterus, 636, 636f
Retrograde pyelography (RP), 457, 457f
Retrolental fibroplasia (RLF), 616

Retroversion, 666
Retroversion position of the uterus, 636, 636f
Retrovirus, 364
Reverse transcriptase, 364
Reye syndrome, 544
RF (rheumatoid factor), 179
Rh factor, 340, 676
Rh negative, 340
Rh positive, 340
Rhabdomyoma, 209
Rhegmatogenous retinal detachment, 615
Rheumatic heart disease, 312
Rheumatism, 209
Rheumatoid arthritis, 167, 167f
Rheumatoid factor (RF), 179
Rheumatologist, 209
Rheumatology, 209
Rhinoplasty, 407
Rhinorrhea, 407
Rhinoscopy, 417
Rhinovirus, 407
Rhodopsin, 597
Rhonchus, 407
Rhytidoplasty, 118
Ribosomes, 63f, 63t
RICE (Rest Ice Compression Elevation), 202
Rickets, 168
Rickettsioses, 80, 80f
Right atrium, 278–279, 279f, 280f
Right bronchus, 386, 387f
Right hypochondriac region, 72, 73f
Right iliac (inguinal) region, 72, 73f
Right lower quadrant (RLQ), 73, 73f
Right lumbar region, 72, 73f
Right upper quadrant (RUQ), 72, 73f
Right ventricle, 279–280, 279f, 280f
Right-sided or right-ventricular heart failure, 304
Right-ventricular ejection fraction (RVEF), 304
Rigor mortis, 209
Ringworm, 124, 124f
RLF (retrolental fibroplasia), 616
Rods, 593, 597
Rogaine® (minoxidil), 131
ROM (range of motion), 200
Root
hair, 98
tongue, 226
tooth, 227, 229f
word (see Word roots)

Root canal, 227
Rorschach Inkblot Test, 723
Rosacea, 119, 119f
Roseola, 119, 119f
Rotation, 147f, 210
Rotator cuff, 210
Route of administration, 89
RP (retrograde pyelography), 457, 457f
RPR (rapid plasma reagin), 712
RSV (respiratory syncytial virus) infection, 407
Rubella, 120, 120f
    congenital syndrome, 677
Rubella (German measles) titer, 676
Rugae, 230, 230f
Rupture of the membranes (sign of impending labor), 647
Ruptured disk, 536
RV (residual volume), 387
RVEF (right-ventricular ejection fraction), 304

S
SA node (sinoatrial node), 282, 283f
Saccule, 563t, 567–568
Sacral curve, 148, 148f
Sacral spinal nerves, 519, 521f
Sacrum, 148, 148f
SAD (seasonal affective disorder), 737, 737f
Sagittal plane, 69, 69f
Saliva, 227, 233, 234
Salivary glands, 224t, 225f, 227, 233, 233f
    primary functions/description, 224t
Salmonellosis, 235
Salpingectomy, 666
Salpingitis, 666
Salpingooophorectomy, 666
Sarcoidosis, 407
Sarcolemma, 210
SARS (severe acute respiratory syndrome), 407
SBAR technique, 28
SCA (sudden cardiac arrest), 296
Scabies, 120, 120f
Scala tympani, 566
Scala vestibuli, 566
Scapular, 168
Scapulohumeral muscles, 210
Scar, 121
SCC (squamous cell carcinoma), 123, 123f
Schiötz tonometer, 618f

Schizophrenia, 736
Schultze mechanism of placental expulsion, 648
Schwann cells, 512
Sciatica, 544
Sclera, 593t, 594f, 597
Scleritis, 616
Scleroderma, 121
Sclerostomy, 609
Sclerotherapy, 126
Scoliosis, 162f, 168, 168f
Scratch (epicutaneous) or prick test, 132
Scrotum, 686, 686t, 687f, 688
Seasonal affective disorder (SAD), 737, 737f
Sebaceous (oil) glands, 95t, 97, 99
Seborrhea, 121
Seborrheic keratosis, 121, 121f
Sebum, 97, 99, 121
Secondary hemostasis, 338
Secondary sexual characteristics, 688
Secretin, 469t, 476
Secretion
    function of epithelial tissue, 66
    function of skin, 97
    tubular, 431, 432f
Secretory phase, 644
Sedatives, 551
Sediment, 449
Segmentectomy, 403
Seizures, 534, 534f
Selective laser trabeculoplasty (SLT), 609
Sella turcica, 469
Semen, 686t
Semen test, 712
Semicircular canals, 563t, 565, 568, 573
Semilunar, 312
Seminal vesicles, 686t, 687f, 690, 691f
Seminiferous tubules, 688, 688f
Sensation, 66, 97
Sensory neurons, 511
Sensory neuropathy, 485
Sensory receptors, 97
Sensory root, 518f, 519
Sepsis, 364
Septicemia, 364
Septum, 312
    heart, 278
    nasal, 381, 382f
Sequela, 19
Seroconversion, 364
Serosa, fallopian tube, 636

Serotonin, 467t, 469, 737
Serotonin-norepinephrine reuptake inhibitors (SNRIs), 742
Serum, 364
Serum creatinine, 457
Severe acute respiratory syndrome (SARS), 407
Sex determination, 638
Sexual disorders, 737
Sexual dysfunction, 737
Sexual masochism, 737
Sexual sadism, 737
Sexually transmitted infections (STIs), 79, 691, 692t–693t, 693f
Shaft, hair, 98
Shaking palsy, 544
Sheath, nerve fiber, 512
Shift-work sleep disorder, 545
Shingles, 537
Shingrix, 537
Shock, 312
Sialadenitis, 256
Sickle cell disease, 355, 355f
Sickle cell hemoglobin, 355
Side effect, 88
Sideropenia, 364
Siderosis, 405
Sight, 598–599
Sigmoid colon, 232, 232f
Sigmoidoscope, 256
Sign, 20
Silent ischemia, 307
Silent letters, 5
Silicosis, 405
Simmonds disease, 493
Sims patient position, 208t
Sinoatrial (SA), 314
Sinoatrial node (SA node), 282, 283f
Sinus (bone marking), 145
Sinusitis, 407
Situation, in SBAR technique, 28
Skeletal muscle, 67, 187f, 187t, 188–189, 188f, 189t, 190f, 191
    classification of, 191
    direction and action of selected, 189t
    relaxants, 215
Skeletal system, 139–185
    abbreviations and acronyms, 179–180
    anatomy and physiology, 140–150, 140t, 141f
    bones, 140–145, 140t, 142t, 143f–145f
    differences in male and female pelvis, 149–150, 149f

    joints and movement, 146, 146f–147f
    vertebral column, 148–149, 148f, 149f
    diagnostic and laboratory tests, 176–179
    drug highlights, 174–175
    fractures, 150, 150f–151f
    functions of, 142f
    medical vocabulary, 155–171
        combining forms, 155
        medical word list, 156–171
        word roots, 156
    Practical Application, 184
Skeletal traction, 170f
Skin, 95t. See also Integumentary system
    accessory structures of, 98–100, 99f
    aging, 98, 126
    aging and, 98
    functions of, 95–97
    layers of, 97–98, 97f
    of newborns, 97
    rejuvenation and resurfacing treatment modalities, 126
    true, 98
Skin signs, 122, 122f
Skin tags, 103
Sleep, 544
Sleep apnea, 394
Sleep problems, 545
Sleeve lobectomy, 403
Slipped disk, 536
SLT (selective laser trabeculoplasty), 609
Small intestine, 224t, 225f, 231, 231f
    primary functions/description, 224t
Smegma, 689
Smooth muscle, 67, 187t, 188f, 191
Snellen eye chart, 625
SNRIs (serotonin-norepinephrine reuptake inhibitors), 742
SOAP: Chart Note, 26–27
SOAP: Chart Note Analysis
    cardiovascular system, 333–334
    female reproductive system, 682–683
    male reproductive system, 717–718
Sociopath, 736
Soft palate, 226f, 227, 227f
Somatic symptom disorder (SSD), 738

Somatostatin, 468t, 472
Somatotrophic, 85
Somatotropin hormone (STH), 467t, 493
Somesthetic area, 515
Somnambulism, 545
Spasm, muscle, 203
Spasticity, 210
Spelling, 5–7
  building medical words, 6–7
  plural endings, 7
  prefixes and suffixes frequently misspelled, 6
  silent letters, 5
Sperm, 689, 690f
Spermatic cord, 688f, 689
Spermatid, 706
Spermatocele, 703f, 706
Spermatogenesis, 690, 706
Spermatozoa, 686, 688, 690f, 706
Spermicide, 706
Sphenoidal sinus, 382, 383f
Sphygmomanometer, 287, 288f, 314
Spider veins, 124, 124f, 314
Spinach, mood boost from, 721
Spinal, 168
Spinal cavity, 71f, 72
Spinal cord, 509t, 510f, 517–518, 518f
Spinal fusion, 169, 545
Spinal injury, as erectile dysfunction cause, 702
Spinal nerves, 509t, 518f, 519, 521t
Spinal tap, 554f
Spine (bone marking), 145
Spiral fracture, 151f
Spirochetal, 80
Spirometer, 408, 408f
Spleen, 336t, 342f, 344
Splenomegaly, 256, 364
Splint, 168
Spondylodesis, 169
Spondylosyndesis, 545
Spongy bone, 143, 144f, 165
Sprain, 169
Spur, 169
Sputum, 408
Squamous cell carcinoma (SCC), 123, 123f
Squamous epithelium, of the vagina, 640
SSD (somatic symptom disorder), 738
Stanford-Binet Intelligence Scale, 723

Stapedectomy, 578
Stapes (stirrup), 563t, 564t, 565, 565f
Stem cells, 65, 364
STEMI (ST-segment elevation myocardial infarction), 301
Stent, 314, 314f
Sterile, 449
Sternal, 169
Sternocleidomastoid, 7, 210
Sternotomy, 169
Steroids, 55, 493
Stethoscope, 314
STH (somatotropin hormone), 467t, 493
Stimulants, 743
STIs (sexually transmitted infections), 79, 691, 692t–693t, 693f
Stoma, 245, 245f
Stomach, 224t, 225f, 230, 230f
  primary functions/description, 224t
Stomatitis, 257
Stool, 232
  culture, 266
  meconium, 232
Strabismus, 617, 617f
Strain, 210
Stratum basale, 95t, 96f, 98
Stratum corneum, 95t, 96f, 98
Stratum granulosum, 95t, 96f, 98
Stratum lucidum, 95t, 98
Stratum spinosum, 95t, 96f, 98
Stress fracture, 151f
Stress test, 327
Striae, 123, 123f
Striated muscle. See Cardiac muscle; Skeletal muscle
Stridor, 408
Stroke, 545–546, 546f
Structural unit, 68
ST-segment elevation myocardial infarction (STEMI), 301
Styes, 595, 617, 617f
Subclavicular, 169
Subconcussive impacts, 530
Subcostal, 169
Subcutaneous, 123
Subcutaneous tissue, 95t, 97f, 98
Subdural, 547
Subjective, in SOAP chart note, 27
Subligual, 257
Subligual drug administration, 257f

Sublingual salivary glands, 233, 233f
Submandibular salivary glands, 233, 233f
Submaxilla, 169
Substance abuse, 738
  as erectile dysfunction cause, 702
Subungual, 123
Sudden cardiac arrest (SCA), 296
Sudoriferous glands, 95t
Suffixes
  adjective, 37t
  compound, 34
  definition, 4, 34
  diminutive, 38t
  frequently misspelled, 6
  general use, 34, 35t
  grammatical, 37, 37t–38t
  medical vocabulary, 51–55
    combining forms, 51
    medical word list, 51–55
    word roots, 51
  noun, 37t
  overview of, 34
  for pathological conditions, 38, 38t–39t
  for surgical and diagnostic procedures, 40, 40t–41t
Suicide, 738
Sulcus
  bone marking, 145
  cerebrum, 515
Sundowning, 547
Superficial, 85
Superficial (directional term), 70f
Superfoods, 721
Superior (directional term), 70f, 70t
Superior colliculi, 517
Superior palpebrae, 594
Supination, 147f
Supine patient position, 208t
Suprarenals. See Adrenal glands (suprarenals)
Surfactant, 388
Surgery, as erectile dysfunction cause, 702
Surgical menopause, 657
Surgical procedures, suffixes for, 40, 40t–41t
Suspensory ligaments, ovary, 639, 639f
Sweat glands, 95t, 97, 99–100
Sweat test (chloride), 132
Symmetrical seizures, 534
Sympathectomy, 547

Sympathetic division, 522, 522f, 523
Sympathetic fibers, 523
Sympathetic ganglia, 523
Sympathetic trunk, 523
Sympathomimetics
Symphysis, 169
Symphysis pubis, 169, 640
Synapse, 512
Synaptic cleft, 512
Synarthrosis, 146
Syndrome, 20
Synergism, 210
Synergist skeletal muscle, 191
Synovial joint, 146
Synovitis, 210
Syphilis, 693f, 693t
Systemic, 85
Systems, 67, 68f
Systole, 314
Systolic blood pressure, 287, 288t
Systolic failure, 304

T

T cells (T lymphocytes), 344, 347–348, 347t
  human immunodeficiency virus (HIV) infection of, 352, 352f
T score, 177
T₃. See Triiodothyronine (T₃)
T₄. See Thyroxine (T₄)
Tachycardia, 302, 315
Tachypnea, 408
TAH (total abdominal hysterectomy), 657
Tailbone. See Coccyx
Taste, sensation of, 226
Taste buds, 226
TAT (Thematic Apperception Test), 723
Taut, 124
TB. See Tuberculosis (TB)
TCAs (tricyclic antidepressants), 743
Tdap vaccine, 92, 404
TDP-43, 532
Teeth, 224t, 227–229, 228f, 229f
  deciduous (primary), 227, 228f
  permanent (secondary), 227, 228f
  primary functions/description, 224t
  structure of, 227–229, 229f
Telangiectasia, 124, 124f, 314
Telangiectasis, 315, 315f
Temporal lobe, 515, 516f

Temporal pulse checkpoint, 285f, 285t
Tendinitis, 169
Tendons, 140, 140t, 187t, 189, 190f, 192, 210, 210f
Tennis elbow, 170
Tenodesis, 211
Tenodynia, 211
TENS (transcutaneous electrical nerve stimulation), 547
Tension, relief of, 200
Testes, 465t, 466f, 468t, 476, 686t, 687f, 688, 688f
Testicles. See Testes
Testicular, 706
Testosterone, 468t, 475, 476, 493, 688
    therapeutic use, 711
Tetany, 211, 471, 471f
Tetracyclines, 583
Tetralogy of Fallot, 281
Tetraplegia, 544
Thalamus, 514f, 514t, 517
Thalassemia, 365
Thallium-201 stress test, 327
Thank you, in AIDET communication, 28
Therapeutic use, of drugs, 88
Thermoanesthesia, 124
Thermography, 178
Thermometer, 20
Thermotherapy, 202
Thiazide diuretics, 454
Thoracic cavity, 71f, 72
Thoracic cavity, transverse section through, 278f
Thoracic curve, 148, 148f
Thoracic spinal nerves, 519, 521f
Thoracic vertebrae, 148, 148f
Thoracocentesis, 408, 408f
Thoracoplasty, 409
Thoracotomy, 409
Threatened (spontaneous abortion type), 653, 653f
Three-day measles, 120
Throat. See Pharynx
Thrombectomy, 365
Thrombin, 337, 365
Thrombocytes (platelets), 337–339, 337t, 338f
    clotting, 338–339, 339f
Thrombokinase, 337
Thrombolytic agents, 323
Thrombophlebitis, 315, 315f
Thromboplastin, 365
Thrombosis, 316, 338, 365, 365f
Thrombus, 315, 316f, 546
Thymectomy, 493

Thymitis, 494
Thymoma, 366
Thymopoietin, 469t, 476
Thymosin, 469t, 476
Thymus, 336t, 342f, 344–345, 466f, 469t, 476, 476f
    aging and, 348
    in newborns, 345
Thyroid, 494
Thyroid cartilage, 384, 385, 385f
Thyroid gland, 465t, 466f, 467t–468t, 470, 471f, 494, 494f
Thyroid hormones, 468t, 470, 498
Thyroid scan, 500, 500f
Thyroidectomy, 494, 494f
Thyroiditis, 488, 494
Thyroid-stimulating hormone (TSH), 467t
Thyrotoxicosis, 495
Thyrotropin-releasing hormone (TRH), 467
Thyroxine (T$_4$), 467t, 470, 495
Thyroxine (T$_4$) test, 500
TIA (transient ischemic attack), 545
Tibial, 170
Tic disorder, 739
Tick bite, 160f
Tidal volume (TV), 390, 417
Tinea, 111, 124, 124f
Tinnitus, 578
Tip, tongue, 226
Tissues, 65–67, 66f
    nervous system, 510–512
TJA (total joint arthroplasty), 156
TLC (total lung capacity), 387, 390, 417
Toenails, 99
Tomatoes, mood boost from, 721
Tongue, 225f, 226, 226f
    black hairy, 241, 241f
    taste buds, 226
Tonicity, 192, 211
Tonography, 617
Tonometer, 618, 618f
Tonometry, 624
Tonsillitis, 409
Tonsillectomy, 366
Tonsils, 336t, 342f, 344, 345f, 383, 384f
Toothache, 246
Topical, 85
TORCH panel, 677
Torsion, 211
Torso, 73
Torticollis, 211

Total abdominal hysterectomy (TAH), 657
Total calcium test, 500
Total cholesterol, 326
Total hip prosthesis, 209f
Total joint arthroplasty (TJA), 156
Total lung capacity (TLC), 387, 390, 417
Touch, sense of, 97
Tourette syndrome, 739
Toxemia, 655
Toxic shock syndrome (TSS), 666
Toxoplasmosis screen, 677
Trachea, 380t, 381f, 386, 386f
Tracheal, 409
Tracheostomy, 409, 409f
Tracheotomy, 409
Traction, 170, 170f
Tractional retinal detachment, 615
Tracts, 512
Transcutaneous electrical nerve stimulation (TENS), 547
Transfusion, 366
Transient ischemic attack (TIA), 545
Transurethral incision of the prostate (TUIP), 699
Transurethral microwave thermotherapy (TUMT), 699
Transurethral needle ablation (TUNA), 699
Transurethral resection of the prostate (TURP or TUR), 699
Transverse colon, 232, 232f
Transverse fracture, 150f
Transverse plane, 69, 69f
Transvestism, 737
Trauma, 55, 55f
Treadmill test, 327
Trendelenburg patient position, 208t
TRH (thyrotropin-releasing hormone), 467
Triage, 20
Triceps, 211
Trichiasis, 618
Trichomoniasis, 693
Trichomycosis, 125
Tricuspid, 316
Tricuspid (right atrioventricular) valve, 279, 280f, 281, 281f
Tricyclic antidepressants (TCAs), 743
Trifocal, 618
Trigeminal nerve, 520f, 521t
Trigger points, 201

Triglycerides, 316, 326
Trigone, urinary bladder, 430, 430f
Triiodothyronine (T$_3$), 468t, 470
Triiodothyronine uptake (T$_3$U), 500
Trimester, 644
Trochanter (bone marking), 145
Trochlear nerve, 520f, 521t
True skin, 98
True vocal cords, 384
Trunk, 73–74
TSH (thyroid-stimulating hormone), 467t
TSS (toxic shock syndrome), 666
Tubal pregnancy, 656, 656f
Tubercle (bone marking), 145
Tuberculosis (TB), 410
Tuberculosis (TB) blood tests, 132
Tuberculosis (TB) skin test, 131, 131f, 417
Tuberosity (bone marking), 145
Tubular reabsorption, 431, 432f
Tubular secretion, 431, 432f
Tubule, renal, 427–429, 428f–429f
Tummy tuck, 117
Tumors, 19
Tuning fork, 578, 578f
Turgor, 55
TV (tidal volume), 390, 417
Tympanectomy, 579
Tympanic, 579
Tympanic cavity, 564–565
Tympanic membrane (eardrum), 563t, 564t, 565, 565f
Tympanitis, 579
Tympanoplasty, 579
Type 1 diabetes mellitus (DM), 472
Type 2 diabetes mellitus (DM), 472
Tzanck test, 132

U

Ulcer, 125, 125f
    medications, 262
    peptic ulcer disease (PUD), 254, 254f
Ulcerative colitis (UC), 252, 257
Ulnar, 170
Ulnocarpal, 170
Ultrafast CT scan, 327
Ultrasound/ultrasonography, 327
    brain, 555
    Doppler, 655, 655f
    endocrine system, 500

fetus, 638, 638*f*, 655, 655*f*, 677, 677*f*
gallbladder, 266
kidneys, 457
liver, 266, 266*f*
ocular, 624
during pregnancy, 677, 677*f*
Umami, 226
Umbilical cord, 647
Umbilical hernia, 251
Umbilical region, 72, 73*f*
Unclassified seizures, 534
Unconscious, 55
Underdosing, 89
Unilateral, 85
Unilateral seizures, 534
Unmyelinated fibers, 512
Unstable angina, 301
Unstriated muscle. *See* Smooth muscle
Upper gastrointestinal (UGI) endoscopy, 266
Urease test, 265
Uremia, 449
Ureteroplasty, 449
Ureterostomy, 450
Ureters, 425*t*, 426*f*–427*f*, 429, 450
Urethra, 425*t*, 426*f*–427*f*, 430, 430*f*–431*f*, 450, 686*t*, 687*f*, 691, 691*f*
Urethral stricture, 450
Urethroperineal, 450
Urge incontinence, 431
Urgency, 450, 698
Uric acid blood test, 179
Urinalysis, 432, 433*t*, 678
Urinary bladder, 425*t*, 426*f*–427*f*, 430, 430*f*–431*f*
Urinary meatus, 430
Urinary system, 424–463
  abbreviations and acronyms, 457–458
  anatomy and physiology, 425–431, 425*t*, 426*f*
    kidneys, 425–429, 425*t*, 426*f*–429*f*
    ureters, 425*t*, 426*f*–427*f*, 429
    urethra, 425*t*, 426*f*–427*f*, 430, 430*f*–431*f*
    urinary bladder, 425*t*, 426*f*–427*f*, 430, 430*f*–431*f*
  diagnostic and laboratory tests, 455–457
  drug highlights, 454–455
  medical vocabulary, 436–450
    combining forms, 436
    medical word list, 437–450
    word roots, 436

Practical Application, 462–463
urinalysis, 432, 433*t*
urine, 431, 432*f*, 433*t*
Urinary tract antibacterials, 455
Urinary tract antiseptics, 455
Urinary tract infections (UTIs), 431
Urination, 430, 450
Urine
  analysis of, 432
  culture, 456
  in fetus, 429, 431
  formation of, 431, 432*f*
  normal and abnormal constituents, 433*t*
Urobilin, 450
Urochrome, 450
Urogenital (UG) system, 425
Urologist, 450
Urology, 450
Urticaria, 113, 113*f*
Uterine body, 634
Uterine fibroid, 667, 667*f*
Uterine leiomyoma, 667
Uterine tubes, 636. *See also* Fallopian tubes
Uterine wall, 636
Uterus, 4, 633*t*, 634*f*–636*f*, 636, 638*f*
  abnormal positions of, 636, 636*f*
  anteflexion position of, 634, 635*f*
  involution of, 646
UTIs (urinary tract infections), 431
Utricle, 563*t*, 567–568
Uveal, 618
Uveitis, 618
Uvula, 226*f*, 227

V

Vaccine, 53, 346
  DTaP, 53, 92, 404
  HPV, 692*t*
  meningococcal, 539
  MMR (measles, mumps, rubella), 115, 120
  pneumococcal, 406
  shingles, 537
  Tdap, 92, 404
Vagina, 633*t*, 634*f*–635*f*
Vaginal discharge increase (sign of impending labor), 647
Vaginitis, 667
Vagotomy, 547

Vagus nerve, 520*f*, 521*t*
Valve replacement surgery, 316
Valves
  heart, 280*f*, 281–282, 281*f*
  in lymphatic vessels, 343*f*
Valvuloplasty, 316
Varicella, 125, 125*f*
Varicocele, 703*f*, 707
Varicose veins, 317, 317*f*
Vas deferens, 686*t*, 687*f*, 688*f*, 689
Vascular disease, as erectile dysfunction cause, 702
Vascular system of the heart, 282, 282*f*
Vascularized lymph node transfer (VLNT), 361
Vasculitis, 366, 366*f*
Vasectomy, 6, 707, 707*f*
Vasoconstrictive, 317
Vasodilators, 317, 321
Vasopressin (VP), 467*t*, 495
Vasopressors, 321
Vasospasm, 317
VC (vital capacity), 387, 390, 417
VDRL (venereal disease research laboratory) test, 712
Vectors, 79
Veins, 285, 286*f*
  primary functions/description, 275*t*
  spider, 314
  varicose, 317, 317*f*
Venereal disease research laboratory (VDRL) test, 712
Venipuncture, 317
Ventilator, 410
Ventral, 85
Ventral (directional term), 69, 70*f*
Ventral cavity, 69, 72
Ventral rami, 519
Ventral root, 518*f*, 519
Ventricles
  brain, 519
  heart, 278–280, 279*f*, 280*f*
Ventricular, 317
Ventricular folds, 384
Ventriculogram, 547
Venules, 287, 287*f*
Vermiform, 258
Vernix caseosa, 97, 647
Verruca, 125
Vertebrae, 148
Vertebral column, 148–149, 148*f*, 149*f*, 171
Vertex, 85
Vertigo, 579
  drugs to treat, 583
Vesicle, 122*f*

Vesiculitis, 707
Vestibular membrane (Reissner membrane), 566
Vestibule, 563*t*, 565, 567–568, 573, 640, 640*f*
Vestibulocochlear (acoustic) nerve, 520*f*, 521*t*
Villi, intestinal, 231
Viral load, 372
Virilism, 495
Virus, 78–79, 78*f*
  antiviral agents, 130
Visceral, 85
Visceral muscle. *See* Smooth muscle
Vision, 593, 598–599
Vision problems, 599
Visual acuity, 596
Visual acuity tests, 625, 625*f*
Vital capacity (VC), 387, 390, 417
Vitiligo, 125
Vitreous, 594*f*, 597
VLDL (very-low-density lipoproteins), 308
VLNT (vascularized lymph node transfer), 361
Vocal cords, 384
Voice box, 384, 402, 577. *See also* Larynx
Volumes, lung, 390
Voluntary, 211
Voluntary muscle, 67. *See also* Skeletal muscle
Volvulus, 258, 258*f*
Voyeurism, 737
Vulva, 633*t*, 640, 640*f*

W

Wart, 125, 125*f*
Water, 60
Wechsler Adult Intelligence Scale-Revised (WAIS-R), 723
Weight loss (sign of impending labor), 647
West Nile virus, 79
Wet mount or wet prep (vaginal smear), 678
Wheal, 122*f*
Wheeze, 410
White blood cells (WBCs). *See* Leukocytes
White blood count (WBC), 372
White matter, 512–513
Whole grains, mood boost from, 721
Whooping cough, 92–93, 404
Windpipe, 386

Word roots
blood and lymphatic system, 351
cardiovascular system, 291
definition, 3
digestive system, 239
endocrine system, 481
eye, 601
female reproductive system, 652
human body organization, 81
integumentary system, 102
male reproductive system, 697
medical terminology, 11
mental health, 726
muscular system, 195
nervous system, 526
respiratory system, 393
skeletal system, 156
suffixes and prefixes, 51
urinary system, 436
Word structure, fundamentals of, 2–4
World Health Organization Collaborating Centre (WHOCC) for Drug Statistics Methodology, 87
Wound, 126
Wound culture, 132

X
Xanthoderma, 126
Xanthoma, 126
Xenograft, 105
Xenophthalmia, 618
Xeroderma, 126
Xerophthalmia, 618
Xerosis, 126
Xiphoid, 171
X-ray, 178, 178*f*

Y
Yolk sac, 638

Z
Zika virus, 540
Zoonoses, 80
Zoophila, 737
Zostavax, 537
Zygote, 636*f*, 637